Exploring Retrovirology

Exploring Retrovirology

Editor: Adeline Foley

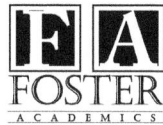

FA FOSTER
A C A D E M I C S

www.fosteracademics.com

www.fosteracademics.com

FA
FOSTER
ACADEMICS

Cataloging-in-Publication Data

Exploring retrovirology / edited by Adeline Foley.
       p. cm.
Includes bibliographical references and index.
ISBN 978-1-63242-839-4
1. Retroviruses. 2. Virology. 3. Virus diseases. 4. Medical virology. 5. Medical microbiology. I. Foley, Adeline.
QR414.5 .E97 2019
616.019--dc23

Foster Academics,
118-35 Queens Blvd., Suite 400,
Forest Hills, NY 11375, USA

ISBN 978-1-63242-839-4 (Hardback)

Contents

Permissions

List of Contributors

Index

Preface

Over the recent decade, advancements and applications have progressed exponentially. This has led to the increased interest in this field and projects are being conducted to enhance knowledge. The main objective of this book is to present some of the critical challenges and provide insights into possible solutions. This book will answer the varied questions that arise in the field and also provide an increased scope for furthering studies.

The study of retroviruses is known as retrovirology. Retroviruses are those types of RNA viruses, which insert a copy of their genome into the DNA of the cells of the organism that they invade. Such insertion changes the genome of the host cell. Those viruses are generally classified as single-stranded positive-sense RNA viruses. Once they enter the cytoplasm of the host cell, the viruses use their own reverse transcriptase enzyme to produce DNA from their RNA genomes. The virions of a retrovirus constitute of enveloped particles, which are 100 nm in diameter. The main virion components include envelope, RNA and proteins. The study of retrovirus has applications in clinical gene therapy for the long-term correction of genetic defects, such as in stem and progenitor cells. Gammaretroviral and lentiviral vectors are used for gene therapy as they mediate stable genetic modification of treated cells. These have been used in many clinical trials as treatment options for various diseases. This book is a compilation of chapters that discuss the most vital concepts and emerging trends in the field of retrovirology. The various studies that are constantly contributing towards evolution of this discipline are examined in detail. This book includes contributions of experts and scientists, which will provide innovative insights into this field.

I hope that this book, with its visionary approach, will be a valuable addition and will promote interest among readers. Each of the authors has provided their extraordinary competence in their specific fields by providing different perspectives as they come from diverse nations and regions. I thank them for their contributions.

Editor

Foamy virus zoonotic infections

Delia M. Pinto-Santini[1], Carolyn R. Stenbak[2] and Maxine L. Linial[3]*

Abstract

Background: Foamy viruses (FV) are ancient complex retroviruses that differ from orthoretroviruses such as human immunodeficiency virus (HIV) and murine leukemia virus (MLV) and comprise a distinct subfamily of retroviruses, the Spumaretrovirinae. FV are ubiquitous in their natural hosts, which include cows, cats, and nonhuman primates (NHP). FV are transmitted mainly through saliva and appear nonpathogenic by themselves, but they may increase morbidity of other pathogens in coinfections.

Conclusions: This review summarizes and discusses what is known about FV infection of natural hosts. It also emphasizes what is known about FV zoonotic infections A large number of studies have revealed that the FV of NHP, simian foamy viruses (SFV), are transmitted to humans who interact with infected NHP. SFV from a variety of NHP establish persistent infection in humans, while bovine foamy virus and feline foamy virus rarely or never do. The possibility of FV recombination and mutation leading to pathogenesis is considered. Since humans can be infected by SFV, a seemingly nonpathogenic virus, there is interest in using SFV vectors for human gene therapy. In this regard, detailed understanding of zoonotic SFV infection is highly relevant.

Keywords: Foamy virus, Simian foamy virus, Retrovirus, Nonhuman primates, Zoonoses

Background

Many human pandemics, including those caused by HIV-1, a retrovirus, and influenza A, an orthomyxovirus, originated from zoonotic infections. It is thought that simian foamy viruses (SFV) are more frequently transmitted from nonhuman primate (NHP) hosts to humans than are other retroviruses, and as a result, SFV zoonotic transmissions have been monitored for several decades (previously reviewed in [1–3]). We provide an updated overview of foamy virus (FV) zoonotic transmission and its implications for human health.

Based on viral molecular properties, retroviruses (Retroviridae) have been subdivided into two subfamilies, the Orthoretrovirinae, including alphaviruses, gammaviruses, and lentiviruses, and the Spumaretrovirinae, including foamy viruses [4]. FV apparently existed before their closest relatives Orthoretrovirinae and Hepadnaviridae (hepatitis B viruses) [5]. Spumaretrovirinae are endemic in many mammalian hosts including cats, cows,

horses, bats and NHP, but not in humans. The prototype foamy virus (PFV) was originally thought to be a human virus since it was isolated from a human nasopharyngeal cancer cell line [6]. Once the PFV genome was sequenced, and compared to the sequence of a chimpanzee SFV it became clear that PFV was of chimpanzee origin [7]. All current evidence indicates that PFV is the result of a chimpanzee FV zoonotic infection in the Kenyan from whom the nasopharyngeal cancer cell line was derived.

All NHP species examined to date, including New World monkeys (NWM), Old World monkeys (OWM) and apes, are infected by SFV [8]. Thus far, there is no observed pathogenicity associated with SFV infection in any natural host. FV transmission occurs mainly through saliva and all natural hosts are known to share saliva via biting, grooming and/or food sharing. Other natural transmission routes, if they exist, have not been identified. However, it has been shown that blood transfusion from an infected to an uninfected nonhuman primate does lead to infection [9]. Thus, in natural or research settings, exposure of uninfected animals to a large amount of infected blood could lead to infection. As seen

*Correspondence: mlinial@fredhutch.org
[3] Division of Basic Sciences, Fred Hutchinson Cancer Research Center, 1100 Fairview Ave. N., A3-205, Seattle, WA 98109, USA
Full list of author information is available at the end of the article

in natural hosts, humans zoonotically infected with SFV show no signs of associated disease.

Foamy virus genome structure and replication

FV are complex retroviruses that share *gag*, *pol* and *env* genes with orthoretroviruses. However, there are many distinct features of FV that are reminiscent of hepatitis B virus (HBV) and other Hepadnaviridae. For example, the FV Pol protein (polymerase or reverse transcriptase) is translated from its own AUG, rather than as part of a Gag-Pol fusion protein as is the case for orthoretroviruses [10]. Secondly, completion of reverse transcription occurs within the virion, prior to infection of a new host cell, making the functional FV genome double-stranded DNA rather than single-stranded RNA [11]. Because of these features, which are unique among retroviruses, FV have been classified as a separate subfamily of Retroviridae.

The prototype foamy virus (PFV) genome is shown in Fig. 1a. The *gag*, *pol* and *env* genes are arranged in that order from the 5′ end of the genome. The long terminal repeat at the 5′ end of the provirus (5′LTR) contains the viral promoter and enhancers that drive transcription of the *gag*, *pol* and *env* mRNAs. The *pol* and *env* mRNAs originate from the 5′LTR and are spliced (Fig. 1b). In addition, PFV contains an internal promoter (IP) that controls transcription of RNAs encoding the accessory proteins Tas and Bet. PFV mRNAs and proteins are shown in Fig. 1b, c, respectively. Tas is the transcriptional activator required for transcription from the 5′LTR. Tas also up-regulates transcription from the IP, but a basal level of transcription of *tas* and *bet* mRNAs from the IP occurs in the absence of Tas. As the Tas protein accumulates, the 5′LTR is activated [12]. Although the second non-structural protein, Bet, is highly expressed, its function is still not well understood [13–19]. Naturally-infected NHP produce antibodies that react strongly with both Gag and Bet proteins when assayed by Western blot, and the presence of anti-Gag and anti-Bet antibodies has proved useful for the detection of FV infections in vivo.

In HIV and other orthoretroviruses, the Gag precursor protein is cleaved into at least 3 Gag proteins, Matrix

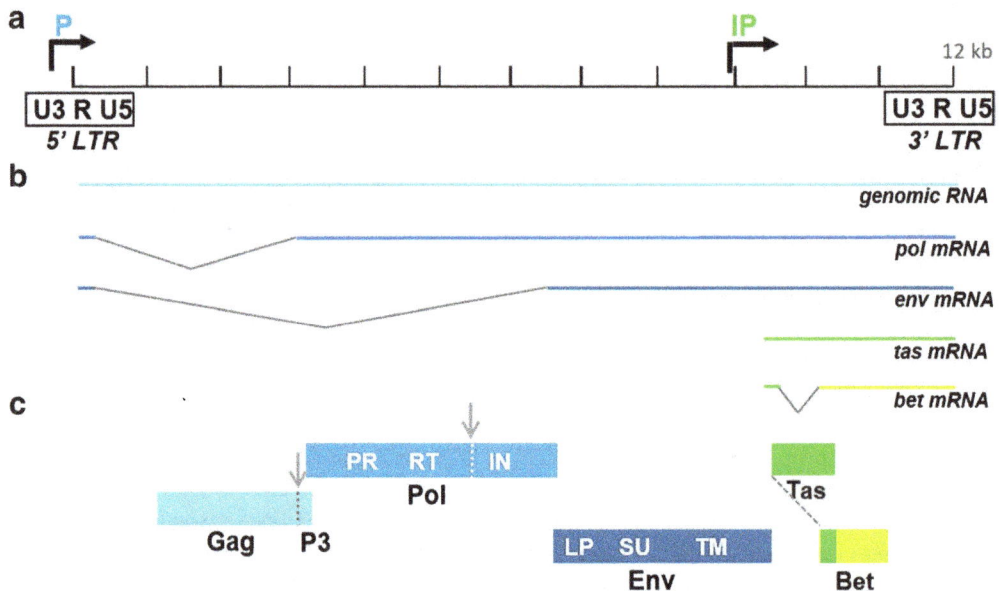

Fig. 1 The Prototype Foamy Virus (PFV) genome, RNA transcripts, and protein products. **a** The molecular clone PFV-13 is depicted (Genbank accession no. U21247; 11,954 bp). The proviral long terminal repeats (LTR) are indicated at the 5′ and 3′ ends of the genome. Each LTR is composed of U3, R and U5 sequences. The U3 sequences are from the 3′ end of the viral RNA genome and the U5 sequences are from the 5′ end of the viral RNA genome. The R sequences are repeat sequences that are created during reverse transcription. Horizontal arrows indicate the location of the two viral promoters. The 5′ LTR promoter is blue and indicated as "P" while the internal promoter is green and indicated as "IP". **b** The five major PFV mRNAs are shown. The first three mRNAs, including the unspliced genomic RNA and the spliced *pol* (polymerase) and *env* (envelope glycoprotein) mRNAs, are expressed from the 5′ LTR promoter and colored different shades of blue. The full-length unspliced RNA (light blue) serves as both the viral genome and the mRNA for the Gag (viral capsid) protein. The two smaller PFV mRNAs encoding the accessory proteins Tas (transactivator) and Bet proteins originate from the IP and are colored dark and light green, respectively. **c** The shaded boxes indicate the major PFV protein products, Gag, Pol and Env, as well as Tas and Bet. Viral protease-mediated cleavage sites within Gag and Pol are indicated with dashed lines and vertical arrows. The C-terminal P3 domain, released upon Gag cleavage, is indicated. The Pol protein contains PR, the protease domain, RT, the reverse transcriptase domain, and IN, the integrase domain. The Env protein is comprised of LP, leader peptide domain, SU, surface domain and TM, transmembrane domain

(MA), Capsid (CA) and Nucleocapsid (NC). The MA protein is myristylated and is required for interaction with the Envelope glycoproteins (Env) and for infectivity. The CA protein is the major virion structural protein, while the NC protein interacts with the RNA genome and is involved in its encapsidation. In contrast to HIV, FV Gag is not cleaved into MA, CA and NC, yet it does contain domains with functional similarity to each of the three mature HIV Gag proteins. Although they serve the same function, the NC domains of orthoretroviruses and foamy viruses are very different at the sequence level. Overall, the amino (N) terminus of the FV Gag protein is more similar to the Gag proteins of orthoretroviruses than is the C terminus, reviewed in [20]. The only cleavage of FV Gag occurs close to the C terminus, releasing a ca. 3 kDa peptide, P3 (Fig. 1c). When a mutation was made that removed the FV Gag cleavage site so that only the full-length Gag protein was produced, the virus was not infectious [21]. It is possible that cleavage is required to change the conformation of the cleaved Gag protein and thus its function, but this has not been demonstrated. It is not known whether the P3 peptide itself plays any role in replication. Since only about half of the synthesized Gag proteins are ultimately cleaved, this results in the presence of a Gag doublet in Western blots.

Retroviruses are known to have a high mutation rate. However, FV are unusual in that their genomes are highly conserved between individuals of the same species and over time, compared to those of orthoretroviruses [22]. Mutations in retroviral genomes are largely attributed to an error-prone reverse transcriptase (RT). The fidelity of PFV RT has been examined in vitro and in cell culture. Recombinant PFV RT was found to have a nucleotide substitution rate very similar to that of recombinant HIV-1 RT in vitro [23]. However, point mutations during replication were less frequent in PFV compared to HIV-1 in cell culture, suggesting a higher fidelity for PFV RT than for HIV-1 RT in vivo [18]. The basis for the lower in vivo mutation rate of PFV RT is unknown.

While a higher fidelity RT would support the genome stability observed for FV, Gartner et al. [18] also found that PFV recombination through template switching was a frequent event. This is important because, like an error-prone RT, recombination can also contribute to virus evolution. Sequence analyses of the *gag* and *env* genes in SFV-infected Old World monkeys (OWM) has identified recombinant viruses, supporting the idea that recombination also occurs in natural infections [24, 25]. Template switching and recombination during reverse transcription, along with the documented cross-species transmission of FV in NHP, leads to the concern that viral recombination between FV of different host species could occur in a co-infected animal [26]. There is

evidence for co-infection with more than one SFV species [27, 28], but no evidence to date of humans infected with more than one SFV species, nor for humans infected with a recombinant SFV derived from more than one species. However, it is possible that FV recombination events could occur similar to those that led to the emergence of the retroviral human pathogen HIV [29].

Cells productively infected by all retroviruses, including foamy viruses, synthesize a large amount of viral mRNAs that encode the viral proteins. These mRNAs include genomic length mRNAs that encode the Gag protein. For each packaged genomic RNA, there are thousands of *gag* mRNAs. Thus, RT-PCR from infected cells detects primarily mRNA, which is indicative of active viral replication. FV, like all orthoretroviruses, package genomic RNA into viral particles. However, in the case of FV, reverse transcription occurs within viral particles as they bud from cells [11] leading to DNA genomes in the particles.

PFV replicates in many primary cells and established cell lines, irrespective of the species from which the cells were isolated. In tissue culture cells in which viral replication is robust, the virus often induces cytopathic effects (CPE). However, human hematopoietic cell lines can be infected by PFV after co-culturing with infected adherent cells, and in these cells the virus can replicate to high titers without CPE [30]. In naturally infected hosts, such as macaques or *Cercopithecus*, SFV replication is seen only in specialized cell types such as superficial differentiating epithelial cells of the oral mucosa [31, 32]. Infected NHP typically have low levels of latent proviral DNA in most tissues, while SFV RNA is detected only in the oral mucosa. Buccal swabs from natural hosts can therefore be used to isolate viral RNA and obtain sequences of actively replicating FV. PCR detection of FV DNA in PBMC is often used to identify infected individuals and determine proviral DNA sequences. FV establishes lifelong, persistent infection and can be transmitted efficiently within natural host populations primarily through saliva, which contains infectious viruses (reviewed in [4]). Viral RNA is never seen in PBMC freshly obtained from infected animals [31, 32] but latently-infected PBMC obtained from FV positive animals will produce virus when stimulated to divide in tissue culture [33].

Given the lack of pathogenicity in natural and human hosts, as well as stable integration of the viral genome into host chromosomes, FV are of interest as vectors for gene therapy applications (reviewed in [34]). FV have additional advantageous features for their use as vectors, including a functional DNA genome which might increase virion stability and a large genome size which allows for insertion of up to 9 Kb of DNA. FV vectors have successfully been used to treat genetic diseases in dogs [35] and are under development to treat human diseases. There is interest in creating viral vectors that encode factors inhibitory to HIV replication [36]. Unlike lentiviral vectors, which can be self-inactivating if they encode anti-HIV factors, FV vectors are not affected by anti-HIV proteins, making them a better choice for such approaches. Because FV are retroviruses, which undergo mutation and recombination, FV vectors should be carefully monitored for genetic changes that could be deleterious to hosts.

Foamy virus natural infections

Foamy viruses have been isolated from many different animal hosts (Table 1). FV are ancient viruses that have coevolved with their natural hosts. The genomic sequence of an ancient relative of land animals, the coelacanth, was published in 2012 [37]. Remarkably, the genomic sequence revealed an endogenous foamy virus suggesting that foamy viruses have existed for at least 400 million years and that they are the oldest known eukaryotic viruses still extant. A comparison of the phylogenetic trees of foamy viruses and their primate hosts reveals congruence both in branching order and divergence time [8]. This indicates that FV have coevolved with nonhuman primates for at least 60 million years, essentially from the beginning of primate evolution.

As mentioned above, foamy viruses are mainly transmitted through saliva by biting, grooming and other means, such as sharing food. It is thus not surprising that the natural hosts for foamy viruses have life styles that include transfer of saliva between individuals. FV have been found in nonhuman primates and cats, which groom and bite members of their individual species. FV have also been described in cows, horses and at least one bat species (*Rhinolophus affinis*) [38]. Cows and horses share food sources with their herd members, for example, by chewing the same cud. Less is known about saliva transfer between bats. However, most bats are highly social and live in large groups, often sharing food. Bat social grooming has also been reported [39]. These behaviors likely lead to intra-species bat FV transmission. Bat FV is called CFV for chiropteran foamy virus [40].

Although there is no evidence for perinatal FV transmission, FV transmission from mothers to offspring occurs, most likely through breastmilk [4, 47]. In natural FV hosts such as cats, cows and NHP, juveniles do not appear to be productively infected and only become so as they mature [48–51]. A detailed study was done in Australia examining bovine foamy virus (BFV) transmission in herds of cattle [48]. The authors examined animals of different ages both for antibodies against BFV and for latent infection of PBMC. PBMC latent infection was defined by the ability of these cells to produce BFV after cocultivation with susceptible bovine cells (CLAB). Calves less than 6 months old, born to BFV positive mothers, were BFV antibody positive but CLAB negative while breastfeeding. Thus, the anti BFV antibodies in the calves were likely maternal. Early after weaning, when calves were separated from adults and pastured with other animals of similar ages and the same sex, anti BFV antibodies were no longer detected in the calves. However, by 18 months of age, the animals began producing BFV antibodies and became CLAB positive, indicative of SFV replication and viral spread to PBMC. A simple interpretation of these data is that newborn calves received both anti-BFV antibodies and virus from their mothers, but did not produce significant amounts of virus before weaning. After weaning and loss of maternal BFV antibodies, the calves began to produce their own anti-BFV antibodies caused by the onset of BFV replication and virus spread. Whether calves younger than 18 months old were unable to support BFV replication, or were protected from virus spread by maternal anti-BFV antibodies, remains unknown. From other studies, in adult macaques, it is known that PBMC containing latent SFV proviruses can transit to the oral mucosa, where susceptible superficial differentiating epithelial cells, once infected, can produce infectious SFV [9]. As discussed below, we favor the hypothesis that the calves were latently infected with maternal BFV but unable to support viral replication.

Table 1 Foamy viruses and their natural hosts

Designation	Full name	Natural host	Original report
BFV	Bovine foamy virus	Cow	Malmquist et al. (1969) [41]
EFV	Equine foamy virus	Horse	Tobaly-Tapiero et al. (2000) [42]
FFV	Feline foamy virus	Domestic cat	Riggs et al. (1969) [43]
CFV	Chiropteran foamy virus	Bat	Wu et al. (2012) [38]
SFV	Simian foamy virus	Nonhuman primate (NHP)	Johnston et al. (1961) [44], Stiles et al. (1964) [45], Rogers et al. (1967) [46]
PFV (SFVpsc_huHSRV.13) [40]	Prototype foamy virus	Chimpanzee	Achong et al.(1971) [6]

A similar picture emerged when a population of captive baboons was studied at a biomedical research foundation [52]. In this facility, infant baboons remained with their mothers for approximately 1 month, and then were removed to individual cages in a nursery without contact with other baboons. The infant baboons were initially SFV antibody positive but the antibody titers waned over the next 6 months. During the first 6 months, PBMC from the infant baboons were SFV PCR negative. PBMC from most juvenile baboons tested (ages not given, but presumably older than 6 months) were also SFV PCR negative. All adult baboons tested (5 years of age or older) were SFV antibody positive, and their PBMC were now SFV PCR positive, despite no interactions with other baboons. The only baboon-baboon interactions were with their mothers during their first month of life, which is when they became infected by SFV. As infants, the baboons acquired SFV maternal antibodies which should have prevented viral production and spread. Although the SFV antibodies waned, no juveniles showed signs of infection, which became evident only when the baboons reached adulthood. As in the cow study, a simple interpretation is that young baboons do not support productive SFV replication and spread. Longitudinal studies done in breeding facilities for *Macaca tonkeana* [53] and *Macaca fascicularis* [54] also showed that SFV infection increases with age and is not seen in animals younger than 6 months of age. Consistent with these results, studies in South and South East Asia showed that SFV antibody production increases with age in free-ranging macaques [51]. These authors had limited data on the SFV PCR status of the juvenile macaques but the data are consistent with PBMC SFV PCR-positivity increasing with age. A likely explanation for these findings is that over time more PBMC transit to the oral mucosa, the site of viral replication, where they become latently infected.

In summary, available data indicate that juvenile FV natural hosts are rarely, if ever, productively infected by FV. Only young adults and adult animals are productively infected. The extent of latent infection of PBMC, if it occurs at all, is at undetectable levels in juvenile animals. Either young juveniles lack host factor(s) required for FV replication or they have an inhibitory factor(s). This enigmatic point, that the time of initial exposure to FV does not coincide with ability to detect proviral DNA in PBMC by PCR or productive infection in the oral mucosa, must be considered when studying FV zoonotic infections.

Much less is known about SFV transmission in New World monkeys (NWM). An initial study, including three captive and four wild monkeys in Costa Rica, found that all seven NWM were SFV positive as detected by PCR [55]. The ages of these NWM were not reported. A study in Brasil [56] found SFV infections in 14 NWM genera including, howler monkeys (5 spp.), spider monkeys (2 spp.), owl monkeys (5 spp.), marmosets (10 spp.), capuchins (6 spp.), squirrel monkeys (3 spp.) and tamarins (9 spp.). Another Brazilian study [57], using both Western blot and PCR assays, found that SFV prevalence increases with age in different species of captive capuchin monkeys. Surprisingly, in wild NWM the SFV prevalence in sexually mature animals was somewhat lower than that in sexually immature animals (48 vs. 61%, respectively). These results indicate that sexual transmission of FV in NWM is unlikely.

In NHP, cross-species FV transmission occurs naturally. For example, in the Ivory Coast, SFV from Western red colobus monkeys was found in chimpanzees, which are predators of the colobus monkeys [27]. Similarly, chimpanzees are predators of *Cercopithecus* monkeys and a *Cercopithecus* SFV was detected in a wild chimpanzee in Equatorial Africa [28]. Phylogenetic analysis has revealed that cross-species and cross-genera transmissions of SFV also occur in NWM [56, 57, 26]. For example, several species of Cebus monkeys cohabit the same areas and SFV cross-species transmission was observed [26]. Such cross-species transmission may occur because of aggressive behaviors rather than predator–prey relationships. Cross-species transmission events in wild NHP could result in generation of new recombinant SFV strains. This is of concern since in the case of lentiviruses only mildly pathogenic SIV were found in African monkeys. After chimpanzees acquired several SIV strains through predation, recombination led to formation of SIVcpz which is somewhat pathogenic in chimpanzees and ultimately led to HIV in humans [29, 58].

FV infected gorillas and chimpanzees have been studied in Cameroon and Gabon [25]. Sequence analyses of the viral *env* genes revealed that there are at least two *env* strains in gorillas and chimpanzees. The data is consistent with recombination within species leading to viral strain differences, although not all the viral parental strains could be identified. Zoonotically infected humans living near chimpanzees and gorillas were found to be infected with the *env* recombinant viruses. However, there was no evidence for further viral recombination in the infected humans.

In addition to natural transmission of SFV in both free-living NHP and captive NHP in zoos and research laboratories, SFV can also be transferred by blood transfusion in research settings, as has been shown in *Macaca fascicularis* and *Macaca mulatta* [9, 59]. These studies in macaques have led to concerns that SFV could be transmitted to humans through blood transfusion from humans who have been in contact with NHP. In fact, it would be surprising if SFV were not transmitted via blood transfusion in humans, since latently infected

PBMC would be present in the blood from an SFV infected donor.

Viral coinfections in SFV natural hosts

Although there is no evidence that FV alone causes clinical disease, there is some indication that it may act as a cofactor in some other pathogenic infections. For example, several studies in macaques indicate that foamy viruses and lentiviruses interact in coinfected hosts. In one study, Murray et al. examined SFV replication in macaques that had been immunosuppressed as a consequence of infection with simian immunodeficiency virus (SIV) [60]. While in healthy macaques SFV replication was confined to the oral mucosa, in SIV immunosuppressed macaques SFV replication was also seen in the small intestine (jejunum). The jejunum is a major site of CD4+ T cell depletion upon SIV infection, but SFV replication was not seen in other tissues in which the number of CD4+ T cells was diminished. Choudhary et al. infected macaques with a laboratory created SIV strain (SIVmac239), highly pathogenic to macaques, and compared macaques naturally infected with SFV to uninfected animals [61]. The authors found that the SIVmac239 strain was more pathogenic in the SFV positive macaques. Specifically, in the SFV positive/SIV positive macaques the SIV viral load was higher, there were fewer CD4+ T cells, and a higher death rate was observed. Although the molecular basis for the SFV/SIV interaction is not known, this could have implications for HIV infected humans (see below).

Foamy virus zoonotic infections

There are many situations in which humans come into contact with FV infected animals. Humans contact domestic cats, which in many countries are kept as pets. Most humans rarely contact cows, unless they live on a farm or work as a cattle farmer, but bovine products are widely consumed. Humans also contact horses in many situations. Interactions with NHP are frequent in research labs, breeding colonies and zoos, but can also occur with pet monkeys, which are often the smaller NWM species. In many parts of the world, such as Africa, Asia and South and Central America, humans often cohabit areas with NHP. Additionally, bush meat hunting is frequent in Africa. Thus, there are many interactions that could possibly lead to zoonotic transmission of feline foamy virus (FFV), bovine foamy virus (BFV), equine foamy virus (EFV) and simian foamy virus (SFV). A number of research groups have studied both the prevalence of antibodies to different FV species in humans as well as FV human persistent infections, as assayed by PCR.

Non-primate hosts

In two studies, veterinarians who work with domestic cats were tested for FFV antibodies. In the first study 175 veterinarians were tested by ELISA and none were found to be FFV antibody positive [62]. A limitation of this study is that veterinarians were not interviewed about their exposure to cats through bites or scratches. In a second and more complete study, Butera et al. [63] examined 204 veterinarians for FFV antibodies using Western blots. Half of the veterinarians in this study reported > 17 years working with cats, and most of the veterinarians reported having cats as pets during their lifetime. In the year preceding the study, almost all participants had received cat bites, scratches or needle exposures to cat fluids. However, none of the subjects were FFV antibody positive. Therefore, there is currently no evidence for zoonotic transmission of FFV.

Since many humans consume bovine products, such as milk and beef, introduction of BFV into humans is also of interest. Unlike the case of FFV there are reports of BFV antibody positive humans. In one study veterinarians, dairy cow caretakers and cattle owners were screened for BFV antibodies. About 7% of the subjects were BFV antibody positive, indicating some exposure to the virus. However, none of these individuals were PCR positive for BFV DNA in PBMC [64]. In a more recent study, three groups of humans were screened for BFV antibodies. It was found that 7% of immunosuppressed patients, 38% of people who interact with cattle and 2% of the general population were BFV antibody positive. There was one BFV PCR positive subject in each group. Each short PCR product showed high homology to an US BFV isolate (M. Materniak-Kornas, personal communication). These data indicate that persistent BFV zoonotic infection is not common.

At present there is no published data showing CFV or EFV transmission to humans.

Primate hosts

In contrast to the cases of FFV and BFV, there are many reports of zoonotic transmission of SFV. Interestingly, as discussed above, the original FV isolate, which was called HFV (human foamy virus), was isolated from a nasopharyngeal cancer cell line obtained from a Kenyan [6].The virus isolated from these cells was later determined to be of chimpanzee origin [7] and was renamed prototype foamy virus (PFV) [65]. PFV is also known as SFVpsc_ huHSRV.13 [40] but will be referred to as PFV herein. Since this original report, there have been many well-documented cases of SFV zoonotic infections, as detailed in Table 2.

In many early studies, evidence for SFV zoonotic transmission was provided by the presence of human

Table 2 Representative SFV zoonotic infection studies

Location	Subjects	No.	No. SFV Ab+ (%)	No. SFV PCR+ (%)	SFV source	References
A. North America						
US and Canada	Lab workers exposed to NHP[a]	231	4 (1.8)	4 (1.8)	3 baboon 1 *Cercopithecus* sp.[c]	Heneine et al. [68]
North America	Zoo keepers working with NHP	133	4 (3)	N/A	Most likely chimpanzee	Sandstrom et al. [69]
Canada	Primate facility workers	46	2 (4.3)	1 (2.2)	1 macaque	Brooks et al. [70]
North America	Res. centers and zoo workers	187	10 (5.3)	9/9 Ab+ tested	8 chimpanzee 1 baboon	Switzer et al. [71]
B. Africa						
Cameroon	Bush meat hunters and butchers	1099	10 (0.9)	3 (0.3)	1 mandrill 1 gorilla 1 *Cercopithecus* sp.	Wolfe et al. [72]
Cameroon	VR[b] near NHP populations	1164	21 (1.8)	4/11 Ab+ tested	3 gorilla 1 chimpanzee	Calattini et al. [73]
	Contact with NHP:					
	– apes	85 29	9 (10.6) 7 (24.1)	9 (10.6) 7 (24.1)	5 gorilla 2 chimpanzee	
	– monkeys	56	2 (3.6)	2 (3.6)	1 mandrill 1 *Cercopithecus* sp.	
Cameroon	General Adult population	1321	26 (2)	2 (0.2)	1 gorilla 1 *Cercopithecus* sp.	Betsem et al. [74]
	People with NHP bites or scratches	198	53 (26.7)	37 (18.6)	31 gorilla 3 chimpanzee 3 *Cercopithecus* sp.	
Gabon	NHP hunters and those interacting with pets[d]	78 10 women 59 men 9 children	19 (24.4)	15 (19.2)	12 gorilla 2 chimpanzee 1 *Cercopithecus* sp.	Mouinga-Ondéme et al. [75]
C. Asia						
Thailand, Indonesia, Nepal and Bangladesh	People sharing NHP habitat	305	8 (2.6)	3 (1)	3 macaques	Jones-Engel et al. [76]
Bangladesh	VR sharing NHP habitat	209	18 (8.6)	12 (5.6)	11 macaques	Engel et al. [77]

[a] Nonhuman primates, [b] village residents

[c] Also known as guenons. This genus is comprised of at least 26 species of Old World monkeys

[d] Includes children

antibodies to SFV using Western blot assays. These early studies used SFV infected human cells to prepare lysates as targets for such antibodies. This led to many false positive results because the human antibodies often reacted to human rather than SFV proteins (reviewed in [50]). Later studies, using PCR assays [66] or more specific serological assays [51, 67] showed that SFV infection of humans was much less widespread than originally claimed. In particular, a study using SFV infected or uninfected monkey cells (Tf cells) eliminated most cross-reactivity issues in Western blot assays [51].

The presence of anti-Gag antibodies could be indicative of either persistent or transient SFV zoonotic infections. Persistent infection is defined by the presence of latent proviruses detected by PCR at least 1 year after initial infection. Transient infections produce anti-SFV antibodies, but do not have detectable levels of integrated provirus over time. In order to conclusively determine persistent infection it is customary to use PCR to detect the presence of integrated SFV provirus in peripheral blood mononuclear cells (PBMC) over time. Since the time of initial infection is not always precisely known, detection of proviral DNA at multiple time points can also indicate persistent infection.

Table 2 includes many of the published reports of SFV zoonoses from Old World monkeys (OWM). Three distinct groups of humans have been studied. The first group includes researchers and technicians who work with nonhuman primates (NHP) in Research Centers and Zoos in North America (Table 2A). The second group includes people in Africa who live in areas cohabited by NHP and also people who are NHP bushmeat hunters and/or butchers (Table 2B). Most of the people in these two groups are occupationally exposed to NHP and therefore could come in contact with NHP saliva and/or blood. The third group includes people in South Asia who cohabit areas with NHP and may or may not be occupationally exposed to NHP in temples (Table 2C).

Old World monkeys—North America

There have been at least four reports of SFV zoonotic infections of humans occupationally exposed to OWM and/or apes in laboratories and zoos in North America (Table 2A). In these studies the percent of SFV antibody positive people ranged from ca. 2–5% [68–71]. In three of these studies [68, 70, 71] the investigators examined the SFV PCR status of 16 SFV antibody positive humans and found that 14 were SFV PCR positive and one was SFV PCR negative. Blood was not available for DNA analysis from one subject. Thus, most of the SFV antibody positive subjects (14/15 or 93%) were persistently infected. Six spouses of these SFV PCR positive lab workers were tested and all were SFV antibody as well as SFV PCR negative [68, 71]. Boneva et al. examined the wives of six SFV positive North American men occupationally exposed to NHP and found that none of them were SFV antibody or PCR positive [78]. Thus, human to human transmission was not detected in North America.

Old World monkeys—Africa

As in North America, people in Africa are exposed to NHP at primate centers, including breeding colonies [79]. Unlike in North America, occupational exposure to NHP occurs in other situations such as hunting and butchering. In this regard, researchers have studied people in Cameroon and Gabon (Central Africa) who bushmeat hunt and people who prepare bushmeat for consumption; therefore, all these study subjects had direct contact with NHP or NHP tissues and/or fluids. In the case of butchers, it is possible that SFV transmission could occur through NHP blood rather than saliva. The researchers found that 11–27% of the individuals tested were SFV antibody positive, of which 72% were SFV PCR positive [72–75] (Table 2B). In contrast, when researchers studied Africans who cohabit areas with NHP, less than 0.5% of people screened were SFV antibody positive [73, 74] (Table 2B). Of these antibody positive people, 16% were persistently infected as detected by PCR. There were also studies done in Western African countries, Democratic Republic of Congo and Ivory Coast. In Ivory Coast, the researchers studied a large number of people some of whom were HIV infected and found that 3 of the people (0.2%) were SFV antibody positive. 2 of the SFV positive

people were HIV positive, demonstrating HIV and SFV co-infection [80]. In the Democratic Republic of Congo over 3000 villagers were screened for SFV infection and 0.5% were found to be SFV antibody positive using Western blots [81]. Compared to the laboratory workers in North America, who presumably take universal precautions, a far greater percent of Africans in direct contact with NHP, primarily hunters, showed exposure to SFV, as measured by antibody production.

In one study the participants were classified by whether they had direct contact with apes or with monkeys [73]. Those who encountered apes were about six times more likely to be SFV infected than those who encountered monkeys. Although the specifics of these encounters are not known, it is likely that ape SFV is more easily zoonotically transmitted than monkey SFV. Since ape bites are deeper than monkey bites, this could result in more efficient transfer of virus in saliva to humans. Consistent with this idea, in two studies where PCR results were obtained, most SFV PCR positive people in Africa were persistently infected with a gorilla SFV [74, 75]. Whether transmission through blood could play a role in more efficient viral transfer from ape to humans has not been examined.

Calattini et al. [73] looked at five spouses and five children of SFV PCR positive subjects in Africa and found that none of the relatives were infected. Betsem et al. [74] examined 30 spouses of SFV PCR positive African subjects and one of the spouses was SFV antibody positive but SFV PCR negative. Because this woman was PCR negative, it was not possible to determine whether the SFV antigen source was her husband or an NHP she independently encountered. Switzer et al. also look at relatives (spouses, parents, siblings and offspring) of 8 SFV antibody positive women in the Democratic Republic of Congo and found no evidence of SFV infection [81]. Overall, no evidence for intra-familial transmission of SFV was found in Africa.

Old World monkeys—Asia

SFV zoonotic transmission has also been studied in Asia (Table 2C). In Asia, there are apes such as gibbons and orangutans but humans who interact with these apes have not been studied. In the areas studied (Thailand, Indonesia, Nepal and Bangladesh) the primary NHP genus is *Macaca* (macaques). In one study people who cohabit areas with macaques in these four countries were analyzed [76]. It was found that 2.6% of the people screened were SFV antibody positive and 1% were SFV PCR positive. Most of the people screened were exposed to macaques in temples. Work then focused on people in Bangladesh, one of the world's most densely populated countries, where a large percentage of the population cohabits areas with macaques. Unlike in Africa, people in Bangladesh do not hunt or consume NHP. In the Bangladesh study, about half of 209 village residents (VR) who were sampled reported having been bitten at least once by a macaque. 8.6% of the 209 VR were SFV antibody positive and 5.6% SFV PCR positive.

In orthoretroviruses, such as murine leukemia virus (MLV), the *env* gene appears to be the most diverse gene [82]. MLV are classified by their host range, which is defined by the receptor binding domain of the Env protein. In contrast, in foamy viruses the *gag* gene sequence is very variable and can be used to define viral strains [24]. The SFV proviruses in Bangladesh macaques were sequenced and six SFV strains were defined based on sequence variation in the *gag* gene. 25% of the adult macaques sampled harbored at least two distinct SFV strains. Humans were found who were also infected with more than one SFV strain. Three humans were coinfected with strain combinations not seen in individual macaques, suggesting that the SFV strains detected were zoonotically transmitted from more than one macaque. This could lead to generation of new recombinant strains in humans, as has been reported to occur in macaques [24]. Such recombination could occur since there is evidence that some SFV replication does occur in humans (see below for discussion). Some of the VR were sampled at two time points (about 1 year apart) and the SFV proviruses were sequenced. In some of these VR, for whom more than one SFV strain was detected by PCR in the initial time point, there were differences in the abundance of strains recovered at the second time [77]. These participants did not report any interactions with NHP between the two time points. Therefore, it is unlikely that they became infected with a different SFV strain between the two sampling times. It is possible that acquired or innate immunity factors could influence the persistence of different SFV strains in humans over time. This requires further study. The difference in abundance of SFV strains over time implies that viral replication does occur in humans. Other evidence for SFV replication in humans is discussed below.

Very little is known about the age at which humans are susceptible to SFV zoonotic infection. The studies in Asia only included adults ages18 or older. One SFV positive 19 year-old Bangladeshi woman reported being severely bitten by a macaque when she was 4 years old. However, as a young adult, macaques did enter her house leaving behind urine and feces. It is likely that she was infected as a child but this has not been validated [76]. Further studies need to be done to determine at what age humans can become persistently infected by SFV. It is also of interest to determine whether there is any age restriction on viral replication as appears to be the case in cows and NHP.

In most of the studies reported in Table 2 the subjects were tested for antibodies to SFV using Western blot or ELISA, and for persistent infection using PCR of DNA extracted from PBMC. There are humans who have been exposed to SFV and who are SFV antibody positive but are not persistently infected, as detected by an SFV PCR assay. People who are SFV PCR positive are of interest because they have the potential to transmit virus to other humans via saliva. It is known that SFV replication occurs in the oral mucosal epithelia cells of NHP [32]. Viral replication would presumably have to occur in the human oral mucosa for efficient FV human to human transmission. When foamy viruses replicate a large amount of viral RNA is produced and can be detected by reverse transcriptase-PCR (RT-PCR). Engel et al. used a sensitive and quantitative RT-PCR assay to look for SFV RNA in buccal swabs from Bangladeshi humans who were persistently infected by macaque SFV, as detected by PCR [77]. Although SFV RNA could easily be detected in macaque buccal swabs using the same assay [83] no SFV RNA could be detected in the human buccal swabs. Similarly, no RNA was detected in buccal swabs from Africans infected by gorilla SFV [84]. These data indicate that SFV replication does not occur in human oral mucosa to the same extent as in NHP oral mucosal tissue. Thus, SFV transfer between humans via saliva is unlikely. PBMC from SFV PCR positive Bangladeshi humans were also assayed for SFV RNA and none was detected [83]. Boneva et al. [78] looked for infectious virus in saliva samples from six SFV positive people in North America. They cultured virus from the saliva of one individual but only in one of four attempts. In this individual PCR analysis of DNA clones from different body sites indicated SFVcpz quasispecies [85]. Thus, there is indirect evidence for SFV replication in this human.

Although there is no direct evidence for SFV replication in humans, as measured by SFV RNA synthesis, several findings can only be explained by some level of SFV viral replication. As cited above, SFV quasispecies was found in a human, with viral DNA sequences varying between tissue compartments [85]. Matsen et al. sequenced proviruses from PBMC obtained from SFV PCR positive humans [86]. Interestingly, evidence for APOBEC3 deamination was found in some proviruses. When SFV proviruses were analyzed in the macaques with which the humans interacted, no evidence of APOBEC3 deamination could be found. Because APOBEC3 deamination occurs during SFV replication, at the single strand DNA synthesis step of reverse transcription, these results suggest that some SFV replication occurs in humans. SFV replication in humans can also be inferred from the large number of human PBMC positive for FV proviral DNA by PCR. Given that about one SFV proviral DNA copy is found per 10^4 PBMC [55] and that the average human has ca. 5×10^9 PBMC, this would require the transfer of about 10^5 infectious SFV particles. This high level of virus is unlikely to be transferred during an NHP bite or scratch. Finally, when samples were taken from SFV-infected humans at different times, the dominant strains differed in the same individual [77]. While this could arise from secondary SFV infection at a time distal from initial infection, there is no evidence for this in the individuals cited. This implies that some strains replicate or persist better than others in different individuals.

In Bangladesh and other South Asian countries, there are ethnically homogenous seminomadic human groups, known as the Bedey. There is a group of Bedey residing in Northeastern Bangladesh who interact more with macaques than do the villagers residing in the same area. This particular Bedey group in Bangladesh trains macaques for performances. These Bedey also earn their livelihoods by performing with these animals. Despite constant interactions with macaques, often leading to bites and scars, these Bedey do not appear to be susceptible to SFV infection. A small number ($n = 45$) of the Northeast Bangladesh Bedey were screened and none of them were SFV antibody positive or SFV PCR positive [87]. These findings suggest that these Bedey constitute a unique human group with high exposure to NHP who may be resistant to SFV infection. The prevalence of SFV in the Bedey performing macaques is nearly as high as that seen in the free-ranging population of macaques in Bangladesh [51]. The SFV viral strains in the performing and free-ranging macaque groups are very similar, based on *gag* sequences [24]. The difference in zoonotic transmission of SFV between Bedey and village residents (VR) who live in the same areas seems compelling. However, as only 45 Bedey were tested, the observed difference in SFV prevalence is not statistically significant (p value < 0.078). Macaque bites often lead to scars and the number of scars in the Bedey and VR were estimated by visual inspection and interviews. There were 152 scars in 269 VR screened, whereas the 45 Bedey had a total of 297 scars (Jones-Engel et al., unpublished results). When the number of SFV PCR positive humans relative to the total number of scars was compared, 12 SFV PCR positive humans per 152 total scars were found in the VR group vs 0 SFV PCR positive humans per 297 total scars in the Bedey group. This difference is statistically significant (p value < 0.0001).

In any human group interacting with OWM, only a fraction of the humans are SFV infected as measured by PCR. Thus, if it can be determined why the Bedey are resistant to SFV infection these results could be extended to other human groups. It is not known why the Bedey

are both SFV antibody and SFV PCR negative, but it could be a result of either acquired or innate immunity. For example, it is known that APOBEC3G can modify SFV genomes in humans [86]. Perhaps the Bedey have very active APOBEC3 genes, which could lead to inactivation of SFV proviruses. Inactivation of proviruses will ultimately shut-down any low level of replication suspected to occur in other humans (innate immunity). Another possibility is that the Bedey have high levels of anti-SFV neutralizing antibodies (acquired immunity). Currently, Western blots only detect anti-SFV Gag antibodies, but not anti-SFV Env antibodies. High levels of anti-SFV Env antibodies could neutralize virus and prevent infection. Until more Bedey are screened, acquired or innate immunity differences between Bedey and VR are merely speculative.

New World monkeys
Table 2 does not include any examples of zoonotic infection by New World monkey (NWM) SFV. In fact, there are currently no reports of such infections. NWM SFV can infect and replicate in human-derived tissue culture cells [88, 55], demonstrating that there is no intrinsic block to replication of NWM SFV in human cells. To date, only a few studies have been published in which NWM SFV zoonotic transmission was examined. In the first published study, a group of primatologists known to have been exposed to NWM was screened by both Western blot and PCR [55]. The nested *pol* PCR assay used could detect SFV DNA in the blood of squirrel, howler and capuchin monkeys as well as from TC cells infected with spider monkey and marmoset SFV. The Western blot antigen used in this study, spider monkey SFV proteins, could be detected using plasma from squirrel monkeys. This antigen was also used to determine whether anti-NWM SFV antibodies could be detected in humans. A total of 69 primatologists were examined and 11.6% (8/69) had antibodies reactive to spider monkey SFV. While all of the 8 NWM SFV seropositive individuals reported some contact with NWM species, only 4 reported direct contacts, such as bites, scratches, or needle sticks. The remaining 4 individuals reported indirect contacts with NWM, including exposure to body fluids. Unlike most OWM SFV-seropositive individuals, NWM SFV-seropositive individuals did not have detectable levels of viral DNA in their blood as assayed by the highly sensitive nested PCR assay which can detect SFV DNA from at least 5 NWM genera. The NWM species that the primatologists interacted with in this study are not known, however the Western blot assay used detects at least spider and squirrel monkey antibodies. Moreover, the PCR assay detects at least, spider, squirrel, capuchin,

marmoset and howler monkey SFV DNA. Thus, the PCR assay can detect more NHP genera than the Western blot assay and the humans who tested NWM SFV Ab positive were SFV PCR negative.

In another published study, 56 people occupationally exposed to NWM in Brazil were screened for NWM SFV infection using both antibody (Western blot) and PCR assays [89]. In this longitudinal study 18% (10/56) of the people sampled were NWM SFV antibody positive at the initial time point, but none of these seropositive people were SFV PCR positive. Six of the 10 seropositive individuals remained seroreactive when screened 2–3 years later. Interestingly three individuals seroreverted, for unknown reasons. In summary, human exposure to NWM SFV occurs and leads to anti-SFV antibody production, however to date there is no evidence of persistent infection of humans with NWM SFV, as detected by PCR.

Viral coinfections in SFV infected humans

Two independent studies in Africa reported a total of four individuals coinfected with SFV and HIV in Cameroon and the Ivory Coast [90, 80]. PBMC DNA was available from two individuals. One was infected with a mandrill SFV and the other one with a guenon SFV. However, there was no mention of the disease outcomes of these coinfected humans relative to humans infected with only HIV.

As discussed above it is known that in macaques there are interactions between foamy virus and lentiviruses that exacerbate the pathogenicity of lentiviruses. Thus, the possibility arises that SFV infection in humans could also augment HIV pathogenicity. Nothing is known about other viral infections, such as CMV, in people who are infected with SFV, but this warrants further study.

Conclusions, speculation and perspectives

Foamy viruses are ancient retroviruses that have apparently existed for at least 400 million years. They predate all other known retroviruses and hepadnaviruses, their closest relatives. Unlike orthoretroviruses, but similar to hepadnaviruses, infectious foamy viruses have functional DNA genomes.

There is much interest in developing SFV as gene therapy vectors for treatment of human diseases. Foamy viruses are retroviruses that permanently integrate into cell genomes and can be used for long-lasting expression of genes of interest. As the functional FV genome is DNA, FV vectors are more likely to be more chemically stable than vectors with RNA genomes, such as orthoretroviruses. These features, combined with a lack of pathogenicity, make SFV promising candidates for development of viral vectors. Foamy viruses are highly

prevalent in their natural hosts, which include bats, cats, cows, horses and NHP. Studies in cows and NHP indicate that foamy virus does not replicate efficiently in juveniles, but latent viral infection seems likely and the viral source is probably of maternal origin, perhaps through breast milk. In the same host species, productive FV infection is detected in almost all adults. Why there is a difference in FV replication between juveniles and adults is not known, but this is an area that should be explored further, especially as it has implications for the development of FV gene therapy vectors for humans.

Zoonotic transmission of SFV is not very widespread because most humans do not interact directly with NHP. However, in those humans who interact directly with Old World monkeys and apes, SFV is rather easily zoonotically transmitted and infected humans do not appear to have any pathology associated with SFV infection. Humans who are SFV Gag antibody positive can be either SFV PCR positive or SFV PCR negative when PBMC DNA is assayed. This indicates that humans who encounter SFV and produce SFV Gag antibodies are not always persistently infected but instead could be transiently infected. A group of humans, the Bedey of Northeastern Bangladesh, frequently interact with macaques and often have scars from macaque bites. Despite these interactions, these Bedey do not appear to be either SFV Gag antibody positive or SFV PCR positive. Understanding human-encoded factors important for establishing SFV persistent infection, which does not seem to occur in these Bedey, is important for the development of optimal gene therapy vectors and may offer new insights into anti-retroviral strategies.

The source of SFV (apes, Old World monkeys or New World monkeys) is an important factor in SFV zoonotic transmission. Humans appear not to be persistently infected by NWM SFV and more susceptible to ape SFV than to OWM SFV infection. This suggests that humans are most sensitive to SFV strains from NHP to which they are more genetically related. It is interesting to speculate as to why humans do not have their own FV, although chimpanzees, the closest NHP relative to humans, do. A likely explanation is that saliva transfer into the blood stream is rarer among adult humans than among adult chimpanzees and other NHP. NHP grooming behaviors, unlike those of humans, routinely involve scratching and biting with saliva transfer. Also, using their opposable thumbs, humans have developed tools that replace biting as an offensive or defensive adult behavior. The paucity of saliva transmission among adult humans might explain the lack of an endemic human FV.

Active foamy virus replication is detected by measuring viral RNA production. To date no viral RNA in either oral mucosal tissue or blood cells has been detected in

SFV-infected humans. However, several lines of evidence suggest that some level of SFV replication must occur in humans. Understanding the timing and location of this undetectable SFV replication in humans will be helpful in monitoring the impact and risk of zoonotic infections.

Although SFV is not known to be pathogenic in humans, nothing has been done to determine whether SFV infections in humans can exacerbate other viral infections. In macaques, SFV infection can accelerate disease by pathogens such as lentiviruses. Macaques infected with a modified SIV in research settings are sicker and die sooner if they are also naturally SFV infected. It is possible that humans who are SFV positive are also prone to accelerated disease by human pathogenic viruses but this has not been studied. Given the number of people interacting with NHP around the world, this is an area of concern.

As some humans are coinfected with more than one SFV strain, they should be closely monitored for the appearance of recombinant SFV strains, as well as for any pathological consequences of infection. Lentiviruses are not highly pathogenic in their natural hosts, but recombination has been shown to generate strains that are pathogenic in accidental hosts such as humans. Understanding the determinants of SFV zoonotic transmission is critical as there are concerns that SFV could emerge as a new human pathogen.

All viruses require transmission in order to survive, and in this respect, foamy viruses could be considered "perfect" viruses. In natural populations foamy viruses spread efficiently to reach very high prevalence rates. Many viruses induce symptoms deleterious to the host in order to be efficiently transmitted. For example, nasopharyngeal viruses often induce runny noses, sneezing and coughing to aid in their transmission. Foamy viruses are mainly transmitted through saliva, and all natural hosts have saliva transfer as part of their regular life style. Thus, foamy viruses do not need to induce any pathological symptoms to aid in their transmission.

In summary, foamy viruses are the most ancient retroviruses and have a long history of coevolution with their natural hosts. Viral transmission occurs efficiently within natural populations to establish life-long, non-pathogenic infections. Zoonotic transmission of SFV can also lead to persistent infection in humans, although less frequently than is seen in natural hosts. Given their unique genomic features and lack of pathogenicity in humans, SFV continue to show promise as vectors for the treatment of life-threatening diseases.

Authors' contributions

DMPS and MLL researched and wrote the sections on Old World monkey foamy viruses as well as bovine and feline foamy viruses. CRS researched and wrote the section about New World monkey foamy viruses. All authors read and approved the final manuscript.

Author details

[1] Division of Basic Sciences, Fred Hutchinson Cancer Research Center, Seattle, WA, USA. [2] Biology Department, Seattle University, Seattle, WA, USA. [3] Division of Basic Sciences, Fred Hutchinson Cancer Research Center, 1100 Fairview Ave. N., A3-205, Seattle, WA 98109, USA.

Acknowledgements

The authors thank Dr. William Mason for his insightful comments during the writing process. We also thank Dr. Julie Overbaugh for critical reading of the manuscript. Finally, Dr. Magdalena Materniak-Kornas provided important information about BFV zoonotic infections.

Competing interests

The authors declare that they have no competing interests.

Funding

DMPS and MLL thank Fred Hutchinson Cancer Research Center for financial support.

References

1. Khan AS. Simian foamy virus infection in humans: prevalence and management. Expert Rev Anti-infect Ther. 2009;7(5):569–80.
2. Switzer WM, Heneine W. Foamy virus infection of humans. In: Liu D, editor. Molecular detection of human viral pathogens. Boca Raton: CRC Press; 2011.
3. Rua R, Gessain A. Origin, evolution and innate immune control of simian foamy viruses in humans. Curr Opin Virol. 2015;10:47–55.
4. Linial ML. Foamy viruses. In: Knipe DM, Howley PM, editors. Fields virology. 5th ed. Philadelphia: Wolters Kluwer/Lippincott Williams & Wilkins; 2007. p. 2245–63.
5. Rethwilm A, Bodem J. Evolution of foamy viruses: the most ancient of all retroviruses. Viruses. 2013;5(10):2349–74.
6. Achong BG, Mansell WA, Epstein MA, Clifford P. An unusual virus in cultures from a human nasopharyngeal carcinoma. J Natl Cancer Inst. 1971;46:299–307.
7. Herchenroder O, Renne R, Loncar D, Cobb EK, Murthy KK, Schneider J, et al. Isolation, cloning, and sequencing of simian foamy viruses from chimpanzees (SFVcpz): high homology to human foamy virus (HFV). Virology. 1994;201:187–99.
8. Switzer WM, Salemi M, Shanmugam V, Gao F, Cong ME, Kuiken C, et al. Ancient co-speciation of simian foamy viruses and primates. Nature. 2005;17(434):376–80.
9. Khan AS, Kumar D. Simian foamy virus infection by whole-blood transfer in rhesus macaques: potential for transfusion transmission in humans. Transfusion. 2006;46(8):1352–9.
10. Yu SF, Baldwin DN, Gwynn SR, Yendapalli S, Linial ML. Human foamy virus replication—a pathway distinct from that of retroviruses and hepadnaviruses. Science. 1996;271(5255):1579–82.

11. Yu SF, Sullivan MD, Linial ML. Evidence that the human foamy virus genome is DNA. J Virol. 1999;73(2):1565–72.

12. Meiering CD, Rubio C, May C, Linial ML. Cell-type-specific regulation of the two foamy virus promoters. J Virol. 2001;75(14):6547–57.

13. Meiering CD, Linial ML. Reactivation of a complex retrovirus is controlled by a molecular switch and is inhibited by a viral protein. Proc Natl Acad Sci USA. 2002;99(23):15130–5.

14. Russell RA, Wiegand HL, Moore MD, Schafer A, McClure MO, Cullen BR. Foamy virus Bet proteins function as novel inhibitors of the APOBEC3 family of innate antiretroviral defense factors. J Virol. 2005;79(14):8724–31.

15. Lochelt M, Romen F, Bastone P, Muckenfuss H, Kirchner N, Kim YB, et al. The antiretroviral activity of APOBEC3 is inhibited by the foamy virus accessory Bet protein. Proc Natl Acad Sci USA. 2005;102:7982–7.

16. Delebecque F, Suspene R, Calattini S, Casartelli N, Saib A, Froment A, et al. Restriction of foamy viruses by APOBEC cytidine deaminases. J Virol. 2006;80(2):605–14.

17. Perkovic M, Schmidt S, Marino D, Russell RA, Stauch B, Hofmann H, et al. Species-specific Inhibition of APOBEC3C by the prototype foamy virus protein bet. J Biol Chem. 2009;284(9):5819–26.

18. Gartner K, Wiktorowicz T, Park J, Mergia A, Rethwilm A, Scheller C. Accuracy estimation of foamy virus genome copying. Retrovirology. 2009;6(1):32.

19. Vasudevan A, Perkovi-ç M, Bulliard Y, Cichutek K, Trono D, Haussinger D, et al. Prototype foamy virus Bet impairs the dimerization and cytosolic solubility of human APOBEC3G. J Virol. 2013;87(16):9030–40.

20. Linial ML, Fan H, Hahn B, Lower R, Neil J, Quackenbush S, et al. Retroviridae. In: Fauquet CM, Mayo MA, Maniloff J, Desselberger U, Ball LA, editors. Virus taxonomy, 7th report of the International Committee on taxonomy of viruses. London: Elsevier/Academic Press; 2004.

21. Enssle J, Fischer N, Moebes A, Mauer B, Smola U, Rethwilm A. Carboxy-terminal cleavage of the human foamy virus gag precursor molecule is an essential step in the viral life cycle. J Virol. 1997;71(10):7312–7.

22. Schweizer M, Schleer H, Pietrek M, Liegibel J, Falcone V, Neumann-Haefelin D. Genetic stability of foamy viruses: long-term study in an African green monkey population. J Virol. 1999;73(11):9256–65.

23. Boyer PL, Stenbak CR, Hoberman D, Linial ML, Hughes SH. In vitro fidelity of the prototype primate foamy virus (PFV) RT compared to HIV-1 RT. Virology. 2007;367(2):253–64.

24. Feeroz M, Soliven K, Small C, Engel G, Pacheco M, Yee J, et al. Population dynamics of rhesus macaques and associated foamy virus in Bangladesh. Emerg Microbes Infect. 2013;22(2):e29.

25. Richard L, Rua R, Betsem E, Mouinga-Ondeme A, Kazanji M, Leroy E, et al. Cocirculation of two env molecular variants, of possible recombinant origin, in gorilla and chimpanzee simian foamy virus strains from Central Africa. J Virol. 2015;89(24):12480–91.

26. Ghersi BM, Jia H, Aiewsakun P, Katzourakis A, Mendoza P, Bausch DG, et al. Wide distribution and ancient evolutionary history of simian foamy viruses in New World primates. Retrovirology. 2015;12(1):1–19.

27. Leendertz FH, Zirkel F, Couacy-Hymann E, Ellerbrok H, Morozov VA, Pauli G, et al. Interspecies transmission of simian foamy virus in a natural predator-prey system. J Virol. 2008;82(15):7741–4.

28. Liu W, Worobey M, Li Y, Keele BF, Bibollet-Ruche F, Guo Y, et al. Molecular ecology and natural history of simian foamy virus infection in wild-living chimpanzees. PLoS Pathog. 2008;4:e1000097.

29. Gao F, Bailes E, Robertson DL, Chen Y, Rodenburg CM, Michael SF, et al. Origin of HIV-1 in the chimpanzee Pan troglodytes troglodytes. Nature. 1999;397(6718):436–41.

30. Yu SF, Stone J, Linial ML. Productive persistent infection of hematopoietic cells by human foamy virus. J Virol. 1996;70(2):1250–4.

31. Falcone V, Leupold J, Clotten J, Urbanyi E, Herchenröder O, Spatz W, et al. Sites of simian foamy virus persistence in naturally infected African green monkeys: latent provirus is ubiquitous, whereas viral replication is restricted to the oral mucosa. Virology. 1999;257:7–14.

32. Murray SM, Picker LJ, Axthelm MK, Hudkins K, Alpers CE, Linial ML. Replication in a superficial epithelial cell niche explains the lack of pathogenicity of primate foamy virus infections. J Virol. 2008;82(12):5981–5.

33. Neumann-Haefelin D, Rethwilm A, Bauer G, Gudat F, zur Hausen H. Characterization of a foamy virus isolated from cercopithecus aethiops lymphoblastoid cells. Med Microbiol Immunol. 1983;172(2):75–86.

34. Trobridge GD. Foamy virus vectors for gene transfer. Expert Opin Biol Ther. 2009;9(11):1427–36.

35. Bauer TR, Allen JM, Hai M, Tuschong LM, Khan IF, Olson EM, et al. Successful treatment of canine leukocyte adhesion deficiency by foamy virus vectors. Nat Med. 2007; (**advanced online publication**).

36. Nalla AK, Trobridge GD. Prospects for foamy viral vector anti-HIV gene therapy. Biomedicines. 2016;4(2):8.

37. Han GZ, Worobey M. An endogenous foamy-like viral element in the coelacanth genome. PLoS Pathog. 2012;8(6):e1002790.

38. Wu Z, Ren X, Yang L, Hu Y, Yang J, He G, et al. virome analysis for identification of novel mammalian viruses in bat species from Chinese provinces. J Virol. 2012;86(20):10999–1012.

39. Carter GLL. Social grooming in bats: are vampire bats exceptional? PLoS ONE. 2015;10(10):e0138430.

40. Khan AS, Bodem J, Buseyne F, Gessain A, Johnson W, Kuhn JH, et al. Spumaretroviruses: updated taxonomy and nomenclature. Manuscript in preparation 2017.

41. Malmquist WA, Van der Maaten MJ, Boothe AD. Isolation, immunodiffusion, immunofluorescence, and electron microscopy of a syncytial virus of lymphosarcomatous and apparently normal cattle. Cancer Res. 1969;29(1):188–200.

42. Tobaly-Tapiero J, Bittoun P, Neves M, Guillemin MC, Lecellier CH, Puvion-Dutilleul F, et al. Isolation and characterization of an equine foamy virus. J Virol. 2000;74(9):4064–73.

43. Riggs JL, Oshirls LS, Taylor DO, Lennette EH. Syncytium-forming agent isolated from domestic cats. Nature. 1969;222(199):1190–1.

44. Johnston P. A second immunological type of simian foamy virus: monkey throat infections and unmasking by both types. J Infect Dis. 1961;109:1–9.

45. Stiles GE, Bittle JL, Cabasso UJ. Comparison of simian foamy virus strains including a new serological type. Nature. 1964;201:1350–3.

46. Rogers N, Basnight M, Gibbs CJ Jr, Gajdusek DC. Latent viruses in chimpanzees with experimental kuru. Nature. 1967;216:446–9.

47. Blasse A, Calvignac-Spencer S, Merkel K, Goffe AS, Boesch C, Mundry R, et al. Mother-offspring transmission and age-dependent accumulation of simian foamy virus in wild chimpanzees. J Virol. 2013;28:5193–204.

48. Johnson RH, de la Rosa J, Abher I, Kertayadnya IG, Entwistle KW, Fordyce G, et al. Epidemiological studies of bovine spumavirus. Vet Microbiol. 1988;16(1):25–33.

49. Winkler IG, Löchelt M, Flower RL. Epidemiology of feline foamy virus and feline immunodeficiency virus infections in domestic and feral cats: a seroepidemiological study. J Clin Microbiol. 1999;37(9):2848–51.

50. Meiering CD, Linial ML. Historical perspective of foamy virus epidemiology and infection. Clin Microbiol Rev. 2001;14:165–76.

51. Jones-Engel L, Steinkraus KA, Murray SM, Engel GA, Grant R, Aggimarangsee N, et al. Sensitive assays for simian foamy viruses reveal a high prevalence of infection in commensal, free-ranging, Asian monkeys. J Virol. 2007;81:7330–7.

52. Broussard SR, Comuzzie AG, Leighton KL, Leland MM, Whitehead EM, Allan JS. Characterization of new simian foamy viruses from African nonhuman primates. Virology. 1997;237(2):349–59.

53. Calattini S, Wanert F, Thierry B, Schmitt C, Bassot S, Saib A, et al. Modes of transmission and genetic diversity of foamy viruses in a Macaca tonkeana colony. Retrovirology. 2006;3(1):23.

54. Hood S, Mitchell JL, Sethi M, Almond NM, Cutler KL, Rose NJ. Horizontal acquisition and a broad biodistribution typify simian foamy virus infection in a cohort of Macaca fascicularis. Virol J. 2013;10:326.

55. Stenbak CR, Craig KL, Ivanov SB, Wang X, Soliven KC, Jackson DL, et al. New World simian foamy virus infections in vivo and in vitro. J Virol. 2014;88:982–91.

56. Muniz CP, Troncoso LL, Moreira MA, Soares EA, Pissinatti A, Bonvicino CR, et al. Identification and characterization of highly divergent simian foamy viruses in a wide range of new world primates from Brazil. PLoS ONE. 2013;8:e67568.

57. Muniz CP, Jia H, Shankar A, Troncoso LL, Augusto AM, Farias E, et al. An expanded search for simian foamy viruses (SFV) in Brazilian New World primates identifies novel SFV lineages and host age-related infections. Retrovirology. 2015;14(12):94.

58. Sharp PM, Hahn BH. The evolution of HIV-1 and the origin of AIDS. Philos Trans R Soc Lond B Biol Sci. 2010;365(1552):2487–94.

59. Brooks JI, Merks HW, Fournier J, Boneva RS, Sandstrom PA. Characterization of blood-borne transmission of simian foamy virus. Transfusion. 2007;47(1):162–70.

60. Murray SM, Picker LJ, Axthelm MK, Linial ML. Expanded tissue targets for foamy virus replication with simian immunodeficiency virus-induced immunosuppression. J Virol. 2006;80:663–70.

61. Choudhary A, Galvin TA, Williams DK, Beren J, Bryant MA, Khan AS. Influence of naturally occurring simian foamy viruses (SFVs) on SIV disease progression in the Rhesus macaque (*Macaca mulatta*) model. Viruses. 2013;5(6):1414–30.

62. Winkler IG, Lochelt M, Levesque JP, Bodem J, Flügel RM, Flower RL. A rapid streptavidin-capture ELISA specific for the detection of antibodies to feline foamy virus. J Immunol Methods. 1997;207(1):69–77.

63. Butera ST, Brown J, Callahan ME, Owen SM, Matthews AL, Weigner DD, et al. Survey of veterinary conference attendees for evidence of zoonotic infection by feline retroviruses. J Am Vet Med Assoc. 2000;217(10):1475–9.

64. Kehl T, Tan J, Materniak M. Non-simian foamy viruses: molecular virology, tropism and prevalence and zoonotic/interspecies transmission. Viruses. 2013;5:2169–209.

65. Linial ML, Fan H, Hahn B, Lower R, Neil J, Quackenbush SL, et al. Retroviridae. In: Fauquet CM, Mayo MA, Maniloff J, Desselberger U, Ball LA, editors. Virus taxonomy, VIIIth report of the ICTV. London: Elsevier/Academic Press; 2004. p. 421–40.

66. Schweizer M, Turek R, Hahn H, Schliephake A, Netzer KO, Eder G, et al. Markers of foamy virus infections in monkeys, apes, and accidentally infected humans—appropriate testing fails to confirm suspected foamy virus prevalence in humans. AIDS Res Hum Retrovir. 1995;11(1):161–70.

67. Ali M, Taylor GP, Pitman RJ, Parker D, Rethwilm A, Cheingsongpopov R, et al. No evidence of antibody to human foamy virus in widespread human populations. AIDS Res Hum Retrovir. 2009;12(15):1473–83.

68. Heneine W, Switzer WM, Sandstrom P, Brown J, Vedapuri S, Schable CA, et al. Identification of a human population infected with simian foamy viruses. Nat Med. 1998;4(4):403–7.

69. Sandstrom PA, Phan KO, Switzer WM, Fredeking T, Chapman L, Heneine W, et al. Simian foamy virus infection among zoo keepers. Lancet. 2000;355(9203):551–2.

70. Brooks JI, Rud EW, Pilon RG, Smith JM, Switzer WM, Sandstrom PA. Cross-species retroviral transmission from macaques to human beings. Lancet. 2002;360(9330):387–8.

71. Switzer WM, Bhullar V, Shanmugam V, Cong ME, Parekh B, Lerche NW, et al. Frequent simian foamy virus infection in persons occupationally exposed to nonhuman primates. J Virol. 2004;78(6):2780–9.

72. Wolfe ND, Switzer WM, Carr JK, Bhullar VB, Shanmugam V, Tamoufe U, et al. Naturally acquired simian retrovirus infections in central African hunters. Lancet. 2004;363(9413):932–7.

73. Calattini S, Betsem EB, Froment A, Mauclere P, Tortevoye P, Schmitt C, et al. Simian foamy virus transmission from apes to humans, rural Cameroon. Emerg Infect Dis. 2007;13(9):1314–20.

74. Betsem E, Rua R, Tortevoye P, Froment A, Gessain A. Frequent and recent human acquisition of simian foamy viruses through apes' bites in central Africa. PLoS Pathog. 2011;7(10):e1002306.

75. Mouinga-Ondeme A, Caron M, Nkoghe D, Telfer P, Preston M, Saib A, et al. Cross-species transmission of simian foamy virus to humans in rural Gabon, Central Africa. J Virol. 2012;86(2):1255–60.

76. Jones-Engel L, May CC, Engel GA, Steinkraus KA, Schillaci MA, Fuentes A, et al. Diverse contexts of zoonotic transmission of simian foamy viruses in Asia. Emerg Infect Dis. 2008;14(8):1200–8.

77. Engel GA, Small CT, Soliven K, Feeroz MM, Wang X, Hasan K, et al. Zoonotic simian foamy virus in Bangladesh reflects diverse patterns of transmission and co-infections among humans. Emerg Microbes Infect. 2013;2(9):e58.

78. Boneva RS, Switzer WM, Spira TJ, Bhullar VB, Shanmugam V, Cong ME, et al. Clinical and virological characterization of persistent human infection with simian foamy viruses. AIDS Res Hum Retrovir. 2007;23:1330–7.

79. Mouinga-Ondeme A, Betsem E, Caron M, Makuwa M, Salle B, Renault N, et al. Two distinct variants of simian foamy virus in naturally infected mandrills (*Mandrillus sphinx*) and cross-species transmission to humans. Retrovirology. 2010;7(1):105.

80. Switzer WM, Tang S, Zheng H, Shankar A, Sprinkle PS, Sullivan V, et al. Dual simian foamy virus/human immunodeficiency virus type 1 infections in persons from Cote d'Ivoire. PLoS ONE. 2016;11(6):e0157709.

81. Switzer W, Ahuka-Mundeke S, Tang S, Shankar A, Wolfe N, Heneine W, et al. Simian foamy virus (SFV) infection from multiple monkey species in women from the Democratic Republic of Congo. Retrovirology. 2012;. https://doi.org/10.1186/1742-4690-9-100.

82. Bamunusinghe D, Naghashfar Z, Buckler-White A, Plishka R, Baliji S, Liu Q, et al. Sequence diversity, intersubgroup relationships, and origins of the mouse leukemia gammaretroviruses of laboratory and wild mice. J Virol. 2016;90(8):4186–98.

83. Soliven K, Wang X, Small CT, Feeroz MM, Lee EG, Craig KL, et al. Simian foamy virus infection of rhesus macaques in Bangladesh: relationship of latent proviruses and transcriptionally active viruses. J Virol. 2013;87(24):13628–39.

84. Rua R, Betsem E, Gessain A. Viral latency in blood and saliva of simian foamy virus-infected humans. PLoS ONE. 2013;8(10):e77072.

85. Switzer WM, Shanmugam V, Bhavalkar-Potdar V, Folks TM, Boneva RS, Chapman LE, et al. Virus recovery from the oral mucosa and evidence of viral quasispecies and tissue compartmentalization in an SFcpz-infected person. In: Fourth international conference on foamy viruses, 2002. p. 12.

86. Matsen FA, Small CT, Soliven K, Engel GA, Feeroz MM, Wang X, et al. A novel Bayesian method for detection of APOBEC3-mediated hypermutation and its application to zoonotic transmission of simian foamy viruses. PLoS Comput Biol. 2014;10(2):e1003493.

87. Craig KL, Hasan MK, Jackson DL, Engel GA, Soliven K, Feeroz MM, et al. A seminomadic population in Bangladesh with extensive exposure to macaques does not exhibit high levels of zoonotic simian foamy virus infection. J Virol. 2015;89(14):7414–6.

88. Pacheco B, Finzi A, McGee-Estrada K, Sodroski J. Species-specific inhibition of foamy viruses from South American monkeys by New World Monkey TRIM5α proteins. J Virol. 2010;84:4095–9.

89. Muniz CP, Cavalcante LTF, Jia H, Zheng H, Tang S, Augusto AM, et al. Zoonotic infection of Brazilian primate workers with New World simian foamy virus. PLoS ONE. 2017;12(9):e0184502.

90. Switzer W, Garcia A, Yang C, Wright A, Kalish M, Folks T, et al. Coinfection with HIV-1 and simian foamy virus in West Central Africans. J Infect Dis. 2008;197(10):1389–93.

2

Nomenclature for endogenous retrovirus (ERV) loci

Robert J. Gifford[1]* ◉, Jonas Blomberg[2], John M. Coffin[3], Hung Fan[4], Thierry Heidmann[5], Jens Mayer[6], Jonathan Stoye[7], Michael Tristem[8] and Welkin E. Johnson[9]*

Abstract

Retroviral integration into germline DNA can result in the formation of a vertically inherited proviral sequence called an endogenous retrovirus (ERV). Over the course of their evolution, vertebrate genomes have accumulated many thousands of ERV loci. These sequences provide useful retrospective information about ancient retroviruses, and have also played an important role in shaping the evolution of vertebrate genomes. There is an immediate need for a unified system of nomenclature for ERV loci, not only to assist genome annotation, but also to facilitate research on ERVs and their impact on genome biology and evolution. In this review, we examine how ERV nomenclatures have developed, and consider the possibilities for the implementation of a systematic approach for naming ERV loci. We propose that such a nomenclature should not only provide unique identifiers for individual loci, but also denote orthologous relationships between ERVs in different species. In addition, we propose that—where possible—mnemonic links to previous, well-established names for ERV loci and groups should be retained. We show how this approach can be applied and integrated into existing taxonomic and nomenclature schemes for retroviruses, ERVs and transposable elements.

Keywords: Retrovirus, Nomenclature, Endogenous, Taxonomy, Classification

Background

Retroviruses (family *Retroviridae*) are characterized by a replication cycle in which the viral RNA genome is reverse-transcribed and integrated into the nuclear genome of the host cell. The principal determinants of the retroviral replication cycle are the enzymes reverse transcriptase (RT) and integrase (IN) [1]. These enzymes allow the conversion of single stranded viral RNA into double-stranded DNA, followed by integration of viral DNA into the nuclear genome of the infected cell to form the 'provirus'. As a chromosomal insertion, the integrated provirus has a life-long association with the infected cell, and survives as long as that cell (or its progeny). When integration occurs in a germ cell (i.e. gametes or early embryo), the resultant provirus can be vertically

inherited as a host allele (see Fig. 1). Such a provirus is called an endogenous retrovirus (ERV). Unless silenced or inactivated (e.g., by methylation [2] or mutation), ERV proviruses retain the potential to give rise to additional germline copies—either by infection of, or retrotransposition within further germ cells [3–5]. Selective forces operating at the level of the host population determine the fate of individual ERV loci. By far the most likely outcome for any newly generated ERV locus is that it will be purged from the gene pool. Despite this, however, vertebrate genomes typically contain thousands of ERV loci that have been genetically 'fixed'—i.e. they occur in all members of the species [6].

Studies over recent years have revealed the profound impact that ERVs have exerted on vertebrate evolution. For example, more of the human genome (~ 8%) is made up of the remnants of past retroviral infections than of sequences encoding the proteins necessary for life (~ 1–2%) [7]. Moreover, ERVs are not—as was once believed—mere 'junk DNA'—some encode intact proteins that have been co-opted or exapted to perform

*Correspondence: robert.gifford@glasgow.ac.uk; welkin.johnson@bc.edu
[1] MRC-University of Glasgow Centre for Virus Research, Glasgow, UK
[9] Biology Department, Boston College, Chestnut Hill,
Massachusetts 02467, USA
Full list of author information is available at the end of the article

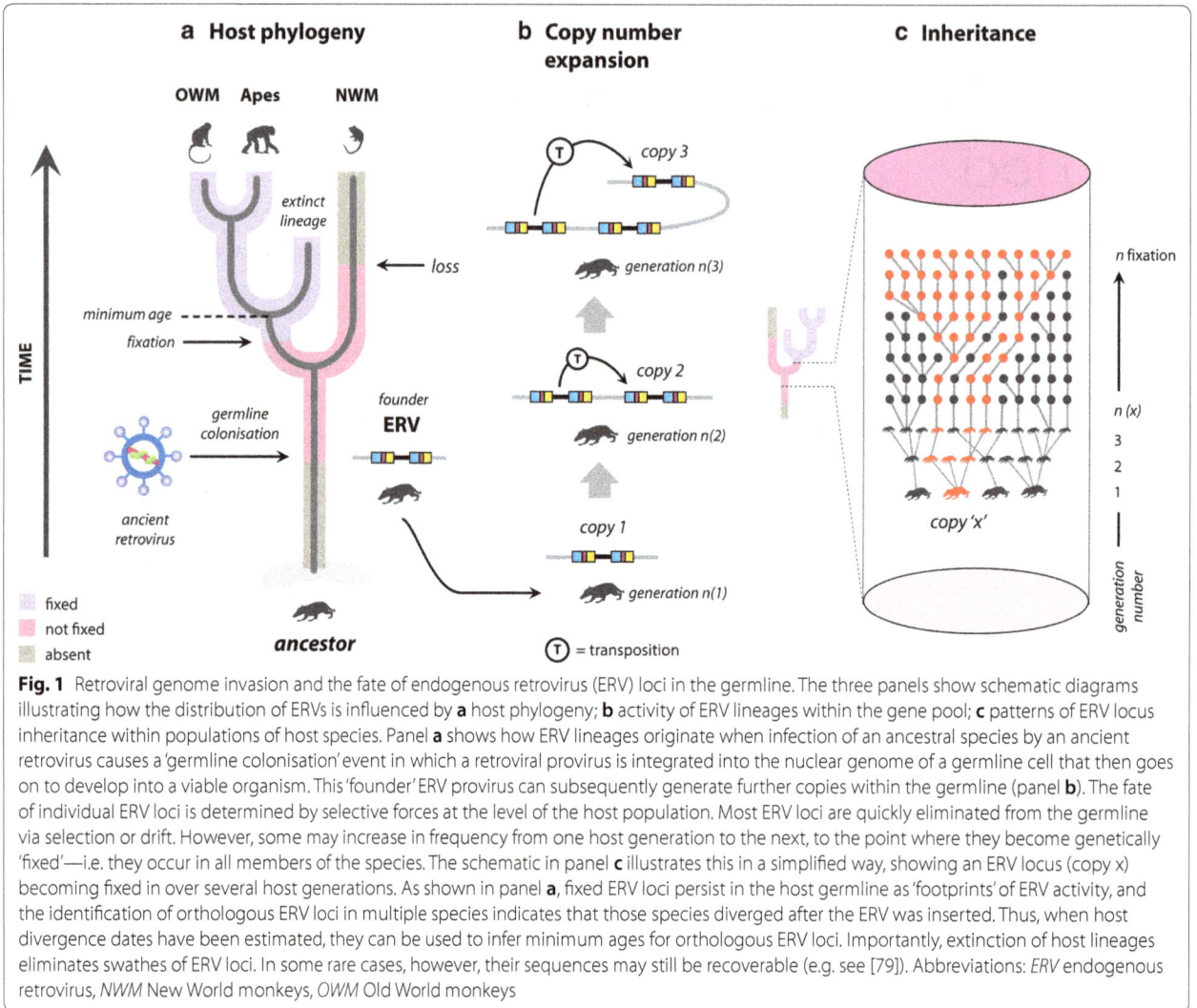

Fig. 1 Retroviral genome invasion and the fate of endogenous retrovirus (ERV) loci in the germline. The three panels show schematic diagrams illustrating how the distribution of ERVs is influenced by **a** host phylogeny; **b** activity of ERV lineages within the gene pool; **c** patterns of ERV locus inheritance within populations of host species. Panel **a** shows how ERV lineages originate when infection of an ancestral species by an ancient retrovirus causes a 'germline colonisation' event in which a retroviral provirus is integrated into the nuclear genome of a germline cell that then goes on to develop into a viable organism. This 'founder' ERV provirus can subsequently generate further copies within the germline (panel **b**). The fate of individual ERV loci is determined by selective forces at the level of the host population. Most ERV loci are quickly eliminated from the germline via selection or drift. However, some may increase in frequency from one host generation to the next, to the point where they become genetically 'fixed'—i.e. they occur in all members of the species. The schematic in panel **c** illustrates this in a simplified way, showing an ERV locus (copy x) becoming fixed in over several host generations. As shown in panel **a**, fixed ERV loci persist in the host germline as 'footprints' of ERV activity, and the identification of orthologous ERV loci in multiple species indicates that those species diverged after the ERV was inserted. Thus, when host divergence dates have been estimated, they can be used to infer minimum ages for orthologous ERV loci. Importantly, extinction of host lineages eliminates swathes of ERV loci. In some rare cases, however, their sequences may still be recoverable (e.g. see [79]). Abbreviations: *ERV* endogenous retrovirus, *NWM* New World monkeys, *OWM* Old World monkeys

physiological functions in host species, and even ERVs that are relatively degraded in terms of their coding capacity can perform important functions as components of gene regulatory networks [8–13].

ERV sequences also provide a unique source of retrospective information about retroviruses that circulated millions of years ago, and can therefore be used to explore the long-term history of evolutionary interaction between retroviruses and their hosts [14, 15]. Until quite recently, most investigations of this nature have of necessity been theoretical or comparative, but in recent years 'investigators have utilized gene synthesis to 'repair' the mutated genes of ERVs and study their biological properties in vitro [16–25].

New vertebrate genome sequences are becoming available for study on an almost daily basis, providing a deluge

of novel ERV data to drive further investigations of ERVs. There is therefore an urgent need for a unified system of nomenclature for ERV loci, not only to assist genome annotation, but also to facilitate research on ERVs and their impact on the genome biology and evolution of host species.

Insights into ERV biology in the genomic era

Modern genomics has allowed investigations of ERVs across a wide range of vertebrate whole genome sequences [26]. Together, these have provided a number of important insights into the general biology of ERV lineages that should be taken into consideration when constructing a nomenclature system.

Firstly, phylogenetic studies in humans and other species have shown that the multitudes of ERV sequences found in vertebrate genomes derive from a relatively small number of initial founder events [27, 28], and that distinct vertebrate lineages contain characteristic sets of ERVs that reflect their specific histories of; (1) retroviral germline invasion; (2) ERV copy number expansion; (3) and ERV locus fixation (see Fig. 1). However, establishing precisely the number of distinct retroviral germline invasion events that have occurred in the evolution of a host lineage is difficult. Significant germline invasions by retroviruses can presumably occur without any ERVs being fixed in descendant species, and even those ERV groups that do get fixed may be comprised entirely of partial and/or low copy number sequences that are problematic to detect. Moreover, even for the subset of ERVs that are detectable, phylogenetic approaches may not allow the number of separate invasion events to be determined with confidence—particularly when multiple invasions involving relatively similar viruses have occurred in the distant past. For example, estimates for the number of distinct germline invasion events that gave rise to the ERVs found in the human genome vary widely, from ~34 to ~80 [10, 73].

Secondly, it is clear from genomic studies that the vast majority of ERVs no longer encode functional proteins. Retroviral proviruses typically possess three principal coding domains (*gag*, *pol* and *env*), flanked at either side by long terminal-repeat sequences (the 5′ and 3′ LTRs) that are identical at the time of integration [29] (Fig. 2). A non-coding sequence containing a tRNA-specific primer-binding site (PBS) is usually present between the end of the 5′ LTR and the first codon of the *gag* gene. Without the purifying selection provided by replication, however, ERV sequences undergo mutational decay. Frequently, internal coding sequences are completely deleted through recombination between 5′ and 3′ LTRs, leaving behind a 'solo LTR' [30]. Indeed, solo LTR numbers are typically orders of magnitude more common than loci containing internal coding regions [31]. Other rearrangements of ERV genomes can also arise through processes such as LINE1-mediated retrotransposition, recombination, and deletion (Fig. 2b) [3]. Recombination can generate a diversity of 'mosaic' ERV forms [6], and can lead to genes and LTR sequences being 'swapped' between retroelement lineages [32].

Finally, comparative genomic studies have shown that in many cases, homologous ERV sequences are present at the same genomic locus in multiple species genomes. Since retroviral integration—while not random—is not site-specific [33, 34], such 'orthologous' ERV loci can be assumed to have been generated before the species they are found in diverged. Thus, if host divergence dates are known, they can be used to infer minimum ages to be

inferred for individual ERV loci, and by extension the founding colonization events that generated ERV lineages [35]. In higher primates, for example, comparative studies show that most integration events are extremely ancient, having occurred after the separation between New World monkeys (Platyrrhini) and Old World monkeys (Catarrhini) but before the split between Old World monkeys and hominoids (*Hominoidae*) around 30–45 million years ago (Mya) [36]. It should be noted, however, that fixed ERV loci may significantly predate the divergence times of the host species they occur in. Furthermore, as shown in Fig. 1, fixed ERV loci can be much younger than the ERV lineage they belong to, and due to different patterns of inheritance in descendant hosts, ERVs can end up being fixed in one set of descendant species, and lost from another.

Existing ERV nomenclature schemes and history of their development

Existing nomenclature systems for ERVs have developed in a haphazard manner reflecting their history of discovery. ERVs were first discovered in the 1960s by virtue of the genetically controlled expression of viral antigens of replication-competent ERVs in chickens and mice [37]. These viruses were closely related to exogenous oncogenic viruses, prompting a decades long search for disease-associated ERVs in other species, especially man [38, 39]. Infectious human counterparts, however, have remained elusive.

Laboratory techniques employed to identify ERVs have included virus isolation by co-cultivation with cells from a variety of species [40], hybridization under low stringency conditions with retroviral probes followed by cloning [41, 42], and PCR with primers directed to conserved regions of RT [42–46]. These studies formed the initial context of ERV nomenclature schemes, but in more recent years, ERV nomenclature has been increasingly influenced by in silico mining of vertebrate genome sequences, based either on sequence similarity or predicted features of proviruses such as nearby LTRs.

Originally, endogenous proviruses were named after the most closely related exogenous retrovirus, such as murine leukemia virus (MLV), as well as subgroups, like xenotropic MLV (XMV) [47]. A common approach to naming ERVs in different species has been to add one or two letters before the designation ERV to indicate the species in which they were initially identified; thus, HERV indicates an ERV first seen in human DNA, and MERV or MuERV implies one originally found in the genomes of murine species [e.g. house mouse (*Mus musculus*)]. HERVs have been further classified on the basis

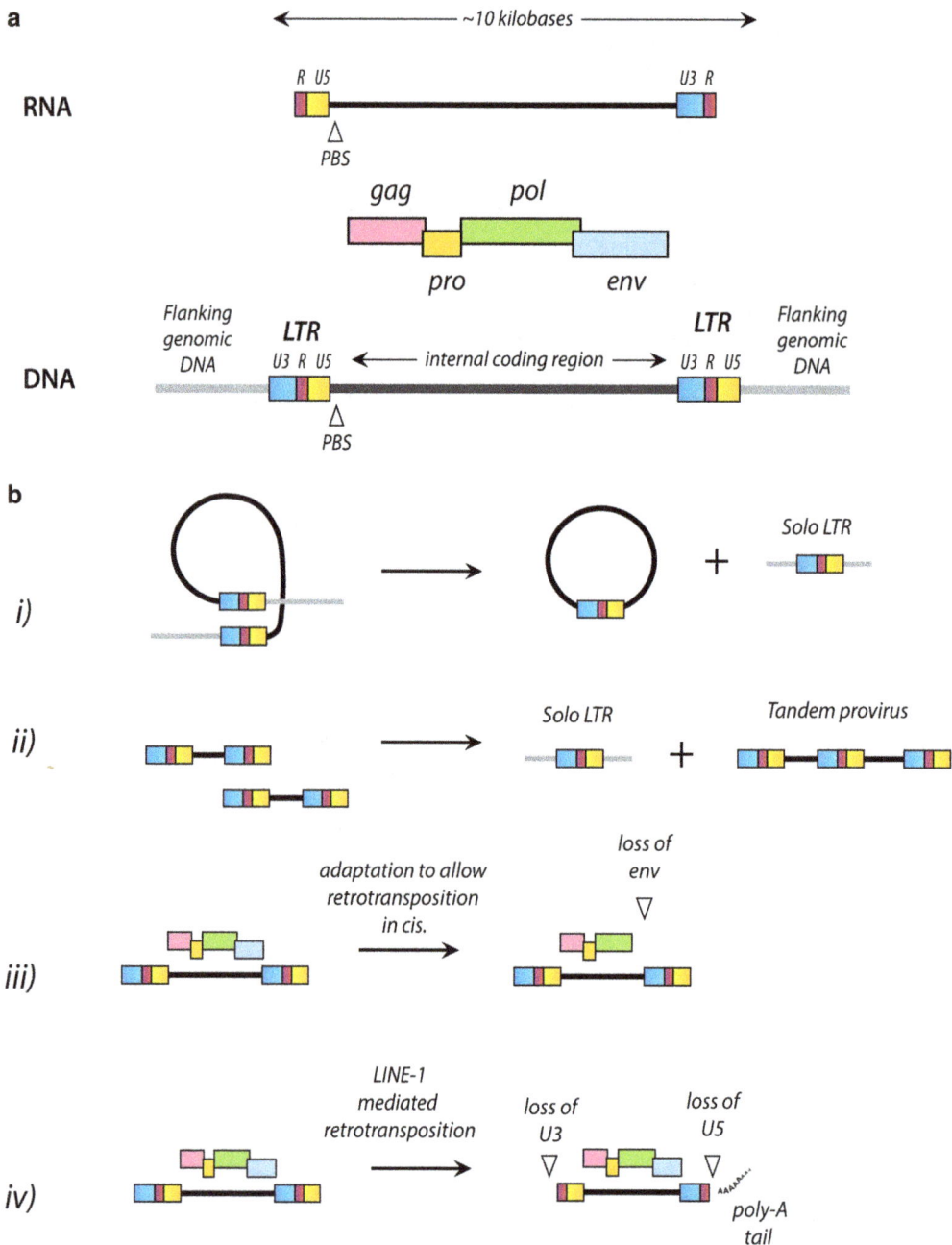

Fig. 2 Genomic structure of ERV sequences. Panel **a** shows a schematic representation of a generalised retroviral provirus. The four coding domains found in all exogenous retroviruses are indicated. The precise organization of these domains varies among retrovirus lineages, and some viruses also encode additional genes. The long terminal repeat (LTR) sequences are comprised of three distinct subregions that are named according to their organization in the genomic RNA: unique 3′ region (U3), repeat region (R), and unique 5′ region (U5). Panel **b** shows a schematic representation of processes that modify ERV sequences. (1) Recombination between the two LTRs of a single provirus resulting in the formation of a solo LTR. (2) Recombination between the 3′ and 5′ LTRs of a given provirus leading to a tandem duplicated provirus. (3) Adaptation to intracellular retrotransposition, resulting in the loss of the envelope gene. (4) LINE1-mediated retrotransposition, resulting in loss of the 5′ U3 sequence, and the 3′ U5 sequence. Variants with larger 5′ truncations may also occur. Poly-A tails at the 3′ end and L1-typical target site duplications flanking the retrotransposed sequence are usually found for these forms. Figure partly adapted from [80]

of the tRNA that binds to the viral primer binding site (PBS) to prime reverse transcription (see Fig. 2a). Hence HERV-K implies a provirus or ERV lineage that use a lysine tRNA, no matter their relationship to one another. In some cases the PBS sequence was not available when novel elements were first discovered leading to the names based on neighboring genes (e.g. HERV-ADP [48]), clone number (e.g. HERV-S71 [49]), or amino acid motifs (e.g. HERV-FRD [42]). Additional designations based on the probe used for cloning, and sub-divisions based on sequence identity or phylogenetic reconstructions, have also been used [50].

The somewhat arbitrary manner in which these nomenclatures have evolved has created a number of anomalies. The first concerns the use of the initial letter(s) to designate species of origin. This presents difficulties with proviruses that were integrated prior to the divergence of their host species. Many of the ERVs present in humans and chimpanzees fall into this category—thus related proviruses in both species genomes can end up with quite different names (e.g. HERVxxx and CERVyyy) despite the fact that proviruses in the two species will be more closely related to one another (identical at the time of integration) than their paralogous siblings within the same phylogenetic grouping. This problem becomes even more acute when considering specific proviruses shared among multiple species (i.e., when the same integrated provirus has been inherited by two or more descendant species). A further difficulty arises when what would appear to be the generic name for ERVs from one species becomes the trivial name for a discrete lineage of proviruses within that species, as has occurred with the MLV-related PERVs (porcine endogenous retroviruses) of pigs [51].

The use of tRNA primer specificity as a basis for sub-classification is problematic because there are a number of instances where this sequence does not reflect the overall relationship between distinct ERV lineages. For example, the HERV-K(HML-5) group appears to use a $tRNA_{Met}$ as primer while the other HERV-K lineages use $tRNA_{Lys}$ [52]. Even very recently integrated proviruses, such as endogenous MLVs, can be found to use different tRNA primers. The frequent convergent evolution implied by these examples, and the limited number of tRNAs available, makes primer usage an unsuitable basis for retroviral taxonomy.

At the level of individual ERV lineages, it is necessary to distinguish among specific proviruses at discrete chromosomal locations (i.e. between different but related ERV loci), and several different systems have developed for this purpose. Most commonly, individual proviruses are simply numbered; e.g. as

$Xmv1$, HERV-K 108, etc. In the case of HERVs, some investigators have chosen to use cytogenetic designations to distinguish among related proviruses [53, 54], as in HERV-K 11q22 (located on the q-arm, chromosomal band 22, of human chromosome 11). The need for this kind of locus-level ERV annotation is far more urgent now that large numbers vertebrate genomes have been sequenced. Indeed, in genomes that have been sequenced to a high degree of coverage, it is now feasible to identify and annotate the majority of ERVs using purely in silico approaches.

The most comprehensive source of repetitive element annotations is REPBASE [55]. REPBASE annotations, which include but are not limited to ERVs, are based on sequence similarity to a set of consensus elements. As such, the naming conventions used within REPBASE may not necessarily reflect phylogenetic relationships between ERVs. Also, REPBASE annotations distinguish LTRs and internal regions, but do not provide any further breakdown of the genomic features found within ERV proviruses. Software tools have also been developed specifically to assist in the identification and characterization of ERVs (for instance, see [56–58]), and these, more focused systems can be used to map ERVs to a fine scale of detail, demarcating genes, protein domains, and functional RNA sequences [6, 59]. Unfortunately, however, there is currently no straightforward way to link the ERV annotations generated by distinct systems with one another, or with the taxonomic groupings of ERVs that have been defined in broad-based phylogenetic studies [27, 28, 45, 60–62].

Integrating ERV classification with retrovirus taxonomy

A further problem is aligning ERV classification—which so far has been derived in large part from systems of repetitive element annotation—with retroviral taxonomy as agreed by the International Committee for Virus Taxonomy (ICTV). The *Retroviridae* family is grouped into the order *Ortervirales* (retro-transcribing viruses) [63], and comprises two sub-families, *Orthoretrovirinae* (orthoretroviruses) and *Spumaretrovirinae* (spumaviruses or 'foamy viruses'). *Spumaretrovirinae* is currently a monogeric subfamily, whereas the *Orthoretrovirinae* comprises six exogenous genera. Endogenous representatives have now been identified for the majority of retroviral genera (Table 1). Some of these ERVs group robustly within the diversity of exogenous representatives in phylogenetic trees. Others group basal to contemporary isolates, but exhibit genomic or phylogenetic characteristics that argue for their inclusion within a particular genus (e.g. the presence of characteristic genomic features such

Table 1 Retroviral genera and their endogenous representatives

Genus	Type species	Endogenous representative[a]	
Alpharetrovirus	ALV	ALV	[37]
Betaretrovirus	MMTV	MMTV	[74]
Gammaretrovirus	MLV	MLV	[75]
Deltaretrovirus	HTLV-1	MinERVa	[66]
Epsilonretrovirus	WDSV	*none*[b]	
Lentivirus	SRLV-A	RELIK	[64]
Spumaretrovirus	SFV	SloEFV	[65]

ALV avian leukosis virus, *MMTV* mouse mammary tumour virus, *MLV* murine leukemia virus, *HTLV* human T cell leukemia virus, *WDSV* walleye dermal sarcoma virus, *SRLV-A* small ruminant lentivirus A, *SFV* simian foamy virus, *MinERVa* *Miniopterus* endogenous deltaretrovirus, *RELIK* rabbit endogenous lentivirus K, *SloEFV* sloth endogenous foamy virus

[a] First reported endogenous representative shown, with citation

[b] No ERVs have been identified that group robustly within the *Epsilonretrovirus* genus. However, distantly related, 'epsilon-like' elements have been described, such as the MER65/HERV-Lb elements found in the human genome [6, 76–78]

as accessory genes and nucleotide composition biases) [64–66].

However, most ERV lineages are more problematic to place in current taxonomic systems, and as a consequence, many have become known by the relatively arbitrary names they have been assigned within repetitive element classification systems. In these systems, ERVs form part of a larger assemblage of LTR-retroelements [55, 67, 68] characterised by their "paired LTR" structure. TE classification systems conventionally group ERVs into three 'classes' (I, II and III), based on relatedness to the exogenous *Gammaretrovirus*, *Betaretrovirus* and *Spumaretrovirus* genera respectively. Individual ERV lineages (i.e. groups of ERVs that are assumed to derive from a single germline invasion event) have historically been referred to as 'families'. This is problematic as the terms 'class' and 'family' have specific, taxonomic meanings and their use in this context is incompatible with existing retroviral taxonomy.

Taxonomy should ideally follow phylogeny [69]. Since the overwhelming evidence from genomic studies indicates that endogenous retroviruses derive from ancient exogenous retroviruses, integration of ERVs into retroviral classification schemes is both feasible and logical, following this principle. Any novel system of classification for ERVs should therefore take into account the phylogenetic relationships of ERVs to exogenous viruses. In addition, it seems likely that integration of ERV nomenclature with exogenous retroviral taxonomy will require the definition of new groups to represent lineages that existed as exogenous retroviruses in the past but now exist only as ERV "fossils" (i.e., extinct lineages).

ERV nomenclature proposal

It is clear that a standard system of nomenclature is required. Such a system would greatly facilitate communication and reproduction of results. For example, it could be used to provide unambiguous lists of loci in methods sections of manuscripts, or for the purposes of reproducing or comparing results of different studies. Ideally, a nomenclature system would provide a stable foundation for the development of increasingly accurate and finely detailed annotations. In addition, it could be used to nurture the establishment of a unified taxonomic system for retroviruses and ERVs.

We therefore propose that ERV loci be assigned standard, unique IDs composed of three elements, each separated by a hyphen, as shown in Fig. 3. The first element is a classifier that identifies the element as an ERV. The second element is itself comprised of two subcomponents—one denoting the lineage of retroviruses that the ERV belongs to, and the second being a numeric ID that uniquely identifies the specific ERV locus within that taxonomic group. The third element identifies the host lineage in which the ERV insertion occurs. The host lineage component may specify a species (i.e. we suggest using well-established abbreviations, such as HomSap for *Homo sapiens*). Alternatively, a higher taxonomic rank may be used to refer to the entire set of orthologous insertions that occurs in an order, family or genus. Examples of how these IDs would be applied to specific ERV loci are shown in Table 2.

Applying the proposed ERV nomenclature in practice

There are a number of contingencies pertaining to way that each of the individual elements within the ID is defined. Firstly, only sequences that disclose robust phylogenetic evidence of having been directly derived from an exogenous retrovirus should receive the classifier 'ERV' in the first ID element. Thus, loci belonging to the ancient mammalian lineage ERV-L would be included (even though none of the canonical ERV-L sequences encode an *env* gene) because the ERV-L RT has been shown to group robustly within the diversity of the family

Category - Taxonomic group . Numeric ID - Species ID

ERV - K(HML.2) . 113 - Hsa

Fig. 3 Proposed ERV ID structure. The proposed ID consists of three components separated by hyphens. The second component consists of two subcomponents, separated by a period, that identify (1) the group the ERV belongs to, and (2) the unique numeric ID of the locus. The third component identifies the species or species group in which the element(s) being referred to occur

Table 2 Application of the proposed nomenclature to example ERV loci

Example description	Locus ID
ERV-L insertion identified in all eutherian mammals[a]	ERV-L.1-*Eutheria*
Human copy of ERV-L.1-*Eutheria*	ERV-L.1-*Homo sapiens*
	ERV-L.1-HomSap*
	ERV-L.1-Hsa*
	L.1-Hsa**
HERV.K (HML2) 113	ERV-K(HML2).113-*Hsa*[b]
Chimpanzee ortholog of HERV.K (HML2) 113	ERV-K(HML2).113-Ptr
All copies of HERV.K (HML2) 113 found in great apes (*Hominidae*)	ERV-K(HML2).113-*Hominidae*
Human copy HERV-K(HML2) 4q35.2	ERV-K(HML2).4352-*Hsa*[c]
Polytropic murine leukemia virus ERV 1 (Pmv-1) in mouse	ERV-Pmv.1-Mus musculus
Xenotropic murine leukemia virus ERV 8 (Xmv-8) in mouse	ERV-Xmv.8-Mmu
Mouse mammary tumour virus (MMTV) locus 9 (Mtv9)	ERV-MMTV.8-Mmu
Xmv-8 in inbred mouse strain C57L	ERV-Xmv.8-Mmu.C57L
Copy 2 of rabbit endogenous lentivirus K (RELiK) in rabbit	ERV-RELiK.2-*Oryctolagus cuniculus*
	ERV-RELiK.2-OryCun*
Copy 2 of rabbit endogenous lentivirus K (RELiK) in hare	ERV-RELiK.2-*Lepus europaeus*
	ERV-RELiK.2-LepEur*
	RELiK.2-OryCun**
Macaque copy #183 of an unclassified Betaretrovirus-like virus	ERV-AB.183-*Macaca mulatta*
Peregrine falcon copy #25 of avian 'Betaretrovirus-like lineage 3'	ERV-AB3.25-*Falco peregrinus*
Use of trailing element to indicate alternative alleles of a polymorphic insertion	ERV-K(HML2).113-Hsa.a[d]
	ERV-K(HML2).113-Hsa.b[d]
Use of trailing element to indicate alternative genome structures of a polymorphic insertion	ERV-K(HML2).113-Hsa.provirus[d]
	ERV-K(HML2).113-Hsa.LTR[d]

*Alternative versions using an abbreviation to designate the host species component of the ID

**A shorter form of the ID can be used when it is clear from the context—or from the lineage component of the ID—that an ERV is being referred to

[a] For reference, see [35]

[b] We propose that where established numeric IDs are already in use, they should be preserved, as is the case for many representatives of the well researched HERV-K(HML2) lineage

[c] In this example, an ID is assigned to an ERV locus that has only previously been referred to via its cytogenetic location—a numeric ID is therefore proposed that preserves a mnemonic link to this cytogenetically-based identifier, without preserving the information about cytogenetic location. This follows a principle of our proposal wherein the numeric ID component of the overall ERV ID can retain mnemonic links to previous IDs, but all auxiliary information associated with ERV loci is obtained from a database via a unique ID, rather than encoded into the ID itself

[d] However, where it aids discussion such information can be appended to the ERV ID stem (e.g. to distinguish distinct alleles and genome structures)

Retroviridae [70]. By contrast, other LTR-retroelements that do not disclose an unambiguous link to retroviruses are excluded. These include, for example, the mammalian apparent retrotransposon (MaLR) elements, which are comprised of LTR-bounded internal sequences containing little or no similarity to retroviruses. Initially, the 'ERV' classifier should be reserved for clearly proviral elements that contain recognisable coding domains in their internal regions, and can be placed within a phylogeny of elements that can itself be placed within the *Retroviridae* family. Subsequently, solo LTR loci can be incorporated if: (1) they are allelic variants, and some proviral alleles also occur at the same locus; (2) they fall within a clade of LTR elements that is demonstrably associated with a particular lineage of ERV proviruses.

Since ERV sequences included in our classification scheme must by definition demonstrate phylogenetic links to exogenous retroviruses, it follows they can be integrated into a unified taxonomic scheme with a rational phylogenetic basis. This taxonomic scheme would provide the basis for assigning the 'lineage' component of the ID. Figure 4 illustrates a proposal for a unified scheme that integrates the classification of exogenous and endogenous retroviruses with minimal disruption to the existing schemas used for each. Within our proposed scheme, ERV loci should ideally be assigned IDs wherein the lineage component accurately reflects their position in such a unified schema. As discussed earlier, some ERVs exhibit phylogenetic and genomic characteristics that clearly identify them as endogenous representatives of contemporary virus groups (Table 1). However, the vast majority of ERVs fall outside the diversity defined by exogenous isolates. Thus, additional taxonomic groups would need to be created before the proposed nomenclature could be applied. These might be relatively broad to begin with—for example, the schema shown in Fig. 4 includes three 'placeholder' groups designed to act as temporary 'bins' for ERV loci that cannot be confidently placed within the existing taxonomic system approved by the ICTV. These groups correspond to three major divergences in orthoretroviral RT sequences [71], and are labelled as follows: *Spumavirus*-related (S), *Gammaretrovirus /Epsilonretrovirus*-related (GE), and *Alpharetrovirus/ Betaretrovirus*-related (AB). Placeholder groups are reserved for ERVs that do not group within the diversity of established genera. Within these broad groups, additional subgroupings representing well-established ERV lineages can then be recognized. Wherever possible, ERVs should be assigned IDs that identify them at

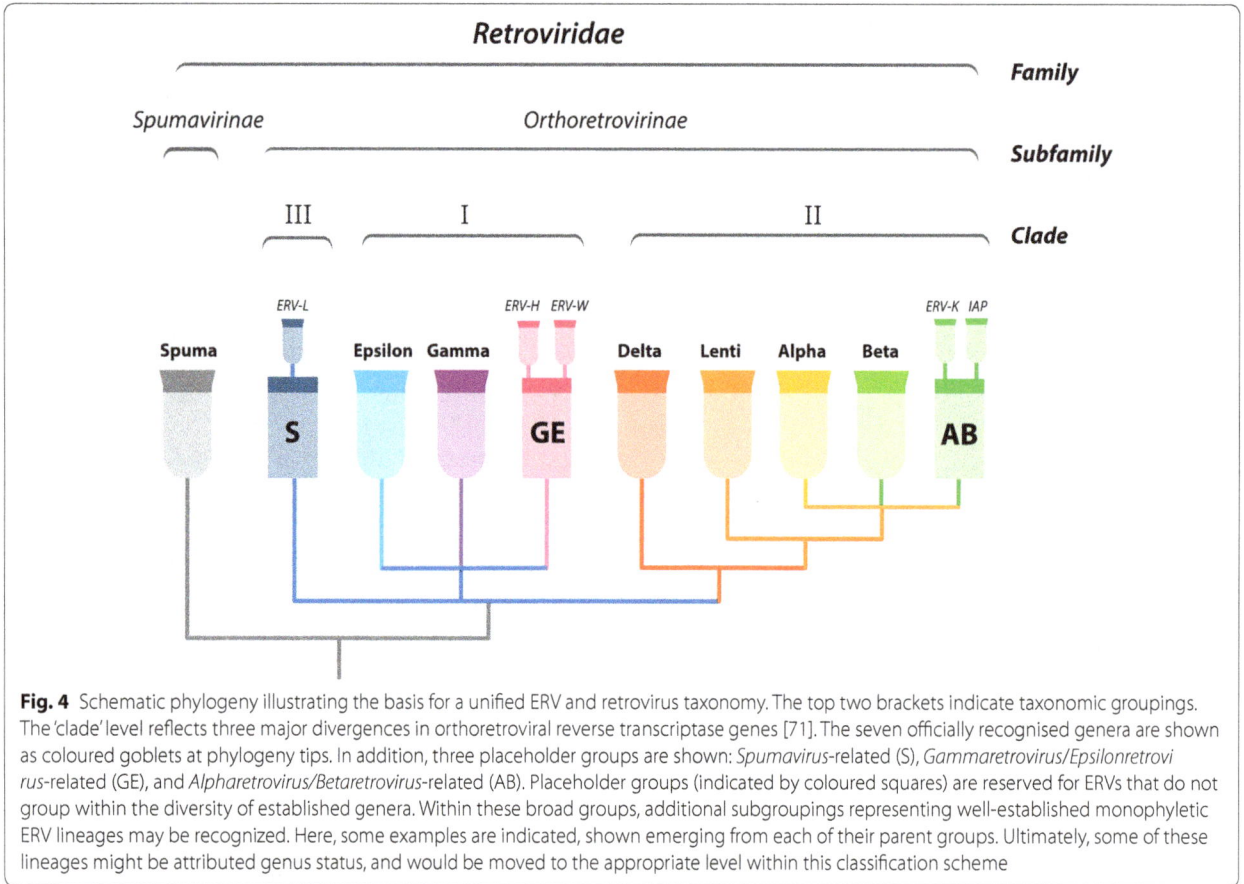

Fig. 4 Schematic phylogeny illustrating the basis for a unified ERV and retrovirus taxonomy. The top two brackets indicate taxonomic groupings. The 'clade' level reflects three major divergences in orthoretroviral reverse transcriptase genes [71]. The seven officially recognised genera are shown as coloured goblets at phylogeny tips. In addition, three placeholder groups are shown: *Spumavirus*-related (S), *Gammaretrovirus/Epsilonretrovirus*-related (GE), and *Alpharetrovirus/Betaretrovirus*-related (AB). Placeholder groups (indicated by coloured squares) are reserved for ERVs that do not group within the diversity of established genera. Within these broad groups, additional subgroupings representing well-established monophyletic ERV lineages may be recognized. Here, some examples are indicated, shown emerging from each of their parent groups. Ultimately, some of these lineages might be attributed genus status, and would be moved to the appropriate level within this classification scheme

the level of individual lineages (i.e. monophyletic lineages of ERV sequences estimated to derive from a single germline colonisation event), or at the level of viral species for ERVs that show close relationships to exogenous viruses, such as some of those found in the mouse genome (see Table 2). Ultimately, some of the ERV lineages that lack exogenous counterparts might be recognised as fossil representatives of extinct lineages, and attributed genus status within the unified taxonomic scheme shown in Fig. 4.

With regard to the numeric ID component, each taxonomic level referenced by the nomenclature would require its own discrete numbering system, entirely independent of all other taxonomic levels, and within which numeric IDs are only assigned once. Inevitably, the taxonomic designations may be subject to a limited amount of change over time, since ERVs are often identified before their phylogenetic relationships are fully resolved. Similarly, the piecemeal task of identifying orthologs would be expected to cause ongoing adjustments to numeric IDs (e.g. as it becomes clear that an ERV in one species is orthologous to an ERV detected in another). Providing each adjustment generates a new key

that is unique within the given taxonomic group, this can be accommodated.

Some ERV lineages have become known by particular names, and within these lineages, certain loci are also often known by particular numbers. We therefore propose that where ERV lineages or loci have established names or IDs that are well established and widely used, a mnemonic link to these should, where expedient, be retained. The examples shown in Table 2 illustrate how the proposed ID structure can support this.

The development of a consistent ERV nomenclature that uniquely identifies ERV loci would establish a basis for stably linking these loci to a wide range of relevant auxiliary information, such as cytogenetic location, or information about the genetic sub-structure of proviral insertions. This would compensate for the loss of such information from the ID itself, which would occur in some cases as a consequence of the standardization (see Table 2). Clearly, however, any auxiliary information attached to IDs would need to be collated and archived in a systematic way (i.e. using a database). Furthermore, ongoing maintenance of the nomenclature itself will be necessary, and a system of governance and oversight would need to be developed through which updates—e.g. addition, subtraction or merging of ERV loci, or reclassification of ERVs based on updated taxonomy—can be coordinated. An important aspect of nomenclature implementation will be the development of benchmarking procedures through which competing annotations can be assessed, as discussed more broadly for TEs in [72].

Conclusions

In this review, we have provided an account of how ERV nomenclature has developed, identifying the idiosyncrasies that have been generated in current nomenclature systems as a consequence of their historical development. We propose a novel, rational approach to naming ERV loci that is designed to unambiguously identify individual ERV loci, while accommodating as far as possible the contingencies and idiosyncrasies of ERV annotation. In addition, the proposed system allows for seamless integration into existing schemes for classification of transposable elements and viruses [55, 63, 67, 69, 73].

Abbreviations

ERV: endogenous retrovirus; LTR: long terminal repeat; NWM: New World monkey; OWM: Old World monkey; PBS: primer binding site; tRNA: transfer RNA; HERV: human endogenous retrovirus; MLV: murine leukemia virus; ICTV: International Committee for Virus Taxonomy.

Author's contributions

RJG, JB, JM, HF, TH, JM, JS, MT, and WEJ wrote the manuscript. All authors read and approved the final manuscript.

Author details
[1] MRC-University of Glasgow Centre for Virus Research, Glasgow, UK. [2] Department of Medical Sciences, Uppsala University, Uppsala, Sweden. [3] Department of Molecular Biology and Microbiology, Tufts University, Boston, MA, USA. [4] Department of Molecular Biology and Biochemistry and Cancer Research Institute, University of California, Irvine, CA 92697, USA. [5] Department of Molecular Physiology and Pathology of Infectious and Endogenous Retroviruses, CNRS UMR 9196, Institut Gustave Roussy, 94805 Villejuif, France. [6] Department of Human Genetics, Center of Human and Molecular Biology, Medical Faculty, University of Saarland, Homburg, Germany. [7] The Francis Crick Institute, Mill Hill Laboratory, The Ridgeway, Mill Hill, London, UK. [8] Imperial College London, Silwood Park Campus, Buckhurst Road, Ascot, Berkshire SL5 7PY, UK. [9] Biology Department, Boston College, Chestnut Hill, Massachusetts 02467, USA.

Acknowledgements
Concepts for this nomenclature proposal were developed over several years in the retrovirus subcommittee of the International Committee on the Taxonomy of Viruses. We thank all members of the subcommittee for their contribution.

Competing interests
The authors declare that they have no competing interests.

Funding
In June 2014 a meeting was held in Missillac, France sponsored by a grant from the Borchard Foundation (awarded to HF) at which the final nomenclature system was developed. We thank the Foundation for its generous support of this effort. RJG was supported by a grant from the UK Medical Research Council (No. MC_UU_12014/10).

References
1. Vogt PK. Historical introduction to the general properties of retroviruses. In: Coffin JM, Hughes SH, Varmus HE, editors. Retroviruses. New York: Cold Spring Harbour Laboratory Press; 1997.
2. Maksakova IA, Mager DL, Reiss D. Keeping active endogenous retroviral-like elements in check: the epigenetic perspective. Cell Mol Life Sci. 2008;65(21):3329–47.
3. de Parseval N, Heidmann T. Human endogenous retroviruses: from infectious elements to human genes. Cytogenet Genome Res. 2005;110(1–4):318–32.
4. Belshaw R, et al. High copy number in human endogenous retrovirus families is associated with copying mechanisms in addition to reinfection. Mol Biol Evol. 2005;22(4):814–7.
5. Ribet D, et al. An infectious progenitor for the murine IAP retrotransposon: emergence of an intracellular genetic parasite from an ancient retrovirus. Genome Res. 2008;18(4):597–609.
6. Vargiu L, et al. Classification and characterization of human endogenous retroviruses; mosaic forms are common. Retrovirology. 2016;13:7.
7. Lander ES, et al. Initial sequencing and analysis of the human genome. Nature. 2001;409(6822):860–921.
8. Jern P, Coffin JM. Effects of retroviruses on host genome function. Annu Rev Genet. 2008;42:709–32.
9. Varela M, et al. Friendly viruses: the special relationship between endogenous retroviruses and their host. Ann N Y Acad Sci. 2009;1178:157–72.
10. Rowe HM, Trono D. Dynamic control of endogenous retroviruses during development. Virology. 2011;411(2):273–87.
11. Dupressoir A, Lavialle C, Heidmann T. From ancestral infectious retroviruses to bona fide cellular genes: role of the captured syncytins in placentation. Placenta. 2012;33(9):663–71.
12. Stoye JP. Studies of endogenous retroviruses reveal a continuing evolutionary saga. Nat Rev Microbiol. 2012;10(6):395–406.
13. Wolf G, Greenberg D, Macfarlan TS. Spotting the enemy within: targeted silencing of foreign DNA in mammalian genomes by the Kruppel-associated box zinc finger protein family. Mob DNA. 2015;6:17.
14. Feschotte C, Gilbert C. Endogenous viruses: insights into viral evolution and impact on host biology. Nat Rev Genet. 2012;13(4):283–96.
15. Gifford RJ. Viral evolution in deep time: lentiviruses and mammals. Trends Genet. 2012;28(2):89–100.
16. Dewannieux M, et al. Identification of an infectious progenitor for the multiple-copy HERV-K human endogenous retroelements. Genome Res. 2006;16(12):1548–56.
17. Lee YN, Bieniasz PD. Reconstitution of an infectious human endogenous retrovirus. PLoS Pathog. 2007;3(1):e10.
18. Perez-Caballero D, et al. Tetherin inhibits HIV-1 release by directly tethering virions to cells. Cell. 2009;139(3):499–511.
19. Soll SJ, Neil SJ, Bieniasz PD. Identification of a receptor for an extinct virus. Proc Natl Acad Sci USA. 2010;107(45):19496–501.
20. Brady T, et al. Integration target site selection by a resurrected human endogenous retrovirus. Genes Dev. 2009;23(5):633–42.

21. Goldstone DC, et al. Structural and functional analysis of prehistoric lentiviruses uncovers an ancient molecular interface. Cell Host Microbe. 2010;8(3):248–59.

22. Dewannieux M, et al. The mouse IAPE endogenous retrovirus can infect cells through any of the five GPI-anchored Ephrin A proteins. PLoS Pathog. 2011;7(10):e1002309.

23. Lemaitre C, et al. The HERV-K human endogenous retrovirus envelope protein antagonizes Tetherin antiviral activity. J Virol. 2014;88(23):13626–37.

24. Blanco-Melo D, Gifford RJ, Bieniasz PD. Reconstruction of a replication-competent ancestral murine endogenous retrovirus-L. Retrovirology. 2018;15(1):34.

25. Blanco-Melo D, Gifford RJ, Bieniasz PD. Co-option of an endogenous retrovirus envelope for host defense in hominid ancestors. Elife. 2017;6:e22519.

26. Johnson WE. Endogenous retroviruses in the genomics era. Annu Rev Virol. 2015;2(1):135–59.

27. Tristem M. Identification and characterisation of novel human endogenous retrovirus families by phylogenetic screening of the human genome mapping project database. J Virol. 2000;74:3715–30.

28. Bénit L, Dessen P, Heidmann T. Identification, phylogeny, and evolution of retroviral elements based on their envelope genes. J Virol. 2001;75(23):11709–19.

29. Coffin JM. Structure and classification of retroviruses. In: Levy JA, editor. The retroviridae. New York: Plenum Press; 1992. p. 19–49.

30. Sverdlov ED. Perpetually mobile footprints of ancient infections in human genome. FEBS Lett. 1998;428(1–2):1–6.

31. Belshaw R, et al. Rate of recombinational deletion among human endogenous retroviruses. J Virol. 2007;81(17):9437–42.

32. Lober U, et al. Degradation and remobilization of endogenous retroviruses by recombination during the earliest stages of a germ-line invasion. Proc Natl Acad Sci USA. 2018;115(34):8609–14. https://doi.org/10.1073/pnas.1807598115.

33. Bushman F, et al. Genome-wide analysis of retroviral DNA integration. Nat Rev Microbiol. 2005;3(11):848–58.

34. Kvaratskhelia M, et al. Molecular mechanisms of retroviral integration site selection. Nucleic Acids Res. 2014;42(16):10209–25.

35. Lee A, et al. Identification of an ancient endogenous retrovirus, predating the divergence of the placental mammals. Philos Trans R Soc Lond B Biol Sci. 2013;368(1626):20120503.

36. Bannert N, Kurth R. The evolutionary dynamics of human endogenous retroviral families. Annu Rev Genomics Hum Genet. 2006;7:149–73.

37. Weiss RA. The discovery of endogenous retroviruses. Retrovirology. 2006;3:67.

38. Löwer R. The pathogenic potential of endogenous retroviruses: facts and fantasies. Trends Microbiol. 1999;7(9):350–6.

39. Voisset C, Weiss RA, Griffiths DJ. Human RNA "rumor" viruses: the search for novel human retroviruses in chronic disease. Microbiol Mol Biol Rev. 2008;72(1):157–96.

40. Weiss RA, et al. Induction of avian tumor viruses in normal cells by physical and chemical carcinogens. Virology. 1971;46(3):920–38.

41. Dunwiddie CT, et al. Molecular cloning and characterization of gag-, pol-, and env-related gene sequences in the ev- chicken. J Virol. 1986;59(3):669–75.

42. Seifarth W, et al. Retrovirus-like particles released from the human breast cancer cell line T47-D display type B- and C-related endogenous retroviral sequences. J Virol. 1995;69(10):6408–16.

43. Medstrand P, Blomberg J. Characterization of novel reverse transcriptase encoding human endogenous retroviral sequences similar to type A and type B retroviruses: differential transcription in normal human tissues. J Virol. 1993;67(11):6778–87.

44. Cordonnier A, Casella JF, Heidmann T. Isolation of novel human endogenous retrovirus-like elements with foamy virus-related pol sequence. J Virol. 1995;69(9):5890–7.

45. Herniou E, et al. Retroviral diversity and distribution in vertebrates. J Virol. 1998;72(7):5955–66.

46. Gifford R, et al. Evolution and distribution of class II-related endogenous retroviruses. J Virol. 2005;79(10):6478–86.

47. Stoye JP, Coffin JM. The four classes of endogenous murine leukemia virus: structural relationships and potential for recombination. J Virol. 1987;61(9):2659–69.

48. Lyn D, et al. The polymorphic ADP-ribosyltransferase (NAD+) pseudogene 1 in humans interrupts an endogenous pol-like element on 13q34. Genomics. 1993;18(2):206–11.

49. Werner T, et al. S71 is a phylogenetically distinct human endogenous retroviral element with structural and sequence homology to simian sarcoma virus (SSV). Virology. 1990;174(1):225–38.

50. Subramanian RP, et al. Identification, characterization, and comparative genomic distribution of the HERV-K (HML-2) group of human endogenous retroviruses. Retrovirology. 2011;8:90.

51. Takeuchi Y, et al. Host range and interference studies of three classes of pig endogenous retrovirus. J Virol. 1998;72(12):9986–91.

52. Lavie L, et al. Human endogenous retrovirus family HERV-K(HML-5): status, evolution, and reconstruction of an ancient betaretrovirus in the human genome. J Virol. 2004;78(16):8788–98.

53. Hughes JF, Coffin JM. Evidence for genomic rearrangements mediated by human endogenous retroviruses during primate evolution. Nat Genet. 2001;29(4):487–9.

54. Macfarlane C, Simmonds P. Allelic variation of HERV-K(HML-2) endogenous retroviral elements in human populations. J Mol Evol. 2004;59(5):642–56.

55. Jurka J, et al. Repbase update, a database of eukaryotic repetitive elements. Cytogenet Genome Res. 2005;110(1–4):462–7.

56. Sperber GO, et al. Automated recognition of retroviral sequences in genomic data–RetroTector. Nucleic Acids Res. 2007;35(15):4964–76.

57. Sperber G, et al. RetroTector online, a rational tool for analysis of retroviral elements in small and medium size vertebrate genomic sequences. BMC Bioinform. 2009;10(Suppl 6):S4.

58. Lerat E. Identifying repeats and transposable elements in sequenced genomes: how to find your way through the dense forest of programs. Heredity (Edinb). 2010;104(6):520–33.

59. Grandi N, et al. Contribution of type W human endogenous retroviruses to the human genome: characterization of HERV-W proviral insertions and processed pseudogenes. Retrovirology. 2016;13(1):67.

60. Hayward A, Cornwallis CK, Jern P. Pan-vertebrate comparative genomics unmasks retrovirus macroevolution. Proc Natl Acad Sci USA. 2015;112(2):464–9.

61. Hayward A, Grabherr M, Jern P. Broad-scale phylogenomics provides insights into retrovirus-host evolution. Proc Natl Acad Sci USA. 2013;110(50):20146–51.

62. Xu X, et al. Endogenous retroviruses of non-avian/mammalian vertebrates illuminate diversity and deep history of retroviruses. PLoS Pathog. 2018;14(6):e1007072.

63. Krupovic M, et al. Ortervirales: new virus order unifying five families of reverse-transcribing viruses. J Virol. 2018;92(12):e00515–8.

64. Katzourakis A, et al. Discovery and analysis of the first endogenous lentivirus. Proc Natl Acad Sci USA. 2007;104(15):6261–5.

65. Katzourakis A, et al. Macroevolution of complex retroviruses. Science. 2009;325(5947):1512.

66. Farkasova H, et al. Discovery of an endogenous Deltaretrovirus in the genome of long-fingered bats (Chiroptera: Miniopteridae). Proc Natl Acad Sci USA. 2017;114(12):3145–50.

67. Wicker T, et al. A unified classification system for eukaryotic transposable elements. Nat Rev Genet. 2007;8(12):973–82.

68. Kapitonov VV, Jurka J. A universal classification of eukaryotic transposable elements implemented in Repbase. Nat Rev Genet. 2008;9(5):411–2.

69. Blomberg J, et al. Classification and nomenclature of endogenous retroviral sequences (ERVs): problems and recommendations. Gene. 2009;448(2):115–23.

70. Bénit L, et al. ERV-L elements: a family of endogenous retrovirus-like elements active throughout the evolution of mammals. J Virol. 1999;73(4):3301–8.

71. Llorens C, Fares MA, Moya A. Relationships of gag-pol diversity between Ty3/Gypsy and retroviridae LTR retroelements and the three kings hypothesis. BMC Evol Biol. 2008;8:276.

72. Hoen DR, et al. A call for benchmarking transposable element annotation methods. Mob DNA. 2015;6:13.

73. Seberg O, Petersen G. A unified classification system for eukaryotic transposable elements should reflect their phylogeny. Nat Rev Genet. 2009;10(4):276.

74. Green RG, Moosey MM, Bittner JJ. Serial transmission of the milk agent of mouse mammary carcinoma. Proc Soc Exp Biol Med. 1946;61:362.

75. Gross L. A filterable agent, recovered from Ak leukemic extracts, causing salivary gland carcinomas in C3H mice. Proc Soc Exp Biol Med. 1953;83(2):414–21.

76. Brown K, Emes RD, Tarlinton RE. Multiple groups of endogenous epsilon-like retroviruses conserved across primates. J Virol. 2014;88(21):12464–71.

77. Sverdlov ED, editor. Retroviruses and Primate Genome Evolution. Austin, TX: Landes Bioscience; 2005. p. 186–203.

78. Oja M, et al. Self-organizing map-based discovery and visualization of human endogenous retroviral sequence groups. Int J Neural Syst. 2005;15(3):163–79.

79. Greenwood AD, et al. Evolution of endogenous retrovirus-like elements of the woolly mammoth (*Mammuthus primigenius*) and its relatives. Mol Biol Evol. 2001;18(5):840–7.

80. Stoye JP. Endogenous retroviruses: still active after all these years? Curr Biol. 2001;11(22):R914–6.

3

HIV-1 protease with leucine zipper fused at N-terminus exhibits enhanced linker amino acid-dependent activity

Fu-Hsien Yu and Chin-Tien Wang[*]

Abstract

Background: HIV-1 protease (PR) activation is triggered by Gag-Pol dimerization. Premature PR activation results in reduced virion yields due to enhanced Gag cleavage. A p6* transframe peptide located directly upstream of protease is believed to play a modulating role in PR activation. Previous reports indicate that the C-terminal p6* tetra-peptide prevents premature PR activation triggered by a leucine zipper (LZ) dimerization motif inserted in the deleted p6* region. To clarify the involvement of C-terminal p6* residues in mitigating enhanced LZ-incurred Gag processing, we engineered constructs containing C-terminal p6* residue substitutions with and without a mutation blocking the p6*/PR cleavage site, and created other Gag or p6* domain-removing constructs. The capabilities of these constructs to mediate virus maturation were assessed by Western blotting and single-cycle infection assays.

Results: p6*-PR cleavage blocking did not significantly reduce the LZ enhancement effect on Gag cleavage when only four amino acid residues were present between the p6* and PR. This suggests that the potent LZ dimerization motif may enhance PR activation by facilitating PR dimer formation, and that PR precursors may trigger sufficient enzymatic activity without breaking off from the PR N-terminus. Enhanced LZ-induced activation of PR embedded in Gag-Pol was found to be independent of the Gag assembly domain. In contrast, the LZ enhancement effect was markedly reduced when six amino acids were present at the p6*-PR junction, in part due to impaired PR maturation by substitution mutations. We also observed that a proline substitution at the P3 position eliminated the ability of p6*-deleted Gag-Pol to mediate virus maturation, thus emphasizing the importance of C-terminal p6* residues to modulating PR activation.

Conclusions: The ability of HIV-1 C-terminal p6* amino acid residues to modulate PR activation contributes, at least in part, to their ability to counteract enhanced Gag cleavage induced by a leucine zipper substituted for a deleted p6*. Changes in C-terminal p6* residues between LZ and PR may affect PR-mediated virus maturation, thus providing a possible method for assessing HIV-1 protease precursor activation in the context of virus assembly.

Keywords: HIV-1, Gag-Pol, P6pol, Protease maturation, Virus maturation, Gag cleavage

Background

The HIV-1 retrovirus contains three major genes (gag, pol and env) and several accessory genes [1]. HIV-1 pol encodes viral enzymes such as protease (PR), reverse transcriptase (RT) and integrase (IN), while gag encodes viral structural proteins. Both Pol and Gag are translated from the same mRNA template. Pol is translated as a Gag-Pol fusion protein associated with a ribosome shift during Gag translation that occurs at a 5% frequency, leading to a Gag-Pol versus Gag expression ratio of approximately 1:20 [2]. Pr160gag-pol and Pr55gag are transported to plasma membranes, where Pr55gag molecules assemble into virus particles [3]; Pr160gag-pol is incorporated into these particles via Pr55gag interaction [4–7]. During or after virus budding, activated PR auto-cleaves from Gag-Pol and mediates virus maturation

*Correspondence: chintien@ym.edu.tw
Department of Medical Research, Taipei Veterans General Hospital and Institute of Clinical Medicine, National Yang-Ming University School of Medicine, 201, Sec. 2, Shih-Pai Road, Taipei 11217, Taiwan

through the proteolytic processing of Pr55gag and Pr160gag-pol [8]. Pr55gag cleavage yields four main products: matrix (p17; MA), capsid (CA; p24), nucleocapsid (NC; p7) and C-terminal p6 [9]. Two spacer peptides—SP1 (or p2) and SP2 (or p1)—respectively separate NC from CA and p6. Pr160gag-pol cleavage generates RT and IN in addition to the Gag proteins MA, CA and NC. PR-mediated virus maturation is necessary for viral infectivity acquisition [10, 11].

It is generally believed that Gag-Pol dimerization triggers PR activation [3]. In agreement with this assumption, mutations upstream or downstream of PR may significantly reduce PR-mediated Gag cleavage efficiency due to inadequate Gag-Pol dimerization [12–16]. In contrast, the promotion of PR activation as a result of enhanced Gag-Pol dimerization or Gag-PR dimer interaction likely triggers premature or enhanced Pr55gag cleavage, resulting in markedly reduced virus production. [17–19]. Accordingly, preventing premature PR activation is central to virus assembly.

Within Gag-Pol, truncated p1-p6gag is replaced with a transframe region referred to as p6* or p6pol. Located directly adjacent to the PR N-terminus, p6* has been described as playing a role in modulating PR activation even though it lacks a specific structure. Mature HIV-1 PR has a dimeric form, and the removal of p6* from PR precursor is essential for PR to be fully functional [20–23]. Mutations that block p6*-PR cleavage markedly impede PR-mediated virus maturation, implying a suppressive effect of p6* on PR activation [22, 23]. Molecular models suggest that p6* may prevent early PR maturation by inducing instability in the folded PR dimer structure [24–27]. However, virus assembly-associated evidence in support of this assumption is limited, since deletion analysis of p6* function has the potential to compromise virus assembly due to an overlap of p6* with the p6gag budding domain.

To investigate p6* function without affecting the p6gag coding region, we engineered an HIV-1 virus-producing vector by placing the pol coding sequence at the PR-inactivated C-terminus. This construct, designated Dp6*PR, was capable of assembling and processing virus particles in a manner similar to that of wild-type (wt). Replacement of p6* with a leucine-zipper (LZ) dimerization domain has been shown to eliminate virus production as a result of enhanced Gag cleavage, but as few as four C-terminal p6 residues remaining between LZ and PR significantly counteract the LZ enhancement effect [28]. These observations provide supporting evidence that p6* may contribute to the prevention of premature PR activation, but it remains unknown whether a correlation exists between the ability of C-terminal p6* residues to counteract LZ enhancement and their ability to modulate

PR maturation. Further, it is unknown whether specific amino acids must be present between LZ and PR in order to counteract the LZ enhancement effect.

To study these questions, we engineered multiple constructs to further analyze the role of C-terminal p6* residues in counteracting LZ enhancement and modulating PR activation. Our results indicate that an HIV-1 PR precursor containing a leucine zipper (LZ) motif linked at the N-terminus eliminated virus particle production associated with enhanced Gag cleavage, suggesting that the HIV-1 PR precursor is capable of exhibiting enhanced enzymatic activity. C-terminal p6* residue substitutions can subvert the Gag cleavage enhancement effect induced by a LZ substitution for p6*, likely the result of interference with PR maturation. While p6*-deleted Gag-Pol (Δp6*fs) containing the last two remaining C-terminal p6* residues was still capable of producing infectious virions following co-expression with Pr55gag, a single amino acid residue change at the deleted p6* region completely removed the ability of Δp6*fs to mediate virus maturation. Our results confirm the importance of C-terminal p6* residues for the spatiotemporal modulation of PR activity, and provide a virus assembly system for studying HIV-1 protease precursor activation by manipulating linker residues between fused peptides and PR.

Methods
Plasmid construction
The parental HIV-1 proviral sequence in this study is HXB2 [29]. The HIV-1 proviral plasmid HIVgpt is considered the backbone of all expression constructs [30]. The constructs used in this research were mostly derived from Dp6*PR, DPR, DWzPR, DWz/PR and DWz//PR. As described previously [31], Dp6*PR contains p6* domain between an inactivated and an active PR. DPR contains BamHI-linked duplicate PR pairs, with the proximal PR was inactivated. DWzPR, DWz/PR and DWz//PR contain leucine zipper replacements of p6* with two, four and six C-terminal p6* residues remaining in the p6*/PR junction, respectively [28]. PSHL and PIDL substitutions for the four C-terminal p6* residues in DWz/PR yielded DWz/PSHL/PR and DWz/PIDL/PR [28]. Primers used for engineering the designated mutations were listed in Table 1.

V/P, as described previously was created by changing amino acid residues at p6*-PR cleavage site from Phe/Pro into Val/Pro [32]. BamHI-containing forward primers were used to amplify the p6* C-terminal coding fragment containing the desired mutation DWzPRV/P, DWz/PRV/P, DWz//PRV/P or DWz/PANF/PR (Table 1). V/P or HIVgpt served as a template and the reverse primer (nt.3116-90) sequence was 5′-TACATACAAAT-CATCCATGTTATTGATA-3′. Amplified fragments

Table 1 Primer sequences used for plasmid construction

Constructs	Forward primer (5′–3′)[a]
DWzPR	5′ CTGT<u>GGATCCT</u>**AACTTC**CCTCAGGTAACGTTATGGCAA 3′-nt 2273
DWz/PR	5′ CG<u>GGATCC</u>T**TCCTTTAACTTC**CCTCAGGTCACGTTATGG 3′-nt 2270
DWz//PR	5′ CG<u>GGATCC</u>T**ACTGTATCCTTTAACTTC**CCTCAGGTCACGTTATGG 3′-nt 2270
DWzPRV/P	5′ CG<u>GGATCC</u>T**AACGTT**CCTCAGATCACGTTATGG 3′-nt 2270
DWz/PRV/P	5′ CG<u>GGATCC</u>T**TCCTTTAACGTT**CCTCAGATCACGTTATGG 3′-nt 2270
DWz//PRV/P	5′ CG<u>GGATCC</u>T**ACTGTATCCTTTAACGTT**CCTCAGATCACGTTATGG 3′-nt 2270
DWz/PSHL/PR	5′ CG<u>GGATCC</u>T**CCCTCTCACCTC**CCTCAGGTCACTCTTTGG 3′-nt 2270
DWz/PIDL/PR	5′ CG<u>GGATCC</u>T**CCCATTGACCTC**CCTCAGGTCACTCTTTGG 3′-nt 2270
DWz/PANF/PR	5′ CG<u>GGATCC</u>T**CCCGCTAACTTC**CCTCAGGTCACTCTTTGG 3′-nt 2270
p6*PSHL	nt 2221-5′ CCGATCGACAAGGAACTGTA**CCCTCTCACCTC**CCTCAG 3′-nt 2258
p6*PIDL	nt 2221-5′ CCGATCGACAAGGAACTGTA**CCCATTGACCTC**CCTCAG 3′-nt 2258
p6*PANF	nt 2221-5′ CCGATCGACAAGGAACTGTA**CCCGCTAACTTC**C 3′-nt 2254

[a] The numbers at the 3′ and/or 5′ ends denote HIV-1 proviral DNA nucleotide positions. Nucleotides corresponding to mutated amino acid residues are shown in boldface. Most of the primers contain BamHI sites (underlined) to facilitate cloning

were digested with BamHI and EcoRV, and subcloned into pBRClaSal/DPR [28]. BamHI-flanking leucine zipper coding fragments derived from PRWzPR [28] were inserted into each pBRClaSal/DPR recombinant, yielding DWzPRV/P, DWz/PRV/P, DWz//PRV/P and DWz/PANF/PR, respectively.

p6*PSHL, p6*PIDL and p6*PANF were constructed by megaprimer PCR method [33] using a forward primer containing the desired mutation (Table 1) and a reverse primer 5′-GGTACAGTCTCAATAGGGCTAATG-3. HIVgpt serves as a template. The amplified fragments were digested with ApaI and BclI, and subcloned into a plasmid cassette pBRCla-Sal that contains HIV-1 coding sequence (from ClaI-nt.831 to SalI-nt.5786). Each mutation-containing pBRCla-Sal cassette was then digested with SpeI and SalI, and ligated into HIVgpt, yielding p6*PSHL, p6*PIDL and p6*PANF.

p6*PSHL, p6*PIDL and p6*PANF were digested with BglII and EcoRV and ligated into DPR digested with BamHI and EcoRV, yielding Dp6*PSHL, Dp6*PIDL/PR and Dp6*PANF/PR, respectively.

GPfs has the Gag and Pol in the same reading frame due to a deletion of the frame shift signal [34]. DWzPR and DWz/PR were digested with BclI. The BclI-flanking fragment containing WzPR and Wz/PR mutations were ligated into PR-inactivated GPfs (fsd) digested with BclI, yielding fsdWzPR and fsdWz/PR. Recombination of fsd-WzPR and a Gag-deleted fsd [34] generated construct fsdWzPRΔGag.

Cell culture and transfection

293T and HeLa cells were maintained in DMEM supplemented with 10% fetal calf serum. Confluent 293T cells were trypsinized, split 1:10 and seeded onto 10-cm plates 18–24 h before transfection. For each construct, 293T cells were transfected with 20 μg of plasmid DNA by the calcium phosphate precipitation method, with the addition of 50 μM chloroquine to enhance transfection efficiency. Culture media and cells were harvested for protein analysis at 48–72 h post-transfection. When pGAG was co-transfected with the Gag-Pol expression constructs at a DNA ratio of 1:1 or 10 to 1, 10 or 15 μg of pGAG were used with the addition of pBlueScript plasmid DNA to a final quantity of 20 μg DNA. The cells and media were harvested for protein analysis 48–72 h post-transfection.

Single-cycle infection assays

293T cells were either co-transfected with 10 μg wt or each of the mutant HIVgpt plus 5 μg of the VSV-G protein expression plasmid pHCMV-G [35], or co-transfected with 1 μg of the GPfs or the p6*-deleted GPfs plasmid with 10 μg pGAG plus 5 μg pHCMV-G. At 48 h after transfection, virus-containing supernatants were collected, filtered, diluted, and used to infect HeLa cells. Aliquots of the same filtered supernatants and cell samples were prepared and subjected to Western blot. Adsorption of virions is allowed to proceed in the presence of 4 μg/ml polybrene. Twenty-four hours after infection, cells were trypsinized, split into dishes, and refed with medium containing drug selection cocktail [36]. Selected drug resistant colonies were fixed and stained with 50% methanol containing 0.5% methylene blue. Numbers of drug-resistant colonies were converted into titers (cfu/ml). Infectivity was expressed as the ratio of the mutant titer to the titer of wt, and normalized to Gag protein levels in parallel experiments.

Western immunoblot analysis

Culture media from transfected 293T cells were filtered through 0.45-μm pore-size and then centrifuged through 2 ml 20% sucrose in TSE (10 mM Tris–HCl, pH 7.5, 100 mM NaCl, 1 mM EDTA) containing 0.1 mM phenylmethylsulfonyl fluoride (PMSF) at 4 °C for 40 min at $274,000 \times g$. Viral pellets and cell lysates mixed with sample buffer were then subjected to SDS-10% PAGE or 4–12% Bis–Tris gradient gels (NuPage Bis–Tris Mini Gels; Thermo Fisher Scientific) followed by immunoblotting analysis as previously described [37]. HIV-1 Gag proteins were probed with an anti-p24gag monoclonal antibody (mouse hybridoma clone 183-H12-5C) from ascites. For HIV-1 RT detection, the primary antibody was rabbit antiserum or a mouse anti-RT monoclonal antibody [38, 39]. Cellular β-actin was detected using a mouse anti-β-actin monoclonal antibody (Sigma). The secondary antibody was either a sheep anti-mouse or a donkey anti-rabbit horseradish peroxidase (HRP)-conjugated antibody (Jackson ImmunoResearch). An enhanced chemiluminescence (ECL) detection system (SuperSignal West Pico Chemiluminescent Substrate; Thermo Fisher Scientific) was used to detect membrane-bound proteins.

Statistical analysis

Differences between control (wt) and experimental (mutant) groups were assessed using Student's t-tests. Data are expressed as mean $\pm$ standard deviation. Significance was defined as $*p < 0.05$, $**p < 0.01$, $***p < 0.001$.

Results

p6*-PR cleavage blocking does not significantly mitigate leucine zipper-induced Gag cleavage enhancement

In a previous study we reported that an HIV-1 mutant (DWzPR) containing a LZ dimerization motif adjacent to and upstream of PR was not capable of producing virions due to the strong enhancement of Gag cleavage [28]. DWzPR is derived from Dp6*PR by replacing a deleted p6* with LZ, but retaining the last two C-terminal p6* residues at the LZ/PR junction (Fig. 1a). We observed that this LZ replacement of p6* led to the elimination of virus assembly, likely due to premature PR activation triggered by the LZ. Based on our prior finding that the DWzPR virus assembly defect is PR activity-dependent, and since p6*-PR cleavage is required for fully active PR, we postulated that blocking p6*-PR cleavage within the LZ/PR junction might help restore DWzPR-associated virus production by reducing PR activity. To test this possibility, we substituted Val for the last C-terminal p6* residue (Phe) at the LZ/PR junction of DWzPR and designated the resulting construct as DWzPRV/P (Fig. 1a; note that p6*-PR cleavage site residues were changed from F/P to V/P). Our data indicate that DWzPR virus yields were

still hardly detected following the Val substitution unless it was accompanied by treatment with an HIV-1 PR inhibitor (Fig. 1b middle panel, lane 4 vs. lane 5). These results suggest that (a) the blocking of p6*-PR cleavage exerted no major impacts on LZ-induced Gag cleavage enhancement, and (b) a HIV-1 PR precursor containing a LZ motif fused at the N-terminus exhibited enhanced enzymatic activity.

As a control, Val substitution for Phe (referred to as a V/P mutation) significantly reduced virus processing efficiency when tested in a wild-type (wt) HIV-1 Gag/Gag-Pol expression vector (Fig. 1c, middle panel, lanes 2 and 6). Constructs with either four or six remaining C-terminal p6* residues at the LZ/PR junction (DWz/PR or DWz//PR) exhibited particle assembly and processing profiles similar to that of the wt (Fig. 1c middle panel, lanes 4 and 5). While the V/P mutation exerted no major impacts on wt virus production, it significantly reduced DWz/PR and DWz//PR virus yields in addition to impairing virus maturation (Fig. 1c middle panel lanes 4–5 vs. 8–9 and panels d and e). The capacity of the C-terminal p6* tetra-peptide to counteract the LZ enhancement effect and modulate PR activation was subject to weakening by the V/P mutation. This may account, at least in part, for the decreased virus assembly and processing efficiency of DWz/PRV/P and DWz//PRV/P (Fig. 1c middle panel, lanes 8 and 9).

Specific C-terminal p6* residues are required to modulate PR maturation

Our results support the proposal that the C-terminal p6* tetra-peptide plays a central role in mitigating PR maturation, likely due to the absence of an intact C-terminal p6* tetra-peptide, which lets LZ dictate the PR maturation process and trigger premature PR activation. To test this hypothesis, we inserted substitution mutations at the C-terminal p6* tetra-peptide without affecting the p6gag amino acid residues. Given our observation of DWzPR exhibiting Gag cleavage enhancement, the last two C-terminal p6* residues (NF) remaining at the LZ/PR junction might be required for PR activation. We therefore engineered a DWz/PANF/PR construct by replacing SF with PA (Fig. 2a). Both the DWz/PSHL/PR and DWz/PIDL/PR constructs contain substitutions for all four C-terminal p6* residues. We found that DWz/PANF/PR displayed a virus assembly and processing profile similar to that of DWz/PR (Fig. 2b, lane 4 vs. 1), but evidence from statistical analyses suggest that its virus particle processing was not as efficient as that of DWz/PR (Fig. 2b, d). Whereas DWz/PIDL/PR exhibited readily detected virus-associated p24gag and mature PR, DWz/PSHL/PR had virus-associated Gag or PR mostly present in unprocessed or incompletely processed precursor forms

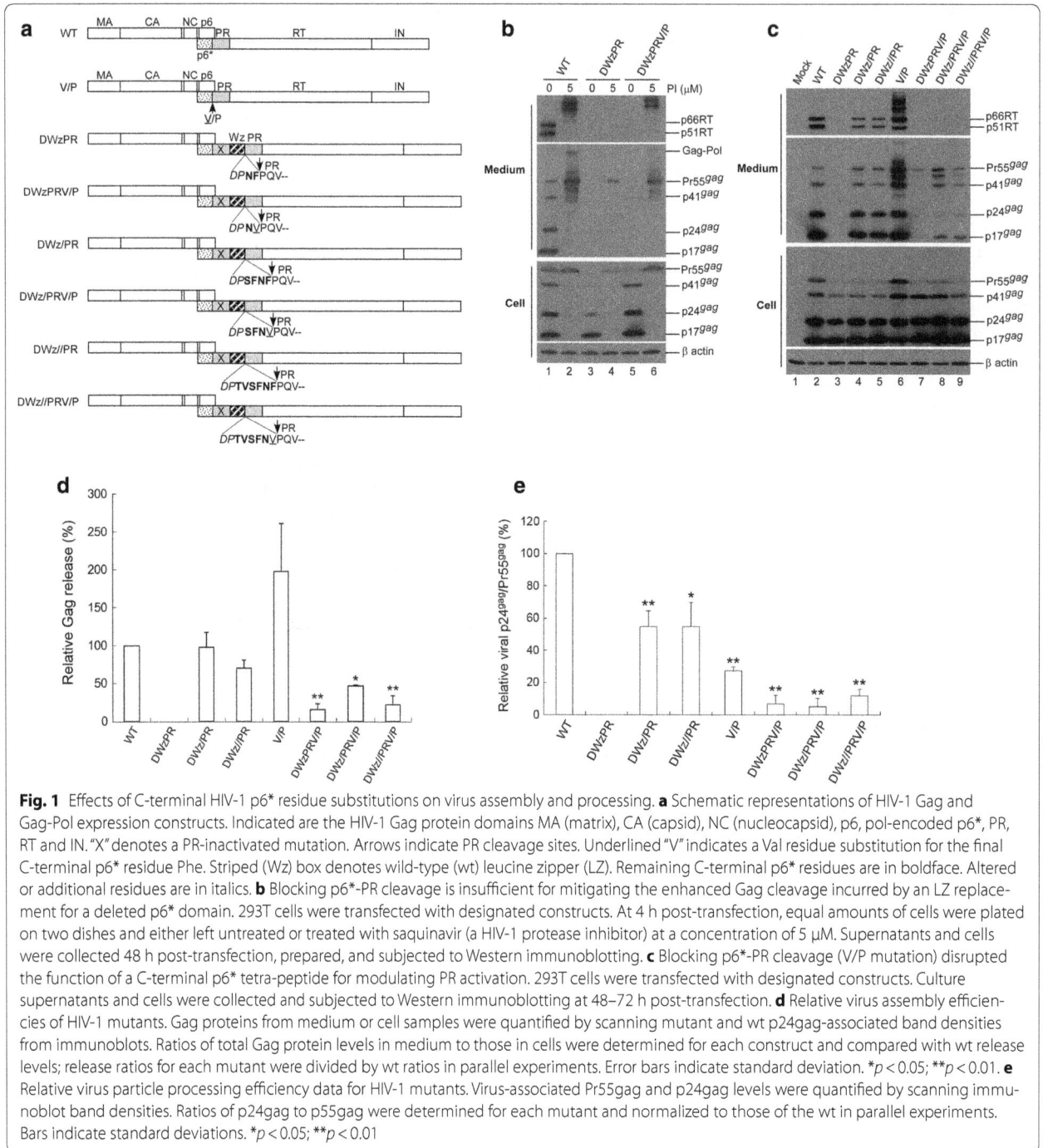

Fig. 1 Effects of C-terminal HIV-1 p6* residue substitutions on virus assembly and processing. **a** Schematic representations of HIV-1 Gag and Gag-Pol expression constructs. Indicated are the HIV-1 Gag protein domains MA (matrix), CA (capsid), NC (nucleocapsid), p6, pol-encoded p6*, PR, RT and IN. "X" denotes a PR-inactivated mutation. Arrows indicate PR cleavage sites. Underlined "V" indicates a Val residue substitution for the final C-terminal p6* residue Phe. Striped (Wz) box denotes wild-type (wt) leucine zipper (LZ). Remaining C-terminal p6* residues are in boldface. Altered or additional residues are in italics. **b** Blocking p6*-PR cleavage is insufficient for mitigating the enhanced Gag cleavage incurred by an LZ replacement for a deleted p6* domain. 293T cells were transfected with designated constructs. At 4 h post-transfection, equal amounts of cells were plated on two dishes and either left untreated or treated with saquinavir (a HIV-1 protease inhibitor) at a concentration of 5 μM. Supernatants and cells were collected 48 h post-transfection, prepared, and subjected to Western immunoblotting. **c** Blocking p6*-PR cleavage (V/P mutation) disrupted the function of a C-terminal p6* tetra-peptide for modulating PR activation. 293T cells were transfected with designated constructs. Culture supernatants and cells were collected and subjected to Western immunoblotting at 48–72 h post-transfection. **d** Relative virus assembly efficiencies of HIV-1 mutants. Gag proteins from medium or cell samples were quantified by scanning mutant and wt p24gag-associated band densities from immunoblots. Ratios of total Gag protein levels in medium to those in cells were determined for each construct and compared with wt release levels; release ratios for each mutant were divided by wt ratios in parallel experiments. Error bars indicate standard deviation. *$p < 0.05$; **$p < 0.01$. **e** Relative virus particle processing efficiency data for HIV-1 mutants. Virus-associated Pr55gag and p24gag levels were quantified by scanning immunoblot band densities. Ratios of p24gag to p55gag were determined for each mutant and normalized to those of the wt in parallel experiments. Bars indicate standard deviations. *$p < 0.05$; **$p < 0.01$

(Fig. 2b, lane 3 vs. lane 2). Similar effects on virus processing were observed when PSHL, PIDL or PANF mutations were cloned into Dp6*PR (Fig. 2c). Western blot data indicate a strong correlation between the virus processing efficiencies of the mutants and their virus-associated mature PR levels. Although Dp6*PANF/PR and DWz/PANF/PR both exhibited relatively low processing

efficiency, no statistical significance was noted when compared with their Dp6*PR and DWZ/PR prototypes (Fig. 2d).

To confirm our conclusions, we tested PIDL, PSHL and PANF substitution mutations in a wt HIVgpt backbone (Fig. 3a). Results indicate that neither PIDL nor PANF mutations significantly affected virus infectivity

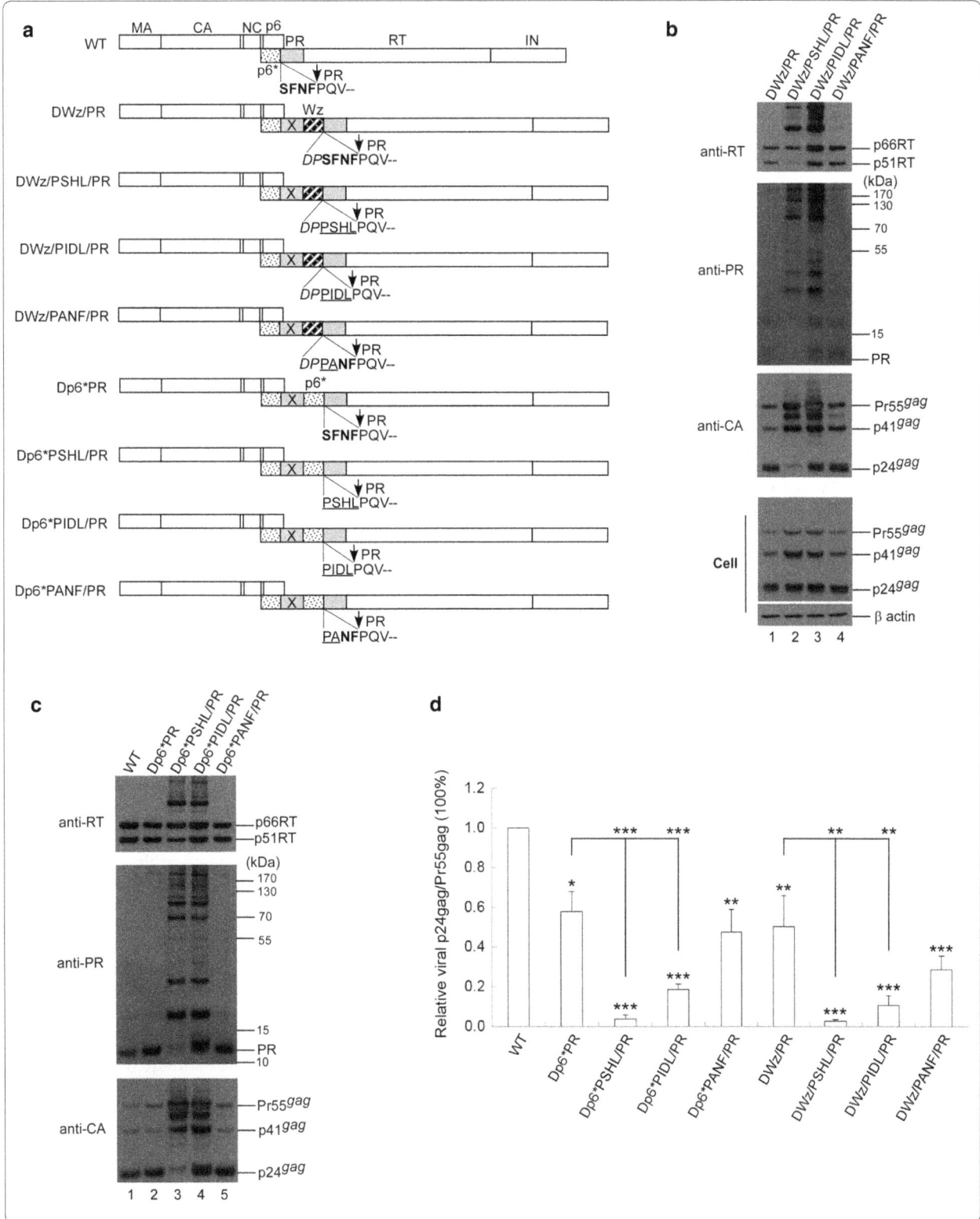

in single cycle infection assays, although both mutations reduced virus processing efficiency (Fig. 3b–d). The data also show that PANF exerted a weaker impact on virus processing and infectivity compared to PIDL. In contrast, the PSHL mutation significantly impaired both virus processing and infectivity (Fig. 3c, d). Combined, these results suggest that specific C-terminal p6* residues, especially the last two, are essential for modulating PR activation.

A single amino acid residue change eliminated the ability of p6*-deleted Gag-Pol to mediate virus maturation

The above conclusions agree with our past observations of HIV-1 Gag-Pol (Δp6*fs) with most p6* deleted, but with the final two C-terminal p6* residues still capable of mediating virus maturation, although less efficiently than wt Gag-Pol [40]. To determine if additional changes at C-terminal p6* residues affect the ability of Δp6*fs to mediate Gag processing, we engineered p6*-deleted constructs with two, four or six C-terminal p6* residues remaining at the p6*/PR junction (respectively designated Δp6*fsPR, Δp6*fs/PR and Δp6*fs//PR). All three contained an additional Pro residue insertion in the deleted p6* region due to cloning procedures (Fig. 4a). All of the p6*-deleted Gag-Pol mutants and wild-type GPfs were co-transfected with a Pr55gag expression vector designated pGAG. Unsurprisingly, virus production was almost completely blocked when each construct was co-expressed with equal amounts of pGAG (10 µg each), presumably due to enhanced Gag cleavage from over-expressed PR activity. The only exception was Δp6*fsPR, which produced significant amounts of mostly unprocessed or incompletely processed virus-associated Gag (Fig. 4b middle panel, lane 7). All constructs other than Δp6*fsPR were capable of producing readily detectable virus-associated p24gag and p66/51RT when co-expressed with pGAG at a plasmid DNA ratio of 1:10 (Fig. 4b, c). In contrast, Δp6*fsPR co-expression with pGAG consistently yielded virions that mostly contained incomplete or unprocessed Gag and RT-associated Gag-Pol (Fig. 4b, lane 4, and Fig. 4c, lane 6). These data suggest

that Δp6*fsPR is profoundly defective in auto-processing and the *in trans* processing of virus particles.

In another test designed to determine whether the p6*-deleted Gag-Pol mutants mediated virus maturation and produced infectious virions, each Gag-Pol construct was co-expressed with pGAG plus a VSV-G envelope expression plasmid. Culture supernatants were collected for protein analysis and used to infect HeLa cells. Our data indicate that with the exception of Δp6*fsPR, all p6*-deleted Gag-Pol mutants were capable of producing infectious virions with infectivity levels of approximately 20–40% relative to wt GPfs (Fig. 4d). The third N-terminal PR residue at Δp6*fsPR (Val instead of Ile) apparently does not account for the virus processing defect, since a Val/Ile polymorphism was found at this position. Further, both Δp6*fs/PR and Δp6*fs//PR containing a Val polymorphism were capable of mediating virus particle maturation. Δp6*fsPR contains an inserted proline adjacent to the last two C-terminal p6* residues. Although Δp6*fs/PR and Δp6*fs//PR both contain the same proline insertion at the p6*-deleted region, both were still found to be capable of mediating virus maturation. The four remaining C-terminal p6* residues within Δp6*fs/PR and Δp6*fs//PR might prevent the Pro insertion from interfering with PR activation.

Enhanced PR activation due to the LZ replacement of p6* is Gag domain-independent

Given the contribution that Gag makes to PR activation by promoting Gag-Pol dimerization, we hypothesized that Gag removal from DWzPR might impair Gag-Pol dimerization, thereby mitigating the LZ enhancement effect on PR activation and reducing both Gag-Pol auto-cleavage and Gag cleavage efficiency. To test this idea, we engineered GPfs versions of DWzPR with a Gag deletion (fsdWzPRΔGag) and without one (fsdWzPR) (Fig. 5a). GPfs and a GPfs version of DWz/PR (designated fsdWz/PR) served as controls. Each construct was co-expressed with D25, a PR-inactivated Gag/Gag-Pol expression plasmid. According to our results, both fsdWzPR and fsdWzPRΔGag produced barely detectable

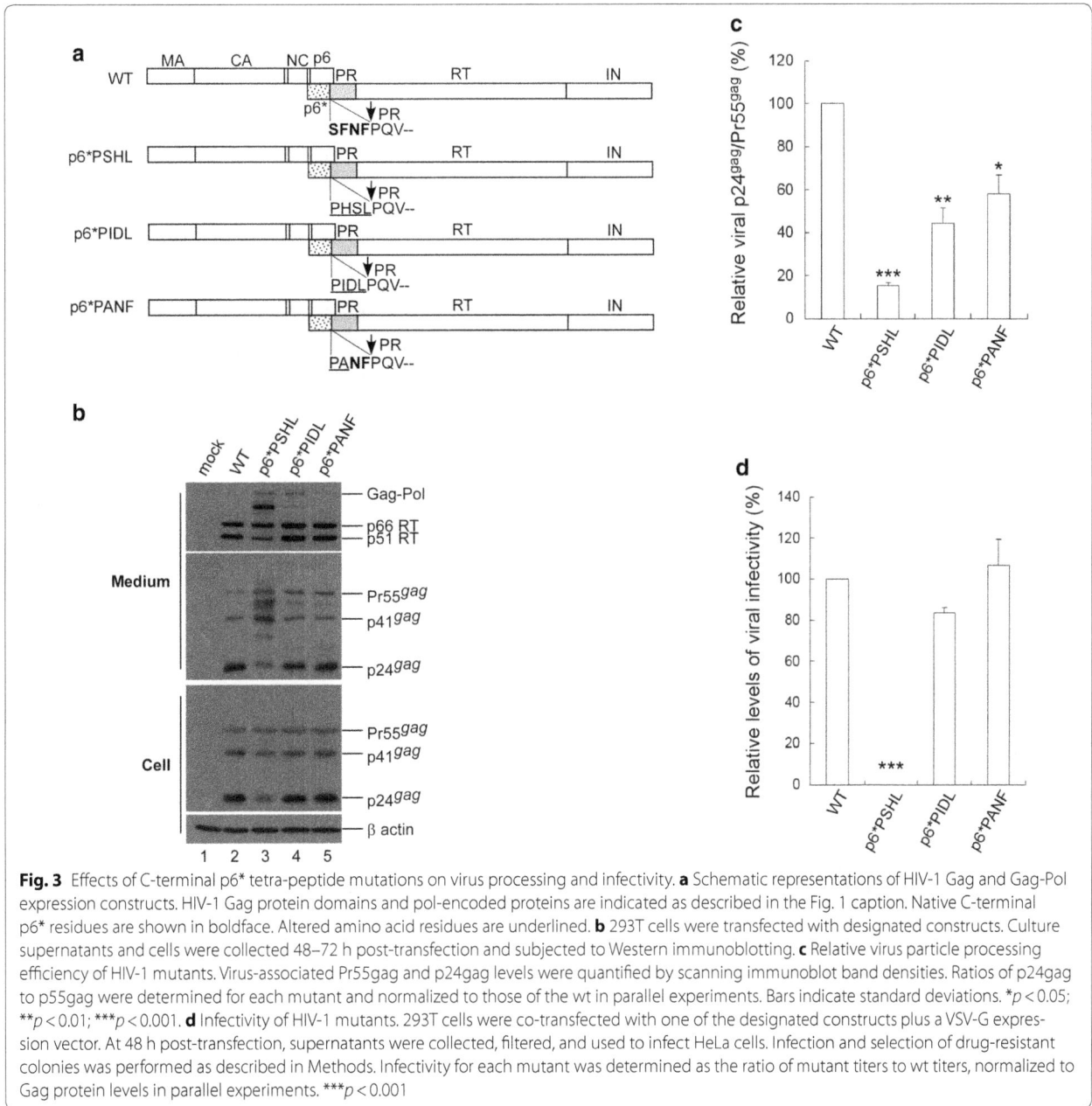

Fig. 3 Effects of C-terminal p6* tetra-peptide mutations on virus processing and infectivity. **a** Schematic representations of HIV-1 Gag and Gag-Pol expression constructs. HIV-1 Gag protein domains and pol-encoded proteins are indicated as described in the Fig. 1 caption. Native C-terminal p6* residues are shown in boldface. Altered amino acid residues are underlined. **b** 293T cells were transfected with designated constructs. Culture supernatants and cells were collected 48–72 h post-transfection and subjected to Western immunoblotting. **c** Relative virus particle processing efficiency of HIV-1 mutants. Virus-associated Pr55gag and p24gag levels were quantified by scanning immunoblot band densities. Ratios of p24gag to p55gag were determined for each mutant and normalized to those of the wt in parallel experiments. Bars indicate standard deviations. $*p < 0.05$; $**p < 0.01$; $***p < 0.001$. **d** Infectivity of HIV-1 mutants. 293T cells were co-transfected with one of the designated constructs plus a VSV-G expression vector. At 48 h post-transfection, supernatants were collected, filtered, and used to infect HeLa cells. Infection and selection of drug-resistant colonies was performed as described in Methods. Infectivity for each mutant was determined as the ratio of mutant titers to wt titers, normalized to Gag protein levels in parallel experiments. $***p < 0.001$

virus-associated p24gag when co-transfected with D25 at a DNA ratio of 1:10 (Fig. 5b middle panel, lanes 3 and 5). In contrast, virus-associated p24gag was readily detected in fsdWz/PR-plus-D25 co-transfection samples although at a much lower level compared to Pr55gag and p41gag (Fig. 5b, lane 7). Incorporated Gag-Pol deficiency due to premature or enhanced Gag-Pol auto-cleavage might result in insufficient virus processing. The over-expression of fsdWzPRΔGag and other GPfs mutants led to the complete blocking of virus assembly (Fig. 5b, lanes 4, 6 and 8).

Virus-associated Gag-Pol molecules detected in medium were likely from D25 (Fig. 5b, upper panel). It is possible that D25 Gag-Pol competes with other Gag-Pol mutants in terms of viral incorporation. There is also the possibility that D25 PR-defective Gag-Pol interferes with the ability of incorporated Gag-Pol mutants to mediate virus particle processing. This may partly explain the relatively lower levels of virus-associated p24gag that we observed in fsdWz/PR co-transfection samples (Fig. 5b middle panel lane 7). To study these possibilities, Gag-Pol mutants were co-expressed with pGAG. Results indicate

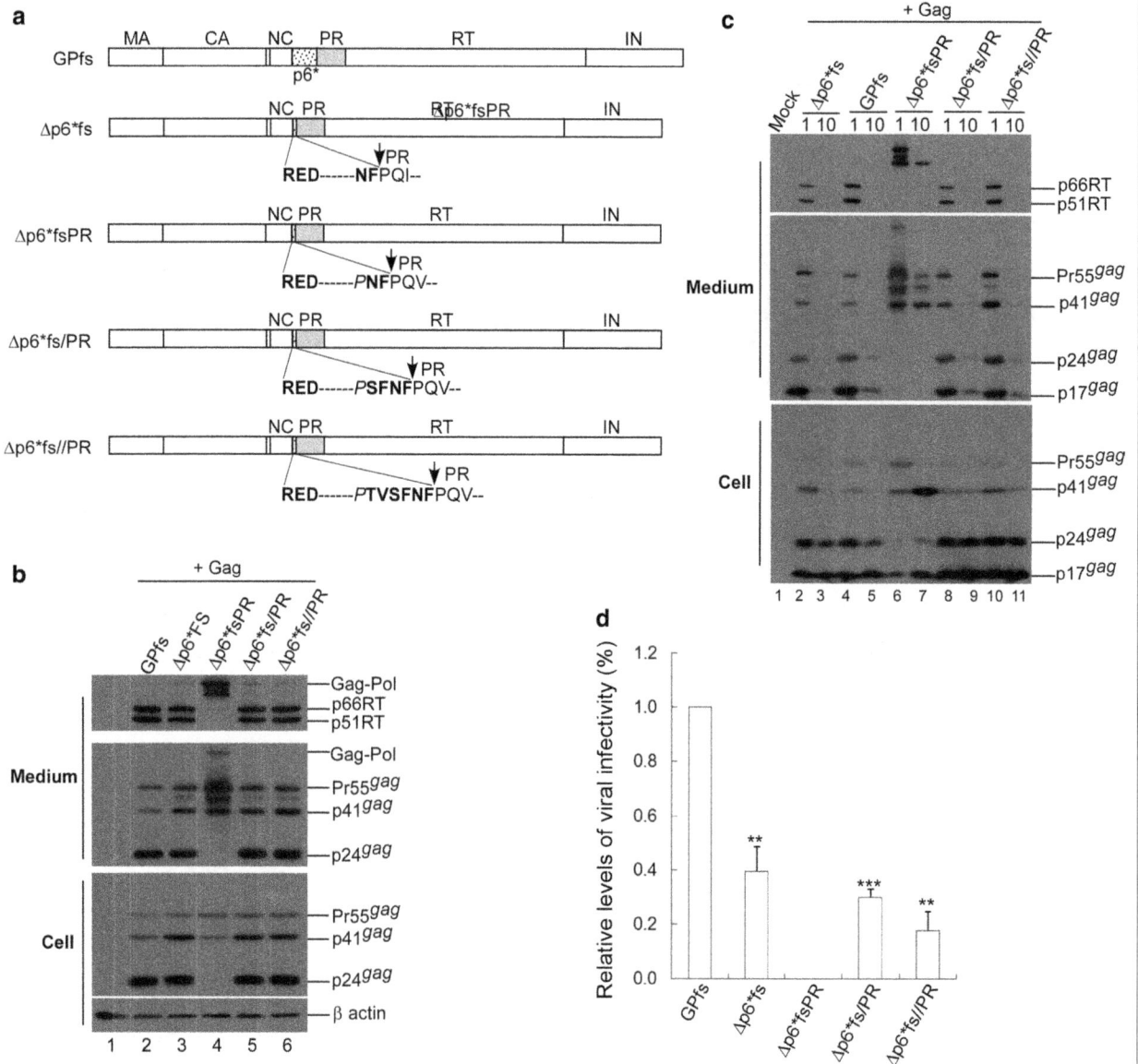

Fig. 4 Effects of C-terminal p6* residue substitutions on the capability of p6*-deleted Gag-Pol mutants to mediate virus maturation. **a** Schematic representations of HIV-1 Gag-Pol expression constructs with deletions of most p6* coding sequences. HIV-1 Gag domains, pol-encoded p6*, PR, RT and IN are indicated. All constructs contain a frame shift (fs) mutation forcing gag and pol into the same reading frame. Dashed lines denote deleted p6* regions. Remaining N-terminal and C-terminal p6* residues are indicated in boldface. Altered or foreign residues are in italics. **b, c** 293T cells were co-transfected with 10 μg of an HIV-1 Pr55gag expression plasmid (pGAG) and 1 or 10 μg (panel **b**) or 1 μg (panel **c**) of the designated Gag-Pol expression construct. At 48 h post-transfection, cells and supernatants were collected and analyzed by Western immunoblotting. Membrane-bound proteins were initially probed with anti-RT serum, stripped, and probed again with anti-p17MA and anti-p24CA monoclonal antibodies. Indicated are HIV-1 Gag-Pol, 66/51RT, Pr55gag, p41gag, p24gag and p17gag positions. **d** A single amino acid change blocked the capability of p6*-deleted Gag-Pol to confer virus infectivity. 293T cells were co-transfected with 10 μg of an HIV-1 Pr55gag expression vector (pGAG) and 1 μg of one of the designated constructs plus 5 μg of a VSV-G expression vector. At 48 h post-transfection, supernatants were collected, filtered, and used to infect HeLa cells. Infectivity for each Gag-Pol construct was determined as the ratio of mutant titers to wt Gag-Pol titers, normalized to virus-associated p24gag protein levels in parallel experiments. $**p < 0.01$; $***p < 0.001$

that virus-associated RT and p24gag were both readily detected in wt GPfs or fsdWz/PR co-transfection samples (Fig. 5c). In contrast, virus-associated RT and p24gag were both barely detectable in fsdWzPR co-transfection samples, likely due to a Gag-Pol incorporating defect (Fig. 5c, lane 3).

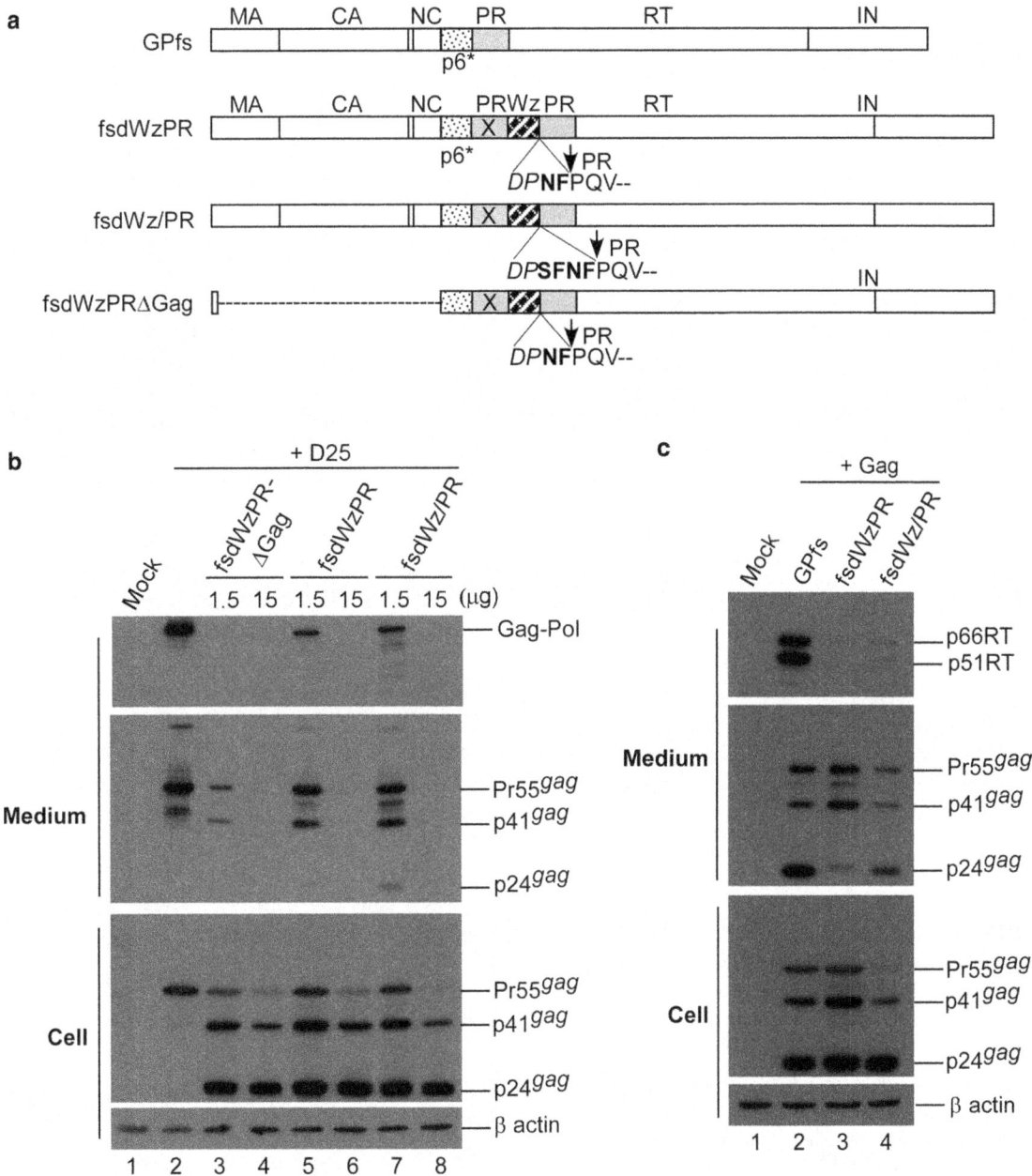

Fig. 5 Enhanced Gag-Pol auto-cleavage reduces virus yields and Gag-Pol viral incorporation. **a** Schematic representations of HIV-1 Gag-Pol expression constructs in a gag-pol frame shift (fs) mutation backbone are as described in the Fig. 4 caption. Striped (Wz) box denotes leucine zipper (LZ). Dashed line indicates deleted Gag coding sequence. "X" denotes a PR-inactivated mutation. Remaining C-terminal p6* residues are in boldface. Altered or additional residues are shown in italics. **b, c** Leucine zipper-induced Gag-Pol auto-cleavage enhancement leads to reductions in virion yields and Gag-Pol packaging. Indicated amounts of designated plasmids were co-expressed with 15 μg of an HIV-1 protease-defective (D25) Gag/Gag-Pol expression vector (panel b) or co-expressed with pGAG (panel c) at a DNA ratio of 1:10. Culture supernatants and cells were collected at 48–72 h post-transfection and subjected to Western immunoblotting. Indicated are HIV-1 Gag-Pol, 66/51RT, Pr55gag, p41gag and p24gag positions

Combined, these results suggest that an LZ replacement for p6* leads to enhanced Gag-Pol auto-cleavage and associated Gag-Pol incorporation deficiency, and that Gag removal does not reduce the LZ enhancement effect on PR activation.

Discussion

Even though the removal of p6* from PR precursor is necessary for PR to be fully functional, the enhancement effect of LZ on PR-mediated Gag processing was not significantly compromised by blocking p6*-PR cleavage.

Further, we noted that DWz/PRV/P, DWz//PRV/P and other constructs with substitution mutations at the remaining C-terminal p6* tetra-peptide were all capable of producing readily detectable virus-associated Gag, although with processing defects for some of the mutants (Figs. 1, 2). These results suggest that the enhancement of PR activation by LZ may be reduced when as few as six amino acid residues, whether native or foreign, are present between LZ and PR. The hexa-peptide between LZ and PR may serve as a spacer that prevents the potent LZ dimerization motif from facilitating PR dimer formation. Additionally, substitutions at the C-terminal p6* tetra-peptide might interfere with PR maturation, thereby contributing, at least in part, to reduced Gag processing efficiency.

As a result of blocked cleavage at the PR-RT site, HIV-1 PR-RT fusion is capable of mediating virus processing and supporting virus replication [41]. In contrast, p6* appears to be capable of inhibiting PR maturation, and therefore must be removed for PR to be fully active. However, DWzPR virus yields were not significantly restored when p6*-PR cleavage was blocked, suggesting that HIV-1 PR precursors containing a LZ motif fused at the N-terminus may exhibit markedly enhanced enzymatic activity even when free mature PR is not released. Theoretically, PR-associated products with LZ linked at the PR N-terminus may exist in DWzPRV/P transfectant samples due to blocked cleavage at p6*/PR. Since attempts to detect these PR-associated products were unsuccessful, we believe PR may access putative cryptic cleavage sites within the LZ in addition to being self-degrading. Regardless, our findings suggest that PR precursors containing foreign peptides fused at the N-terminus are still capable of being functionally active. Specifically, PR activity may be significantly enhanced when a potent dimerization motif is present at the PR N-terminus.

Although C-terminal p6* substitutions with either PIDL or PANF residues exerted no major impacts on HIVgpt virus infectivity according to single-round infection assays, they did reduce virus processing efficiency (Fig. 3). These data agree with an earlier report that substitutions for C-terminal p6* residues can impair PR maturation, resulting in a virus processing defect [20]. Negative effects of C-terminal p6* tetra-peptide substitution mutations on virus processing become increasingly noticeable when tested with a Dp6*PR backbone (Fig. 2c), presumably due to PR function perturbation by an upstream inactivated PR copy.

According to single-cycle infection assays, Δp6*fs generated mature infectious virions. In contrast, Δp6*fsPR (with only one amino acid difference from Δp6*fs in the linker region) was completely blocked in terms of mediating virus maturation (Fig. 4). Δp6*fs has a Leu at the

P3 position, while Δp6*fsPR has a foreign Pro insertion at P3. Pro residues were barely detected at the P3 position flanking the PR cleavage site (i.e., the third amino acid residue immediately upstream from the PR substrate cleavage site). Leu was one of several amino acids found at the P3 position [42]. This raises the possibility of P3-Pro disrupting PR maturation, thereby blocking the ability of Δp6*fsPR to mediate virus processing. Even though they both contain a Pro insertion in the deleted p6* region, Δp6*fs/PR and Δp6*fs//PR were still capable of mediating virus maturation, likely due to the containment of an intact C-terminal p6* tetra-peptide SFNF at the p6*/PR junction. This agrees with our observations involving DWz/PR and DWz//PR, both of which contain an intact C-terminal p6* tetra-peptide and are capable of counteracting the LZ enhancement of PR activation.

In addition to containing only four residues between LZ and PR, DWzPR has a Pro at the P3 position, which might contribute to its failure to counteract the LZ enhancement effect on PR-mediated Gag cleavage. C-terminal p6* residues might inhibit PR maturation by destabilizing the structure of the folded PR dimer [43]. The absence of regulated PR dimer structure folding due to mutations at C-terminal p6* residues might allow the potent LZ dimerization motif to facilitate or exert a synergetic effect on Gag-Pol or PR dimer formation via PR dimer stabilization. PR is consequently prematurely activated, resulting in a significant enhancement of Gag processing as was observed for DWzPR and DWzPRV/P.

In conclusion, our findings suggest that an HIV-1 PR precursor containing an N-terminally extended peptide can function efficiently without liberating free mature PR. HIV-1 PR precursor activity might be manipulated via the altering of peptide residues adjacent to the PR N-terminus.

Authors' contributions

CTW designed this project and wrote the manuscript. FHY performed the experiment and helped with the data analysis. Both authors read and approved the final manuscript.

Acknowledgements

We thank K.J. Huang and Y.R. Lin for materials and reagents. We also thank the following individuals from the National Institutes of Health AIDS Research and Reference Reagent Program for their assistance in obtaining the following reagents: Stephen Hughes for MAb21 anti-RT monoclonal antibodies and D. Bailey and Mark Page for HIV-1 PR antiserum.

Competing interests

The authors declare that they have no competing interests.

Funding

This work was supported by Grants V104C-056 and V105C-036 from the Taipei Veterans General Hospital and by Taiwan Ministry of Science and Technology Grants 104-2320-B-010-035, 105-2320-B-010-023 and 106-2320-B-010-017-MY2.

References

1. Petropoulos C. Retroviral taxonomy, protein structures, sequences, and genetic maps. In: Coffin JM, Hughes SH, Varmus HE, editors. Retroviruses. New York: Cold Spring Harbor Laboratory Press; 1997.
2. Jacks T, Power MD, Masiarz FR, Luciw PA, Barr PJ, Varmus HE. Characterization of ribosomal frameshifting in HIV-1 gag-pol expression. Nature. 1988;331:280–3.
3. Freed EO. HIV-1 assembly, release and maturation. Nat Rev Microbiol. 2015;13:484.
4. Huang M, Martin MA. Incorporation of Pr160(gag-pol) into virus particles requires the presence of both the major homology region and adjacent C-terminal capsid sequences within the Gag-Pol polyprotein. J Virol. 1997;71:4472–8.
5. Smith AJ, Srinivasakumar N, Hammarskjöld ML, Rekosh D. Requirements for incorporation of Pr160gag-pol from human immunodeficiency virus type 1 into virus-like particles. J Virol. 1993;67:2266–75.
6. Srinivasakumar N, Hammarskjöld ML, Rekosh D. Characterization of deletion mutations in the capsid region of human immunodeficiency virus type 1 that affect particle formation and Gag-Pol precursor incorporation. J Virol. 1995;69:6106–14.
7. Park J, Morrow CD. The nonmyristylated Pr160gag-pol polyprotein of human immunodeficiency virus type 1 interacts with Pr55gag and is incorporated into viruslike particles. J Virol. 1992;66:6304–13.
8. Lee SK, Potempa M, Swanstrom R. The choreography of HIV-1 proteolytic processing and virion assembly. J Biol Chem. 2012;287:40867–74.
9. Swanstrom R, Wills JW. Synthesis, assembly, and processing of viral proteins. In: Coffin JM, Hughes SH, Varmus HE, editors. Retroviruses. New York: Cold Spring Harbor Laboratory Press; 1997.
10. Pettit SC, Moody MD, Wehbie RS, Kaplan AH, Nantermet PV, Klein CA, Swanstrom R. The p2 domain of human immunodeficiency virus type 1 Gag regulates sequential proteolytic processing and is required to produce fully infectious virions. J Virol. 1994;68:8017–27.
11. Peng C, Ho BK, Chang TW, Chang NT. Role of human immunodeficiency virus type 1-specific protease in core protein maturation and viral infectivity. J Virol. 1989;63:2550–6.
12. Liao WH, Wang CT. Characterization of human immunodeficiency virus type 1 Pr160 gag-pol mutants with truncations downstream of the protease domain. Virology. 2004;329:180–8.
13. Louis JM, Nashed NT, Parris KD, Kimmel AR, Jerina DM. Kinetics and mechanism of autoprocessing of human immunodeficiency virus type 1 protease from an analog of the Gag-Pol polyprotein. Proc Natl Acad Sci USA. 1994;91:7970–4.
14. Pettit SC, Gulnik S, Everitt L, Kaplan AH. The dimer interfaces of protease and extra-protease domains influence the activation of protease and the specificity of GagPol cleavage. J Virol. 2003;77:366–74.
15. Quillent C, Borman AM, Paulous S, Dauguet C, Clavel F. Extensive regions of pol are required for efficient human immunodeficiency virus polyprotein processing and particle maturation. Virology. 1996;219:29–36.
16. Zybarth G, Carter C. Domains upstream of the protease (PR) in human immunodeficiency virus type 1 Gag-Pol influence PR autoprocessing. J Virol. 1995;69:3878–84.
17. Figueiredo A, Moore KL, Mak J, Sluis-Cremer N, de Bethune MP, Tachedjian G. Potent nonnucleoside reverse transcriptase inhibitors target HIV-1 Gag-Pol. PLoS Pathog. 2006;2:e119.
18. Tachedjian G, Orlova M, Sarafianos SG, Arnold E, Goff SP. Nonnucleoside reverse transcriptase inhibitors are chemical enhancers of dimerization of the HIV type 1 reverse transcriptase. Proc Natl Acad Sci USA. 2001;98:7188–93.
19. Pan YY, Wang SM, Huang KJ, Chiang CC, Wang CT. Placement of leucine zipper motifs at the carboxyl terminus of HIV-1 protease significantly reduces virion production. PLoS One. 2012;7:e32845.
20. Ludwig C, Leiherer A, Wagner R. Importance of protease cleavage sites within and flanking human immunodeficiency virus type 1 transframe protein p6* for spatiotemporal regulation of protease activation. J Virol. 2008;82:4573–84.
21. Partin K, Zybarth G, Ehrlich L, DeCrombrugghe M, Wimmer E, Carter C. Deletion of sequences upstream of the proteinase improves the proteolytic processing of human immunodeficiency virus type 1. Proc Natl Acad Sci USA. 1991;88:4776–80.
22. Tessmer U, Krausslich HG. Cleavage of human immunodeficiency virus type 1 proteinase from the N-terminally adjacent p6* protein is essential for efficient Gag polyprotein processing and viral infectivity. J Virol. 1998;72:3459–63.
23. Paulus C, Ludwig C, Wagner R. Contribution of the Gag-Pol transframe domain p6* and its coding sequence to morphogenesis and replication of human immunodeficiency virus type 1. Virology. 2004;330:271–83.
24. Chatterjee A, Mridula P, Mishra RK, Mittal R, Hosur RV. Folding regulates autoprocessing of HIV-1 protease precursor. J Biol Chem. 2005;280:11369–78.
25. Ishima R, Torchia DA, Louis JM. Mutational and structural studies aimed at characterizing the monomer of HIV-1 protease and its precursor. J Biol Chem. 2007;282:17190–9.
26. Louis JM, Clore GM, Gronenborn AM. Autoprocessing of HIV-1 protease is tightly coupled to protein folding. Nat Struct Biol. 1999;6:868–75.
27. Sadiq SK, Noe F, De Fabritiis G. Kinetic characterization of the critical step in HIV-1 protease maturation. Proc Natl Acad Sci USA. 2012;109:20449–54.
28. Yu F-H, Huang K-J, Wang C-T. C-terminal HIV-1 transframe p6* tetrapeptide blocks enhanced Gag cleavage incurred by leucine zipper replacement of a deleted p6* domain. J Virol. 2017;91:e00103-17.
29. Ratner L, Haseltine W, Patarca R, Livak KJ, Starcich B, Josephs SF, Doran ER, Rafalski JA, Whitehorn EA, Baumeister K, et al. Complete nucleotide sequence of the AIDS virus. HTLV-III. Nature. 1985;313:277–84.
30. Page KA, Landau NR, Littman DR. Construction and use of a human immunodeficiency virus vector for analysis of virus infectivity. J Virol. 1990;64:5270–6.
31. Yu F-H, Chou T-A, Liao W-H, Huang K-J, Wang C-T. Gag-Pol transframe domain p6* is essential for HIV-1 protease-mediated virus maturation. PLoS ONE. 2015;10:e0127974.
32. Chen S-W, Chiu H-C, Liao W-H, Wang F-D, Chen SSL, Wang C-T. The virus-associated human immunodeficiency virus type 1 Gag-Pol carrying an active protease domain in the matrix region is severely defective both in autoprocessing and in trans processing of gag particles. Virology. 2004;318:534–41.
33. Boles E, Miosga T. A rapid and highly efficient method for PCR-based site-directed mutagenesis using only one new primer. Curr Genet. 1995;28:197–8.
34. Chiu H-C, Yao S-Y, Wang C-T. Coding sequences upstream of the human immunodeficiency virus type 1 reverse transcriptase domain in Gag-Pol are not essential for incorporation of the Pr160gag-pol into virus particles. J Virol. 2002;76:3221–31.
35. Yee JK, Friedmann T, Burns JC. Generation of high-titer pseudotyped retrovirus with very broad host range. Methods in Cell Biology. 1994;43:99–112.
36. Chen YL, Ts'ai PW, Yang CC, Wang CT. Generation of infectious virus particles by transient co-expression of human immunodeficiency virus type 1 gag mutants. J Gen Virol. 1997;78(Pt 10):2497–501.
37. Chiang C-C, Wang S-M, Tseng Y-T, Huang K-J, Wang C-T. Mutations at human immunodeficiency virus type 1 reverse transcriptase tryptophan repeat motif attenuate the inhibitory effect of efavirenz on virus production. Virology. 2009;383:261–70.
38. Ferris AL, Hizi A, Showalter SD, Pichuantes S, Babe L, Craik CS, Hughes SH. Immunologic and proteolytic analysis of HIV-1 reverse transcriptase structure. Virology. 1990;175:456–64.
39. Hizi A, McGill C, Hughes SH. Expression of soluble, enzymatically active, human immunodeficiency virus reverse transcriptase in Escherichia coli and analysis of mutants. Proc Natl Acad Sci. 1988;85:1218–22.
40. Chiu H-C, Wang F-D, Chen Y-MA, Wang C-T. Effects of human immunodeficiency virus type 1 transframe protein p6* mutations on viral protease-mediated Gag processing. J Gen Virol. 2006;87:2041–6.
41. Cherry E, Liang C, Rong L, Quan Y, Inouye P, Li X, Morin N, Kotler M, Wainberg MA. Characterization of human immunodeficiency virus type-1 (HIV-1) particles that express protease-reverse transcriptase fusion proteins11. J Mol Biol. 1998;284:43–56.
42. Pettit SC, Simsic J, Loeb DD, Everitt L, Hutchison CA, Swanstrom R. Analysis of retroviral protease cleavage sites reveals two types of cleavage sites and the structural requirements of the P1 amino acid. J Biol Chem. 1991;266:14539–47.

The RNA surveillance proteins UPF1, UPF2 and SMG6 affect HIV-1 reactivation at a post-transcriptional level

Shringar Rao[1,2], Raquel Amorim[1,3], Meijuan Niu[1], Abdelkrim Temzi[1] and Andrew J. Mouland[1,2,3]*

Abstract

Background: The ability of human immunodeficiency virus type 1 (HIV-1) to form a stable viral reservoir is the major obstacle to an HIV-1 cure and post-transcriptional events contribute to the maintenance of viral latency. RNA surveillance proteins such as UPF1, UPF2 and SMG6 affect RNA stability and metabolism. In our previous work, we demonstrated that UPF1 stabilises HIV-1 genomic RNA (vRNA) and enhances its translatability in the cytoplasm. Thus, in this work we evaluated the influence of RNA surveillance proteins on vRNA expression and, as a consequence, viral reactivation in cells of the lymphoid lineage.

Methods: Quantitative fluorescence in situ hybridisation—flow cytometry (FISH-flow), si/shRNA-mediated depletions and Western blotting were used to characterise the roles of RNA surveillance proteins on HIV-1 reactivation in a latently infected model T cell line and primary CD4+ T cells.

Results: UPF1 was found to be a positive regulator of viral reactivation, with a depletion of UPF1 resulting in impaired vRNA expression and viral reactivation. UPF1 overexpression also modestly enhanced vRNA expression and its ATPase activity and N-terminal domain were necessary for this effect. UPF2 and SMG6 were found to negatively influence viral reactivation, both via an interaction with UPF1. UPF1 knockdown also resulted in reduced vRNA levels and viral gene expression in HIV-1-infected primary CD4+ T cells.

Conclusion: Overall, these data suggest that RNA surveillance proteins affect HIV-1 gene expression at a post-transcriptional level. An elucidation of the role of vRNA metabolism on the maintenance of HIV-1 persistence can lead to the development of novel curative strategies.

Keywords: HIV-1 latency, RNA surveillance proteins, HIV-1 genomic RNA stability, Post-transcriptional regulation, Nonsense-mediated mRNA decay, NMD, UPF1, UPF2, SMG6

Background

The implementation of combination antiretroviral therapy (cART) to treat human immunodeficiency virus type 1 (HIV-1) has led the infection to be likened to a chronic condition, with patients on cART having near-normal life expectancy [1]. However, this therapy is not without its drawbacks, such as adverse side effects that lower the adherence rates, the development of drug resistance and its economic repercussions [2–4]. But one of the biggest disadvantages of this therapy is that it is not curative and an infected individual needs to be on cART for the entire duration of their lifetime to effectively suppress viremia. The major hurdle towards an HIV-1 cure is the property of virus to form a stable latent reservoir upon infection that is responsible for the rapid rebound of plasma viral loads when cART is discontinued [5]. This reservoir is primarily composed of resting memory CD4+ T cells along with monocytes and macrophages [6] in peripheral blood and other anatomical compartments such as the gut, lymph nodes and central nervous system. Latency in HIV-1 infection is defined as a reversibly non-productive state of infection which is characterised by the presence

*Correspondence: andrew.mouland@mcgill.ca
[1] HIV-1 RNA Trafficking Laboratory, Lady Davis Institute at the Jewish General Hospital, Montreal, QC H3T 1E2, Canada
Full list of author information is available at the end of the article

of infected cells that do not actively produce viral particles, but retain the ability to do so [7]. Latent cells harbour a replication competent proviral DNA integrated in their genomes [8]. Many research groups have studied the functional aspects of the maintenance of latency in cells by investigating the molecular mechanisms leading to a block at the level of transcription (reviewed in [6, 9, 10]). However, certain studies also highlight that co and post-transcriptional events can also contribute to the maintenance of latency in HIV-1 infected cells [11–13]. These include defective splicing of the genomic viral RNA (vRNA) [14], inhibition of nucleocytoplasmic export of vRNA [13, 15, 16] or an impediment to vRNA translation [17, 18]. Thus, in this work, we investigate the role of the RNA surveillance proteins on the post-transcriptional events that are involved in the maintenance of HIV-1 latency.

RNA surveillance is a host quality control mechanism that identifies and degrades unspliced, aberrantly spliced, intron-containing, upstream open reading frame-containing and premature termination codon (PTC)-containing mRNAs to prevent the accumulation of potentially toxic truncated proteins within the cell (reviewed in [19]). A central player in this mechanism is the Up Frameshift Protein 1 (UPF1), an RNA binding protein that has ATPase and RNA helicase activity [20]. It is a multifunctional protein that has defined roles in DNA repair and replication [21, 22], RNA stability [23–25], telomere metabolism [21] and cell cycle progression [22] (reviewed in [26]). Its most characterised function, however, is its role in nonsense-mediated mRNA decay (NMD) during which UPF1 interacts with a family of proteins such as UPF2, UPF3A and UPF3B, a kinase SMG1 and an endonuclease SMG6 resulting in the degradation of aberrant mRNAs (reviewed in [19, 27]). Although NMD was previously implicated only in the degradation of aberrant mRNA, it is now widely accepted that NMD also targets up to 10% of other physiological mRNAs for degradation in response to cellular needs [19, 28–30], including transcripts that contain long 3'UTRs [31].

In order to promote their survival, viruses have evolved numerous strategies to either evade or manipulate the RNA surveillance pathways (reviewed in [32]). Retroviruses, despite containing long 3'UTRs that are recognised by UPF1, are capable of evading NMD by virtue of the presence of RNA stability elements in their genome [33] (reviewed in [34, 35]). In previous studies, our group has demonstrated that HIV-1 not only evades NMD, it also hijacks UPF1 to form an RNP that promotes vRNA stability and nucleocytoplasmic export [36, 37]. This effect may be exerted during the rapid, co-transcriptional association of UPF1 with vRNA during transcription [38]. UPF2, another protein involved in NMD, has been shown to block nucleocytoplasmic export of the vRNA

by binding to UPF1 and preventing its nucleocytoplasmic shuttle [37]. Once in the cytoplasm, UPF1 assembles in another distinct RNP on the vRNA resulting in not only the increased stability of the vRNA, but also in its enhanced translation leading to increased levels of the HIV-1 structural protein pr55^{Gag} viral production [36]. Additionally, UPF1 interacts with vRNA in an RNA length-dependent manner and this could contribute to its incorporation into progeny HIV-1 virions [38–41]. Therefore, there is substantial evidence to show that UPF1 can affect vRNA metabolism at different levels.

In this study, we investigated the ability of UPF1 and its associated proteins UPF2 and SMG6 to influence the HIV-1 gene expression and, as a consequence, viral reactivation at a post-transcriptional level by overexpression and siRNA-mediated knockdown studies in cells of the lymphoid lineage. We employed a fluorescence in situ hybridisation/flow cytometry (FISH-Flow) to monitor vRNA expression levels and viral protein production in a latently-infected T cell line. We observed that these proteins can modulate the HIV-1 gene expression and thus the post-transcriptional maintenance of HIV-1 latency. We have also identified the domains responsible for these effects on viral reactivation by mutational studies. Importantly, we also demonstrate a direct effect of UPF1 on vRNA expression in primary HIV-1 infected CD4+ T cells.

Results

FISH-Flow can be used to monitor vRNA levels and viral reactivation in J-Lat cells

UPF1 has previously been demonstrated to affect vRNA metabolism at three distinct stages: overall vRNA stability, the nucleocytoplasmic export of the vRNA, and vRNA translation in the cytoplasm [36, 37]. Therefore, we employed the FISH-Flow technique using probes against the GagPol region of the vRNA in latently infected J-Lat 10.6 cells to monitor both the transcriptional as well as translational products of the HIV-1 provirus. This technique has previously been employed to assess ongoing HIV-1 replication, to quantify the size of the inducible latent reservoir in HIV-infected individuals, to determine the kinetics of latency reversal and to characterize the specific cell subpopulations of CD4+ T cells that transcribe HIV-1 RNA [17, 42–44] (reviewed in [45, 46]). Using this technique, it is possible to distinguish between cells that contain both vRNA and viral proteins, and cells that only contain untranslated vRNA, thus differentiating between the transcription-competent and translation-competent viral reservoir [45, 46]. Cells can then also be seeded on a coverslip to determine the sub-cellular localisation of the vRNA using laser scanning confocal microscopy (LCSM). This comprehensive analysis enables us to investigate how UPF1 influences viral reactivation and to distinguish between an effect on vRNA expression, export or translation. J-Lat 10.6 cells, a well-established model of studying HIV-1 latency and reactivation [88, 47, 48], and primary CD4+ T cells are used in this study. The J-Lat cells have a GFP reporter in the *nef* open reading frame of the virus to monitor viral gene expression and, thus, viral reactivation. The cells can be reactivated by treatment with phorbol myristate acetate (PMA) or TNFα (Additional file 1: Figure S1A). To assess whether the FISH-Flow technique can be used in the J-Lat cell model to measure reactivation, cells were either mock treated with dimethyl sulfoxide (DMSO) or treated with PMA to reactivate the cells. PMA is a protein kinase C agonist and is a strong activator of cellular transcription and was the latency reversing agent of choice because it leads to maximal reactivation of the J-Lat 10.6 cells [49]. We also validated the PMA treatment did not affect the baseline expression levels of our proteins of interest: UPF1, UPF2 and SMG6 (Additional file 1: Figure S1B–D). Jurkat cells were used as a negative, uninfected control to determine the specificity of the FISH-Flow technique. Upon treatment with PMA, 60.89 ($\pm$11.35)% of J-Lat cells produced GFP indicating viral protein production and reactivation (Fig. 1a, b). Efficient GagPol mRNA staining was also observed in 63.78 ($\pm$15.16)% of PMA-treated cells. (PE channel, Fig. 1a, b). It is also important to note that 4.79 ($\pm$2.44)% of PMA-treated cells contained vRNA but not GFP, representing the transcription-competent viral reservoir as previously described [45, 46]. The 2.48 ($\pm$1.17) of PMA-treated cells that were GFP+ but did not contain vRNA represent the cells that are generating multiply-transcripts but not full length transcripts, since the GFP codon is present on the *nef* open reading frame [88]. The uninduced J-Lat cells contained some residual vRNA and GFP production, with 2.59 ($\pm$1.76)% of cells expressing GFP and 0.27 ($\pm$0.11)% of cells expressing vRNA (Fig. 1a, b). Although the vRNA is the unspliced genomic viral RNA whereas GFP is generated from the multiply spliced viral RNA, GFP was used as a marker for viral reactivation rather than intracellular p24 due to the efficiency of measuring viral reactivation at a single cell level by Flow cytometry due to the stability of GFP. The levels of pr55^{Gag}, coded for by the vRNA, can be measured by Western blot to further correlate effects vRNA transcription and translation, if necessary. Jurkat cells did not show any vRNA+ cells, indicating that this technique is highly specific (Fig. 1a). Cells from each of these conditions were seeded onto coverslips and observed by laser scanning confocal microscopy (Fig. 1c) to view the subcellular localisation of the vRNA. Therefore, the FISH-Flow technique is an efficient method to monitor viral reactivation at the transcriptional and translational levels in J-Lat cells.

UPF1 knockdown attenuates HIV-1 proviral reactivation

In previous studies conducted by our group, we observed that UPF1 knockdown lead to reduced vRNA stability in the nucleus and in the cytoplasm of cell [36]. Thus, we hypothesised that the depletion of UPF1 can reduce vRNA expression at a post-transcriptional level and thereby inhibit viral reactivation. To evaluate the effect of UPF1 levels on proviral reactivation, J-Lat cells were either transfected with a non-silencing siRNA (siNS) or with siRNA against UPF1 (siUPF1). In each of these conditions, cells were either left uninduced (DMSO) or treated with PMA to reactivate the cells. The percentage of reactivation in the form of GFP production was monitored by flow cytometry and the cell lysates were subjected to Western blotting to validate UPF1 knockdown using antibodies against UPF1, pr55^{Gag} and actin. Treatment of cells with siUPF1 resulted in a 68.9 ($\pm$29.9)% decrease in UPF1 protein levels as measured by Western blot, demonstrating the efficiency of siUPF1 treatment (Additional file 1: Figure S2A). UPF1 knockdown had no significant effect on viral reactivation in the uninduced condition (Fig. 2a). However, upon reactivation with PMA, UPF1 knockdown lead to a 35.3 ($\pm$8.4)% decrease in viral reactivation as compared to the siNS condition (Fig. 2a), which correlated with reduced pr55^{Gag} levels observed by Western blots (Fig. 2b). In order to determine if this decrease in viral reactivation was due to an effect on the vRNA levels or due to inefficient nucleocytoplasmic export or translation of the vRNA, we also conducted FISH-Flow analyses in each of the above reactions. The levels of vRNA were also quantified by RT-qPCR. Upon treatment with PMA, UPF1 knockdown lead to a 23.5 ($\pm$4.8)% decrease in the number of vRNA expressing cells as compared to the siNS treated cells (Fig. 2c, d) as well as a 72.6 ($\pm$0.1)% decrease in the levels of vRNA as quantified by RT-qPCR (Fig. 2e). Of these vRNA expressing cells, a knockdown of UPF1 also led to a 28.0 ($\pm$11.8)% decrease in per cell vRNA levels as measured median fluorescence intensity (MFI) of the vRNA channel (PE) as compared the vRNA in the siNS treated cells (Additional file 1: Figure S2B). This is in accordance with our previous work where we demonstrated that a knockdown of UPF1 resulted in a decrease in vRNA stability [36]. The reduction in vRNA levels as quantified by RT-qPCR in the siUPF1 condition is more dramatic than the reduction of GFP production in the same condition, possibly due to increased stability of GFP as compared to the vRNA. It is also important to note that these detrimental effects of UPF1 knockdown on vRNA levels is specific to the vRNA, since no significant differences were observed in the % of cell expressing a housekeeping mRNA RPL13A and the MFI of the RPL13A mRNA channel measured by FISH-Flow, or

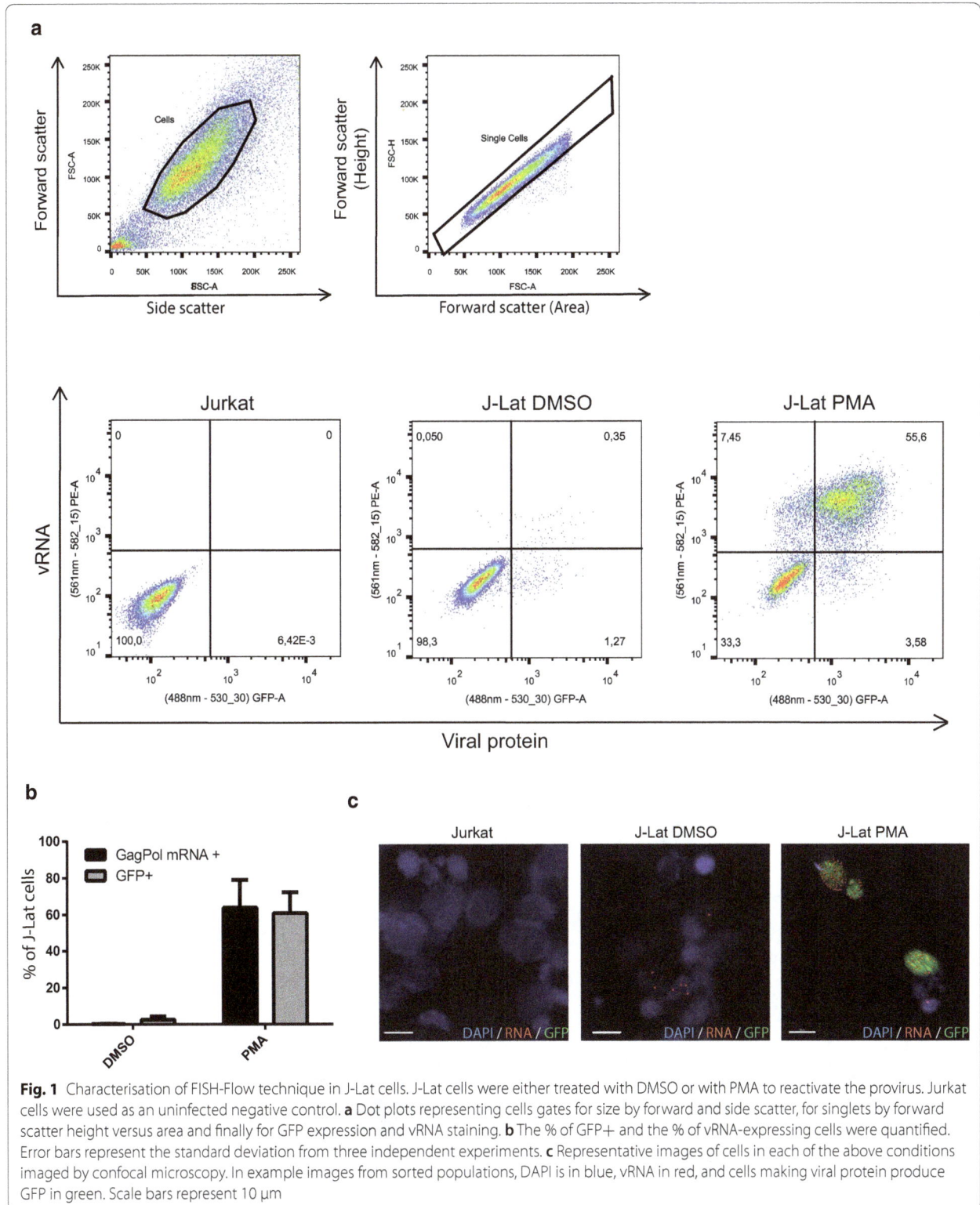

Fig. 1 Characterisation of FISH-Flow technique in J-Lat cells. J-Lat cells were either treated with DMSO or with PMA to reactivate the provirus. Jurkat cells were used as an uninfected negative control. **a** Dot plots representing cells gates for size by forward and side scatter, for singlets by forward scatter height versus area and finally for GFP expression and vRNA staining. **b** The % of GFP+ and the % of vRNA-expressing cells were quantified. Error bars represent the standard deviation from three independent experiments. **c** Representative images of cells in each of the above conditions imaged by confocal microscopy. In example images from sorted populations, DAPI is in blue, vRNA in red, and cells making viral protein produce GFP in green. Scale bars represent 10 μm

in the relative levels of housekeeping mRNA GAPDH measured by RT-qPCR (Additional file 1: Figure S2C–E). However, in these experimental conditions, we can not differentiate between cells that have successful knockdown of UPF1 and non-transfected cells. Therefore, to partially overcome this caveat, we also stained the cells with a UPF1 mRNA probe and, using FISH-Flow analysis, we delineated between UPF1 high vs.

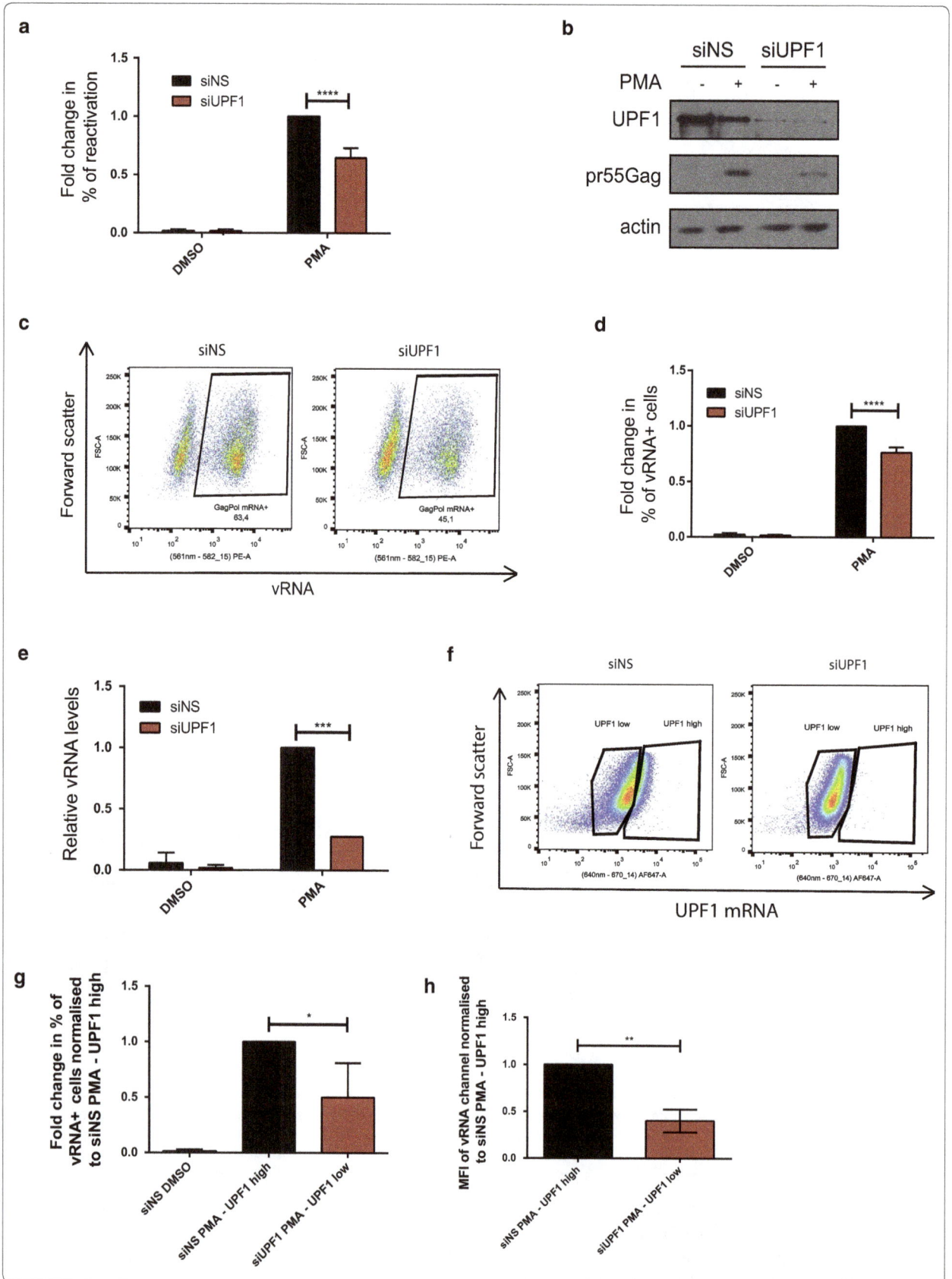

UPF1 low cells (Fig. 2f). Using this gating strategy, it was observed that the UPF1 low population of the siUPF1-PMA treated cells showed a 50.5 (± 31.07) reduction in the % of vRNA-expressing cells as compared to the UPF1 high population of the siNS-PMA condition (Fig. 2g). Of these vRNA expressing cells, a knockdown of UPF1 also led to a 1.66 fold reduction in the median fluorescence intensity (MFI) of the vRNA channel (PE) as compared the vRNA in the siNS treated cells (Fig. 2h). Since UPF1 has previously characterised roles in nuclear export [37], we determined if a knockdown of UPF1 resulted in increased nuclear retention of the vRNA. Cellular fractionation was performed and the vRNA present in whole cell, cytoplasmic and nuclear fractions were quantified by RT-PCR (Additional file 1: Figure S3A, B). A decrease is vRNA levels was observed in all fractions, thus implying that in these experimental conditions, UPF1 is acting on vRNA expression rather than on nuclear export (Additional file 1: Figure S3A, B). Taken together, these data suggest that a knockdown of UPF1 leads to attenuated

HIV-1 proviral reactivation in J-Lat cells at a post-transcriptional level, by reducing vRNA levels and thus, viral reactivation and protein production.

UPF1 overexpression enhances HIV-1 proviral reactivation by enhancing vRNA levels

UPF1 overexpression has been shown to enhance vRNA stability, nucleocytoplasmic export and translation in previous studies [36, 37]. Therefore, we hypothesised that UPF1 overexpression could enhance proviral reactivation. J-Lat cells were either mock transfected or transfected with FLAG-UPF1. They were then either left uninduced (DMSO) or reactivated with PMA. We employed the FISH-Flow technique using probes against the vRNA as well as UPF1 mRNA to gate for UPF1-overexpressing populations (Fig. 3a). The percentage of reactivation was monitored by flow cytometry and the cell lysates were subjected to Western blotting to validate UPF1 overexpression using antibodies against UPF1, pr55^{Gag} and actin (Fig. 3b, c). UPF1 overexpression resulted in a 21.3

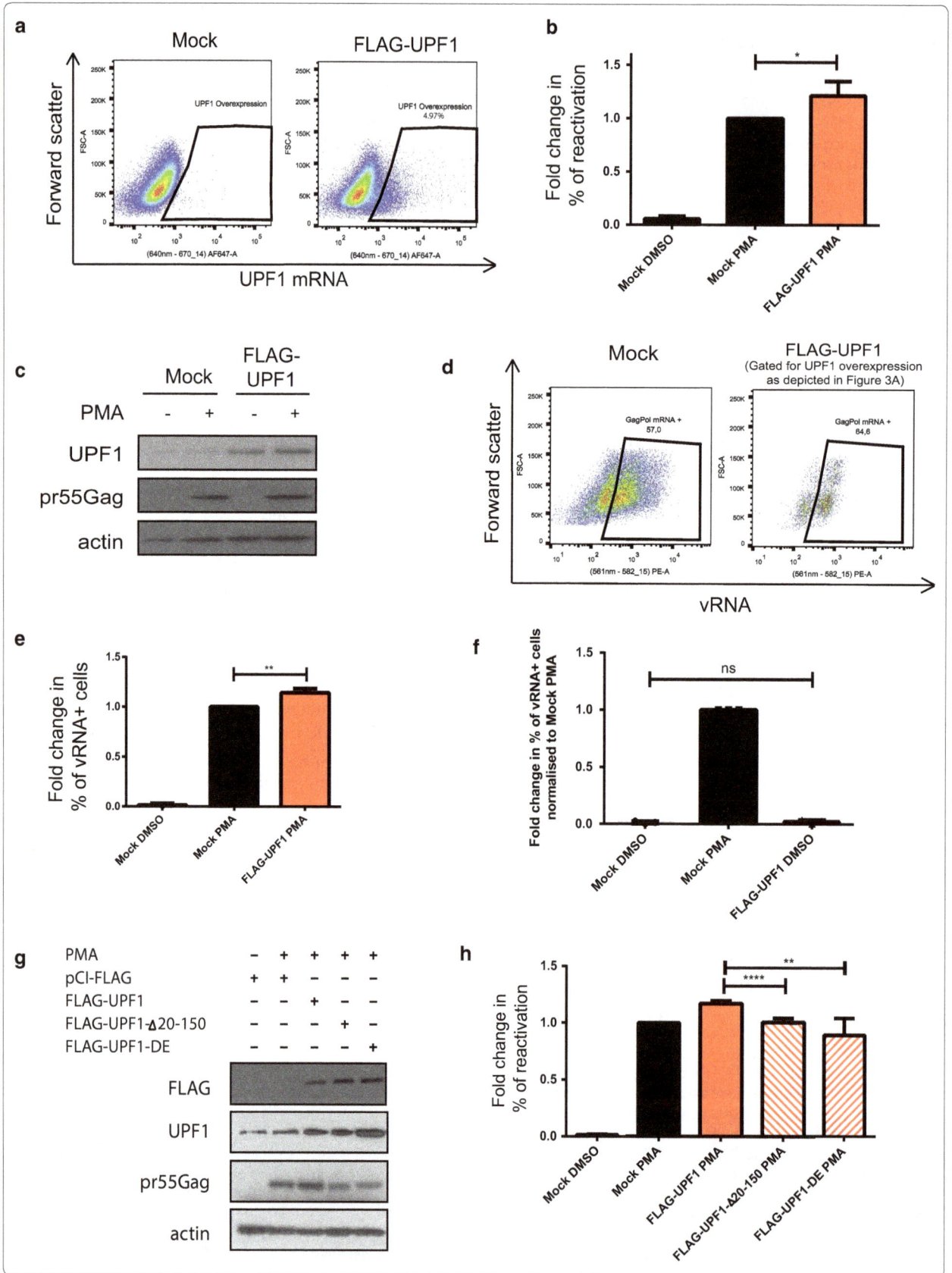

($\pm$ 13.5)% increase in viral reactivation upon PMA treatment as compared to the mock-transfected condition (Fig. 3b). UPF1 overexpression also led to a 14.4 ($\pm$ 4.2)% increase in vRNA levels in the UPF1 overexpressing cells and compared to the mock transfected cells (Fig. 3d, e). UPF1 overexpression in uninduced condition shows no increase in % of vRNA cells as demonstrated by FISH-Flow (Fig. 3f), indicating that UPF1 alone is unable to activate transcription of the provirus and PMA is necessary for transcription to take place. UPF1 overexpression also does not result in a change in the % of vRNA+/GFP- cells as compared to mock treated cells (Additional file 1: Figure S3C). This implies that enhanced viral reactivation upon UPF1 overexpression is due to an effect on vRNA levels rather than an increase in the translation of the transcriptional-competent reservoir. Hence, UPF1 overexpression enhances proviral reactivation at a post-transcriptional level by modestly increasing the expression of the vRNA, thereby resulting in enhanced viral reactivation. This is consistent with our previous work where we demonstrated that an overexpression of UPF1 results in enhanced vRNA stability [36].

In order to determine which domain of UPF1 is responsible for enhancing vRNA expression, we either mock transfected cells, or transfected them with FLAG-UPF1 or other constructs of UPF1 that contain deletions in the N-terminal region (FLAG-UPF1-Δ20-150), deletions in the C-terminal (FLAG-UPF1-1-1074), mutations in the RNA helicase domain of UPF1 (FLAG-UPF1-RR857AA), mutations leading to a deficiency in UPF2 binding ability (FLAG-UPF1-LECY) or mutations in the ATPase region of UPF1 (FLAG-UPF1-DE). These cells were then treated with PMA and the % of reactivation was monitored by flow cytometry (Additional file 1: Figure S4A). The ability of UPF1 overexpression to enhance viral reactivation was lost when the FLAG-UPF1-Δ20-150 construct, which contains an N-terminal deletion or the FLAG-UPF1-DE,

that has impaired ATPase activity, were used (Fig. 3g, h). The overexpression of these UPF1 mutants resulted in reactivation at levels comparable to the mock transfected cells treated with PMA. These results indicate that the N-terminal domain and ATPase activity of UPF1 are necessary for its mild effect on enhancing vRNA expression and are consistent with our previous work [36].

UPF2 overexpression attenuates HIV-1 reactivation via an interaction with UPF1

Previous work from our lab has demonstrated that UPF2 is excluded from the HIV-1 RNP and that its overexpression can block UPF1-mediated nucleocytoplasmic export of vRNA [37]. UPF2 is also known to bind UPF1 with a high affinity [50]. For these reasons, we hypothesised that when UPF2 is present in excess it can sequester UPF1 in the cytoplasm resulting in reduced UPF1 being bound to vRNA. J-Lat cells were either mock transfected or transfected with FLAG-UPF2 and cells were either left uninduced (DMSO) or treated with PMA. The percentage of reactivation in the form of GFP production was monitored by flow cytometry and the cell lysates were subjected to Western blotting to validate UPF2 overexpression using antibodies against UPF2, pr55^{Gag} and actin. Upon reactivation with PMA, UPF2 overexpression resulted in a 25.95 ($\pm$ 16.8)% decrease in viral reactivation (Fig. 4a) and viral protein production (Fig. 4b). To differentiate between UPF2 overexpressing cells from the whole population and to see if it has any effect on vRNA levels, we conducted FISH-Flow using probes against UPF2 mRNA and vRNA (Fig. 4c). Upon reactivation with PMA, UPF2 overexpression led to a 57.36 ($\pm$ 27.83) decrease in the percentage of vRNA expressing cells as compared to the mock transfected cells (Fig. 4d, e). Therefore, an overexpression of UPF2 resulted in a modest, albeit statistically significant ($p < 0.05$) decrease in viral reactivation due to a reduction in vRNA expression.

(See figure on next page.)
Fig. 4 UPF2 overexpression inhibits the reactivation of HIV-1 in J-Lat cells. J-Lat 10.6 cells were either mock transfected or transfected with Flag-UPF2 and were uninduced (DMSO) or reactivated (PMA). **a** Reactivation, monitored by GFP production, was quantified by flow cytometry and the percentages of reactivation were normalised to the mock-PMA reactivated condition. Error bars represent the standard deviation from three independent experiments with at least 10,000 cells counted per treatment. Asterisks represent statistically significant difference between groups (Two-way ANOVA; $p < 0.05$). **b** Cell lysates were run on SDS-PAGE gels and UPF2 and pr55^{Gag} protein levels were detected by Western Blotting. **c** Gating strategy to detect UPF2 overexpressing cells by detecting UPF2 mRNA levels by FISH-Flow. **d** Of the UPF2-mRNA expressing cells gated for in (**c**), the % of vRNA expressing cells were quantified. Error bars represent the standard deviation from three independent experiments. Asterisks represent statistically significant difference between groups (One-way ANOVA; $p < 0.05$). **e** Example dot plot depicting vRNA expression in mock transfected and UPF2 overexpressing populations using FISH-Flow technique. **f** J-Lat cells were mock transfected or transfected with FLAG-UPF2 or FLAG-UPF2-1-1096. Cell lysates were run on acrylamide gels and UPF2 and pr55^{Gag} protein levels were detected by Western Blotting. **g** J-Lat cells were mock transfected, transfected with FLAG-UPF2 or co-transfected with FLAG-UPF1 or FLAG-UPF1-LECY. Cell lysates were run on acrylamide gels and UPF2, UPF1 and pr55^{Gag} protein levels were detected by Western Blotting. **h** Reactivation in the form of GFP expression was quantified in cells transfected as in (**f**) and (**g**) and the percentages of reactivation were normalised to the mock-PMA reactivated condition. Error bars represent the standard deviation from three independent experiments with at least 10,000 cells counted per treatment. Asterisks represent statistically significant difference between groups (One-way ANOVA; $p < 0.0001$)

a

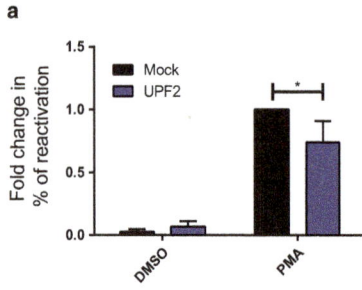

b

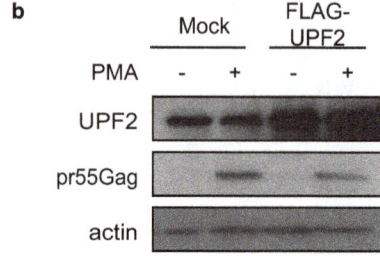

c

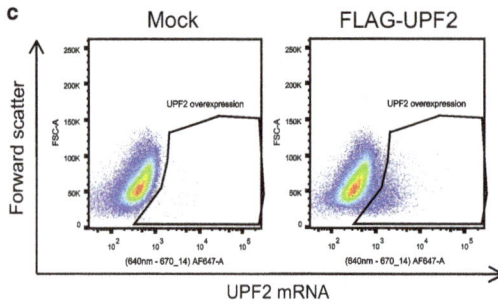

d

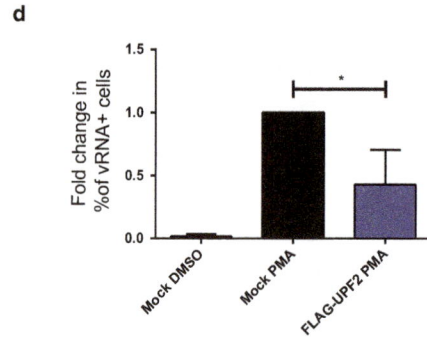

e

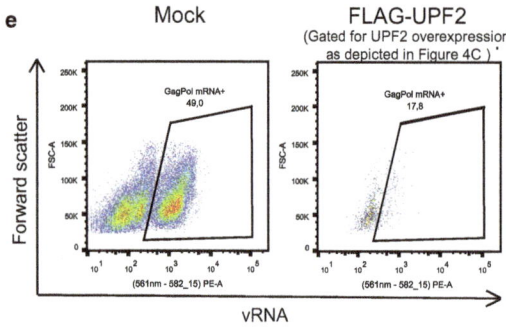

f

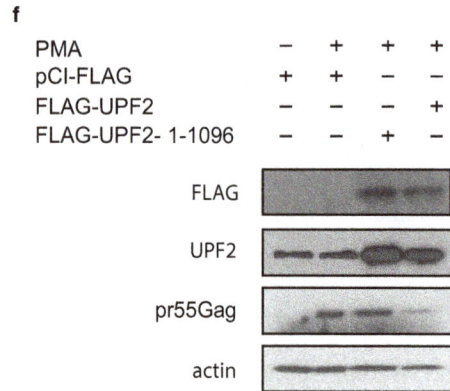

g

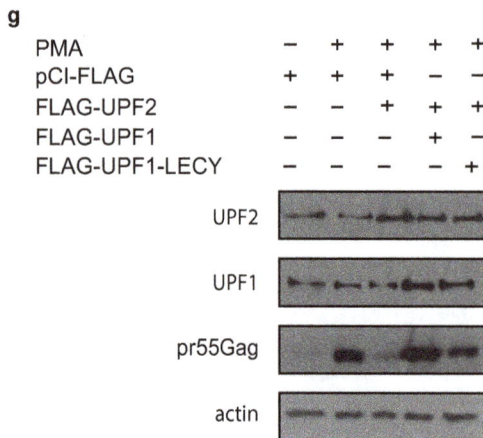

h

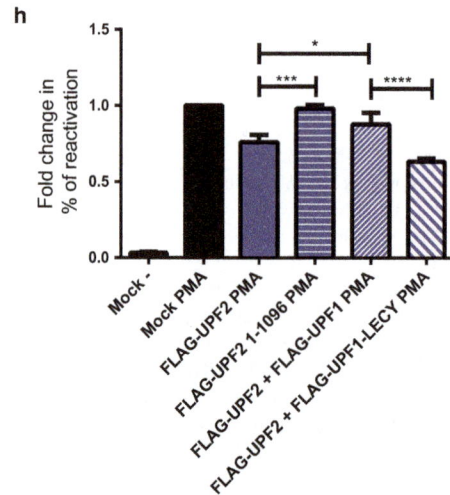

In order to determine if this detrimental effect of UPF2 on vRNA levels is an indirect effect due to its binding to UPF1, we transfected cells with a mutant of UPF2 that does not bind to UPF1 [37, 51, 89] (FLAG-UPF2-1-1096) and compared the % of reactivation in the mock transfected cells, the UPF2 expressing cells and the UPF2-1-1096-expressing cells. It was observed that when UPF2 loses the ability to bind UPF1, there is a loss of its inhibitory effect on reactivation, with reactivation at levels comparable to the mock treated cells (Fig. 4f, h). We also co-transfected FLAG-UPF2 with either FLAG-UPF1 or with FLAG-UPF1-LECY that contains a mutation in the UPF2 binding site and monitored the % of reactivation. UPF1 coexpression is able to rescue the deleterious effect of UPF2 on viral reactivation, but not when in contains a mutation to the UPF2-binding site (Fig. 4g, h). This indicates that the deleterious effect of UPF2 on viral reactivation is a result of its binding to UPF1 which is sequestered and unable to exert a positive effect on vRNA expression, consistent with previous reports [37].

SMG6 overexpression is detrimental to HIV-1 proviral reactivation

UPF1 is an integral member of a network of proteins involved in NMD, including UPF2, UPF3A, UPF3B, SMG6, SMG5, SMG7 and SMG1. SMG6 is the endonuclease involved in the final step of the degradation of aberrant RNA in NMD [52, 53] and has a direct influence on RNA levels. Thus, to evaluate the roles of SMG6 in proviral reactivation, we either mock transfected J-Lat cells or transfected them with HA-SMG6 and either left them uninduced or reactivated them with PMA. The percentage of reactivation in the form of GFP production was monitored by flow cytometry (Fig. 5a) and the cell lysates were subjected to Western blotting to validate SMG6 overexpression using antibodies against SMG6, pr55^{Gag} and actin (Fig. 5b). Overexpression of

SMG6 resulted in a 21.2 ($\pm$9.1)% decrease in reactivation (Fig. 5a). Furthermore, upon reactivation with PMA, FISH-Flow analyses revealed a small but significant decrease (7.6$\pm$4.1%) in the percentage of vRNA expressing cells upon SMG6 overexpression as compared to the mock-transfected cells (Fig. 5c, d). Of the vRNA present upon SMG6 overexpression, there was a 1.25-fold decrease in the median fluorescence intensity (Fig. 5e). Thus, SMG6 is detrimental to vRNA expression and attenuates PMA-induced proviral reactivation.

SMG6 contains an exon junction binding domain (EBM) [54], a 14-3-3-like domain that binds to phosphorylated UPF1 [55] and a PilT N-terminus (PIN) domain [56] that possesses the endonuclease activity [56–58]. In order to determine which of these domains are responsible for the negative effect on vRNA levels, we transfected J-Lat cells with plasmids that express SMG6 with mutations in each of the aforementioned domains; HA-SMG6-mEBM, HA-SMG6-m14-3-3 and HA-SMG6-mPIN respectively. These cells were reactivated with PMA and the percentage of reactivation was monitored using flow cytometry. While the overexpression of HA-SMG6 and the exon junction binding mutant HA-SMG6-mEBM attenuated proviral reactivation, the overexpression of HA-SMG6-m14-3-3 and HA-SMG6-mPIN displayed reactivation levels similar to the mock transfected cells (Fig. 5f, g). Thus, these results demonstrate that both, the binding of SMG6 to phosphorylated UPF1 and its endonuclease activity are necessary for its inhibitory effect on vRNA levels (Fig. 5f, g).

SMG6 knockdown increases vRNA expression, but does not affect viral reactivation

To determine the effect of SMG6 depletion on HIV-1 proviral reactivation, we conducted siRNA mediated knockdown studies. J-Lat cells were either transfected with a non-silencing siRNA (siNS) or with siRNA against SMG6 (siSMG6) and cells were either left uninduced

(See figure on next page.)

Fig. 5 SMG6 overexpression leads to attenuated reactivation of HIV-1. **a** J-Lat 10.6 cells were either mock transfected or transfected with HA-SMG6 and were uninduced (DMSO) or reactivated (PMA). Reactivation, monitored by GFP production, was quantified by flow cytometry and the percentages of reactivation were normalised to the mock-PMA reactivated condition. Error bars represent the standard deviation from three independent experiments with at least 10,000 cells counted per treatment. Asterisks represent statistically significant difference between groups (Two-way ANOVA; $p < 0.01$). **b** Cell lysates were run on acrylamide gels and SMG6 and pr55^{Gag} protein levels were detected by Western Blotting. **c** Example dot plot depicting vRNA expression in mock PMA and SMG6 PMA conditions using FISH-Flow technique. **d** The % of vRNA expressing cells were quantified. Error bars represent the standard deviation from three independent experiments. Asterisks represent statistically significant difference between groups (One-way ANOVA; $p < 0.05$). **e** MFI of the vRNA signal were quantified. Asterisks represent statistically significant difference between groups (student's t-test; $p < 0.05$). **f** J-Lat cells were mock transfected or transfected with HA-SMG6, HA-SMG6-mEBM, HA-SMG6-m14-3-3 or HA-SMG6-mPIN and reactivated with PMA. Cell lysates were run on acrylamide gels and SMG6 and pr55^{Gag} protein levels were detected by SDS-PAGE followed by Western Blotting. **g** Reactivation in the above conditions was quantified and the percentages of reactivation were normalised to the mock PMA reactivated condition. Error bars represent the standard deviation from three independent experiments with at least 10,000 cells counted per treatment. Asterisks represent statistically significant difference between groups (One-way ANOVA; $p < 0.05$)

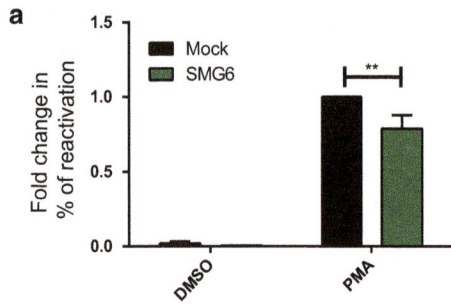

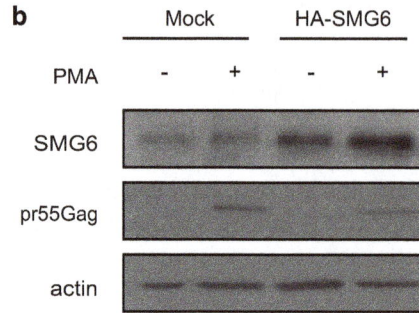

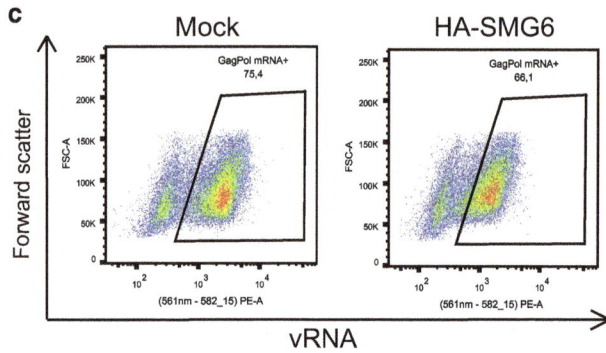

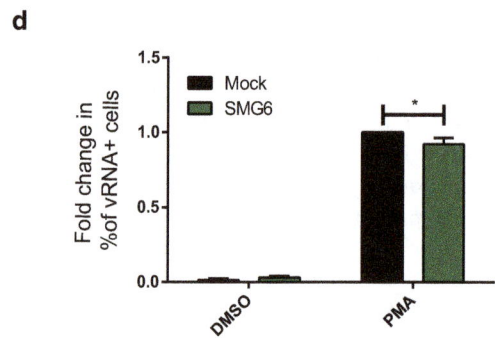

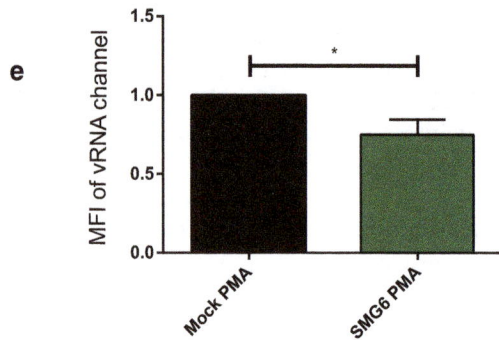

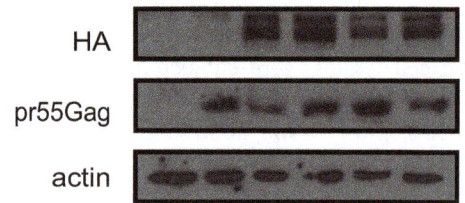

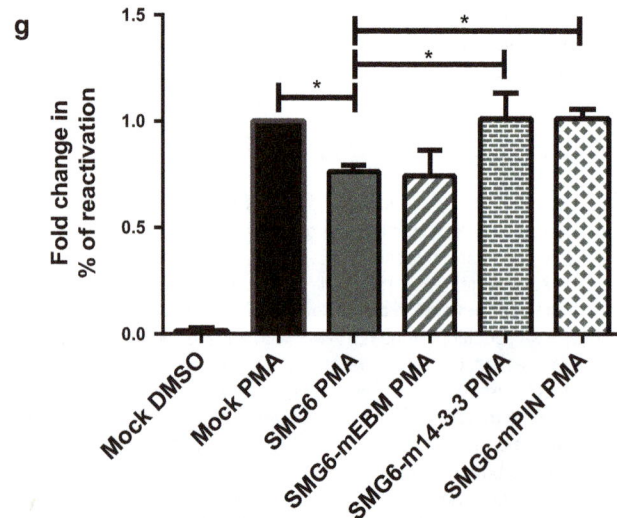

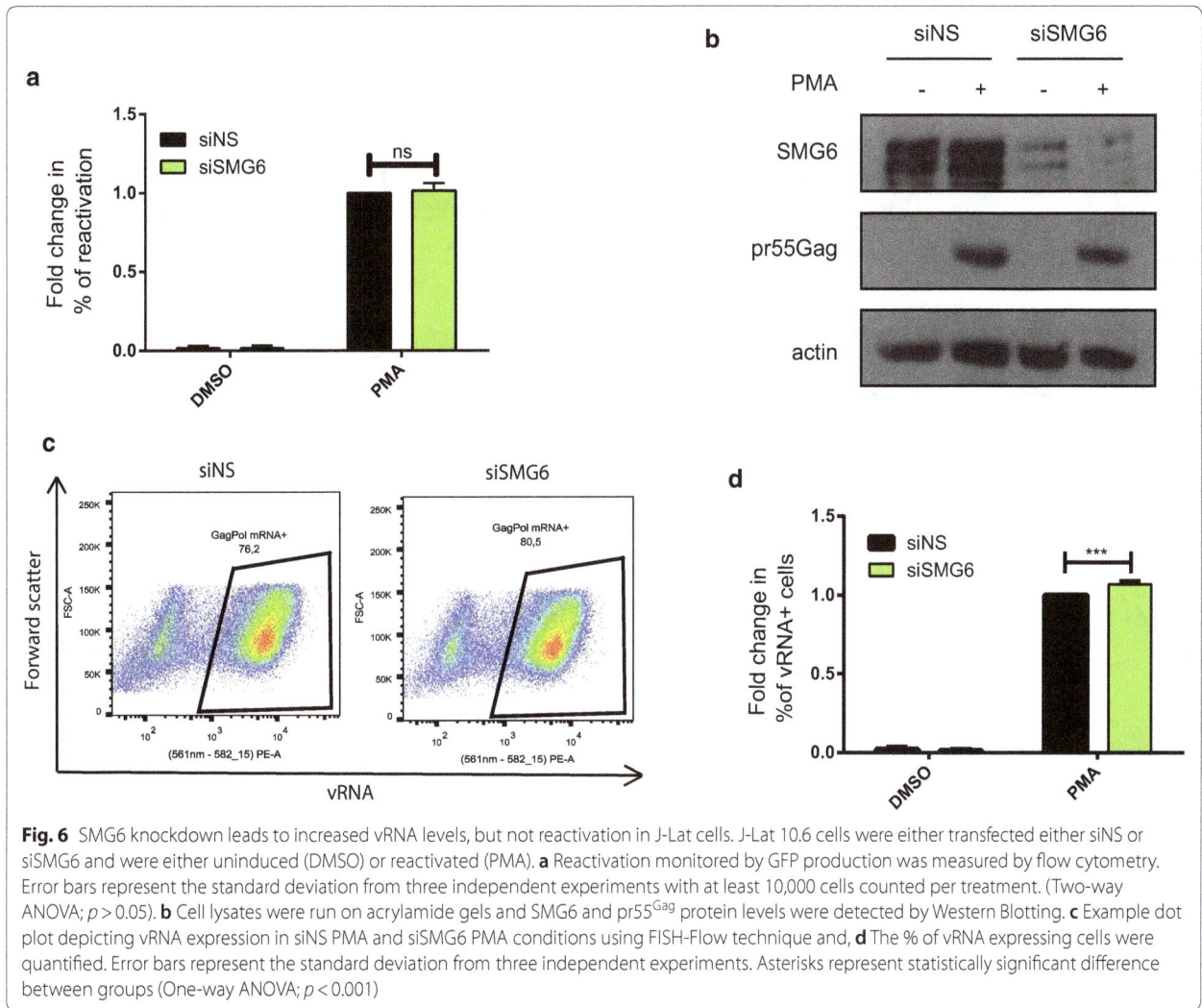

Fig. 6 SMG6 knockdown leads to increased vRNA levels, but not reactivation in J-Lat cells. J-Lat 10.6 cells were either transfected either siNS or siSMG6 and were either uninduced (DMSO) or reactivated (PMA). **a** Reactivation monitored by GFP production was measured by flow cytometry. Error bars represent the standard deviation from three independent experiments with at least 10,000 cells counted per treatment. (Two-way ANOVA; $p > 0.05$). **b** Cell lysates were run on acrylamide gels and SMG6 and pr55^{Gag} protein levels were detected by Western Blotting. **c** Example dot plot depicting vRNA expression in siNS PMA and siSMG6 PMA conditions using FISH-Flow technique and, **d** The % of vRNA expressing cells were quantified. Error bars represent the standard deviation from three independent experiments. Asterisks represent statistically significant difference between groups (One-way ANOVA; $p < 0.001$)

(DMSO) or treated with PMA to reactivate the cells. The percentage of reactivation in the form of GFP production was monitored by flow cytometry and the cell lysates were subjected to Western blotting to validate SMG6 knockdown using antibodies against SMG6, pr55^{Gag} and actin. A knockdown of SMG6 did not have a significant effect on viral reactivation at the level of protein production (Fig. 6a, b). However, upon reactivation with PMA and using FISH-Flow using probes against vRNA, SMG6 knockdown resulted in a small but significant increase ($6.9 \pm 1.8\%$) in the total number of vRNA expressing cells as compared to the siNS condition (Fig. 6c, d). This further illustrates that SMG6 is detrimental to vRNA expression.

UPF1 knockdown impairs vRNA expression in primary HIV-1 infected CD4+ T cells

UPF1 enhances vRNA expression and, as a consequence, viral reactivation in J-Lat cells. UPF2 and SMG6 are

detrimental to vRNA expression, both, via interactions with UPF1. We also assessed the effects of UPF1, UPF2 and SMG6 overexpression on TNFα-induced reactivation of J-Lat cells and observed comparable results (Additional file 1: Figure S4B). However, whether these effects of UPF1 on vRNA expression and pr55^{Gag} expression were also observed in primary CD4+ T cells was yet to be determined. In order to address this question, we conducted shRNA-mediated knockdown of UPF1 in primary CD4+ T cells and observed the effects on vRNA levels and pr55^{Gag} expression upon HIV-1 infection by FISH-Flow. Negatively selected CD4+ T cells from three donors were activated with phytohemagglutinin (PHA). They were then transduced with shUPF1-containing lentiviral particles. Lentiviral particles containing a scrambled sequence were used as a negative control (shNS). The cells were infected with HIV-1 24 h post transduction by spinoculation. Cells were collected 6 days post infection and FISH-Flow was conducted to monitor vRNA

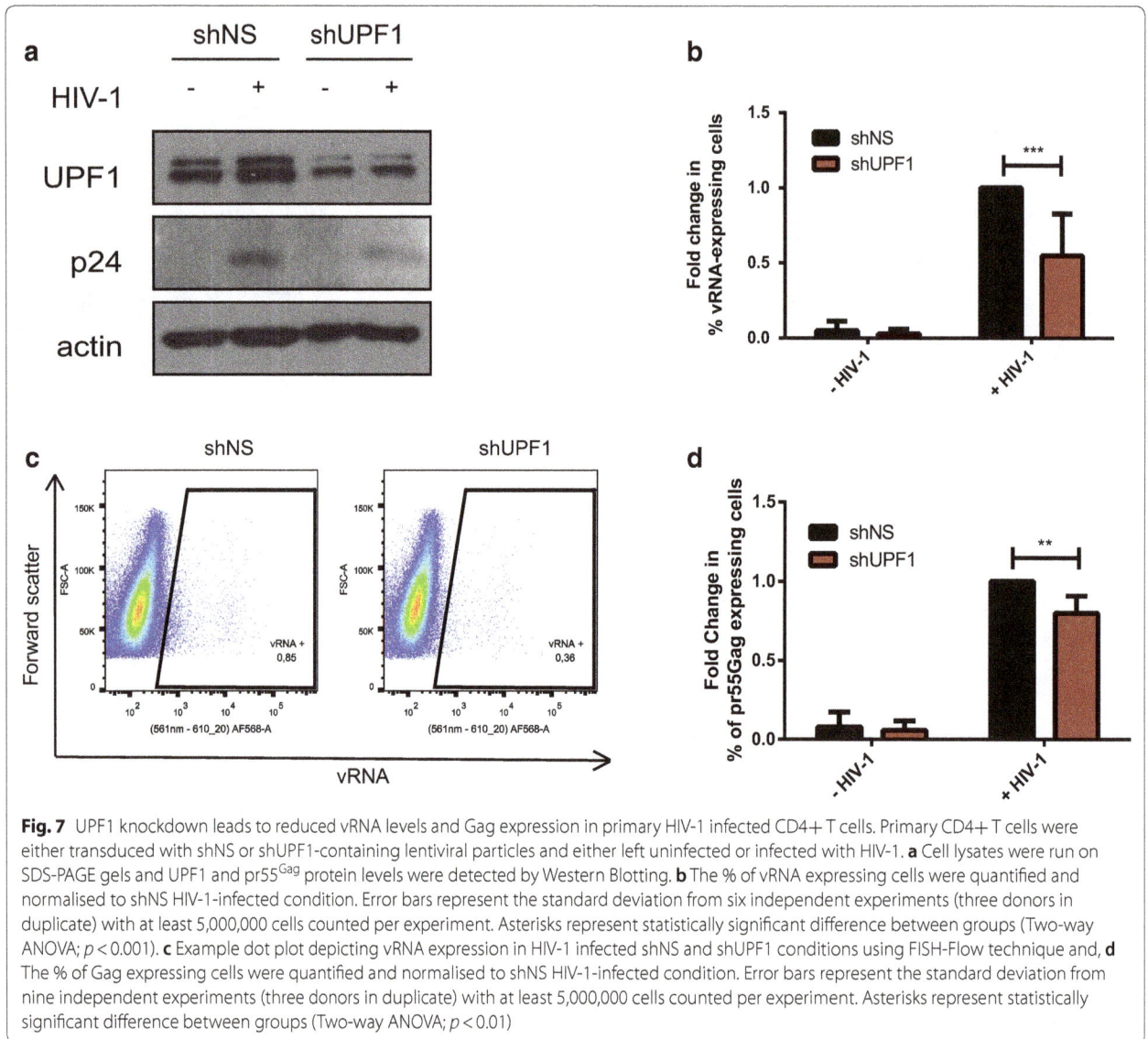

Fig. 7 UPF1 knockdown leads to reduced vRNA levels and Gag expression in primary HIV-1 infected CD4+ T cells. Primary CD4+ T cells were either transduced with shNS or shUPF1-containing lentiviral particles and either left uninfected or infected with HIV-1. **a** Cell lysates were run on SDS-PAGE gels and UPF1 and pr55^{Gag} protein levels were detected by Western Blotting. **b** The % of vRNA expressing cells were quantified and normalised to shNS HIV-1-infected condition. Error bars represent the standard deviation from six independent experiments (three donors in duplicate) with at least 5,000,000 cells counted per experiment. Asterisks represent statistically significant difference between groups (Two-way ANOVA; $p < 0.001$). **c** Example dot plot depicting vRNA expression in HIV-1 infected shNS and shUPF1 conditions using FISH-Flow technique and, **d** The % of Gag expressing cells were quantified and normalised to shNS HIV-1-infected condition. Error bars represent the standard deviation from nine independent experiments (three donors in duplicate) with at least 5,000,000 cells counted per experiment. Asterisks represent statistically significant difference between groups (Two-way ANOVA; $p < 0.01$)

and intracellular pr55^{Gag} levels. Cell lysates were also subjected to Western blotting to validate UPF1 knockdown (Fig. 7a). In humans, UPF1 has two isoforms and both isoforms are detected in primary CD4+ T cells [90] (Additional file 1: Figure S5A). However, in J-Lat cells, only the larger one is expressed at high enough levels to be detected by the UPF1 antibody (Additional file 1: Figure S5A). shUPF1 treatment in primary T cells resulted in a 53.8 (± 4.5)% decrease in UPF1 protein levels as compared to the shNS-treated cells (Additional file 1: Figure S5B). Results from three independent donors demonstrated that a knockdown of UPF1 resulted in a 45.16 (± 27.9)% decrease in vRNA levels as compared to the mock treated cells (Fig. 7b, c). This also corresponded with 20.1 (± 10.9)% reduced intracellular pr55^{Gag} staining

(Fig. 7d). Therefore, UPF1 also enhances vRNA levels and promotes viral gene expression in primary CD4+ T cells.

Discussion

The 'active viral reservoir' has been defined as the HIV-1 infected cells that contain viral RNA species but do not produce infectious viral particles [59, 60] and this highlights the post-transcriptional maintenance of HIV-1 latency. Latently-infected resting CD4+ cells T cells have been demonstrated to contain cell-associated unspliced and multiply spliced HIV-1 RNA [11, 61]. In these cells, the vRNA was sequestered within the nucleus and could be efficiently rescued through the overexpression of the host protein polypyrimidine tract binding protein (PTB), suggesting that latency can be reversed at a post-transcriptional level [61]. Two characterised primary T cell models of latency have also demonstrated a post-transcriptional block to HIV-1 reactivation, either by sequestration of the vRNA in the nucleus or splicing defects [14, 16, 62]. In addition, microRNAs have been implicated in the maintenance of HIV-1 latency (reviewed in [18]), providing another example of how post-transcriptional events can affect proviral reactivation. In the quest for an HIV-1 cure, the importance of investigating the contribution of post-transcriptional events and vRNA metabolism in the maintenance of HIV-1 latency is being recognised [63–65]. One HIV-1 cure strategy is the 'shock and kill' approach which involves reactivating the latent provirus by small molecules (shock) and then to eliminating the virus (kill) using intensive cART and/or immunomodulators [66]. Numerous compounds are under investigation as candidates for latency-reversing agents (LRAs) which promote the transcription of the provirus (reviewed in [67, 68]). So far, the use of LRAs have limited ability to decrease the size of the viral reservoir, with only two reports of successful reduction in reservoir size [7, 69, 70]. The shortcomings of current LRAs is highlighted in a recent study using FISH-Flow in which CD4+ T cells from HIV-1 infected patients were reactivated with the LRAs romidepsin or PMA/ionomycin and only 2–10% of cells that expressed vRNA produced viral proteins [17]. Therefore, the LRAs might be more effective if used in combination with drugs that affect vRNA metabolism at a post-transcriptional level. By modulating the activities of the RNA surveillance proteins or creating small molecules that mimic their activity, we can increase the stability of the vRNA to facilitate reactivation of these latent cells so that they are visible to the immune system and can be targeted by host immune responses and antiretrovirals. Alternatively, we can also apply this study to create novel long-lasting antiretrovirals by designing small molecules to inhibit the binding of UPF1 to vRNA thereby decreasing vRNA stability and reducing viral production.

Using FISH-Flow, this study demonstrates that the RNA surveillance proteins UPF1, SMG6 and UPF2 can affect HIV-1 gene expression, and thus viral reactivation at a post-transcriptional level. Although the effects of UPF1, UPF2 and SMG6 overexpression on modulating viral latency are modest (Figs. 3b, 4a and 5a), these effects nevertheless provide novel evidence of the contribution of post-transcriptional events in viral reactivation from latency. UPF1 was demonstrated to be a positive regulator of viral reactivation in the J-Lat 10.6 latent T cell model. Notably, we also demonstrate a direct effect of UPF1 on enhancing vRNA levels and viral gene expression in primary CD4+ T cells. The overexpression of the ATPase mutant of UPF1 (FLAG-DE-UPF1) did not lead

to enhanced reactivation of HIV-1 in J-Lat cells (Fig. 3g, h), indicating that the ATPase activity is responsible for enhanced vRNA expression and viral reactivation. This is in concordance with our previous work where we showed that this UPF1 construct was unable to upregulate vRNA levels and enhance vRNA stability [36]. This ATPase mutant has impaired RNA-binding capacity [71]. To exert its positive effects on vRNA metabolism, UPF1 needs to be able to bind to the vRNA and subsequently lead to the assembly of distinct RNPs that promote vRNA stability, export and translation [37]. An impairment of RNA binding capability could lead to a dissociation of UPF1 from the vRNA, thereby providing another possible explanation why no enhanced viral reactivation was observed when the ATPase mutant of UPF1 was used.

The HIV-1 vRNA metabolism is controlled by numerous cis-acting RNA sequences [72], such as the cis-repressive sequences or instability sequences (INS) [73]. UPF1 contains two zinc fingers that have been implicated to bind to INSs [74] and thus, could promote vRNA stability. The FLAG-UPF1-Δ20-150 construct contains a deletion in the zinc finger motif [36] that could lead to impaired binding to the HIV-1 INS. In agreement with our previous studies where we demonstrate that an overexpression of FLAG-UPF1-Δ20-150 does not lead to enhanced vRNA expression levels [36]; here we demonstrated that, in the context of reversal from viral latency, an overexpression of FLAG-UPF1-Δ20-150 does not lead to enhanced proviral reactivation (Fig. 3g, h), most likely due to impaired binding of UPF1 to the vRNA due to the loss of a zinc finger motif.

We have also previously shown that UPF2 is excluded from HIV-1 RNPs through antagonistic interactions with the viral or host proteins such as Rev or Staufen1 [37]. The binding of UPF2 to UPF1 has been reported to induce a conformational change in UPF1 that stimulates its RNA helicase activity and dampens its RNA binding capability, thereby hampering its binding to the vRNA [75, 76]. UPF2 also binds to UPF1 with high affinity [77] and this could limit the availability of UPF1 to bind to the vRNA. Our data reinforce the hypothesis that UPF2 is detrimental to vRNA metabolism, as we observed that overexpression of UPF2 resulted in reduced vRNA expression and viral reactivation (Fig. 4a–e). This deleterious effect is likely a result UPF2 binding to UPF1 and its sequestration, since viral reactivation was restored to levels similar to control cells when the UPF2 mutant deficient in UPF1 binding was used (Fig. 4f–h). In accordance with our work, a previous report using an shRNA library in J-Lat 5A8 cells showed that shRNAs against UPF1 were disenriched in the reactivated population as compared to the latent population, indicating that it exerts a positive effect on the reactivation of the HIV-1 provirus

[78]; whereas shRNAs against UPF2 were enriched in the reactivated population, indicating that UPF2 promotes that maintenance of latency in J-Lat cells [78].

SMG6 is the endonuclease responsible for cleaving mRNAs that are targeted for NMD [52, 53]. Both SMG6 and UPF1 have been reported to be present at transcription sites [79] and SMG6 interacts with UPF1 in a phospho-dependent [55] and a phospho-independent manner [90]. Furthermore, because of its endonuclease activity, SMG6 could have a direct effect on UPF1-bound mRNA levels, such as the vRNA. Our observation that an overexpression of SMG6 results in a decrease of vRNA expression and, consequently, decreased viral reactivation, suggests that SMG6 is detrimental to vRNA stability (Fig. 5a–g). Using mutational studies, we identified that the binding of SMG6 via its 14-3-3 like domain to phosphorylated UPF1 as well its endonuclease activity via its PIN region is necessary to downregulate the viral reactivation (Fig. 5f, g).

Recent transcriptome analyses have demonstrated that UPF1 binds promiscuously to all cellular RNAs; both, canonically identified NMD targets as well as to non-NMD targets and long non-coding RNAs [39, 80–83]. The marker for a cellular NMD target has been revealed to be the RNA's binding to phosphorylated UPF1 [19, 84]. UPF1 interacts with the PIK-related protein kinase SMG1, SMG8, SMG9, and the two translation termination factors eRF1 and eRF3 to form a decay inducing complex called the SURF [85, 86]. The phosphorylation of UPF1 by SMG1 is necessary for mRNA decay and creates an N-terminal binding platform for SMG6 that cleaves the targeted mRNAs [52, 53, 55]. Hyperphosphorylated UPF1 has been also shown to attract downstream NMD machinery with higher affinity [87]. Therefore, we can speculate that in the context of the interaction between UPF1 and the vRNA, the hyperphosphorylation of UPF1 would be detrimental to vRNA stability due to increased recruitment of SMG6 and other mRNA decay factors. The ATP deficient UPF1 mutant FLAG-UPF1-DE has also been demonstrated to be hyperphosphorylated and assembles complexes with SMG6 on both target and non-target mRNAs [83]. This could provide another possible explanation why the overexpression of the ATPase defective UPF1 did not result in enhanced viral reactivation (Fig. 3g, h). Further investigation is required to elucidate the roles of the phosphorylation status of UPF1 on proviral reactivation.

Conclusion

In this manuscript, we provide evidence that the RNA surveillance proteins UPF1, UPF2 and SMG6 can affect vRNA expression and thus, the maintenance of HIV-1 latency. These findings can be applied to bolster the reactivation of the HIV-1 provirus to effectively decrease the size of the viral reservoir using a shock and kill approach or can be harnessed to create a novel set of antiretrovirals.

Methods

Cell culture

J-Lat 10.6 cells (J-Lat full-length clone 10.6; NIH AIDS Reagent Program) are a Jurkat derived T cell line that is latently infected with HIV-1 in which the *nef* sequence was replaced with a green fluorescent protein (GFP) coding sequence [88]. J-Lat latent proviruses were reactivated by adding 20 ng/mL of phorbol 12-myristate 13-acetate (PMA) (Sigma-Aldrich) to the culture media for 24 h. In case of reactivation with TNFα, 10 ng/ml TNFα (Sigma-Aldrich) was added to the culture media for 24 h. Reactivation of cells was quantified by measuring GFP expression by flow cytometry. All cell cultures were maintained in RPMI 1640 (Life Technologies) supplemented with 10% fetal bovine serum (Hyclone) and 1% penicillin/streptomycin (Life Technologies) at 37 °C and 5% CO_2. HEK293T cells were purchased from the American Type Culture Collection (ATCC). TZM-bl HeLa cell line was obtained from NIH AIDS Reference and Reagent Program. Both of these cells lines were grown in Dulbecco's modified Eagle medium (DMEM, Invitrogen) containing 10% fetal bovine serum (HyClone) and 1% penicillin–streptomycin (Invitrogen). PBMCs were isolated from leukophoresed blood collected from healthy donors. All subjects provided informed consent for participating in this study. The research ethics boards of the recruiting sites, the Centre Hospitalier de l'Universite de Montreal and McGill University Health Centre approved this study. PBMCs were isolated by density-gradient centrifugation using lymphocyte separation medium (Corning). CD4+ T cells were negatively selected using the EasySep human T cell enrichment kit according to manufacturer's protocol (StemCell). Negatively selected CD4+ T cells were maintained in RPMI 1640 (Life Technologies) supplemented with 10% fetal bovine serum (Hyclone) and IL-2 (Sigma-Aldrich). CD4+ T cells were activated by treating them with 10ug/ml PHA (Sigma-Aldrich) for 72 h.

Antibodies

Mouse anti-p24 was obtained from NIH AIDS Reagents Program; rabbit antisera to UPF1 and UPF2 were generously supplied by Jens Lykke-Andersen (University of California, San Diego, CA, USA); rabbit anti-EST1A (SMG6) and mouse anti-actin were purchased from Abcam; rabbit anti-FLAG was purchased from

Sigma-Aldrich; mouse anti-HA was purchased from Roche; mouse anti-GAPDH was purchased from Techniscience; mouse anti-nucleolin was purchased from Santa-Cruz Biochemistry; KC57-FITC was purchased from Beckman Coulter; horseradish peroxidase-conjugated secondary antibodies were purchased from Rockland Immunochemicals.

Plasmids

The plasmids pCI-FLAG, FLAG-UPF1, FLAG-UPF1-Δ20-150, FLAG-UPF1-1-1074, FLAG-UPF1-RR857AA, FLAG-UPF1-LECY, FLAG-UPF1-DE, FLAG-UPF2 and FLAG-UPF2-1-1096 were described previously [36, 37, 89]. HA-SMG6, HA-SMG6-mEBM, HA-SMG6-m14-3-3 and HA-SMG6-mPIN were a kind gift from Dr. Oliver Muhlemann and are previously described [90]. pNL4.3 was obtained from NIH AIDS Reagents Program.

Gene silencing

Custom siRNA duplexes were synthesised by Qiagen. The target sequence for UPF1 was 5′-AAGATGCAGTTC CGCTCCATT-3′ and for SMG6 was 5′-GCTGCAGGT TACTTACAAG-3′. The siNS used in this study is a commercially available non-silencing control duplex with target sequence 5′-AATTCTCCGAACGTGTCACGT′-3′.

Transfections

J-Lat or Jurkat T cells were transfected with either 1 µg of plasmid DNA or 20 nM of siRNA per 1×10^6 cells using the Neon Transfection System (Thermo Fisher Scientific) according to manufacturer's protocols using the following electroporation parameters: three pulses of 1350 V and 10 ms at a cell density of 1×10^7/mL. J-Lat cells were reactivated 24 h after transfection. HEK293T cells were transfected using JetPrime transfection reagent according to manufacturer's protocol using 1ul of Jetprime (Polyplus) for 1ug of plasmid DNA.

Viral transduction

psPAX2, pMD2.G and the pLKO-shNS lentiviral control plasmid containing scrambled non-target shRNA used as a negative control were kind gifts from Dr. Marc Fabian (McGill University). pLKO-shUPF1 (TRCN0000022254) expression vector containing shRNA to UPF1 was obtained from the McGill genetic perturbation service. HEK293T cells were plated in 10 cm-dishes plates and were co-transfected with either shNS or shUPF1 expressing lentivirus, psPAX2 and pMD2.G. Supernatants were collected 48 h post-transfection, passed through a 0.45-µm filter (Pall) and supplemented with 5 µg/ml polybrene

(Sigma-Aldrich). The viral particles were added to the primary CD4+ T cells (1 ml of supernatant per 10,000,000 cells) and incubated for 16 h, following which they were infected with HIV-1.

HIV-1 virus production and infection

NL4.3 virus particles were prepared by transfection of HEK293T cells with HIV-1 NL4-3 provirus-encoding plasmid pNL4.3 using the JetPrime transfection reagent. The supernatants were collected 48 h post transfection, filtered through a 0.45-µm filter (Pall) and centrifuged at 20,000 r.p.m. for 1 h at 4 °C to pellet the virus. Viruses were resuspended in RPMI and stored at −80 °C. The multiplicity of infection (MOI) of viruses were quantified using the X-gal staining assay in TZM-bl cells as described in [91]. CD4+ T cells in RPMI were infected with an MOI of 0.5 NL4.3 viruses by spinoculation at 1800 r.p.m. for 45 min. Following spinoculation, the cells were washed and replenished with complete culture media. Cells were collected 6 days post infection.

Western blotting

Cells were lysed in NP40 lysis buffer (50 mM Tris pH 7.4, 150 mM NaCl, 0.5 mM EDTA, 0.5% NP40). Protein concentration on each cell lysate was quantified by Bradford assay. Equal amounts of protein (20 µg) were separated by SDS-PAGE and transferred to a nitrocellulose membrane (Bio-Rad). Blocking was performed using 5% non-fat milk in Tris-buffered saline (pH 7.4) with 0.1% Tween 20 (TBST) for 1 h at room temperature. Membranes were probed with the indicated primary and corresponding horseradish peroxidase-conjugated secondary antibodies. Proteins were detected using Western Lightning Plus-ECL (PerkinElmer). Signal intensities were scanned by densitometry using ImageJ software (NIH, Bethseda, USA).

FISH-flow

Cells were collected, fixed, permeabilized and subjected to the PrimeFlow RNA assay (Thermo Fisher Scientific) following the manufacturer's instructions and as described in [42, 92]. For intracellular pr55^{Gag} staining in primary CD4+ T cells, KC57-FITC antibody (Beckman Coulter) was used in permeabilisation buffer from the kit at a dilution of 1:50 for 30 min at room temperature, followed by 30 min at 4 °C. For all samples, mRNA was labelled with a set of 40 probe pairs diluted 1:20 in diluent provided in the kit and hybridized to the target mRNA for 2 h at 40 °C. The probes for GagPol, UPF1, UPF2 and SMG6 used had the following catalog numbers: GagPol HIV-1 VF10-10884, UPF1 VA1-3004200, UPF2 VA1-3007897 and SMG6 VA1-3001031. Positive control probes against the house-keeping gene RPL13A (VA1-13100) were included in each experiment. Samples were washed to remove excess probes and stored overnight in the presence of RNAsin. Signal amplification was then performed by sequential 1.5 h, 40 °C incubations with the pre-amplification and amplification mix. Amplified mRNA was labelled with fluorescently-tagged probes for 1 h at 40 °C. Gates were set on the uninfected Jurkat cells, unstimulated J-Lat control or uninfected primary CD4+ T cells where appropriate. Samples were acquired on a BD LSR Fortessa Analyzer. Analysis was performed using the FlowJo V10 software (Treestar).

Confocal microscopy following FISH-flow

Cells that underwent the FISH-Flow assay described above were seeded on 18 mm diameter coverslips and air dried. Coverslips were mounted in ProLong Gold Antifade Reagent with DAPI (Life Technologies). Laser scanning confocal microscopy was performed on a Leica DM16000B microscope equipped with a WaveFX spinning disk confocal head (Quorum Technologies) using a 63X objective lens. Images were acquired with a Hamamatsu ImageEM EM-charges coupled device (CCD) camera and image reconstruction was performed with the Imaris software (v. 8.4.1, Bitplane, Inc.).

RT-qPCR

For data presented in Fig. 2e, total RNA was extracted from cells using Aurum Total RNA Mini kits (Bio-Rad). RT-qPCR analysis of HIV-1 RNA levels was performed as previously described [93, 94]. For data presented in Additional file 1: Figure S2E and Additional file 1: Figure S3B, cellular fractionation was performed as described in [95]. RNA extraction from each fraction were performed using Trizol Reagent (Thermo Fisher Scientific) following manufacturer's instructions. cDNA was obtained using the High-Capacity cDNA Reverse Transcription Kit (Applied Biosystems). cDNA and primers were then added to GoTaq Green Master Mix (Promega). GAPDH was amplified using the primers GAPDH_1 forward 5′-TGA CCACAGTCCATGCCATC-3′ and GAPDH_1 reverse 5′-ATGATGTTCTGGAGAGCCCC-3′ and HIV-1 vRNA using the primers pNL4-3_1 forward 5′-GGGAGCTAG AACGATTCGCA-3′ and pNL4-3_1 reverse 5′-GGA TGGTTGTAGCTGTCCCA-3′. The PCR products were visualised in a 1% agarose gel by staining the DNA with RedSafe Nucleic Acid Staining Solution (iNtRON). Signals were captured using a Gel Doc System and intensities were normalised to the GAPDH signal.

Statistical analysis

All experiments were performed in triplicate, and the data are presented as the mean ± standard deviation (SD). A p value of < 0.05 in a student's t-test, one-way or two-way ANOVA test was considered statistically significant. GraphPad Prism 6 (Graphpad Software Inc.) was used to conduct statistical analyses and create graphs.

Additional file

Additional file 1: Figure S1. A J-Lat cells were treated with TNF-alpha or different concentrations of PMA and the % of GFP positive cells were measured. Example dot plot depicting **B** UPF1 mRNA, **C** UPF2 mRNA and **D** SMG6 mRNA expression in mock transfected cells with and without PMA addition using FISH-Flow technique. **Figure S2.** J-Lat 10.6 cells were either transfected with siNS or siUPF1 and were uninduced (DMSO) or reactivated (PMA). **A** Quantification of UPF1 protein expression by densitometry analysis of Western blots. **B** MFI of the vRNA signal were quantified. Asterisks represent statistically significant difference between groups (student's t-test; $p < 0.05$). **C** The % of RPL13A mRNA expressing cells were quantified. **D** MFI of the PRL13A signal were quantified. **E** Relative GAPDH mRNA levels as measured by RT-PCR. For all graphs, error bars represent the standard deviation from three independent experiments. **Figure S3. A** Cellular fractionation was performed in siNS or siUPF1 treated conditions, with and without PMA treatment. The fractions were run on SDS-PAGE gels and GAPDH and nucleolin protein levels were detected by Western Blotting to confirm fractionation. **B** The relative amounts of vRNA in each fraction were quantified by RT-PCR and normalised to levels of GAPDH mRNA. Error bars represent the standard deviation from three independent experiments. **C** J-Lat cells were mock transfected, transfected with FLAG-UPF1, FLAG-UPF2 or HA-SMG6 and reactivated with PMA. The % of vRNA+/GFP-cells was quantified. Error bars represent the standard deviation from three independent experiments. **Figure S4. A** J-Lat cells were mock transfected, transfected with FLAG-UPF1 or with FLAG-UPF1 mutants and reactivated with PMA. Reactivation in the above conditions was quantified and the percentages of reactivation were normalised to the Mock PMA reactivated condition. Error bars represent the standard deviation from three independent experiments with at least 10000 cells counted per treatment. Asterisks represent statistically significant difference between groups. **B** J-Lat cells were mock transfected, transfected with FLAG-UPF1, FLAG-UPF2 or HA-SMG6 and reactivated with TNF-alpha. Reactivation in the above conditions was quantified and the percentages of reactivation were normalised to the Mock PMA reactivated condition. Error bars represent the standard deviation from three independent experiments with at least 10000 cells counted per treatment. **Figure S5. A** Equal amounts of cell lysates from J-Lat 10.6 and primary CD4+ T cells were subjected to Western blotting and probed for UPF1 and actin. **B** Primary CD4+ T cells were either transduced with shNS or shUPF1-containing lentiviral particles and either left uninfected or infected with HIV-1. Quantification of UPF1 protein expression by densitometry analysis of Western blots.

Authors' contributions

SR, RA and AJM conceived of the study and designed experiments. SR conducted most of the experiments with significant contribution from RA. MN and AT provided technical help and comments on experimental design. SR drafted the manuscript with the support and comments from RA and AJM. All authors read and approved the final manuscript.

Author details

[1] HIV-1 RNA Trafficking Laboratory, Lady Davis Institute at the Jewish General Hospital, Montreal, QC H3T 1E2, Canada. [2] Department of Microbiology and Immunology, McGill University, Montreal, QC H3A 2B4, Canada. [3] Department of Medicine, McGill University, Montreal, QC H3A 0G4, Canada.

Acknowledgements

We thank the late Mark Wainberg, Andreas Kulozik, Niels Gehring, Jens Lykke-Andersen, Oliver Muehlemann, Mark Fabian, blood donors, Jean-Pierre Routy, Mario Legault and the Réseau SIDA et maladie infectieuses of the Fonds de recherche Santé-Québec for generous provision of cells and reagents; Niels Gehring and Nada Hafez for helpful discussions; Daniel Kaufmann, Alan Cochrane, Amy Baxter and Lewis Liu for assay development; Christian Young for technical assistance; and Alessandro Cinti for critical reading of the manuscript.

Competing interests

The authors declare that they have no competing interests.

Funding

This study, S.R. and R.A. were supported by The Canadian HIV Cure Enterprise Team Grant HIG-133050 (to A.J.M.) from the Canadian Institutes of Health Research (CIHR) in partnership with Canadian Foundation for HIV-1/AIDS Research and International AIDS Society and from the Lady Davis Research Institute/Jewish General Hospital. R.A. was funded in part by a Conselho Nacional de Desenvolvimento Científico e Tecnológico Fellowship (Brazil). M.N. was supported by a generous contribution to this project from the Lady Davis Institute/Jewish General Hospital. The funders had no role in study design, data collection and interpretation, or the decision to submit the work for publication.

References

1. Antiretroviral Therapy Cohort C. Life expectancy of individuals on combination antiretroviral therapy in high-income countries: a collaborative analysis of 14 cohort studies. Lancet. 2008;372:293–9.
2. Hoffmann C, Rockstroh JK. HIV 2015/16. Hamburg: Medizin Fokus Verlag; 2015.
3. Al-Dakkak I, Patel S, McCann E, Gadkari A, Prajapati G, Maiese EM. The impact of specific HIV treatment-related adverse events on adherence to antiretroviral therapy: a systematic review and meta-analysis. AIDS Care. 2013;25:400–14.
4. Nakagawa F, Miners A, Smith CJ, Simmons R, Lodwick RK, Cambiano V, Lundgren JD, Delpech V, Phillips AN. Projected lifetime healthcare costs associated with HIV infection. PLoS ONE. 2015;10:e0125018.
5. Chun TW, Moir S, Fauci AS. HIV reservoirs as obstacles and opportunities for an HIV cure. Nat Immunol. 2015;16:584–9.
6. Ruelas DS, Greene WC. An integrated overview of HIV-1 latency. Cell. 2013;155:519–29.
7. Martin AR, Siliciano RF. Progress toward HIV eradication: case reports, current efforts, and the challenges associated with cure. Annu Rev Med. 2016;67:215–28.
8. Chun TW, Finzi D, Margolick J, Chadwick K, Schwartz D, Siliciano RF. In vivo fate of HIV-1-infected T cells: quantitative analysis of the transition to stable latency. Nat Med. 1995;1:1284–90.
9. Mbonye U, Karn J. Transcriptional control of HIV latency: cellular signaling pathways, epigenetics, happenstance and the hope for a cure. Virology. 2014;454–455:328–39.
10. Cary DC, Fujinaga K, Peterlin BM. Molecular mechanisms of HIV latency. J Clin Invest. 2016;126:448–54.
11. Chun TW, Justement JS, Lempicki RA, Yang J, Dennis G Jr, Hallahan CW, Sanford C, Pandya P, Liu S, McLaughlin M, et al. Gene expression and viral prodution in latently infected, resting CD4+ T cells in viremic versus aviremic HIV-infected individuals. Proc Natl Acad Sci USA. 2003;100:1908–13.
12. Sarracino A, Marcello A. The relevance of post-transcriptional mechanisms in HIV latency reversal. Curr Pharm Des. 2017;23:4103–11.
13. Lassen KG, Ramyar KX, Bailey JR, Zhou Y, Siliciano RF. Nuclear retention of multiply spliced HIV-1 RNA in resting CD4+ T cells. PLoS Pathog. 2006;2:e68.
14. Swiggard WJ, Baytop C, Yu JJ, Dai J, Li C, Schretzenmair R, Theodosopoulos T, O'Doherty U. Human immunodeficiency virus type 1 can establish latent infection in resting CD4+ T cells in the absence of activating stimuli. J Virol. 2005;79:14179–88.
15. Saleh S, Solomon A, Wightman F, Xhilaga M, Cameron PU, Lewin SR. CCR7 ligands CCL19 and CCL21 increase permissiveness of resting memory CD4+ T cells to HIV-1 infection: a novel model of HIV-1 latency. Blood. 2007;110:4161–4.
16. Saleh S, Wightman F, Ramanayake S, Alexander M, Kumar N, Khoury G, Pereira C, Purcell D, Cameron PU, Lewin SR. Expression and reactivation of HIV in a chemokine induced model of HIV latency in primary resting CD4+ T cells. Retrovirology. 2011;8:80.
17. Grau-Expósito J, Serra-Peinado C, Miguel L, Navarro J, Curran A, Burgos J, Ocaña I, Ribera E, Torrella A, Planas B, et al. A novel single-cell fish-flow assay identifies effector memory CD4+ T cells as a major niche for HIV-1 transcription in HIV-infected patients. MBio. 2017. https://doi.org/10.1128/mBio.00876-17.
18. Sun B, Yang R, Mallardo M. Roles of microRNAs in HIV-1 replication and latency. Microrna. 2016;5:120–3.
19. Kurosaki T, Maquat LE. Nonsense-mediated mRNA decay in humans at a glance. J Cell Sci. 2016;129:461–7.
20. Bhattacharya A, Czaplinski K, Trifillis P, He F, Jacobson A, Peltz SW. Characterization of the biochemical properties of the human Upf1 gene product that is involved in nonsense-mediated mRNA decay. RNA. 2000;6:1226–35.
21. Chawla R, Redon S, Raftopoulou C, Wischnewski H, Gagos S, Azzalin CM. Human UPF1 interacts with TPP1 and telomerase and sustains telomere leading-strand replication. EMBO J. 2011;30:4047–58.
22. Azzalin CM, Lingner J. The human RNA surveillance factor UPF1 is required for S phase progression and genome stability. Curr Biol. 2006;16:433–9.
23. Kim YK, Furic L, Desgroseillers L, Maquat LE. Mammalian Staufen1 recruits Upf1 to specific mRNA 3'UTRs so as to elicit mRNA decay. Cell. 2005;120:195–208.
24. Ciaudo C, Bourdet A, Cohen-Tannoudji M, Dietz HC, Rougeulle C, Avner P. Nuclear mRNA degradation pathway(s) are implicated in Xist regulation and X chromosome inactivation. PLoS Genet. 2006;2:e94.
25. Maekawa S, Imamachi N, Irie T, Tani H, Matsumoto K, Mizutani R, Imamura K, Kakeda M, Yada T, Sugano S, et al. Analysis of RNA decay factor mediated RNA stability contributions on RNA abundance. BMC Genom. 2015;16:154.
26. Isken O, Maquat LE. The multiple lives of NMD factors: balancing roles in gene and genome regulation. Nat Rev Genet. 2008;9:699–712.
27. Fatscher T, Boehm V, Gehring NH. Mechanism, factors, and physiological role of nonsense-mediated mRNA decay. Cell Mol Life Sci. 2015;72:4523–44.
28. Nickless A, Bailis JM, You Z. Control of gene expression through the nonsense-mediated RNA decay pathway. Cell Biosci. 2017;7:26.
29. McIlwain DR, Pan Q, Reilly PT, Elia AJ, McCracken S, Wakeham AC, Itie-Youten A, Blencowe BJ, Mak TW. Smg1 is required for embryogenesis and regulates diverse genes via alternative splicing coupled to nonsense-mediated mRNA decay. Proc Natl Acad Sci USA. 2010;107:12186–91.
30. Lykke-Andersen S, Jensen TH. Nonsense-mediated mRNA decay: an intricate machinery that shapes transcriptomes. Nat Rev Mol Cell Biol. 2015;16:665–77.
31. Kebaara BW, Atkin AL. Long 3'-UTRs target wild-type mRNAs for nonsense-mediated mRNA decay in Saccharomyces cerevisiae. Nucleic Acids Res. 2009;37:2771–8.
32. Balistreri G, Bognanni C, Muhlemann O. Virus escape and manipulation of cellular nonsense-mediated mRNA decay. Viruses. 2017;9:24.

33. Withers JB, Beemon KL. The structure and function of the rous sarcoma virus RNA stability element. J Cell Biochem. 2011;112:3085–92.

34. Mocquet V, Durand S, Jalinot P. How retroviruses escape the nonsense-mediated mRNA decay. AIDS Res Hum Retrovir. 2015;31:948–58.

35. Toro-Ascuy D, Rojas-Araya B, Valiente-Echeverria F, Soto-Rifo R. Interactions between the HIV-1 unspliced mRNA and host mRNA decay machineries. Viruses. 2016;8:320.

36. Ajamian L, Abrahamyan L, Milev M, Ivanov PV, Kulozik AE, Gehring NH, Mouland AJ. Unexpected roles for UPF1 in HIV-1 RNA metabolism and translation. RNA. 2008;14:914–27.

37. Ajamian L, Abel K, Rao S, Vyboh K, Garcia-de-Gracia F, Soto-Rifo R, Kulozik AE, Gehring NH, Mouland AJ. HIV-1 recruits UPF1 but excludes UPF2 to promote nucleocytoplasmic export of the genomic RNA. Biomolecules. 2015;5:2808–39.

38. Kula A, Guerra J, Knezevich A, Kleva D, Myers MP, Marcello A. Characterization of the HIV-1 RNA associated proteome identifies Matrin 3 as a nuclear cofactor of Rev function. Retrovirology. 2011;8:60.

39. Hogg JR, Goff SP. Upf1 senses 3'UTR length to potentiate mRNA decay. Cell. 2010;143:379–89.

40. Serquina AK, Das SR, Popova E, Ojelabi OA, Roy CK, Gottlinger HG. UPF1 is crucial for the infectivity of human immunodeficiency virus type 1 progeny virions. J Virol. 2013;87:8853–61.

41. Abrahamyan LG, Chatel-Chaix L, Ajamian L, Milev MP, Monette A, Clement JF, Song R, Lehmann M, DesGroseillers L, Laughrea M, et al. Novel Staufen1 ribonucleoproteins prevent formation of stress granules but favour encapsidation of HIV-1 genomic RNA. J Cell Sci. 2010;123:369–83.

42. Baxter AE, Niessl J, Fromentin R, Richard J, Porichis F, Charlebois R, Massanella M, Brassard N, Alsahafi N, Delgado GG, et al. Single-cell characterization of viral translation-competent reservoirs in HIV-infected individuals. Cell Host Microbe. 2016;20:368–80.

43. Martrus G, Niehrs A, Cornelis R, Rechtien A, Garcia-Beltran W, Lutgehetmann M, Hoffmann C, Altfeld M. Kinetics of HIV-1 latency reversal quantified on the single-cell level using a novel flow-based technique. J Virol. 2016;90:9018–28.

44. Baxter AE, Niessl J, Morou A, Kaufmann DE. RNA flow cytometric FISH for investigations into HIV immunology, vaccination and cure strategies. AIDS Res Ther. 2017;14:40.

45. Prasad VR, Kalpana GV. FISHing out the hidden enemy: advances in detecting and measuring latent HIV-infected cells. MBio. 2017;8:e01433.

46. Baxter AE, O'Doherty U, Kaufmann DE. Beyond the replication-competent HIV reservoir: transcription and translation-competent reservoirs. Retrovirology. 2018;15:18.

47. Planelles V, Wolschendorf F, Kutsch O. Facts and fiction: cellular models for high throughput screening for HIV-1 reactivating drugs. Curr HIV Res. 2011;9:568–78.

48. Spina CA, Anderson J, Archin NM, Bosque A, Chan J, Famiglietti M, Greene WC, Kashuba A, Lewin SR, Margolis DM, et al. An in-depth comparison of latent HIV-1 reactivation in multiple cell model systems and resting CD4+ T cells from aviremic patients. PLoS Pathog. 2013;9:e1003834.

49. Brogdon J, Ziani W, Wang X, Veazey RS, Xu H. In vitro effects of the small-molecule protein kinase C agonists on HIV latency reactivation. Sci Rep. 2016;6:39032.

50. Kadlec J, Guilligay D, Ravelli RB, Cusack S. Crystal structure of the UPF2-interacting domain of nonsense-mediated mRNA decay factor UPF1. RNA (New York, NY). 2006;12:1817–24.

51. Clerici M, Mourao A, Gutsche I, Gehring NH, Hentze MW, Kulozik A, Kadlec J, Sattler M, Cusack S. Unusual bipartite mode of interaction between the nonsense-mediated decay factors, UPF1 and UPF2. EMBO J. 2009;28:2293–306.

52. Eberle AB, Lykke-Andersen S, Muhlemann O, Jensen TH. SMG6 promotes endonucleolytic cleavage of nonsense mRNA in human cells. Nat Struct Mol Biol. 2009;16:49–55.

53. Huntzinger E, Kashima I, Fauser M, Sauliere J, Izaurralde E. SMG6 is the catalytic endonuclease that cleaves mRNAs containing nonsense codons in metazoan. RNA. 2008;14:2609–17.

54. Kashima I, Jonas S, Jayachandran U, Buchwald G, Conti E, Lupas AN, Izaurralde E. SMG6 interacts with the exon junction complex via two conserved EJC-binding motifs (EBMs) required for nonsense-mediated mRNA decay. Genes Dev. 2010;24:2440–50.

55. Okada-Katsuhata Y, Yamashita A, Kutsuzawa K, Izumi N, Hirahara F, Ohno S. N- and C-terminal Upf1 phosphorylations create binding platforms for SMG-6 and SMG-5:SMG-7 during NMD. Nucleic Acids Res. 2012;40:1251–66.

56. Glavan F, Behm-Ansmant I, Izaurralde E, Conti E. Structures of the PIN domains of SMG6 and SMG5 reveal a nuclease within the mRNA surveillance complex. EMBO J. 2006;25:5117–25.

57. Takeshita D, Zenno S, Lee WC, Saigo K, Tanokura M. Crystallization and preliminary X-ray analysis of the PIN domain of human EST1A. Acta Crystallogr, Sect F: Struct Biol Cryst Commun. 2006;62:656–8.

58. Takeshita D, Zenno S, Lee WC, Saigo K, Tanokura M. Crystal structure of the PIN domain of human telomerase-associated protein EST1A. Proteins. 2007;68:980–9.

59. Pasternak AO, Lukashov VV, Berkhout B. Cell-associated HIV RNA: a dynamic biomarker of viral persistence. Retrovirology. 2013;10:41.

60. Pasternak AO, Berkhout B. What do we measure when we measure cell-associated HIV RNA. Retrovirology. 2018;15:13.

61. Lassen KG, Bailey JR, Siliciano RF. Analysis of human immunodeficiency virus type 1 transcriptional elongation in resting CD4+ T cells in vivo. J Virol. 2004;78:9105–14.

62. Pace MJ, Graf EH, Agosto LM, Mexas AM, Male F, Brady T, Bushman FD, O'Doherty U. Directly infected resting CD4+ T cells can produce HIV Gag without spreading infection in a model of HIV latency. PLoS Pathog. 2012;8:e1002818.

63. Le Douce V, Janossy A, Hallay H, Ali S, Riclet R, Rohr O, Schwartz C. Achieving a cure for HIV infection: Do we have reasons to be optimistic? J Antimicrob Chemother. 2012;67:1063–74.

64. Deeks SG, Lewin SR, Ross AL, Ananworanich J, Benkirane M, Cannon P, Chomont N, Douek D, Lifson JD, Lo YR, et al. International AIDS society global scientific strategy: towards an HIV cure 2016. Nat Med. 2016;22:839–50.

65. Schwartz C, Bouchat S, Marban C, Gautier V, Van Lint C, Rohr O, Le Douce V. On the way to find a cure: purging latent HIV-1 reservoirs. BCP Biochem Pharmacol. 2017;146:10–22.

66. Deeks SG. HIV: shock and kill. Nature. 2012;487:439–40.

67. Delagreverie HM, Delaugerre C, Lewin SR, Deeks SG, Li JZ. Ongoing clinical trials of human immunodeficiency virus latency-reversing and immunomodulatory agents. Open Forum Infect Dis. 2016;3:ofw189.

68. Darcis G, Van Driessche B, Van Lint C. Preclinical shock strategies to reactivate latent HIV-1: an update. Curr Opin HIV AIDS. 2016;11:388–93.

69. Leth S, Schleimann MH, Nissen SK, Hojen JF, Olesen R, Graversen ME, Jorgensen S, Kjaer AS, Denton PW, Mork A, et al. Combined effect of Vacc-4x, recombinant human granulocyte macrophage colony-stimulating factor vaccination, and romidepsin on the HIV-1 reservoir (REDUC): a single-arm, phase 1B/2A trial. Lancet HIV. 2016;3:e463–72.

70. Guihot A, Marcelin AG, Massiani MA, Samri A, Soulie C, Autran B, Spano JP. Drastic decrease of the HIV reservoir in a patient treated with nivolumab for lung cancer. Ann Oncol. 2018;29:517–8.

71. Cheng Z, Muhlrad D, Lim MK, Parker R, Song H. Structural and functional insights into the human Upf1 helicase core. EMBO J. 2007;26:253–64.

72. Andrew JM, Eric AC, Luc D. Trafficking of HIV-1 RNA: recent progress involving host cell RNABinding proteins. Curr Genomics. 2003;4:237–51.

73. Schwartz S, Felber BK, Pavlakis GN. Distinct RNA sequences in the gag region of human immunodeficiency virus type 1 decrease RNA stability and inhibit expression in the absence of Rev protein. J Virol. 1992;66:150–9.

74. Applequist SE, Selg M, Raman C, Jack HM. Cloning and characterization of HUPF1, a human homolog of the Saccharomyces cerevisiae nonsense mRNA-reducing UPF1 protein. Nucleic Acids Res. 1997;25:814–21.

75. Chakrabarti S, Jayachandran U, Bonneau F, Fiorini F, Basquin C, Domcke S, Le Hir H, Conti E. Molecular mechanisms for the RNA-dependent ATPase activity of Upf1 and its regulation by Upf2. Mol Cell. 2011;41:693–703.

76. Chamieh H, Ballut L, Bonneau F, Le Hir H. NMD factors UPF2 and UPF3 bridge UPF1 to the exon junction complex and stimulate its RNA helicase activity. Nat Struct Mol Biol. 2008;15:85–93.

77. Ohnishi T, Yamashita A, Kashima I, Schell T, Anders KR, Grimson A, Hachiya T, Hentze MW, Anderson P, Ohno S. Phosphorylation of hUPF1 induces formation of mRNA surveillance complexes containing hSMG-5 and hSMG-7. Mol Cell. 2003;12:1187–200.

78. Besnard E, Hakre S, Kampmann M, Lim HW, Hosmane NN, Martin A, Bassik MC, Verschueren E, Battivelli E, Chan J, et al. The mTOR complex controls HIV latency. Cell Host Microbe. 2016;20:785–97.

79. de Turris V, Nicholson P, Orozco RZ, Singer RH, Muhlemann O. Cotranscriptional effect of a premature termination codon revealed by live-cell imaging. RNA. 2011;17:2094–107.

80. Hurt JA, Robertson AD, Burge CB. Global analyses of UPF1 binding and function reveal expanded scope of nonsense-mediated mRNA decay. Genome Res. 2013;23:1636–50.

81. Kurosaki T, Maquat LE. Rules that govern UPF1 binding to mRNA 3′ UTRs. Proc Natl Acad Sci USA. 2013;110:3357–62.

82. Zund D, Gruber AR, Zavolan M, Muhlemann O. Translation-dependent displacement of UPF1 from coding sequences causes its enrichment in 3′ UTRs. Nat Struct Mol Biol. 2013;20:936–43.

83. Lee SR, Pratt GA, Martinez FJ, Yeo GW, Lykke-Andersen J. Target discrimination in nonsense-mediated mRNA decay requires Upf1 ATPase activity. Mol Cell. 2015;59:413–25.

84. Kurosaki T, Li W, Hoque M, Popp MW, Ermolenko DN, Tian B, Maquat LE. A post-translational regulatory switch on UPF1 controls targeted mRNA degradation. Genes Dev. 2014;28:1900–16.

85. Kashima I, Yamashita A, Izumi N, Kataoka N, Morishita R, Hoshino S, Ohno M, Dreyfuss G, Ohno S. Binding of a novel SMG-1-Upf1-eRF1-eRF3 complex (SURF) to the exon junction complex triggers Upf1 phosphorylation and nonsense-mediated mRNA decay. Genes Dev. 2006;20:355–67.

86. Yamashita A, Izumi N, Kashima I, Ohnishi T, Saari B, Katsuhata Y, Muramatsu R, Morita T, Iwamatsu A, Hachiya T, et al. SMG-8 and SMG-9, two novel subunits of the SMG-1 complex, regulate remodeling of the mRNA surveillance complex during nonsense-mediated mRNA decay. Genes Dev. 2009;23:1091–105.

87. Durand S, Franks TM, Lykke-Andersen J. Hyperphosphorylation amplifies UPF1 activity to resolve stalls in nonsense-mediated mRNA decay. Nat Commun. 2016;7:12434.

88. Jordan A, Bisgrove D, Verdin E. HIV reproducibly establishes a latent infection after acute infection of T cells in vitro. EMBO J. 2003;22:1868–77.

89. Serin G, Gersappe A, Black JD, Aronoff R, Maquat LE. Identification and characterization of human orthologues to Saccharomyces cerevisiae Upf2 protein and Upf3 protein (Caenorhabditis elegans SMG-4). Mol Cell Biol. 2001;21:209–23.

90. Nicholson P, Josi C, Kurosawa H, Yamashita A, Muhlemann O. A novel phosphorylation-independent interaction between SMG6 and UPF1 is essential for human NMD. Nucleic Acids Res. 2014;42:9217–35.

91. Xing L, Wang S, Hu Q, Li J, Zeng Y. Comparison of three quantification methods for the TZM-bl pseudovirus assay for screening of anti-HIV-1 agents. J Virol Methods. 2016;233:56–61.

92. Baxter AE, Niessl J, Fromentin R, Richard J, Porichis F, Massanella M, Brassard N, Alsahafi N, Routy JP, Finzi A, et al. Multiparametric characterization of rare HIV-infected cells using an RNA-flow FISH technique. Nat Protoc. 2017;12:2029–49.

93. Wong R, Balachandran A, Mao AY, Dobson W, Gray-Owen S, Cochrane A. Differential effect of CLK SR Kinases on HIV-1 gene expression: potential novel targets for therapy. Retrovirology. 2011;8:47.

94. Duffy S, Cochrane A. Analysis of HIV-1 RNA Splicing. In: Alternative pre-mRNA splicing. Wiley-VCH Verlag GmbH & Co. KGaA; 2012. pp. 438–48.

95. Suzuki K, Bose P, Leong-Quong RY, Fujita DJ, Riabowol K. REAP: a two minute cell fractionation method. BMC Res Notes. 2010;3:294.

Broadly neutralizing antibodies: What is needed to move from a rare event in HIV-1 infection to vaccine efficacy?

Harini Subbaraman, Merle Schanz and Alexandra Trkola[*] ⓘ

Abstract

The elicitation of broadly neutralizing antibodies (bnAbs) is considered crucial for an effective, preventive HIV-1 vaccine. Led by the discovery of a new generation of potent bnAbs, the field has significantly advanced over the past decade. There is a wealth of knowledge about the development of bnAbs in natural infection, their specificity, potency, breadth and function. Yet, devising immunogens and vaccination regimens that evoke bnAb responses has not been successful. Where are the roadblocks in their development? What can we learn from natural infection, where bnAb induction is possible but rare? Herein, we will reflect on key discoveries and discuss open questions that may bear crucial insights needed to move towards creating effective bnAb vaccines.

Background

The potency of the neutralization response to HIV-1 has long been underappreciated, as most of the antibodies identified were type-specific or had only limited breadth [1]. This only changed in the early 2000s, with the discovery of the new classes of potent bnAbs [1, 2]. This positioned bnAb responses as the major goal of vaccine development and in prevention. Despite their potency and breadth, there is no evidence that bnAbs ameliorate disease progression in natural infection, as they are subject to viral escape like any autologous neutralization activity [3–6]. Application of bnAbs as a therapeutic vaccine in established infection is therefore limited to settings where activity over shorter intervals is required. This is similar to what has been discussed in treatment combinations that aim to eliminate the latent HIV-1 reservoir [7]. In prevention, where bnAbs are considered both as a passively administered drug and are intended to be elicited by vaccines, their potential is obvious and has been underscored by numerous animal studies [1, 2, 8]. The virus inoculum that needs to be combatted to prevent transmission is low [9]. bnAbs have a window of opportunity to prevent infection in the absence of an established cellular HIV reservoir and potentially in concert with effector functions of the immune system. However, challenges for the use of bnAbs for prevention remain high. Therapeutically, bnAbs could be selectively applied to patients harboring sensitive strains. In contrast, antibodies elicited by a vaccine and/or used in a prevention setting must be highly potent and have exceptional breadth, targeting a wide spectrum of globally circulating HIV-1 strains.

Discoveries in the last decade have revealed that such elite neutralizing responses occur during natural infection, but are rare [10–14]. Initial hopes that delineation of the epitopes of identified elite bnAbs would allow rapid construction of matching immunogens were not fulfilled. Reverse vaccinology and structure-guided immunogen design based on these elite bnAbs brought much momentum to the field. The most recently developed immunogens are the first that induce Tier-2 neutralizing activity, but none of them has evoked a bnAb response to date [15, 16]. Therefore, natural infection remains the only system in which we can decipher the parameters that drive the evolution of bnAbs. Herein, we review key observations made on the determinants of bnAb development by studying both individual bnAb donors and HIV-1 patient cohorts and mark open questions that need to be addressed.

*Correspondence: trkola.alexandra@virology.uzh.ch
Institute of Medical Virology, University of Zurich, Zurich, Switzerland

The complex interrelation of bnAb maturation and virus escape

Focused efforts to decipher antibody maturation pathways alongside virus evolution have facilitated reconstruction of bnAb development in some individuals [3, 4, 17–23]. It is generally appreciated that a complex interplay between escape virus and Ab response is needed to trigger bnAb evolution [22]. The role of virus diversification, including superinfection, which can precede the emergence of breadth, has been underscored in several studies [3, 5, 20, 22, 24–27]. Whether virus diversification is driving or is, in fact, a consequence of bnAb development remains difficult to dissect, as Env variability also increases in response to bnAb pressure [28–31]. This iterative and circular nature of virus and antibody co-evolution that occurs in natural infection will be difficult to mimic by vaccination. Deciphering cause and consequence, as well as defining minimal necessary components of bnAb development will be key for designing successful vaccine regimens.

Prolonged bnAb maturation does not necessarily lead to improved breadth. The highest frequency of bnAb activity is observed after approximately 3 years of infection [12, 14, 32–34]. However, further prolonged replication does not increase frequencies [12, 14, 32, 33] and can even lead to a decrease or loss of bnAb activity [20]. Hence, while a relatively long exposure to viral antigen is commonly needed in adult HIV-1 infection to mount bnAb responses, continued adaptation of early bnAbs can also lead to "off-track" antibodies that lack breadth but have increased autologous strain specificity [3, 17, 22, 35]. Likewise, continued somatic hypermutation (SHM) will always generate "dead-end" antibodies harboring mutations that impede further development of functional antibodies [3, 17, 36]. SHM observed in isolated bnAbs often includes mutations not required for breadth development [37]. Short bnAb maturation phases with targeted breadth evolution must therefore be an ultimate goal for vaccine design.

Virus escape creates new epitopes that allow bnAb responses to mature [5, 24]. Slow virus escape may be beneficial for bnAb development, as this prolongs exposure to the bnAb-sensitive epitope, thereby extending antigenic stimulation and increasing chances of bnAb maturation [38–40]. Along these lines, partial evasion of virus from bnAbs, as can occur during cell–cell transmission [38, 41–43], allows the bnAb-sensitive virus to persist, ensuring sustained epitope presentation to the maturing antibody.

The virus population is not only shaped by the bnAb lineage, but is also subject to pressure of the vigorous type-specific antibody response each patient mounts. This can, in turn, substantially impact bnAb evolution.

Early bnAb development may be compromised through competitive exclusion by strain-specific antibodies that target the same epitope [44, 45]. Yet, cooperation between different antibody lineages may also facilitate bnAb development by driving the virus into escape mutations that prevent full escape from bnAb lineages [18, 19, 40]. Antibody helper lineages can be strictly strain-specific [40] or mature into bnAbs [19]. Understanding whether the development of multiple bnAb lineages [5] and bnAb/helper [18] tandems are common or rare events will be essential to appreciate (1) their importance and (2) the need to incorporate similar help into vaccination strategies. Of note, recent reports have suggested that passively administered bnAbs may perform antibody helper functions. Therapeutic administration of the bnAb 3BNC117 to viremic individuals enhanced heterologous plasma neutralization breadth beyond escape to 3BNC117 [46]. Passive immunization of newborn macaques with nAbs at sub-neutralizing doses before oral SHIV challenge led to rapid elicitation of an autologous neutralization response and early control of viremia [47].

Factors that drive bnAb development

A range of factors that promote bnAb development has been implicated and several confirmed across different cohorts [6, 11, 12, 14, 32, 33, 48–50] (Tables 1, 2 and Fig. 1). These studies highlight that a combination of partly interdependent factors, which are linked with disease progression, direct bnAb development. Several prominent drivers of bnAb development are linked to persistent antigenic stimulation. The independent impact of viral load, infection length and diversity on bnAb frequency has been demonstrated [12, 14, 33, 48, 49]. These factors act in concert to ensure consistent antigenic stimulation. High viral load was the factor most consistently found to positively influence neutralization breadth across cohorts [6, 11, 12, 14, 32, 33, 48–51]. However, while rates of bnAb activity are significantly higher amongst individuals with high viral load, breadth can also develop in HIV-1 controllers, although commonly at lower frequency [11, 34, 39, 51–53]. Thus, high antigen loads promote bnAb evolution but are certainly not the sole driving force.

Two other parameters linked to extended antigenic stimulation, virus diversity and length of infection, also increase the likelihood of bnAb elicitation [11, 12, 14, 48, 49]. This highlights that exposure to antigen over prolonged periods of time aids bnAb evolution. Env diversification inevitably increases during protracted infection, which is mostly driven by the consecutive rounds of Ab maturation and virus escape. Env diversity must therefore be viewed as both cause and consequence of neutralizing

Table 1 Overview of patient cohort studies investigating viral and disease factors linked with bnAb development

Reference	Number of subjects[a]	Investigated viral and disease factors	Association with breadth	Additional information on investigated parameter
Doria-Rose et al. [11]	103	Viral load	Positive	Contemporaneous
		Infection duration	None	
		Transmission mode	None	
		CD4+ T cell levels	None	Contemporaneous
		History of ART use	None	
Euler et al. [6]	82	Viral load	Positive	Set point
		CD4+ T cell levels	Negative	Set point
		Disease progression	None	
Gray et al. [33]	40	Viral load	Positive	Set point
		CD4+ T cell levels	Negative	6 months post-infection
		CD4+ T cell decline	Positive	Difference between levels pre-infection and at 6 months
Landais et al. [14]	439	Viral load	Positive	Set point
		Infecting subtype	Positive	Subtype C infection
		Infection duration	Positive	
		Transmission mode	None	
		CD4+ T cell levels	Negative	All tested time points beyond 6 months post-infection
Mikkell et al. [32]	38	Viral load	Positive	Contemporaneous
Piantadosi et al. [48]	70	Viral load	Positive	Set point
		Viral diversity	Positive	Env
		CD4+ T cell levels	None	Contemporaneous
		Disease progression	None	
Rusert et al. [12]	4484	Viral load	Positive	Contemporaneous
		Viral diversity	Positive	Pol
		Infecting subtype	None	
		Infection duration	Positive	
		Transmission mode	Weakly positive	Modestly higher bnAb activity in IDUs
		CD4+ T cell levels	Weakly positive	Contemporaneous; modest association with cross-neutralization activity
Sather et al. [49]	39	Viral load	Positive	Average of all tested time points
		Infection duration	Positive	
		CD4+ T cell levels	None	Average of all tested time points
van Gils et al. [50]	35	Viral load	Positive	Set point
		CD4+ T cell levels	Negative	Set point

[a] Indicates total number of subjects included. Specific analyses may have been carried out on subsets of these numbers

antibody maturation. Emerging escape variants may generate new epitopes on Env that engage novel antibody germlines and start a bnAb lineage, as demonstrated for individual donors [5, 24]. The presence of multiple transmitted founder (T/F) viruses as reported for intravenous drug users (IDUs), as well as in superinfection, similarly expose the immune system to high Env diversity. In a recent large cohort study, IDUs showed modestly higher frequency of bnAb activity [12, 54]. Whether this is a result of higher diversity or other factors intrinsic to HIV infection of IDUs remains to be determined. Env diversity has been postulated as a driver of bnAb activity in cases of superinfection [3, 20, 25–27]. Nevertheless, superinfection does not guarantee the development of bnAb activity, as recent studies revealed [55, 56]. Diversity may have a dual role in bnAb development. Highly diverse Env populations may have an increased chance to harbor a specific Env variant that is capable of initiating a bnAb lineage. Continuously increasing Env diversity, on the other hand, provides a means to support bnAb maturation by presenting multiple antigenic variants.

The impact of the infecting virus

As evidenced by the unresolved impact of viral diversity in steering bnAb responses, the overall role of the infecting virus remains to be defined. What are the genetic

Table 2 Overview of patient cohort studies investigating host and immune factors linked with bnAb development

Reference	Number of subjects[a]	Investigated host and immune factors	Association with breadth
Boliar et al. [90]	41	*Total plasma IgG*	*Positive*
		B cell expression of:	
		PD-1	None
		BTLA	None
		Ki67	None
		CD95	None
Cohen et al. [78]	15	*CXCR5$^+$ CD4$^+$ T cells*	*Positive*
		CXCR5$^+$ PD-1$^+$ CD4$^+$ T cells	*Positive*
		CXCR5$^+$ PD-1$^+$ ICOS$^+$ CD4$^+$ T cells	*Positive*
		Plasma CXCL13	*Positive*
		Plasma IL21	None
		Plasma BAFF	None
		Other cytokines and chemokines	None
		CD3$^-$CD19$^+$ CD27$^-$ naïve B cells	None
		CD3$^-$ CD19$^+$ CD27$^+$ memory B cells	None
		Env-specific CD3$^-$ CD19$^+$ CD27$^+$ gp120$^+$ memory B cells	None
		CXCR5 expression on B cells	None
		Expression of activation-associated genes	*Positive*
		Expression of IFN-stimulated genes IFI27 and ISG15	*Positive*
		Expression of *CXCL13* and *RGS13*	*Positive*
Doria-Rose et al. [51]	148	Total CD19$^+$B cells	None
		CD19$^+$IgG$^+$ B cells	None
		CD19$^+$ CD27$^+$ memory B cells	None
		CD19$^+$ CD20$^-$ CD27^{+++} CD38^{+++} plasmablasts	None
		Env-specific CD19$^+$ gp140$^+$ B cells	None
Doria-Rose et al. [11]	103	Ethnicity	None
		Gender	None
		Age	None
		HLA genotype	None
Dugast et al. [53]	163	*Plasma CXCL13*	*Positive*
		Plasma sCD40L	*Positive*
		Plasma RANTES	*Positive*
		Plasma TNF-a	*Positive*
		Plasma IP-10	*Positive*
		Other cytokines and chemokines	None
Havenar-Daughton et al. [81]	228	*Plasma CXCL13*	*Positive*
Kadelka et al. [54]	4281	*IgG1, IgG2 and IgG3 binding to trimeric Env*	*Positive*
		IgG1 binding to Env-gp120	*Positive*
		IgG2 binding to Env-gp120	*Positive*
		IgG3 binding to MPER	*Positive*
		IgG3 binding to p17 and p24	*Positive*

Table 2 (continued)

Reference	Number of subjects[a]	Investigated host and immune factors	Association with breadth
Landais et al. [14]	439	Gender	None
		Age	None
		Geographical origin	None
		Total plasma IgG	*Positive*
		Env-specific IgG binding titer	*Positive*
		Env-specific IgG binding avidity	None
		HLA genotype	*Positive (HLA-A*03)*
		KIR genotype	None
Locci et al. [79]	328	CXCR5$^+$CD4$^+$ T cells	None
		ICOS$^+$PD-1^{+++} CXCR5$^+$ CD4$^+$ T cells	None
		PD-1$^+$ CXCR3$^-$CXCR5$^+$CD4$^+$ memory Tfh cells	*Positive*
		CXCR3$^-$ CXCR5$^+$CD4$^+$ T cells	None
		PD-1$^+$CXCR3$^+$ memory Tfh cells	None
Mabuka et al. [83]	22	*Plasma CXCL13*	*Positive*
		Plasma BAFF	None
		CD19$^+$CD21$^-$CD27$^+$ activated memory B cells	None
		CD19$^+$CD21$^-$CD27$^-$ tissue-like memory B cells	None
		CD19$^+$CD21$^+$CD27$^+$ resting memory B cells	None
		CD19$^+$CD27$^+$CD38^{+++} plasmablasts	None
Mikkell et al. [32]	38	CD4+ and CD8+T cell expression of:	
		Ki67	None
		CD57	None
		CD38	*Positive (CD4+ T cells)*
		PD-1	*Positive (CD4+ T cells)*
		HLADR	None
Moody et al. [75]	239	HLA genotype	None
		Plasma autoantibodies	*Positive*
		PD1$^+$CXCR3$^-$CXCR5$^+$CD4$^+$ resting memory Tfh cells	*Positive*
		CD25$^+$ Foxp3$^+$ CD4$^+$ Treg cells	*Negative*
		CD25$^+$Foxp3$^+$CXCR5$^+$CD4$^+$ follicular Treg cells	None
		PD-1 expression on CD25$^+$ Foxp3$^+$ CD4$^+$ Treg cells	*Positive*
		PD-1 expression on CD25$^+$Foxp3$^+$CXCR5$^+$CD4$^+$follicular Treg cells	*Positive*
		HLA-DR expression on CD4$^+$ Treg cells	*Positive*
		CTLA-4 expression on CD4$^+$ Treg cells	*Positive*
		LAG-3 expression on CD4$^+$ Treg cells	*Positive*
		Genome-wide mutations	None
Ranasinghe et al. [77]	67	*Gag-specific CD4$^+$ responses*	Positive
		Gp41- specific CD4$^+$ responses	Positive
		Gp120-specific CD4$^+$ responses	None

Table 2 (continued)

Reference	Number of subjects[a]	Investigated host and immune factors	Association with breadth
Richardson et al. [82]	23	ADCC	None
		ADCP	None
		ADCD	Positive
		ADCT	Positive
		Fc polyfunctionality	Positive
		FcR binding	Positive
		C1q binding	Positive
		IgG subclass diversity	Positive
		IgG2 binding to trimeric Env, gp120, V3	Positive
		IgG2 binding to p24	Positive
		IgG4 binding to trimeric Env, gp41, V2	Positive
		Plasma CXCL13	Positive
		AID expression in B cells	Positive
Rusert et al. [12]	4484	Ethnicity	Positive (blacks compared to whites)
		Gender	Weakly positive (modestly higher breadth in men)
Sather et al. [49]	39	Env-specific IgG binding titer	None
		Env-specific IgG binding avidity	Positive
		CD8$^+$ T cell levels	None

[a] Indicates total number of subjects included. Specific analyses may have been carried out on subsets of these numbers

determinants of the virus that trigger a bnAb lineage? As discussed above, it is possible that viral diversity can foster bnAb evolution, but whether diversity at the level of the infecting virus (superinfection, multiple T/F viruses) is decisive or not, has not been resolved.

Understanding the role of the T/F viruses may be key [9]. While no large differences in bnAb elicitation have been seen in male to male and heterosexual transmission [11, 12, 14], bnAb activity is found more frequently after mother to child transmission [57, 58] (see section below) and possibly also in IDUs [12]. Whether the transmitted virus or other factors that differ in these settings underlie the elevated chances to develop bnAb responses needs to be dissected. Differential glycosylation, variable loop length and specific motifs linked with certain bnAb specificities may play a role, but could also differ dependent on subtype and transmission mode [59–64]. However, causal relationships between prospective Env features and neutralization breadth remain difficult to establish. This is also true for deciphering Env determinants that trigger germline precursors of bnAb lineages [65–69]. With few exceptions [19, 20, 22], inferred germline versions of bnAbs often lack measurable binding activity to Env probes, which are efficiently recognized by the mature bnAbs [65–67, 69–71]. This suggests that Envs with distinct characteristics are needed for triggering these bnAbs. Intriguingly, some reports suggest that inferred germline ancestors of Abs with non/low

neutralizing activity frequently bind a range of recombinant Envs with high affinity [45, 72]. Larger numbers of bnAbs and non-neutralizing antibodies need to be investigated to confirm this disparity. However, based on their comparative ease to engage diverse Env variants, non/low-neutralizing antibodies may have a selection advantage in the germinal center (GC) reaction.

A main issue that has not been clarified is whether the capacity of a virus to induce a bnAb is (1) restricted to a specific Env variant that is only transiently present and lost upon Env evolution or (2) preserved over prolonged time periods and may even be stable over multiple transmissions. Despite continuous Env evolution, there is emerging proof that some Env traits are stable and evoke similar responses. Clear evidence for this stems from the comparison of bnAb specificities mounted in subtype B infection compared to non-B infection. Non-B infection proved superior in mounting V2-glycan-directed responses [12], which is supported by the fact that none of the isolated potent V2 bnAbs stems from subtype B infection or targets subtype B viruses efficiently [73]. In contrast, subtype B viruses were more effective in mounting CD4bs responses [12]. Thus, while the genetic subtype had no impact on the frequency of bnAb activity, it shaped the specificity of the response. Thus, specific Env features in the respective virus subtypes that direct the immune response towards a certain specificity must exist.

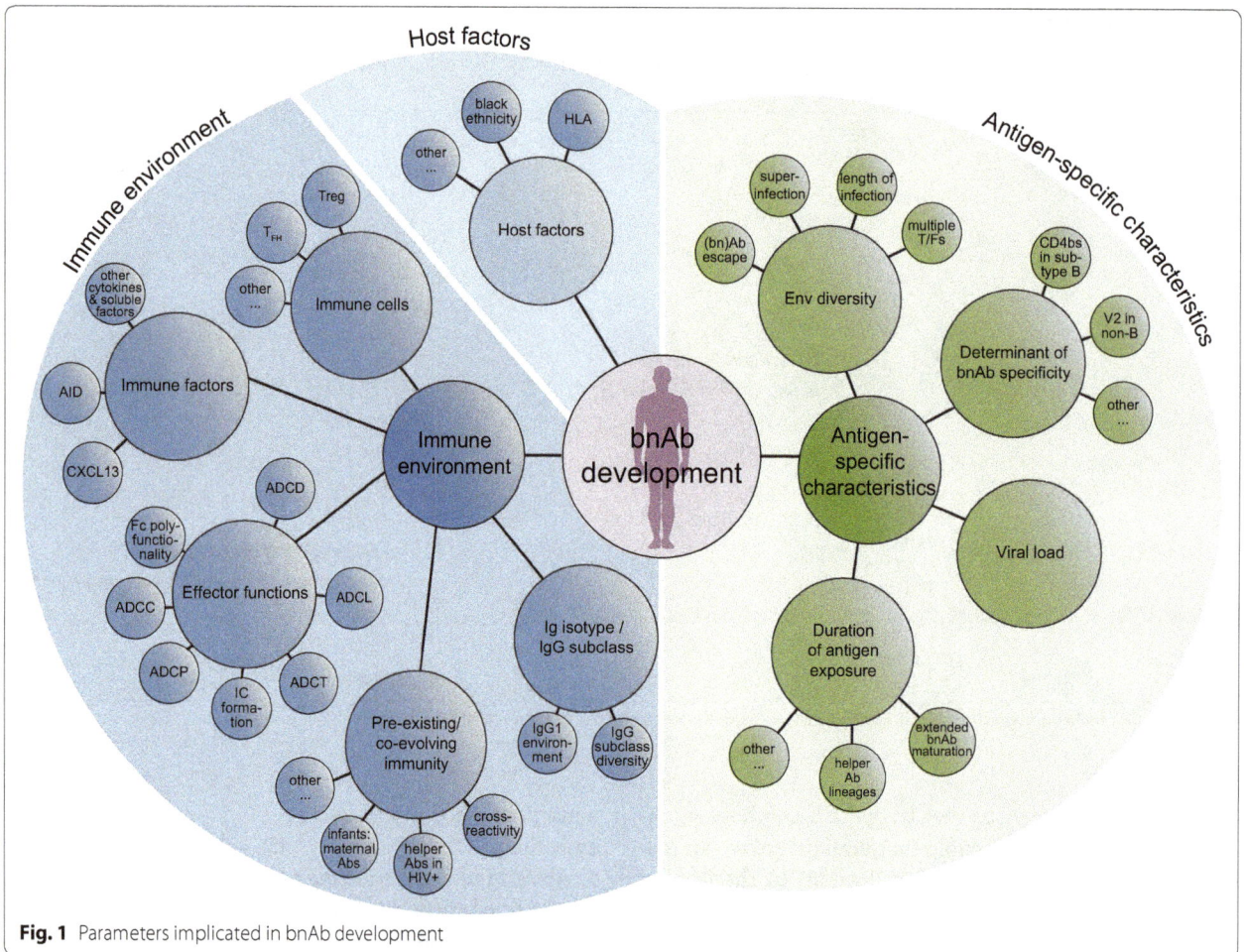

Fig. 1 Parameters implicated in bnAb development

In principle, bnAb development could be facilitated by a range of phenotypic virus features that influence epitope exposure and accessibility. These include, Env conformation and stability, the degree of shielding, and Env density on the virion surface. Unravelling genetic and/or structural Env features that promote or suppress bnAb development will be crucial for vaccine success.

Immune environment

bnAbs often show poly/autoreactivity (reviewed in [74]) and autoantibody frequency has been reported to be high in bnAb-developing individuals [75]. Autoreactivity is particularly strong in the case of MPER bnAbs 2F5 and 4E10, and immune tolerance mechanisms must be overcome for the induction of MPER bnAb responses in humanized mouse models [74]. Therfore, reduced immune control may foster bnAb development in certain cases. An indication that this may occur in natural HIV infection stems from the observation that low CD4$^+$ T cell levels and a high rate of CD4$^+$ T cell decline appear to be linked with broad neutralization

in some cohorts [6, 14, 33, 50]. While the distribution of CD4$^+$ T cell subsets was not assessed directly in most studies, lower CD4$^+$ T cell levels may implicate reduced levels of regulatory CD4$^+$ T cells that may feed into bnAb development. However, a link between low CD4$^+$ T cell levels and neutralization breadth was not observed universally [11, 48, 49, 51]. This may in part be due to the inverse association between CD4$^+$ T cell counts and viral load [76]. With viral load confirmed as an independent determinant of bnAb evolution, assessing the specific effect of CD4$^+$ T cell levels requires cohorts with the power to dissect confounding factors. Controlling for a range of factors, including viral load and infection length, the Swiss 4.5k Screen studying 4484 individuals found only a marginal independent impact of lower CD4$^+$ T cell levels in individuals that mounted low levels of breadth and not those who had potent bnAb activity [12]. Of note, in the same cohort CD4$^+$ T cell levels were found not to correlate with binding antibody responses to gp120, but a strong inverse effect on MPER IgG1 levels was observed [54].

This supports the notion that while MPER antibodies may benefit from a partially impaired immune system, the majority of bnAbs will not benefit from an environment with reduced CD4$^+$ T cells. In fact, a recent study suggests that perturbations in the CD4$^+$ T cell environment are linked with neutralization breadth. bnAb inducers had lower numbers of PD-1^{high} regulatory CD4$^+$ T cells, highlighting a decreased regulatory capacity [75]. Extensive levels of SHM are commonly found in bnAbs. HIV-specific CD4 T cell responses have been linked with neutralization breadth [77] and elevated GC activity in bnAb inducers has been indicated by increased frequency of circulating memory T follicular helper (T$_{FH}$) CD4$^+$ cells, particularly early in infection [75, 78–80]. Likewise, elevated plasma levels of CXCL13, a cytokine involved in B cell migration to the GC, and increased expression of activation-induced cytidine deaminase (AID), the enzyme that orchestrates Ig hypermutation and class switch recombination, was observed in bnAb-inducers [53, 78, 81–83].

What stimulates such beneficial immune environments has not been resolved, but host genetics are implicated by several lines of evidence. A decreased prevalence of the protective allele HLA-B*57 [84] (linked with slower disease progression) and expression of a specific HLA allele (HLA-A*03) [14] have been implicated. Likewise, other HLA variants and SNPs within the MHC complex may directly or indirectly impact bnAb evolution via influencing viral load [11, 14, 75, 84]. As highlighted by CD4bs bnAbs, some bnAb specificities are restricted to a limited set of Ig heavy chain germline alleles, which encode signature features relevant for the specific epitope recognition [71]. Hence, it is possible that the ability to produce these types of antibodies is genetically restricted. However, no overall difference in the immunoglobulin gene repertoires of bnAb inducers and non-neutralizers has been observed to date [85].

In support of a strong genetic influence, individuals with black ethnicity were found to more frequently induce bnAb activity compared to white study participants [12] and have enhanced antibody binding IgG1 responses [54]. Ethnicity-dependent differences in the antibody response to a HIV-1 gp120 immunogen have independently been reported [86]. While the influence of socio-economic factors cannot be excluded, focused studies to reveal a potential genetic determinant are highly warranted. Depending on the genetic determinants identified this may or may not be relevant to vaccines. Nevertheless, their contribution needs to be determined to understand if future HIV bnAb-inducing vaccines can be expected to be effective in the whole population or only in proportions thereof.

Specific antibody signatures are linked with neutralization breadth

With increased knowledge about parameters that are linked with bnAb development in natural infection (Tables 1, 2 and Fig. 1), opportunities to define factors that promote bnAb activity and surrogate markers that predict bnAb evolution are now within reach. An important step towards this came from recent systems serology studies that investigated multiple aspects of the antibody response repertoire in vaccine recipients, non-neutralizers and individuals who developed broad neutralization activity [53, 54, 82, 87–89].

Titer [14] and avidity [49] of IgG binding responses to Env-based antigens have been reported to correlate with neutralization breadth. IgG subclass distribution of the HIV-1 antigen response shows a distinct IgG1-driven pattern in bnAb inducers, suggesting the presence of immune regulatory mechanisms that promote IgG1 responses [54]. In addition, elevated IgG2 and IgG4 responses against HIV antigens in bnAb-inducers compared to non-neutralizers have been observed early in infection [82]. This may in part reflect higher antigen exposure, as IgG2 anti-Env responses are strongly driven by viral load [54]. Diverse parameters that influence the development of neutralization breadth (Tables 1, 2) also impact binding antibody responses to HIV-1 but in an antigen-dependent manner [54], underscoring the complexity of these interrelations. Differential antibody profiles observed in response to HIV-1 Env vaccination regimens [87–89] suggest that modulating the immune response towards patterns that may favor bnAb evolution could be possible. However, this requires detailed knowledge of which antibody features are needed, as well as defined strategies to shift responses in the desired direction.

The importance of effector functions in the protective effect of neutralizing antibodies has been long recognized and both activity of non-neutralizing and neutralizing antibodies in the context of effector functions implicated [53, 91–96]. These include immune complex (IC) formation, antibody dependent complement deposition (ADCD) and lytic (ADCL) activity, antibody dependent cytotoxicity (ADCC), antibody dependent trogocytosis (ADCT) and antibody dependent phagocytosis (ADCP). Increased effector activity of antibodies that bind to Env-expressing infected cells with high affinity, like bnAbs, may deliver superior antiviral activity allowing elimination of infected cells—a goal of HIV-1 cure approaches [94–96].

IgG subtypes differ in their capacity to deliver effector functions and differential glycosylation of the Fc also influences the interaction with Fc receptors and the efficacy of the effector responses [97]. Considerable evidence suggests that steering immune responses towards certain Ig subclasses and/or Fc modifications needs to be evaluated. HIV-1 controllers display antibody subclass profiles that are skewed towards IgG1 or IgG3 responses with the ability to coordinate several effector functions including ADCC and ADCP that suppress viral replication [98–100]. Similarly, immune correlates of protection in the RV144 trial have been linked to antibody effector functions [101, 102]. Systems serology approaches revealed that polyfunctional Fc-effector profiles of anti-Env responses are a critical component of viral control in natural infection [98–100, 103] and distinguish responses to different vaccine regimens [87–89]. When and where Fc effector activity is important, whether improved signaling capacity through immune complex formation or activation of the cell killing mechanism is required, needs to be determined. Common immune determinants that regulate both Fab and Fc mediated activities may be involved, since Fc polyfunctionality and potency early in infection have been associated with the propensity to develop neutralization breadth [82]. Increased levels of ADCD and ADCT were observed early (but not later) in infection in individuals who developed bnAbs [82]. This stresses the complexity in dissecting cause and consequence also in this context. We need to decipher to what extent Fc effector functions actively foster bnAb development and/or develop in parallel (as they depend on the same immune factors) in order to appreciate the importance of stimulating Fc effector environments by vaccination.

HIV-1 infected infants develop bnAbs more frequently, more rapidly and with less SHM

While most bnAbs have high levels of SHM and evolved after prolonged maturation pathways, this seems not to be needed in all settings. A proportion of adults develop bnAb activity comparatively rapidly [12, 20, 22, 32]. In infant HIV infection, bnAb evolution is generally fast and, with more than 70% of cases developing breadth, also substantially more frequent than in adults [57, 58]. Deciphering the underlying causes of slow and rapid bnAb evolution in adults and infants may open new potentials for vaccine design and immunization strategies. The first infant bnAb characterized in detail highlights the potential [104]. In line with a more direct developmental pathway in infants, the N332 glycan-dependent supersite-targeting bnAb BF520.1, isolated from a HIV-1 infected infant 1 year post-infection, has notably low levels of SHM (6.6% nt) and lacks heavy and light chain indels compared to adult V3 glycan region-targeting bnAbs [104]. If conditions that allow rapid development of low SHM bnAbs like BF520.1 prove to be transferrable to other settings this may open immense potential to create an effective bnAb vaccine in adults. Pinpointing the

causative effects will however be challenging. A range of factors differ between adult and infant infection and several may feed into each other. While it seems surprising, the infant immune system appears to provide a better setting for bnAb development. In early life, B cell responses are partially restricted, the Ig germ-line repertoire is not fully developed and the co-stimulatory network is not yet fully functional, leading to compromised B cell responses with lower SHM and heterogeneity [105, 106]. IgG subclass distribution differs markedly in infants with IgG1 and IgG3 levels, the most relevant subclasses for neutralizing HIV responses [54], rising sooner to adult-like concentrations than IgG2 and IgG4 [106, 107].

While antibodies with lower SHM may prove to be common in infants, it is intriguing that bnAbs with low SHM have not been described in adults. Does the adult immune system not favor the development of low SHM bnAbs? A potential scenario could be that cross-reactive antibodies that bind to HIV Env exist in adults. Following the dogma of original antigenic sin [108], instead of priming a de novo antibody response, the evolution of the Env antibody response would be restricted to affinity maturation of a pre-existing cross-reactive antibody. This may limit the response and require more extensive SHM to reach neutralization breadth. Of note, cross-reactivity with unrelated proteins and/or host antigens have been described for several HIV bnAbs [23, 109–111].

Vertical transmission is distinct from all other HIV-1 transmissions, as maternal antibodies are transferred and remain present for prolonged time periods. The role of maternal Abs in influencing transmission risk is still debated [112–115]. Irrespective of their potential in preventing transmission, it is intriguing to speculate that maternal antibodies may function as helper antibodies [19, 40]. The presence of maternal Abs may allow immune-focusing that aids neutralizing antibody development, as described for passive immunization of infant macaques [47]. Influence of maternal antibodies on vaccine responses in infants has been reported [107] and may comprise a number of mechanisms including activation of the immune system through IC formation that aid bnAb evolution. Specific immune-focusing of the infant response could also be envisaged through binding of immunodominant epitopes by maternal antibodies, shielding these from access by infant BCRs and thereby directing the Ab response to other sites without competing for survival signals in the GC reaction. In the setting of HIV-1 infection, this immediately raises the question whether neutralizing or non-neutralizing antibodies or even combinations thereof would be needed to create effective immune-focusing [116].

High viral load—a strong influence on bnAb evolution in adults—is frequent in infant HIV-1 infection in the

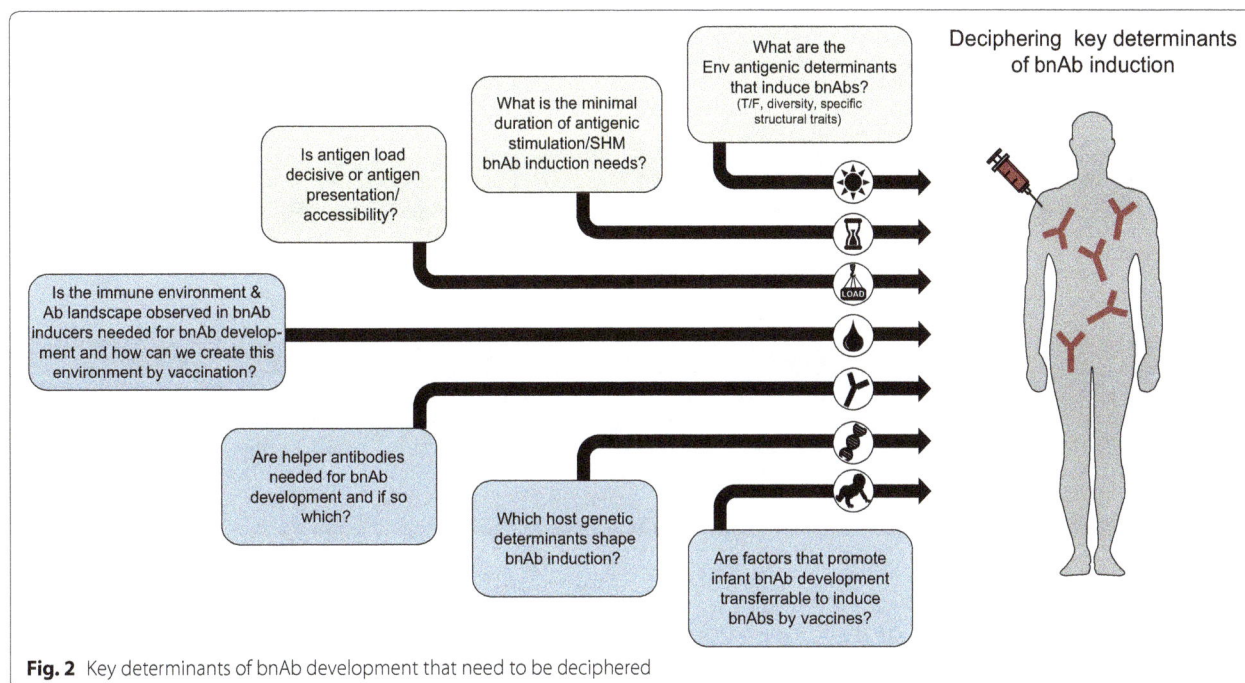

Fig. 2 Key determinants of bnAb development that need to be deciphered

first 2 years of life [117, 118] and may also promote infant bnAb development as seen in adult HIV infection [11, 12, 14, 32, 33, 48–50]. Importantly, vertical transmission may also create bottlenecks that differ from sexual transmission, potentially favoring transmission of phenotypically distinct strains that favor bnAb triggering. Defining the phenotypic properties of T/F viruses from vertical transmission cases that developed Ab breadth is of high relevance. The best case scenario for vaccine design would be that specific Env properties of infant T/F viruses are the underlying cause of the frequent and rapid bnAb evolution in infant HIV infection. Of note, the T/F virus BG505, derived from an infant that developed a bnAb response [119] is the currently most thoroughly studied trimeric Env immunogen and focus of diverse immunization strategies [119, 120].

Conclusion

Detailed analysis of determinants that shape bnAb responses in natural infection have led to the identification of a range of factors that are linked with the development of neutralization breadth. However, so far we lack formal proof for which factors are ultimately causative in bnAb elicitation and which evolve alongside. Delineating the causes and consequences, as well as defining parameters that need to be incorporated into vaccine regimens will be critical. Figure 2 highlights key questions that need to be addressed, based on the current state of the field. Resolving these

topics, ranging from the impact of the Env immunogen and the immune environment in which the bnAb response favorably evolves, to understanding why the infant HIV-1 infection is superior in mounting bnAb responses, will be challenging. However, this is ultimately necessary to move HIV vaccine design forward.

Authors' contributions
HS, MS and AT wrote this article together and give their consent to publication. All authors read and approved the final manuscript.

Acknowledgements
We thank Claus Kadelka and Melissa Robbiani for critical reading.

Competing interests
The authors declare that they have no competing interests.

Funding
Financial support has been provided by the Swiss National Science Foundation (SNF #314730_172790 to AT).

References

1. Burton DR, Hangartner L. Broadly neutralizing antibodies to HIV and their role in vaccine design. Annu Rev Immunol. 2016;34:635–59.

2. Nishimura Y, Martin MA. Of mice, macaques, and men: broadly neutralizing antibody immunotherapy for HIV-1. Cell Host Microbe. 2017;22(2):207–16.

3. Bhiman JN, Anthony C, Doria-Rose NA, Karimanzira O, Schramm CA, Khoza T, Kitchin D, Botha G, Gorman J, Garrett NJ, et al. Viral variants that initiate and drive maturation of V1V2-directed HIV-1 broadly neutralizing antibodies. Nat Med. 2015;21(11):1332–6.

4. Bonsignori M, Liao HX, Gao F, Williams WB, Alam SM, Montefiori DC, Haynes BF. Antibody-virus co-evolution in HIV infection: paths for HIV vaccine development. Immunol Rev. 2017;275(1):145–60.

5. Wibmer CK, Bhiman JN, Gray ES, Tumba N, Abdool Karim SS, Williamson C, Morris L, Moore PL. Viral escape from HIV-1 neutralizing antibodies drives increased plasma neutralization breadth through sequential recognition of multiple epitopes and immunotypes. PLoS Pathog. 2013;9(10):e1003738.

6. Euler Z, van Gils MJ, Bunnik EM, Phung P, Schweighardt B, Wrin T, Schuitemaker H. Cross-reactive neutralizing humoral immunity does not protect from HIV type 1 disease progression. J Infect Dis. 2010;201(7):1045–53.

7. Ferrari G, Pollara J, Tomaras GD, Haynes BF. Humoral and innate antiviral immunity as tools to clear persistent HIV infection. J Infect Dis. 2017;215(suppl_3):S152–9.

8. Pegu A, Hessell AJ, Mascola JR, Haigwood NL. Use of broadly neutralizing antibodies for HIV-1 prevention. Immunol Rev. 2017;275(1):296–312.

9. Joseph SB, Swanstrom R, Kashuba AD, Cohen MS. Bottlenecks in HIV-1 transmission: insights from the study of founder viruses. Nat Rev Microbiol. 2015;13(7):414–25.

10. Hraber P, Seaman MS, Bailer RT, Mascola JR, Montefiori DC, Korber BT. Prevalence of broadly neutralizing antibody responses during chronic HIV-1 infection. Aids. 2014;28(2):163–9.

11. Doria-Rose NA, Klein RM, Daniels MG, O'Dell S, Nason M, Lapedes A, Bhattacharya T, Migueles SA, Wyatt RT, Korber BT, et al. Breadth of human immunodeficiency virus-specific neutralizing activity in sera: clustering analysis and association with clinical variables. J Virol. 2010;84(3):1631–6.

12. Rusert P, Kouyos RD, Kadelka C, Ebner H, Schanz M, Huber M, Braun DL, Hoze N, Scherrer A, Magnus C, et al. Determinants of HIV-1 broadly neutralizing antibody induction. Nat Med. 2016;22(11):1260–7.

13. Simek MD, Rida W, Priddy FH, Pung P, Carrow E, Laufer DS, Lehrman JK, Boaz M, Tarragona-Fiol T, Miiro G, et al. Human immunodeficiency virus type 1 elite neutralizers: individuals with broad and potent neutralizing activity identified by using a high-throughput neutralization assay together with an analytical selection algorithm. J Virol. 2009;83(14):7337–48.

14. Landais E, Huang X, Havenar-Daughton C, Murrell B, Price MA, Wickramasinghe L, Ramos A, Bian CB, Simek M, Allen S, et al. Broadly neutralizing antibody responses in a large longitudinal sub-Saharan HIV primary infection cohort. PLoS Pathog. 2016;12(1):e1005369.

15. Sanders RW, Moore JP. Native-like Env trimers as a platform for HIV-1 vaccine design. Immunol Rev. 2017;275(1):161–82.

16. Pancera M, Changela A, Kwong PD. How HIV-1 entry mechanism and broadly neutralizing antibodies guide structure-based vaccine design. Curr Opin HIV AIDS. 2017;12(3):229–40.

17. MacLeod DT, Choi NM, Briney B, Garces F, Ver LS, Landais E, Murrell B, Wrin T, Kilembe W, Liang CH, et al. Early antibody lineage diversification and independent limb maturation lead to broad HIV-1 neutralization targeting the env high-mannose Patch. Immunity. 2016;44(5):1215–26.

18. Gao F, Bonsignori M, Liao HX, Kumar A, Xia SM, Lu X, Cai F, Hwang KK, Song H, Zhou T, et al. Cooperation of B cell lineages in induction of HIV-1-broadly neutralizing antibodies. Cell. 2014;158(3):481–91.

19. Bonsignori M, Zhou T, Sheng Z, Chen L, Gao F, Joyce MG, Ozorowski G, Chuang GY, Schramm CA, Wiehe K, et al. Maturation pathway from germline to broad HIV-1 neutralizer of a CD4-mimic antibody. Cell. 2016;165(2):449–63.

20. Doria-Rose NA, Schramm CA, Gorman J, Moore PL, Bhiman JN, DeKosky BJ, Ernandes MJ, Georgiev IS, Kim HJ, Pancera M, et al. Developmental pathway for potent V1V2-directed HIV-neutralizing antibodies. Nature. 2014;509(7498):55–62.

21. Wu XL, Zhou TQ, Zhu J, Zhang BS, Georgiev I, Wang C, Chen XJ, Longo NS, Louder M, McKee K, et al. Focused evolution of HIV-1 neutralizing antibodies revealed by structures and deep sequencing. Science. 2011;333(6049):1593–602.

22. Liao HX, Lynch R, Zhou T, Gao F, Alam SM, Boyd SD, Fire AZ, Roskin KM, Schramm CA, Zhang Z, et al. Co-evolution of a broadly neutralizing HIV-1 antibody and founder virus. Nature. 2013;496(7446):469–76.

23. Bonsignori M, Hwang KK, Chen X, Tsao CY, Morris L, Gray E, Marshall DJ, Crump JA, Kapiga SH, Sam NE, et al. Analysis of a clonal lineage of HIV-1 envelope V2/V3 conformational epitope-specific broadly neutralizing antibodies and their inferred unmutated common ancestors. J Virol. 2011;85(19):9998–10009.

24. Moore PL, Gray ES, Wibmer CK, Bhiman JN, Nonyane M, Sheward DJ, Hermanus T, Bajimaya S, Tumba NL, Abrahams MR, et al. Evolution of an HIV glycan-dependent broadly neutralizing antibody epitope through immune escape. Nat Med. 2012;18(11):1688–92.

25. Williams KL, Wang B, Arenz D, Williams JA, Dingens AS, Cortez V, Simonich CA, Rainwater S, Lehman DA, Lee KK, et al. Superinfection drives HIV neutralizing antibody responses from several B cell lineages that contribute to a polyclonal repertoire. Cell Rep. 2018;23(3):682–91.

26. Powell RL, Kinge T, Nyambi PN. Infection by discordant strains of HIV-1 markedly enhances the neutralizing antibody response against heterologous virus. J Virol. 2010;84(18):9415–26.

27. Cortez V, Odem-Davis K, McClelland RS, Jaoko W, Overbaugh J. HIV-1 superinfection in women broadens and strengthens the neutralizing antibody response. PLoS Pathog. 2012;8(3):e1002611.

28. Moore PL, Sheward D, Nonyane M, Ranchobe N, Hermanus T, Gray ES, Abdool Karim SS, Williamson C, Morris L. Multiple pathways of escape from HIV broadly cross-neutralizing V2-dependent antibodies. J Virol. 2013;87(9):4882–94.

29. van Gils MJ, Bunnik EM, Burger JA, Jacob Y, Schweighardt B, Wrin T, Schuitemaker H. Rapid escape from preserved cross-reactive neutralizing humoral immunity without loss of viral fitness in HIV-1-infected progressors and long-term nonprogressors. J Virol. 2010;84(7):3576–85.

30. Wu X, Wang C, O'Dell S, Li Y, Keele BF, Yang Z, Imamichi H, Doria-Rose N, Hoxie JA, Connors M, et al. Selection pressure on HIV-1 envelope by broadly neutralizing antibodies to the conserved CD4-binding site. J Virol. 2012;86(10):5844–56.

31. Sather DN, Carbonetti S, Kehayia J, Kraft Z, Mikell I, Scheid JF, Klein F, Stamatatos L. Broadly neutralizing antibodies developed by an HIV-positive elite neutralizer exact a replication fitness cost on the contemporaneous virus. J Virol. 2012;86(23):12676–85.

32. Mikell I, Sather DN, Kalams SA, Altfeld M, Alter G, Stamatatos L. Characteristics of the earliest cross-neutralizing antibody response to HIV-1. PLoS Pathog. 2011;7(1):e1001251.

33. Gray ES, Madiga MC, Hermanus T, Moore PL, Wibmer CK, Tumba NL, Werner L, Mlisana K, Sibeko S, Williamson C, et al. The neutralization breadth of HIV-1 develops incrementally over four years and is associated with CD4+ T cell decline and high viral load during acute infection. J Virol. 2011;85(10):4828–40.

34. Euler Z, van den Kerkhof TL, van Gils MJ, Burger JA, Edo-Matas D, Phung P, Wrin T, Schuitemaker H. Longitudinal analysis of early HIV-1-specific neutralizing activity in an elite neutralizer and in five patients who developed cross-reactive neutralizing activity. J Virol. 2012;86(4):2045–55.

35. Landais E, Murrell B, Briney B, Murrell S, Rantalainen K, Berndsen ZT, Ramos A, Wickramasinghe L, Smith ML, Eren K, et al. HIV envelope glycoform heterogeneity and localized diversity govern the initiation and maturation of a V2 apex broadly neutralizing antibody lineage. Immunity. 2017;47(5):990–1003.e1009.

36. Doria-Rose NA, Bhiman JN, Roark RS, Schramm CA, Gorman J, Chuang GY, Pancera M, Cale EM, Ernandes MJ, Louder MK, et al. New member of the V1V2-Directed CAP256-VRC26 lineage that shows increased breadth and exceptional potency. J Virol. 2015;90(1):76–91.

37. Klein F, Diskin R, Scheid JF, Gaebler C, Mouquet H, Georgiev IS, Pancera M, Zhou T, Incesu RB, Fu BZ, et al. Somatic mutations of the immunoglobulin framework are generally required for broad and potent HIV-1 neutralization. Cell. 2013;153(1):126–38.

38. Reh L, Magnus C, Kadelka C, Kuhnert D, Uhr T, Weber J, Morris L, Moore PL, Trkola A. Phenotypic deficits in the HIV-1 envelope are associated with the maturation of a V2-directed broadly neutralizing antibody lineage. PLoS Pathog. 2018;14(1):e1006825.

39. Freund NT, Wang H, Scharf L, Nogueira L, Horwitz JA, Bar-On Y, Golijanin J, Sievers SA, Sok D, Cai H, et al. Coexistence of potent HIV-1 broadly neutralizing antibodies and antibody-sensitive viruses in a viremic controller. Sci Transl Med. 2017;9(373):eaal2144.

40. Anthony C, York T, Bekker V, Matten D, Selhorst P, Ferreria RC, Garrett NJ, Karim SSA, Morris L, Wood NT, et al. Cooperation between strain-specific and broadly neutralizing responses limited viral escape and prolonged the exposure of the broadly neutralizing epitope. J Virol. 2017;91(18):e00828–17.

41. Abela IA, Berlinger L, Schanz M, Reynell L, Gunthard HF, Rusert P, Trkola A. Cell-cell transmission enables HIV-1 to evade inhibition by potent CD4bs directed antibodies. PLoS Pathog. 2012;8(4):e1002634.

42. Malbec M, Porrot F, Rua R, Horwitz J, Klein F, Halper-Stromberg A, Scheid JF, Eden C, Mouquet H, Nussenzweig MC, et al. Broadly neutralizing antibodies that inhibit HIV-1 cell to cell transmission. J Exp Med. 2013;210(13):2813–21.

43. Li H, Zony C, Chen P, Chen BK. Reduced potency and incomplete neutralization of broadly neutralizing antibodies against cell-to-cell transmission of HIV-1 with transmitted founder Envs. J Virol. 2017;91(9):e02425–16.

44. Luo SS, Perelson AS. Competitive exclusion by autologous antibodies can prevent broad HIV-1 antibodies from arising. Proc Natl Acad Sci USA. 2015;112(37):11654–9.

45. McGuire AT, Dreyer AM, Carbonetti S, Lippy A, Glenn J, Scheid JF, Mouquet H, Stamatatos L. HIV antibodies. Antigen modification regulates competition of broad and narrow neutralizing HIV antibodies. Science. 2014;346(6215):1380–3.

46. Schoofs T, Klein F, Braunschweig M, Kreider EF, Feldmann A, Nogueira L, Oliveira T, Lorenzi JC, Parrish EH, Learn GH, et al. HIV-1 therapy with monoclonal antibody 3BNC117 elicits host immune responses against HIV-1. Science. 2016;352(6288):997–1001.

47. Ng CT, Jaworski JP, Jayaraman P, Sutton WF, Delio P, Kuller L, Anderson D, Landucci G, Richardson BA, Burton DR, et al. Passive neutralizing antibody controls SHIV viremia and enhances B cell responses in infant macaques. Nat Med. 2010;16(10):1117–9.

48. Piantadosi A, Panteleeff D, Blish CA, Baeten JM, Jaoko W, McClelland RS, Overbaugh J. Breadth of neutralizing antibody response to human immunodeficiency virus type 1 is affected by factors early in infection but does not influence disease progression. J Virol. 2009;83(19):10269–74.

49. Sather DN, Armann J, Ching LK, Mavrantoni A, Sellhorn G, Caldwell Z, Yu X, Wood B, Self S, Kalams S, et al. Factors associated with the development of cross-reactive neutralizing antibodies during human immunodeficiency virus type 1 infection. J Virol. 2009;83(2):757–69.

50. van Gils MJ, Euler Z, Schweighardt B, Wrin T, Schuitemaker H. Prevalence of cross-reactive HIV-1-neutralizing activity in HIV-1-infected patients with rapid or slow disease progression. Aids. 2009;23(18):2405–14.

51. Doria-Rose NA, Klein RM, Manion MM, O'Dell S, Phogat A, Chakrabarti B, Hallahan CW, Migueles SA, Wrammert J, Ahmed R, et al. Frequency and phenotype of human immunodeficiency virus envelope-specific B cells from patients with broadly cross-neutralizing antibodies. J Virol. 2009;83(1):188–99.

52. Scheid JF, Mouquet H, Feldhahn N, Seaman MS, Velinzon K, Pietzsch J, Ott RG, Anthony RM, Zebroski H, Hurley A, et al. Broad diversity of neutralizing antibodies isolated from memory B cells in HIV-infected individuals. Nature. 2009;458(7238):636–40.

53. Dugast A-S, Arnold K, Lofano G, Moore S, Hoffner M, Simek M, Poignard P, Seaman M, Suscovich TJ, Pereyra F, et al. Virus-driven inflammation is associated with the development of bNAbs in spontaneous controllers of HIV. Clin Infect Dis. 2017;64(8):1098–104.

54. Kadelka C, Liechti T, Ebner H, Schanz M, Rusert P, Friedrich N, Stiegeler E, Braun DL, Huber M, Scherrer AU, et al. Distinct, IgG1 driven antibody response landscapes demarcate individuals with broadly HIV-1 neutralizing activity. J Exp Med. 2018;215(6):1589–608.

55. Ronen K, Dingens AS, Graham SM, Jaoko W, Mandaliya K, McClelland RS, Overbaugh J. Comprehensive characterization of humoral correlates of human immunodeficiency virus 1 superinfection acquisition in high-risk Kenyan women. EBioMedicine. 2017;18:216–24.

56. Courtney CR, Mayr L, Nanfack AJ, Banin AN, Tuen M, Pan R, Jiang X, Kong X-P, Kirkpatrick AR, Bruno D, et al. Contrasting antibody responses to intrasubtype superinfection with CRF02_AG. PLoS ONE. 2017;12(3):e0173705.

57. Goo L, Chohan V, Nduati R, Overbaugh J. Early development of broadly neutralizing antibodies in HIV-1-infected infants. Nat Med. 2014;20(6):655–8.

58. Muenchhoff M, Adland E, Karimanzira O, Crowther C, Pace M, Csala A, Leitman E, Moonsamy A, McGregor C, Hurst J, et al. Nonprogressing HIV-infected children share fundamental immunological features of nonpathogenic SIV infection. Sci Transl Med. 2016;8(358):358ra125.

59. Smith SA, Burton SL, Kilembe W, Lakhi S, Karita E, Price M, Allen S, Hunter E, Derdeyn CA. Diversification in the HIV-1 envelope hyper-variable domains V2, V4, and V5 and higher probability of transmitted/founder envelope glycosylation favor the development of heterologous neutralization breadth. PLoS Pathog. 2016;12(11):e1005989.

60. Rademeyer C, Korber B, Seaman MS, Giorgi EE, Thebus R, Robles A, Sheward DJ, Wagh K, Garrity J, Carey BR, et al. Features of recently transmitted HIV-1 clade C viruses that impact antibody recognition: implications for active and passive immunization. PLoS Pathog. 2016;12(7):e1005742.

61. van den Kerkhof TLGM, Feenstra KA, Euler Z, van Gils MJ, Rijsdijk LWE, Boeser-Nunnink BD, Heringa J, Schuitemaker H, Sanders RW. HIV-1 envelope glycoprotein signatures that correlate with the development of cross-reactive neutralizing activity. Retrovirology. 2013;10(1):102.

62. Gnanakaran S, Daniels MG, Bhattacharya T, Lapedes AS, Sethi A, Li M, Tang H, Greene K, Gao H, Haynes BF, et al. Genetic signatures in the envelope glycoproteins of HIV-1 that associate with broadly neutralizing antibodies. PLoS Comput Biol. 2010;6(10):e1000955.

63. Li M, Salazar-Gonzalez JF, Derdeyn CA, Morris L, Williamson C, Robinson JE, Decker JM, Li Y, Salazar MG, Polonis VR, et al. Genetic and neutralization properties of subtype C human immunodeficiency virus type 1 molecular env clones from acute and early heterosexually acquired infections in southern Africa. J Virol. 2006;80(23):11776–90.

64. Hraber P, Korber BT, Lapedes AS, Bailer RT, Seaman MS, Gao H, Greene KM, McCutchan F, Williamson C, Kim JH, et al. Impact of clade, geography, and age of the epidemic on HIV-1 neutralization by antibodies. J Virol. 2014;88(21):12623–43.

65. Xiao X, Chen W, Feng Y, Zhu Z, Prabakaran P, Wang Y, Zhang MY, Longo NS, Dimitrov DS. Germline-like predecessors of broadly neutralizing antibodies lack measurable binding to HIV-1 envelope glycoproteins: implications for evasion of immune responses and design of vaccine immunogens. Biochem Biophys Res Commun. 2009;390(3):404–9.

66. Hoot S, McGuire AT, Cohen KW, Strong RK, Hangartner L, Klein F, Diskin R, Scheid JF, Sather DN, Burton DR, et al. Recombinant HIV envelope proteins fail to engage germline versions of anti-CD4bs bNAbs. PLoS Pathog. 2013;9(1):e1003106.

67. McGuire AT, Hoot S, Dreyer AM, Lippy A, Stuart A, Cohen KW, Jardine J, Menis S, Scheid JF, West AP, et al. Engineering HIV envelope protein to activate germline B cell receptors of broadly neutralizing anti-CD4 binding site antibodies. J Exp Med. 2013;210:655–63.

68. Zhou T, Zhu J, Wu X, Moquin S, Zhang B, Acharya P, Georgiev IS, Altae-Tran HR, Chuang GY, Joyce MG, et al. Multidonor analysis reveals structural elements, genetic determinants, and maturation pathway for HIV-1 neutralization by VRC01-class antibodies. Immunity. 2013;39(2):245–58.

69. Jardine J, Julien JP, Menis S, Ota T, Kalyuzhniy O, McGuire A, Sok D, Huang PS, MacPherson S, Jones M, et al. Rational HIV immunogen design to target specific germline B cell receptors. Science. 2013;340(6133):711–6.

70. Scheid JF, Mouquet H, Ueberheide B, Diskin R, Klein F, Oliveira TY, Pietzsch J, Fenyo D, Abadir A, Velinzon K, et al. Sequence and structural convergence of broad and potent HIV antibodies that mimic CD4 binding. Science. 2011;333(6049):1633–7.

71. Zhou T, Lynch RM, Chen L, Acharya P, Wu X, Doria-Rose NA, Joyce MG, Lingwood D, Soto C, Bailer RT, et al. Structural repertoire of HIV-1-neutralizing antibodies targeting the CD4 supersite in 14 donors. Cell. 2015;161(6):1280–92.

72. Mouquet H, Scheid JF, Zoller MJ, Krogsgaard M, Ott RG, Shukair S, Artyomov MN, Pietzsch J, Connors M, Pereyra F, et al. Polyreactivity increases the apparent affinity of anti-HIV antibodies by heteroligation. Nature. 2010;467(7315):591–5.

73. Yoon H, Macke J, West AP Jr, Foley B, Bjorkman PJ, Korber B, Yusim K. CATNAP: a tool to compile, analyze and tally neutralizing antibody panels. Nucl Acids Res. 2015;43(W1):W213–9.

74. Kelsoe G, Haynes BF. Host controls of HIV broadly neutralizing antibody development. Immunol Rev. 2017;275(1):79–88.

75. Moody MA, Pedroza-Pacheco I, Vandergrift NA, Chui C, Lloyd KE, Parks R, Soderberg KA, Ogbe AT, Cohen MS, Liao HX, et al. Immune perturbations in HIV-1-infected individuals who make broadly neutralizing antibodies. Sci Immunol. 2016;1(1):aag0851.

76. Mellors JW, Munoz A, Giorgi JV, Margolick JB, Tassoni CJ, Gupta P, Kingsley LA, Todd JA, Saah AJ, Detels R, et al. Plasma viral load and CD4+ lymphocytes as prognostic markers of HIV-1 infection. Ann Intern Med. 1997;126(12):946–54.

77. Ranasinghe S, Soghoian DZ, Lindqvist M, Ghebremichael M, Donaghey F, Carrington M, Seaman MS, Kaufmann DE, Walker BD, Porichis F. HIV-1 antibody neutralization breadth is associated with enhanced HIV-specific CD4+ T cell responses. J Virol. 2015;90(5):2208–20.

78. Cohen K, Altfeld M, Alter G, Stamatatos L. Early preservation of CXCR5+ PD-1+ helper T cells and B cell activation predict the breadth of neutralizing antibody responses in chronic HIV-1 infection. J Virol. 2014;88(22):13310–21.

79. Locci M, Havenar-Daughton C, Landais E, Wu J, Kroenke MA, Arlehamn CL, Su LF, Cubas R, Davis MM, Sette A, et al. Human circulating PD-1+CXCR3-CXCR5+ memory Tfh cells are highly functional and correlate with broadly neutralizing HIV antibody responses. Immunity. 2013;39(4):758–69.

80. Yamamoto T, Lynch RM, Gautam R, Matus-Nicodemos R, Schmidt SD, Boswell KL, Darko S, Wong P, Sheng Z, Petrovas C, et al. Quality and quantity of TFH cells are critical for broad antibody development in SHIVAD8 infection. Sci Transl Med. 2015;7(298):298ra120.

81. Havenar-Daughton C, Lindqvist M, Heit A, Wu JE, Reiss SM, Kendric K, Bélanger S, Kasturi SP, Landais E, Akondy RS, et al. CXCL13 is a plasma biomarker of germinal center activity. Proc Natl Acad Sci. 2016;113(10):2702.

82. Richardson SI, Chung AW, Natarajan H, Mabvakure B, Mkhize NN, Garrett N, Abdool Karim S, Moore PL, Ackerman ME, Alter G, et al. HIV-specific Fc effector function early in infection predicts the development of broadly neutralizing antibodies. PLoS Pathog. 2018;14(4):e1006987.

83. Mabuka JM, Dugast AS, Muema DM, Reddy T, Ramlakhan Y, Euler Z, Ismail N, Moodley A, Dong KL, Morris L, et al. Plasma CXCL13 but Not B cell frequencies in acute HIV infection predicts emergence of cross-neutralizing antibodies. Front Immunol. 2017;8:1104.

84. Euler Z, van Gils MJ, Boeser-Nunnink BD, Schuitemaker H, van Manen D. Genome-wide association study on the development of cross-reactive neutralizing antibodies in HIV-1 infected individuals. PLoS ONE. 2013;8(1):e54684.

85. Scheepers C, Shrestha RK, Lambson BE, Jackson KJ, Wright IA, Naicker D, Goosen M, Berrie L, Ismail A, Garrett N, et al. Ability to develop broadly neutralizing HIV-1 antibodies is not restricted by the germline Ig gene repertoire. J Immunol. 2015;194(9):4371–8.

86. Montefiori DC, Metch B, McElrath MJ, Self S, Weinhold KJ, Corey L. Network HIVVT: demographic factors that influence the neutralizing antibody response in recipients of recombinant HIV-1 gp120 vaccines. J Infect Dis. 2004;190(11):1962–9.

87. Chung AW, Kumar MP, Arnold KB, Yu WH, Schoen MK, Dunphy LJ, Suscovich TJ, Frahm N, Linde C, Mahan AE, et al. Dissecting polyclonal vaccine-induced humoral immunity against HIV using systems serology. Cell. 2015;163(4):988–98.

88. Chung AW, Ghebremichael M, Robinson H, Brown E, Choi I, Lane S, Dugast A-S, Schoen MK, Rolland M, Suscovich TJ, et al. Polyfunctional Fc-effector profiles mediated by IgG subclass selection distinguish RV144 and VAX003 vaccines. Sci Transl Med. 2014;6(228):228ra238.

89. Mahan AE, Jennewein MF, Suscovich T, Dionne K, Tedesco J, Chung AW, Streeck H, Pau M, Schuitemaker H, Francis D, et al. Antigen-specific antibody glycosylation is regulated via vaccination. PLoS Pathog. 2016;12(3):e1005456.

90. Boliar S, Murphy MK, Tran TC, Carnathan DG, Armstrong WS, Silvestri G, Derdeyn CA. B-lymphocyte dysfunction in chronic HIV-1 infection does not prevent cross-clade neutralization breadth. J Virol. 2012;86(15):8031–40.

91. Bournazos S, Klein F, Pietzsch J, Seaman MS, Nussenzweig MC, Ravetch JV. Broadly neutralizing anti-HIV-1 antibodies require Fc effector functions for in vivo activity. Cell. 2014;158(6):1243–53.

92. Hessell AJ, Hangartner L, Hunter M, Havenith CEG, Beurskens FJ, Bakker JM, Lanigan CMS, Landucci G, Forthal DN, Parren PWHI, et al. Fc receptor but not complement binding is important in antibody protection against HIV. Nature. 2007;449:101.

93. Huber M, Trkola A. Humoral immunity to HIV-1: neutralization and beyond. J Intern Med. 2007;262(1):5–25.

94. Halper-Stromberg A, Lu CL, Klein F, Horwitz JA, Bournazos S, Nogueira L, Eisenreich TR, Liu C, Gazumyan A, Schaefer U, et al. Broadly neutralizing antibodies and viral inducers decrease rebound from HIV-1 latent reservoirs in humanized mice. Cell. 2014;158(5):989–99.

95. Lu CL, Murakowski DK, Bournazos S, Schoofs T, Sarkar D, Halper-Stromberg A, Horwitz JA, Nogueira L, Golijanin J, Gazumyan A, et al. Enhanced clearance of HIV-1-infected cells by broadly neutralizing antibodies against HIV-1 in vivo. Science. 2016;352(6288):1001–4.

96. Bruel T, Guivel-Benhassine F, Amraoui S, Malbec M, Richard L, Bourdic K, Donahue DA, Lorin V, Casartelli N, Noël N, et al. Elimination of HIV-1-infected cells by broadly neutralizing antibodies. Nat Commun. 2016;7:10844.

97. Lu LL, Suscovich TJ, Fortune SM, Alter G. Beyond binding: antibody effector functions in infectious diseases. Nat Rev Immunol. 2018;18(1):46–61.

98. Ackerman ME, Mikhailova A, Brown EP, Dowell KG, Walker BD, Bailey-Kellogg C, Suscovich TJ, Alter G. Polyfunctional HIV-specific antibody responses are associated with spontaneous HIV control. PLoS Pathog. 2016;12(1):e1005315.

99. Lai JI, Licht AF, Dugast AS, Suscovich T, Choi I, Bailey-Kellogg C, Alter G, Ackerman ME. Divergent antibody subclass and specificity profiles but not protective HLA-B alleles are associated with variable antibody effector function among HIV-1 controllers. J Virol. 2014;88(5):2799–809.

100. Sadanand S, Das J, Chung AW, Schoen MK, Lane S, Suscovich TJ, Streeck H, Smith DM, Little SJ, Lauffenburger DA, et al. Temporal variation in HIV-specific IgG subclass antibodies during acute infection differentiates spontaneous controllers from chronic progressors. Aids. 2018;32(4):443–50.

101. Haynes BF, Gilbert PB, McElrath MJ, Zolla-Pazner S, Tomaras GD, Alam SM, Evans DT, Montefiori DC, Karnasuta C, Sutthent R, et al. Immune-correlates analysis of an HIV-1 vaccine efficacy trial. N Engl J Med. 2012;366(14):1275–86.

102. Tomaras GD, Ferrari G, Shen X, Alam SM, Liao HX, Pollara J, Bonsignori M, Moody MA, Fong Y, Chen X, et al. Vaccine-induced plasma IgA specific for the C1 region of the HIV-1 envelope blocks binding and effector function of IgG. Proc Natl Acad Sci USA. 2013;110(22):9019–24.

103. Ackerman ME, Crispin M, Yu X, Baruah K, Boesch AW, Harvey DJ, Dugast AS, Heizen EL, Ercan A, Choi I, et al. Natural variation in Fc glycosylation of HIV-specific antibodies impacts antiviral activity. J Clin Invest. 2013;123(5):2183–92.

104. Simonich CA, Williams KL, Verkerke HP, Williams JA, Nduati R, Lee KK, Overbaugh J. HIV-1 neutralizing antibodies with limited hypermutation from an infant. Cell. 2016;166(1):77–87.

105. Simon AK, Hollander GA, McMichael A. Evolution of the immune system in humans from infancy to old age. Proc Biol Sci. 1821;2015(282):20143085.

106. Tobin NH, Aldrovandi GM. Immunology of pediatric HIV infection. Immunol Rev. 2013;254(1):143–69.

107. Siegrist CA, Aspinall R. B-cell responses to vaccination at the extremes of age. Nat Rev Immunol. 2009;9(3):185–94.

108. Francis T. On the doctrine of original antigenic sin. Proc Am Philos Soc. 1960;104(6):572–8.

109. Liao HX, Chen X, Munshaw S, Zhang R, Marshall DJ, Vandergrift N, Whitesides JF, Lu X, Yu JS, Hwang KK, et al. Initial antibodies binding to HIV-1 gp41 in acutely infected subjects are polyreactive and highly mutated. J Exp Med. 2011;208(11):2237–49.

110. Liu MF, Yang G, Wiehe K, Nicely NI, Vandergrift NA, Rountree W, Bonsignori M, Alam SM, Gao JY, Haynes BF, et al. Polyreactivity and autoreactivity among HIV-1 antibodies. J Virol. 2015;89(1):784–98.

111. Mouquet H, Scharf L, Euler Z, Liu Y, Eden C, Scheid JF, Halper-Stromberg A, Gnanapragasam PN, Spencer DI, Seaman MS, et al. Complex-type N-glycan recognition by potent broadly neutralizing HIV antibodies. Proc Natl Acad Sci USA. 2012;109(47):E3268–77.

112. Ghulam-Smith M, Olson A, White LF, Chasela CS, Ellington SR, Kourtis AP, Jamieson DJ, Tegha G, van der Horst CM, Sagar M. Maternal but not infant anti-HIV-1 neutralizing antibody response associates with enhanced transmission and infant morbidity. mBio. 2017;8(5):e01373-17.

113. Omenda MM, Milligan C, Odem-Davis K, Nduati R, Richardson BA, Lynch J, John-Stewart G, Overbaugh J. Evidence for efficient vertical transfer of maternal HIV-1 envelope-specific neutralizing antibodies but no association of such antibodies with reduced infant infection. J Acquir Immune Defic Syndr. 2013;64(2):163–6.

114. Lynch JB, Nduati R, Blish CA, Richardson BA, Mabuka JM, Jalalian-Lechak Z, John-Stewart G, Overbaugh J. The breadth and potency of passively acquired human immunodeficiency virus type 1-specific neutralizing antibodies do not correlate with the risk of infant infection. J Virol. 2011;85(11):5252–61.

115. Overbaugh J. Mother-infant HIV transmission: do maternal HIV-specific antibodies protect the infant? PLoS Pathog. 2014;10(8):e1004283.

116. Horwitz JA, Bar-On Y, Lu CL, Fera D, Lockhart AAK, Lorenzi JCC, Nogueira L, Golijanin J, Scheid JF, Seaman MS, et al. Non-neutralizing antibodies alter the course of HIV-1 infection in vivo. Cell. 2017;170(4):637–648. e610.

117. Richardson BA, Mbori-Ngacha D, Lavreys L, John-Stewart GC, Nduati R, Panteleeff DD, Emery S, Kreiss JK, Overbaugh J. Comparison of human immunodeficiency virus type 1 viral loads in Kenyan women, men, and infants during primary and early infection. J Virol. 2003;77(12):7120–3.

118. Shearer WT, Quinn TC, LaRussa P, Lew JF, Mofenson L, Almy S, Rich K, Handelsman E, Diaz C, Pagano M, et al. Viral load and disease progression in infants infected with human immunodeficiency virus type 1. Women and Infants Transmission Study Group. N Engl J Med. 1997;336(19):1337–42.

119. Wu X, Parast AB, Richardson BA, Nduati R, John-Stewart G, Mbori-Ngacha D, Rainwater SM, Overbaugh J. Neutralization escape variants of human immunodeficiency virus type 1 are transmitted from mother to infant. J Virol. 2006;80(2):835–44.

120. Sanders RW, van Gils MJ, Derking R, Sok D, Ketas TJ, Burger JA, Ozorowski G, Cupo A, Simonich C, Goo L, et al. HIV-1 VACCINES. HIV-1 neutralizing antibodies induced by native-like envelope trimers. Science. 2015;349(6244):4223.

Beyond the replication-competent HIV reservoir: transcription and translation-competent reservoirs

Amy E. Baxter[1,2], Una O'Doherty[3*] and Daniel E. Kaufmann[1,2*] (iD)

Abstract

Recent years have seen a substantial increase in the number of tools available to monitor and study HIV reservoirs. Here, we discuss recent technological advances that enable an understanding of reservoir dynamics beyond classical assays to measure the frequency of cells containing provirus able to propagate a spreading infection (replication-competent reservoir). Specifically, we focus on the characterization of cellular reservoirs containing proviruses able to transcribe viral mRNAs (so called transcription-competent) and translate viral proteins (translation-competent). We suggest that the study of these alternative reservoirs provides complementary information to classical approaches, crucially at a single-cell level. This enables an in-depth characterization of the cellular reservoir, both following reactivation from latency and, importantly, directly ex vivo at baseline. Furthermore, we propose that the study of cellular reservoirs that may not contain fully replication-competent virus, but are able to produce HIV mRNAs and proteins, is of biological importance. Lastly, we detail some of the key contributions that the study of these transcription and translation-competent reservoirs has made thus far to investigations into HIV persistence, and outline where these approaches may take the field next.

Keywords: HIV reservoirs, CD4 T cells, Flow cytometry, RNA flow cytometry, Fluorescence in situ hybridization

Background

Despite over 30 years of research and the tremendous successes of combined anti-retroviral therapy (ART), HIV remains a chronic disease for which there is no cure. In individuals receiving ART, the amount of circulating virus in the plasma is brought down to undetectable levels, as measured by current standard clinical assays. However, the virus is able to persist in the form of integrated proviruses in a predominantly CD4 T cell reservoir and will rebound from this cellular reservoir if therapy is discontinued [1–5]. Therefore, a key challenge for the field is how to identify cellular reservoirs of HIV [6], and crucially, how to measure the impact of potential

cure strategies on the replication-competent reservoir [7] as well as defective proviruses capable of expressing HIV proteins [8, 9].

Multiple techniques have been proposed, developed, and successfully utilized to identify the reservoir. Many of these techniques will be discussed in detail elsewhere in this series. Broadly, the majority of approaches focus on either the very early (DNA), or the very late (infectious virus) products of the viral life cycle. This focus has many advantages, but there are key limitations to be considered. For example, common PCR based techniques including the measure of total and integrated HIV DNA [2, 10] vastly overestimate the size of the reservoir due to the high prevalence of integrated, but "defective" proviruses [9, 11, 12]. On the other end of the scale, the Quantitative Viral Outgrowth Assay (Q-VOA), [4, 5, 13] and variants [14–16] may underestimate the size of the reservoir, as not all replication-competent proviruses are inducible with one round of stimulation [11] or able to

*Correspondence: unao@pennmedicine.upenn.edu; daniel.kaufmann@umontreal.ca
[1] CR-CHUM, Université de Montréal, Montréal, QC, Canada
[3] Department of Pathology and Laboratory Medicine, Division of Transfusion Medicine and Therapeutic Pathology, University of Pennsylvania, Philadelphia, PA, USA
Full list of author information is available at the end of the article

propagate in the in vitro conditions required for detection. Crucially, such approaches provide population-level, rather than single-cell level, information allowing only a quantification of the relative size of the reservoir, rather than in-depth reservoir characterization.

With these challenges in mind, we and others have sought a different way of characterizing and understanding HIV persistence (see Fig. 1). For example, while the maintenance of intact, replication-competent viruses is clearly a major barrier to HIV eradication, can transcription or translation-competent proviruses contribute to HIV pathogenesis on ART, and provide key insights into HIV persistence? We suggest that proviruses that may not be fully replication-competent, but that are capable of transcribing viral mRNAs and translating viral proteins, provide an additional dimension to persistence studies; and that the elimination of such proviruses should be considered in the context of a cure. Furthermore, we propose that the in-depth analysis of the cellular HIV reservoir at baseline, i.e. those cells containing proviruses that spontaneously produce viral products in ART-treated individuals in the absence of stimulation or reactivation, enables a deeper understanding and informative quantification of the response to latency reversing agents (LRAs) in the context of "shock/kick and kill" [17] and alternative cure strategies [18–20]. Here, we detail the initial studies of the transcription and translation-competent reservoirs, which have recently overcome issues of specificity and sensitivity, to begin to address these questions.

The approaches we describe uniquely investigate HIV reservoirs at the single-cell level; termed here cellular HIV reservoirs. The use of the word "cellular" distinguishes these measures from the more prevalent population-level analyses utilized in the field. Population-level analysis provide crucial insight into the size and nature of the reservoir; however we and others have demonstrated that studying the reservoir at a single-cell level can provide an additional critical understanding of the heterogeneity of the reservoir.

Lastly, we have avoided the term "latent" when describing these cellular HIV reservoirs since this phrase is commonly used to describe cells containing a provirus that

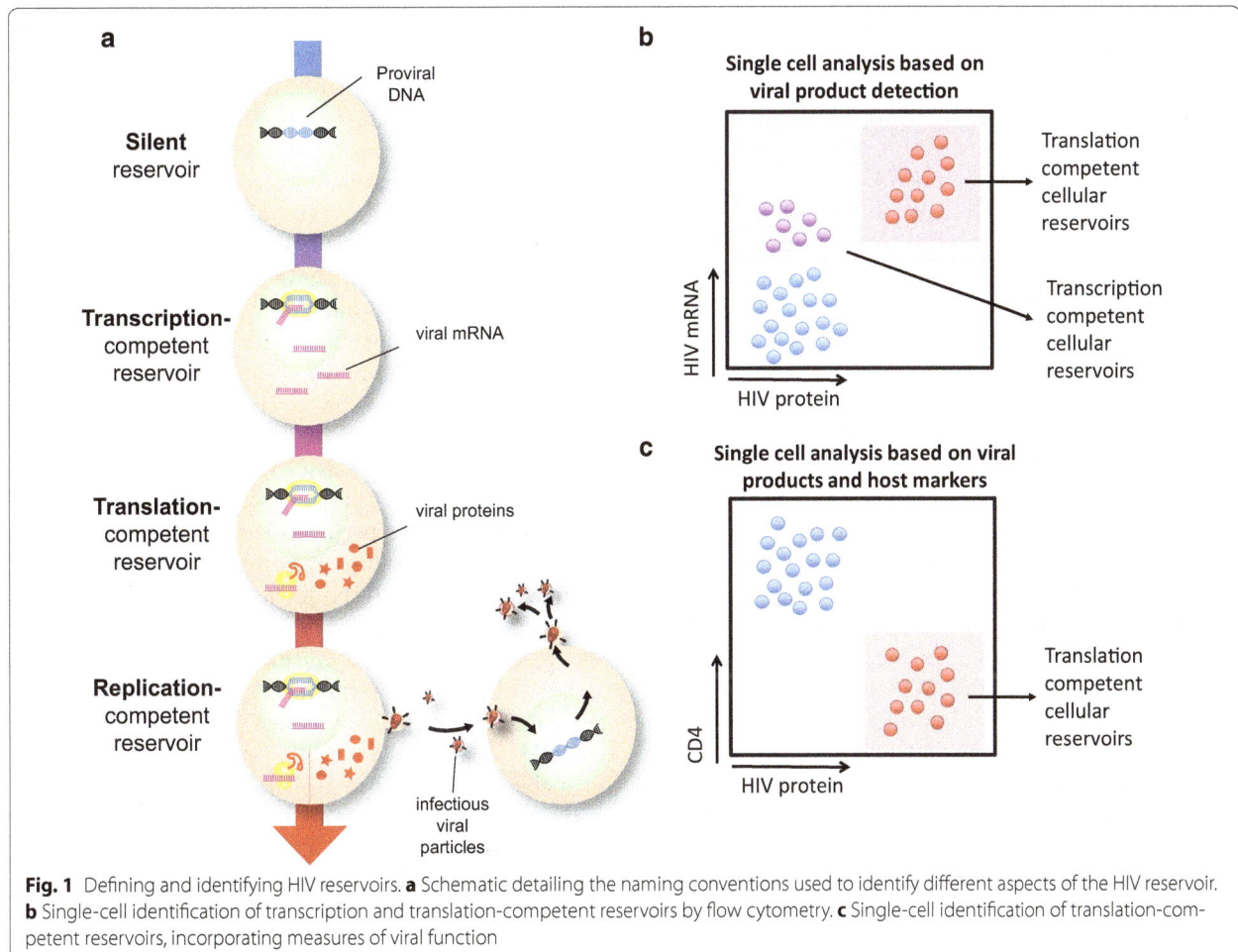

Fig. 1 Defining and identifying HIV reservoirs. **a** Schematic detailing the naming conventions used to identify different aspects of the HIV reservoir. **b** Single-cell identification of transcription and translation-competent reservoirs by flow cytometry. **c** Single-cell identification of translation-competent reservoirs, incorporating measures of viral function

is transcriptionally silent. However, we and others have shown that a rare subset of HIV-infected cells in individuals on long-term ART can express HIV mRNA and proteins in the absence of a spreading infection. By this definition, these cells are not latent at the time of detection, but, as has been suggested, might cycle back to a latent state and thus contribute to the latent HIV reservoir [21, 22].

Summary of HIV transcription and translation

The transcription and translation of the HIV genome has been studied in detail in vitro (reviewed in [23]). Briefly, the first fully spliced transcripts encode the HIV accessory proteins Tat and Rev [23, 24]. Tat is an essential regulatory protein for viral replication, which binds the HIV TAR (Trans-Acting Response element) RNA, inducing transcription [23]. In concert, Rev promotes HIV RNA nuclear export by binding the Rev Responsive Element (RRE) present in partially spliced and unspliced RNA [23]. Thus, as Tat and Rev protein levels increase, partially spliced RNAs are exported. In this manner, other accessory proteins, in addition to HIV Envelope (Env), are made. Lastly, unspliced mRNA forms are exported to the cytoplasm such that Gag and Pol are also translated, and viral particles are produced.

In addition, there are multiple levels of post-transcriptional regulation that can impact expression of viral mRNAs and proteins. These include mRNA splicing, RNA processing by microRNAs and nuclear export, as well as control at the translation level [23, 25]. In the context of HIV latency, these points of regulation remain underexplored [21, 26]. However, such post-transcriptional regulation should be taken into consideration when measuring HIV reservoirs based on detection of transcription or translation products. For example, a cell that is able to transcribe HIV mRNAs may not be able to translate HIV proteins, due to control at the post-transcriptional level [27].

While many studies have probed the control of HIV expression in T cell lines and activated T cells, little is known about the control of HIV expression in more quiescent or resting primary T cells. It is clear that activated T cells are much more effective at producing infectious virus than quiescent cells, producing 100-fold more HIV Gag RNA per provirus [28]. Whether HIV gene regulation has unique differences between resting and activated cells requires more investigation both in vitro and in vivo; primary models suggest that while splice products form in resting cells, the levels of fully and partially spliced mRNAs are ~ 100-fold lower than in activated cells [28]. Thus, further work building on the lessons learned from the study of in vitro latency models is required to determine how HIV expression is controlled in vivo [29].

Measuring transcription-competent cellular reservoirs

Relatively early in the epidemic, prior to the discovery and widespread implementation of potent ART regimens, multiple groups reported the detection of HIV RNA species within CD4 T cells from chronically HIV-infected individuals using PCR-based approaches [30, 31]. The advent of potent ART-induced viral suppression saw the detection of such cell-associated (CA)-RNA applied to the latent HIV reservoir. In the late 2000s, Fischer and colleagues provided a key insight into the significance of this transcription-competent reservoir (Fig. 1a) by monitoring multiple forms of RNA within cells, and measuring the frequency of RNA-expressing cells at limiting dilution in HIV-infected individuals as they began therapy. They observed that HIV CA-RNA measures decayed drastically when compared to HIV DNA measures within the same individual [32], and suggested that ~ 5% of cells containing HIV DNA also expressed HIV RNA in individuals on ART [33]. Importantly, more recent work using a nested PCR approach confirmed that the HIV mRNAs detected predominantly resulted from genuine HIV mRNA transcription, rather than chimeric read-through products transcribed from host promoters [34]. This work clearly demonstrated the relevance of cellular RNA-based measures for investigations in cure strategies, and is discussed in depth elsewhere in this series [35]. As with measures of HIV DNA, most classical CA-RNA measures are based upon modified versions of real-time PCR for various HIV mRNA species [36]. Crucially, therefore, this approach provides population-level information, allowing a quantification of the relative size of the reservoir in HIV-infected individuals, but does not enable an in-depth analysis of the cellular nature of the reservoir. With this in mind, we and others have applied various approaches to detect single cells containing a provirus able to produce HIV RNA species; termed the transcription-competent cellular reservoir.

The first studies of transcription-competent cellular HIV reservoirs were performed in the pre-ART era to investigate key questions regarding HIV pathogenesis. In situ hybridization (ISH) for HIV mRNA was used to identify and describe the persistence of HIV-infected cells in the lymph nodes, in particular in the germinal centers, of HIV-infected infected subjects in the clinically latent stage of disease when plasma viral loads are low [37]. Later, a quantification system was developed to enable the frequencies of these HIV mRNA+ cells to be compared between tissues and between samples from different individuals [38]. In more recent years, this technique has been transferred to the study of SIV in non-human primate models and has provided valuable insights into the pathogenesis of and immune response to

HIV [39, 40]. While powerful, microscopy-based ISH is limited by its relatively low throughput. In the context of chronic, untreated HIV infection, the prevalence of HIV-infected cells is sufficient to enable detection, but still requires laborious analysis of many sections to obtain robust quantitation. However the frequency of such cells is dramatically reduced in ART-treated individuals. Thus, additional, complementary high-throughput techniques were required to investigate very high number of cells to identify these rare events and characterize the cellular reservoir that persisted in individuals on ART.

The late 1990s saw the advent of a new era in immunology; that of multiparametric flow cytometry. This high-throughput approach was soon applied to the study of cellular HIV sanctuaries in HIV-infected, untreated individuals. Patterson and colleagues pioneered an approach based on reverse-transcriptase (RT)-PCR-based amplification and Fluoresence ISH (FISH) detection of intracellular HIV RNA [41], and later a probe-based approach termed SUSHI (simultaneous ultrasensitive subpopulation staining/hybridization in situ, [42–44]). While these approaches provided a key proof of concept for the field, as the authors note, the frequencies of HIV mRNA$^+$ cells detected with these assays are generally higher than would be predicted based on measurements of integrated HIV DNA [41]. This indicates a potential issue with false positive detection that may hamper interpretation of this data.

Building on this pioneering initial work, in recent years a new version of these ISH technologies sought to overcome the issues of high background/nonspecific staining and low signal-to-noise ratios, which limited earlier iterations. In 2012 Wang et al. [45] detailed a microscopy technique known as RNAscope. This approach builds on a branched DNA (bDNA) technique described previously [46], but added additional levels of stringency to reduce off-target binding. Briefly, a series of DNA probes are designed whereby each probe has two sections; the first recognizes the target mRNA and the second forms part of a conserved "tail" sequence. The probes are designed such that pairs of probes which recognize adjacent regions of the target mRNA each contain one half of this conserved tail. Only this combined "tail" sequence can be recognized by a DNA pre-amplifier, which in turn is recognized by a secondary amplifier. This amplified structure is then labeled with a fluorescent probe, or an alkaline phosphatase or horseradish peroxidase (HRP) molecule. The requirement for the two probes (known as a "Z") to bind adjacent to one another in order for the pre-amplifier to bind substantially reduces off-target binding.

Those in the HIV cure field quickly recognized the significance of this approach. The application of this technique to microscopy has been advanced in particular by the Estes laboratory, who have demonstrated the increased sensitivity and high specificity of this assay when compared to alternative ISH approaches (see Table 1 [47, 48]). The low background is particularly striking; the team imaged nearly 70 mm^2 of uninfected tissue from rhesus macaques and identified only two false-positive RNA$^+$ cells [47]. Recently, this group has successfully applied this technology to quantify transcription-competent cellular SIV reservoirs across a broad range of tissues in both untreated and ART-treated animals, confirming the predominance of lymphoid tissues as a key reservoir [49]. While HIV RNA$^+$ cells were identified in untreated subjects, further work is required to determine if such cells can be readily identified in ART-treated individuals.

In parallel, this approach was applied to flow cytometry, and developed by our group and others in collaboration with the company Affymetrix (now part of ThermoFisher) into a commercial RNAflow assay known as PrimeFlow^{TM}. It was quickly utilized for the high-throughput, high-sensitivity detection of cellular mRNAs [50]. Thus far, three groups have reportedly applied this RNAflow technology to the flow-cytometric study of transcription-competent HIV reservoirs (Fig. 1b, Table 1), with variations in terms of the specificity of the assay and therefore applicability of the approach to studying samples directly from HIV-infected, and particularly ART-treated, individuals [51]. While Altfeld and colleagues successfully applied the technique to the detection of in vitro HIV-infected cells and cell lines, they reported that the sensitivity of this iteration was unlikely to be sufficient to detect HIV mRNA-expressing cells directly in HIV-infected subjects [52]. Similarly, we noted that the *GagPol* probes used in this study showed relatively high background (in the range of ~ 1000 *GagPol* mRNA false-positive events per million CD4 T cells in HIV-uninfected donors) precluding the detection of the transcription-competent reservoir in our hands [53, 54].

More recently, however, Grau-Expósito et al. [55] reported a high-sensitivity version of the RNAflow assay which used 50 probes sets designed against the *GagPol* region of the conserved HXB2 genome. While the authors also reported false-positive event detection in HIV-uninfected individuals, this was taken into account by subtracting this "false-positive" detection rate from the frequency of events detected in HIV-infected samples. The group concludes that this allows a data normalization and present data suggesting that this is reproducible between experiments. Indeed, this mathematical approach may enable quantification of the transcription-competent reservoir. However, such an approach relies on the relative stability of the "false-positive" population between experiments, and furthermore

Table 1 Comparison of single-cell approaches to measure the transcription- and translation-competent reservoirs

Cellular reservoir measured	Assay	Assay overview	Advantages	Limitations	Potential applications	Key references
Transcription-competent cellular reservoir	RNAflow cytometry	Detection of cells expressing HIV RNA in suspension by fluorescence in situ hybridisation (FISH) using branched DNA (bDNA) technology	High throughput In depth phenotyping of single cells Highly flexible and adaptable	Background observed in HIV-uninfected individuals Labour intensive (2–3 days protocol) High starting cell number required	LRA screening Reservoir quantification In depth phenotyping of the reservoir Biomarker discovery	[52, 55]
	Simultaneous ultrasensitive subpopulation staining/hybridization in situ (SUSHI)	Detection of cells expressing HIV RNA in suspension by fluorescence in situ hybridisation (FISH)	High throughput	Higher than predicted frequencies of mRNA$^+$ cells observed	Reservoir quantification Phenotyping of single cells, including myeloid cells	[41–44]
	Conventional in situ hybridization	Detection of cells expressing HIV RNA in situ using radiolabelled or enzymatic detection	Tissue level information	Limited cell phenotyping Labour intensive	Reservoir quantification in tissues	[37, 38, 47, 48]
	RNAScope	Detection of cells expressing HIV RNA in situ using branched DNA amplification and detection	Tissue level information Highly sensitive and specific Short assay duration	Limited cell phenotyping	Reservoir quantification in tissues/whole body	[47–49]
Translation-competent cellular reservoir	Fiber optic array scanning technology (FAST)	Antibody-based detection of cells expressing HIV protein and down-regulating CD4, in suspension	Relatively high throughput Short assay duration	Specialized microscopy tools and software required Limited cell phenotyping	LRA screening Reservoir quantification	[62]
	RNAflow cytometry	Concurrent detection of cells expressing HIV RNA by FISH using branched DNA (bDNA) technology, and HIV protein in suspension	High linearity and specificity High throughput In depth phenotyping of single cells Highly flexible and adaptable	Labour intensive (2–3 days protocol) High starting cell number required	LRA screening Reservoir quantification In depth phenotyping of the reservoir Biomarker discovery	[53–55]

this "false-positive" population will still effectively contaminate the true positive HIV-infected population. This contamination therefore precludes an in-depth phenotyping analysis of these rare HIV mRNA$^+$ cells, particularly in samples from ART-treated individuals where the frequencies of mRNA$^+$ cells is close to the limit of detection.

Thus, while this assay shows great promise, the applicability for the detection of transcription-competent cellular reservoirs in samples from treated patients remains unclear. Previous studies using highly-sensitive, limiting dilution RT-PCR demonstrated that low levels of HIV *gag* mRNA could be detected in a subset, only ~ 5%, of HIV DNA-containing cells in subjects on ART [33]. Using a dilution assay, Grau-Expósito et al. demonstrated that the detection of mRNA$^+$ cells was linear down to the lowest dilution tested (50 events per million cells). Accordingly, in samples from untreated HIV-infected individuals, the median frequency of mRNA$^+$ events detected was above this threshold at ~ 165 per million CD4 T cells. However, unsurprisingly, these events were much rarer in samples from ART-treated individuals (~ 6–20 per million CD4 T cells in the absence of stimulation [55]). Therefore further validation may be required to ensure that this approach is linear down to the ranges required for the robust evaluation of cure therapies.

A further key consideration of such flow-cytometric mRNA-based detection assays is the sensitivity of these approaches in terms of the number of mRNA copies that a cell must express to be detected. To address this question, Baxter et al. performed a confocal microscopy analysis of CD4 T cells from a HIV-negative individual, processed with the HIV$^{RNA/Gag}$ assay. They observed a mean of ~ 7 false-positive *GagPol* mRNA spots per cell; providing a conservative detection limit of ~ 20 *GagPol* mRNA copies per cell (+3 standard deviations, [53]). This limit enabled identification of ~ 94% of *GagPol* mRNA$^+$ cells from a HIV-infected individual. Therefore, an HIV-infected cell containing at least 20 copies of HIV mRNA is highly likely to be truly infected (0.15% false positive discovery rate for a Gaussian distribution); however an infected cell with fewer copies of HIV RNA is more likely to be missed. Crucially, the number of spots per cell was closely associated with the total fluorescence intensity of the cell, suggesting this approach enables a relative quantification of mRNA copy number [53].

Importantly, however, this analysis makes the assumption that each "spot" represents one mRNA copy, which may not be accurate. Furthermore, the number of copies required for detection varies according to the number of probe set pairs that bind to each mRNA; thus the selection of probe sets and the heterogeneity of the target mRNA are key variables [54]. In a hypothetical example,

consider two samples. In the first sample, the probe sets and the viral mRNA sequence match perfectly, therefore if 50 probe sets are available, 50 probe sets will bind. In the second sample, there is a high degree of sequence mismatches with the original sequence used to design the probes; although 50 probe sets are available, only ten are able to bind the target mRNA. Therefore, for a cell in the second sample to reach the same total fluorescence intensity as a cell in the first sample, five-times as many mRNA copies may be required. While this is an oversimplification, it demonstrates a key point that these assays may "miss" true HIV-infected cells due to sequence heterogeneity. One potential solution is to design individual probes for each patient after sequencing the patient's virus, but this may be prohibitively costly. Given this point, and those raised above, work in our laboratory and others is ongoing to increase both the specificity and the sensitivity, and therefore the applicability, of these RNA-flow assays to the detection of the transcription-competent cellular reservoirs.

Measuring translation-competent cellular reservoirs

A key consideration in the measurement of transcription-competent reservoirs is that not all of the cells detected as HIV mRNA$^+$ contain proviruses able to produce infectious virions, or even HIV protein (Fig. 1a). Indeed, defective and hypermutated RNAs, including those containing APOBEC-mediated G-to-A hypermutations, have been readily detected in HIV-infected individuals [56–58]. Furthermore, given the high prevalence of defective mRNAs detected following latency reversal/reactivation, it has been hypothesized that RNAs containing major mutations may be more susceptible to reactivation and thus more likely to be detected [57]. Therefore, to add a further level of stringency to these approaches, we and others have focused on the identification of the translation-competent cellular reservoir. We suggest that a cell containing a provirus that is capable of HIV protein translation at a high level is more likely to be replication-competent than a provirus detected only as integrated HIV DNA or capable of producing only HIV RNAs. However, previous reports have indicated that a fraction of "defective" proviruses are capable of producing some HIV proteins, particularly *pol* mutants [8, 58, 59]. Thus, while we acknowledge that not all translation-competent proviruses identified are also replication-competent, we propose that the translation-competent cellular reservoir is substantially enriched for replication competence compared to, for example, the integrated HIV DNA reservoir.

The first compelling evidence that HIV reservoirs could be translating HIV proteins came from in vitro models. HIV Gag protein was used as a target, as this protein is expressed at very high levels in HIV-infected cells and each virion incorporates ~ 5000 Gag particles [60]. HIV Gag was detected in a small fraction of resting T cells after direct infection in vitro (Gag[+], [28]), however this represented only a minority of the cells containing integrated HIV DNA. Whether these Gag[+] cells were an in vitro artifact or had a counterpart in vivo was unclear until recently [53, 55, 61]. The first evidence that HIV Gag could be expressed in resting CD4[+] T cells in vivo came from the sorting of resting HIV Gag[+] non CD4-lineage negative PBMCs from HIV-infected subjects. In the order of ~ 1 Gag[+] cell per million PBMCs were detected from ART-treated individuals [61]. However, this technique was labor intensive and fraught with false positives. While Gag[+] cells were enriched for HIV DNA, only 10% of the sorted Gag[+] cells contained HIV DNA. Thus, this approach provided key evidence that HIV protein expression likely occurred in T cells in ART-treated subjects, but indicated that more sensitive methods were required.

Detection of HIV cellular reservoirs was further advanced by exploiting HIV's ability to downregulate CD4 as a surrogate marker for cellular reservoirs (Fig. 1c) [53, 55, 62]. A well-known function of Nef, Env and Vpu is the downmodulation of CD4 in activated T cell infection [63–68]. In vitro experiments showed that after direct infection of resting CD4[+] T cells a subset of cells with integrated HIV DNA were Gag[+] and negative for surface CD4, suggesting internalization and downregulation of CD4 [62]. Sorted Gag[+]CD4[−] cells contained HIV proviruses by Alu-gag PCR, proving the presence of Gag was not due to bound virions. Moreover, extensive phenotyping confirmed that these were genuine TCRαβ CD4 T cells with internalized CD4. Mutational analysis showed that Nef and Env, but not Vpu, were required for CD4 internalization, suggesting that if an HIV-infected cell downregulates CD4 it is likely that additional HIV open reading frames (including *env*, *nef*, *tat*, and *rev*) are intact and expressed. Thus, to express Gag and to downregulate CD4, a large fraction of the 3′ and 5′ regions of the HIV genome must be intact.

These in vitro experiments suggested that an approach combining detection of Gag protein expression with CD4 downregulation could be used to identify translation-competent cellular reservoirs. However, sorting strategies, while useful for proof of principle, proved impractical. Thus, the O'Doherty lab introduced a different approach (Table 1, [62]). They exploited a rare cell detection technique used in cancer detection, FAST (Fiber-optic Array Scanning Technology [69–71]), to scan up to 20 million cells adhered to a slide, followed with Automated Digital Microscopy to confirm the cellular phenotype. Applying this rationale and technology enabled imaging of high numbers of PBMCs from ART-treated patients, stained for intracellular CD4 and Gag protein. Indeed, they identified Gag[+] cells at low frequencies (0.33–2.7 events per million PBMCs), many of which were CD4[−], or showed punctate internalized CD4 staining. The absence of surface CD4 suggests that indeed, the majority of these cells contain a translation-competent HIV provirus and are distinct from the false-positive Gag[+] events observed in HIV-uninfected individuals [62]. The key strength of FAST combined with Automated Digital Microscopy is the lower false positive rate compared to classical Gag staining by flow cytometry. While FAST has the potential to be high throughput, the technique is still in early development, the confirmation of positive results by Automated Digital Microscopy is time intensive and this technology is not widely available. Therefore, alternative methods to detect the translation-competent cellular reservoir were required.

Combining measures of transcription and translation-competent cellular reservoirs

Combining HIV protein detection with HIV RNA detection provided a key breakthrough to overcome the hurdle of false positive signals, using a high-throughput routinely available technology [52, 53]. These approaches utilize the simultaneous detection of HIV *GagPol* mRNA using the RNAflow technique described above [55], along with concurrent intracellular antibody staining for HIV Gag protein [61], (Fig. 1b, Table 1). While Martrus et al. [52] found that the specificity of this dual-staining approach was also insufficient for the analysis of samples from HIV-infected individuals, Baxter et al. [53, 54] were able to identify translation-competent cellular reservoirs in samples from chronic, untreated HIV-infected individuals and, crucially, in ART-treated individuals following in vitro restimulation. This approach was coined as the HIV[RNA/Gag] assay. As discussed above, key considerations for such assays are the sequence homology between the probes and the target mRNA and the number of probes required. We designed probes against a lab-adapted strain JR-CSF and found that the redundancy afforded by the use of a high number of probe sets (40 total against *gag* and *pol* [53]) was sufficient to overcome the majority of the sequence heterogeneity in primary subject samples. Crucially, the false positive detection rate when protein and mRNA detection was combined was exceptionally low, with only one HIV *GagPol* mRNA[+,] Gag protein[+] (HIV[RNA+/Gag+]) event detected in nearly 8 million CD4 T cells from HIV-negative individuals. In comparison, the high false positive rate based on HIV mRNA or protein expression alone masked the detection of translation-competent cellular reservoirs [54]. Furthermore, this iteration was highly linear and specific;

bringing these two advances together enabled the detection of 0.5–1 $HIV^{RNA+/Gag+}$ events per million CD4 T cells.

Importantly, the high specificity and flow-cytometric basis of this approach enabled multi-parameter, in-depth phenotyping of the translation-competent cellular HIV reservoir that were not previously possible. For example, consistent with observations made by the O'Doherty laboratory [62], cells identified as $HIV^{RNA+/Gag+}$ strongly downregulated CD4. Moreover, $HIV^{RNA+/Gag+}$ cells were enriched in the circulating T follicular helper cell population [53] and cells expressing inhibitory receptors, consistent with previous reports [72–75]. These examples demonstrate the importance of a low false-positive detection in measuring HIV cellular reservoirs.

Lastly, while Grau-Expósito et al. [55] focused on the transcription-competent cellular reservoir, they also identified a subset of mRNA-expressing cells which expressed viral Gag protein, and thus were also able to identify the translation-competent reservoir as a subpopulation of the transcription-competent cellular reservoir. An area of key further interest is to determine what features (viral or host) may distinguish these two different reservoirs.

Taken together, this work demonstrates that the detection of multiple HIV viral products, or the downstream consequences of these products such as loss of CD4 expression, can overcome the issue of false positive events. Furthermore, we suggest that this multi-faceted approach increases the likelihood that a translation-competent cellular reservoir contains a replication-competent provirus. Nonetheless, careful controls for false positive signals are imperative and additional work is required to determine which fraction of the translation-competent cellular reservoir is truly replication-competent.

Why measure transcription and translation-competent cellular reservoirs?
Closing the gap between DNA quantitation and measures of replication-competent virus
A crucial caveat in the measurement of transcription/translation-competent cellular reservoirs is that not all cells detected by these assays may contain a virus able to initiate a spreading infection in vivo: a replication-competent provirus. However, we suggest that the detection of cells containing proviruses able to produce viral mRNA and proteins is biologically and scientifically relevant. Secondly, we propose that the populations of HIV-infected cells detected by these approaches are likely to be highly enriched for replication-competent virus. Thus, measuring the translation-competent cellular reservoir after latency reversal may be an appropriate and informative surrogate for detection of replication-competent

proviruses. Optimistically, such approaches may overcome the gap between the overestimation of the reservoir size measured by DNA-centric techniques and the reported underestimation of the reservoir size by the Q-VOA.

To address this second point, both the Buzon and Kaufmann laboratories observed associations with their measures of the cellular reservoir and DNA-based measures, which commonly overestimate the size of the translation-competent reservoir [76]. Baxter et al. also observed a correlation between levels of integrated HIV DNA and the frequency of the translation-competent cellular reservoir in samples from ART-treated individuals following in vitro stimulation with PMA/ionomycin. Interestingly though, DNA measures and the frequency of $HIV^{RNA+/Gag+}$ cells were not associated at baseline. Importantly, the frequency of the cells detected as transcription/translation-competent cellular reservoirs is substantially lower than the number of copies of HIV DNA detected (~ 160-fold lower [55] and ~ 200-fold lower [53]). This difference suggests that measurement of the transcription/translation-competent cellular reservoirs identify a population that is substantially closer to the replication-competent reservoir than DNA measures.

On the other end of the scale, both groups compared their measures to the Q-VOA, which estimates the replication-competent reservoir at frequencies ~ 1000-fold lower than DNA-based approaches at ~ 1 event per million resting CD4 T cells [76], although this likely represents an underestimation [6]. Interestingly, neither group identified a correlation between the frequency of the transcription/translation-competent reservoirs with the Q-VOA. Crucially, the frequency of events detected were higher than, but in the same order of magnitude as, the IUPM. For example, Baxter et al. [53] identified a median frequency of ~ 4.7 $HIV^{RNA+/Gag\,protein+}$ events per million CD4 T cells following PMA/ionomycin stimulation, compared to a QVOA reading of 1.4 IUPM (Infectious Units per Million) from the same subjects. The similarities between measurements made by IUPM and the translation-competent reservoir after latency reversal further indicate that these measures close in on the true replication-competent reservoir. There are multiple differences between the assays which could explain the lack of a correlation between these two measurement types, including but not limited to the detection of non-replication competent reservoirs within the transcription/translation-competent cellular reservoir population and the stimulation used [11] and the statistical variation predicted by Poisson distribution when detecting exceptionally rare cells [54]. Such differences should be considered when comparing the two assays.

Uncovering a unique aspect of the reservoir

A key rationale behind measuring the transcription- and translation-competent reservoirs is the additional level of detailed, complementary information that can be gained from the study of this form of the reservoir. As discussed above, many of the techniques used to identify the transcription- and/or translation-competent reservoirs provide information at a single-cell level, as they are often flow cytometry or microscopy-based. This means that an individual cell can be probed for multiple parameters of interest in addition to HIV RNA/protein, such as cellular activation, exhaustion or memory markers [52, 53, 55, 62, 77]. In contrast, PCR-based techniques and the Q-VOA provide only population-level comparative information (i.e. population A contains a higher proportion of HIV DNA than population B). This is particularly important to consider in the context of the wide heterogeneity of the cellular reservoir; when assessing cure strategies it is of paramount importance to understand how all subpopulations of the cellular reservoir respond, rather than treating the reservoir as a homogenous entity. For example, while it has previously been reported that both the central, transitional and effector memory T cell populations contain HIV DNA, there are conflicting reports regarding whether replication-competent virus is predominantly localized in the central memory compartment [78], or the effector memory compartment [79]. CD4 T cells expressing exhaustion markers including PD-1, LAG-3 and TIGIT have been shown to be enriched for HIV DNA, but this enrichment is further dependent on the state of CD4 T cell differentiation [75]. Furthermore, expression of multiple inhibitory receptors on CD4 T cells prior to ART has been identified as a predictive biomarker of viral rebound following treatment interruption; this suggests that the expression of such markers may also identify a subpopulation of latently infected cells with a higher proclivity to viral transcription [80]. From only these limited examples, it is apparent that analysis of bulk CD4 memory populations would prevent an understanding of these subtleties. While sorting individual CD4 T cell populations for downstream analysis is possible, this becomes less feasible when analyzing exceedingly rare CD4 T cell subpopulations, and quickly limited in terms of the number of populations that can be concurrently analyzed. As the approaches we have described for the analysis of the transcription- and translation-competent cellular reservoirs, particularly those which are flow cytometry-based, overcome these limitations, these techniques will become increasingly useful for in-depth characterization of the HIV reservoir.

An additional strength of these techniques is the ability to compare in vitro models and validation experiments with in vivo-infected T cells. Spina et al. [81] previously indicated the limitations of latency models to fully recapitulate latency reversal, however we suggest that the lessons learnt from in vitro models can advance in vivo research. For example, the in vitro observations of a rare Gag+ populations in resting CD4 T cells have been supported by the in vivo detection of this population directly in samples from ART-treated individuals [61, 62]. Using the HIV$^{RNA/Gag}$ assay, the in vitro observation of a down-regulation of HLA-Class I on HIV$^{RNA+/Gag+}$ cells was confirmed. In contrast, however, HLA-Class II-expressing CD4 T cells were enriched for both HIV mRNAs and protein only in ex vivo samples [53]. Therefore, such approaches can be used to both investigate HIV biology in vivo, but also to build upon key observations made in in vitro models.

Quantifying the HIV reservoir at the single-cell level in ART-treated subjects

We further suggest that a highly useful aspect of this type of measurement is the ability to quantify the HIV reservoir in ART-treated individuals at the single-cell level (i.e. directly ex vivo in ART-treated subject samples). Such measurements capture a distinct view of the reservoir; this represents the cells from ART-treated individuals that spontaneously reactivate the provirus to produce HIV mRNA, protein, and perhaps viral particles, in the absence of a spreading infection and/or exogenous stimulation [15, 49, 53]. We speculate that the cells containing transcription/translation-competent virus that are producing HIV mRNA and/or protein might revert to a latent state before dying from viral cytotoxicity or immune clearance [22]. Therefore, investigating these cells could provide insight into the single-cell phenotype of the latent reservoir. In addition, plasma sequences identified during viral rebound following treatment interruption match proviruses in cells that were already expressing HIV mRNA before ART was stopped. This indicates that clones of these proviruses likely contributed to the rebound viremia [56]. Thus, defining those single cells that contain transcription/translation-competent viruses and produce viral products during ART may help identify the cell population from which viral rebound may occur.

Furthermore, we propose that quantification of the cellular reservoir in ART-treated individuals in the absence of stimulation can provide a more nuanced understanding of the reactivation of the latent reservoir in response to stimulation. It should be noted that the persistent HIV reservoir in ART-treated individuals has been extensively studied at the population level. As discussed in detail elsewhere in this review series, classical measurements such as cell-associated RNA and integrated DNA have been used to monitor total HIV reservoir size during suppressive ART [36, 82, 83]. Using these approaches, the reservoir is readily quantifiable. In contrast, the detection of alternatively spliced mRNAs by TILDA did not observe spliced mRNA production without in vitro stimulation in all samples studied [84]. Given these differences, we suggest that the quantification of this persistent reservoir at the single cell level could provide key insights. However, such studies have only been conducted in detail recently. Using single-cell RNAflow based approaches, HIV mRNA-expressing CD4 T cells were robustly identified in samples from 2 of 6 virally suppressed ART-treated individuals [55], while HIV$^{RNA+/Gag+}$ CD4 T cells were detected in 8 samples, from a total of 14 [53]. Using the FAST approach, Gag protein^{+} cells were identified in all five of the subjects studied [61], including one individual who was repeatedly sampled over several years. In those samples where translation/transcription competent cellular reservoirs were detected, the frequencies ranged from ~ 10 mRNA^{+} to ~ 1.0 HIV$^{RNA+/Gag+}$ events per million CD4 T cells. Given these frequencies, we postulate that one of the major issues when monitoring this baseline cellular reservoir is the number of cells studied. The lower the total number of cells analyzed in the assay, the lower the probability of detecting the very rare cells infected with HIV [54]. In studies performed by our laboratories we routinely assess two-four million CD4 T cells [53], or six-eighteen million PBMCs [62] to enable detection of these rare cells. The analysis of such a high number of cells is made possible only by the use of the high-throughput approaches, but nonetheless, detection of these rare cells remains challenging requiring significant expertise and is constrained by the size of available clinical samples. While such limitations must be considered, studying the transcription/translation-competent reservoirs can provide additional information regarding the nature of the HIV reservoir at baseline as well as after stimulation.

Detailing a biologically relevant population
We suggest here that the transcription/translation-competent cellular reservoir may contribute to both the persistent reservoir and importantly the pathogenesis of HIV on ART, and are thus biologically relevant. If this is the case, these cells, not only cells containing replication-competent viruses, need to be considered in the context of HIV cure.

T cell exhaustion and ongoing immune activation are characteristic features of chronic infections [85], including HIV [86–89], and are driven in part by exposure to persistent antigen [90]. In the presence of suppressive ART, HIV antigen levels should be low, however, p24 and Env protein products can still be detected in the plasma of HIV-infected individuals under long-term (~ 10 years)

of suppressive therapy [9]. Furthermore, ultrasensitive techniques have detected very low level viremia in ART-treated individuals [91, 92]. Additionally, the ongoing production of HIV proteins from "defective" proviruses has been demonstrated [8, 59, 62]. Such observations have led to the term "zombie" proviruses, as while "defective" proviruses may not be "alive", they still may contribute to HIV pathogenesis on ART [59]. These points indicate that the translation-competent cellular reservoir may contribute to continued antigen presence, either through the production of replication-competent virus in the absence of spreading infection at baseline, or through viral protein production only. Crucially though, the precise role of HIV antigen in the persistence of immune activation remains unclear, particularly as HIV antigens are very unlikely to be the only drivers of ongoing immune dysfunction; products from microbial translocation [93, 94] and concurrent viral infections such as CMV and EBV are likely to contribute [95]. While further work is required to determine the significance of the translation-competent reservoir in regards to T cell dysfunction, we suggest that the clearance of such translation-competent cellular reservoirs may need to be considered in addition to the removal of replication-competent virus in the context of a HIV cure.

In addition to contributing to immune activation, viral protein production, possibly from "defective" proviruses may explain the continued presence of antibodies against HIV [9] and indeed may shape the antibody repertoire. Furthermore, a recent study from the Ho/Siliciano lab suggested that cells expressing viral proteins, even from "defective" proviruses, can be recognized and killed by cytotoxic T lymphocytes (CTL) [58]. In support of this finding, other groups have also reported immune-based clearance of HIV-infected cells measured by loss of HIV/SIV DNA, implying that some expression of defective proviruses must be occurring [96–99]. Accordingly, anti-HIV CTL activity in vitro is strongly correlated with viral DNA levels in vivo [61]. As with the antibody repertoire, it is likely that such interactions may also shape the CTL landscape.

Lessons from the study of transcription/translation-competent reservoirs: an evolving field
The contribution of multiple groups to the study of the transcription/translation-competent reservoirs have provided key insights into the biology of HIV reservoirs, the cellular identity of the reservoir, and the efficiency of cure strategies. A number of groups have reported the association of the size of the transcription/translation-competent reservoirs with subject characteristics and indicators of disease progression in untreated HIV infection. For example the size of these reservoirs is inversely correlated

with both CD4/CD8 ratio and plasma viral load [53, 55]. In ART-treated individuals, the CD4 T cell count and CD4/CD8 ratio are important indicators of the immunological response to therapy. A poor reconstitution of the CD4 T cell compartment is associated with increased morbidity and mortality among ART-treated subjects, and is correlated with a larger latent HIV reservoir [100–102]. In line with this suggestion, the level of integrated HIV DNA has been inversely associated with CD4 T cell count [103] and CD4/CD8 ratio [103–106]. Correspondingly an inverse correlation was also observed between the size of the PMA/ionomycin-inducible translation-competent reservoir and the CD4/CD8 ratio [53]. This suggests that a smaller translation-competent reservoir is also associated with increased immunological recovery in response to ART, indicating the potential clinical significance of this reservoir measure.

The approaches pioneered to investigate the HIV cellular reservoir have raised the possibility that there may be distinctions between the subsets of cells captured as the translation-competent versus the transcription competent reservoir. For example, T cell memory populations, in particular the central memory population, contains the majority of HIV DNA in subject on ART [103]. While Baxter et al. [53] observed a comparable distribution between the central and effector memory subsets of HIV$^{RNA+/Gag+}$ cells, Grau-Expósito et al. [55] observed that the effector memory population contained a significantly higher frequency of mRNA$^+$ cells than all other memory subsets. Furthermore they identified the same enrichment in the baseline transcription-competent reservoir in ART-treated individuals. While further work is required to determine if the discrepancies between the Buzon and Kaufmann lab studies represent a biologically significant difference between the transcription and translation-competent reservoirs, or if this variation is due to experimental/technical or cohort differences, these data demonstrate the variety and detail of information that such techniques can provide.

The power of this single-cell approach is evident in latency reversal studies, where the RNAflow approach allows simultaneous monitoring of HIV mRNA$^+$ cells, and co-expression of HIV Gag protein, in response to stimulation with PMA/ionomycin and clinical LRAs. For example, while romidepsin stimulation resulted in a ~ fourfold increase in the frequencies of mRNA$^+$ cells, the majority of this population did not express Gag protein, in contrast to stimulation with PMA/ionomycin which led to a substantial increase in the frequency of dual expressing CD4 T cells [55]. This difference may be explained simply by the time point studied, as the kinetics of latency reversal are likely to differ between LRAs so the mRNA$^+$ cells may become positive for Gag protein

at a later time point. In support of the former explanation, when the kinetics of latency reversal was monitored in vitro, an mRNA$^+$ population rapidly appeared that became Gag protein$^+$ over 48 h [52]. Alternatively, the authors suggest that romidepsin may be able to stimulate HIV transcription, but not translation [27], as has previously been observed in vitro using alternative approaches for inducible reservoir measurement [15, 107]. While in a small clinical trial, romidepsin infusions increased plasma HIV-1 RNA levels in 5 of 6 participants, it has not been determined whether this increase in plasma RNA represents true de novo production of virus from reactivated latent proviruses [108], as 3 of these subjects were receiving protease inhibitors as part of their ART. Therefore, further work is required to determine the effectiveness of romidepsin as an LRA.

In complementary experiments, Baxter et al. took a different approach and used this technique to address the question: which subsets of CD4 T cells respond to LRAs in vitro by producing HIV mRNA and protein? Cells were stimulated in vitro with the PKC agonists bryostatin or ingenol [109, 110], and the LRA-responsive cells were phenotyped using the memory markers CD27 and CD45RA. Surprisingly, reactivation of HIV RNA and protein expression in response to bryostatin predominantly occurred in the effector memory compartment, despite the central memory population containing high levels of integrated HIV DNA. Curiously, the same polarization was not seen with ingenol, which induced reactivation in all memory compartments [53]. This initial data suggests, critically, that not all populations of HIV-infected CD4 T cells will respond to all LRAs equally. Although further work is required to validate and expand on this results, this supports the requirement for combination therapies to target the entire latent reservoir and again highlights the importance of considering the single-cell heterogeneity of the reservoir in cure strategies.

Future perspectives

The studies presented here demonstrate the power of studying the transcription/translation-competent cellular reservoirs. While these insights are tremendously valuable for the cure field, the level of heterogeneity detected thus far has been considerable. With this in mind, many groups have sought to discover a single marker that can be used to identify and robustly discriminate cells containing replication-competent proviruses. For example, CD32a has recently been identified as a promising biomarker for latently-infected CD4 T cells [111]. Therefore, an immediate question is whether the transcription/translation-competent cellular reservoirs are also enriched for this marker; the first published study to do so observed limited enrichment [55]. However, the ability to analyze expression and co-expression of multiple markers at a single cell level means that the techniques used for the identification of the transcription/translation-competent reservoirs can be utilized for screening approaches. This type of analysis has clear potential for use in the identification of biomarkers for latent HIV-infected cells, which could then be preferentially targeted by cure strategies.

The application of such single-cell measurements to clinical cure research is a key next step in the development of these approaches. For example, this approach has the power to determine whether a particular treatment is effective at clearing latent virus from a specific cellular compartment. It remains to be determined, however, how the size of the transcription/translation-competent reservoir may be associated with positive treatment outcome; specifically, if a reduction in the size of the transcription/translation-competent reservoir is associated with a longer time to rebound, or post-treatment control, following analytic treatment interruption. In line with this, it will be important to determine if the detection of the transcription/translation-competent reservoirs can provide useful information, when compared to classical measures of HIV DNA or RNA at a population level in this context.

While most of the work shown here has focused on CD4 T cell as the predominant reservoir, alternative cell populations, such as macrophages, have been shown to be infected with HIV. The contribution of this population to HIV persistence however remains controversial [112–114]. Interestingly, Jambo et al. [115] were able to use a flow-based FISH approach to identify HIV-infected alveolar macrophages in bronchial lavages from chronically infected individuals. While additional studies are required to confirm these results, this initial study indicates the power of such approaches to study cell populations other than CD4 and opening up the number of questions that can be addressed.

Lastly, in this review we have focused on assays using flow cytometry and microscopy as a readout. However, the field is now moving beyond viral mRNA/protein detection by flow cytometry, for example by combining single cell sorting by FACS with detection of multiple SIV mRNAs (including *tat/rev*, *env*, *gag* and *LTR*) by ultrasensitive PCR. While this initial study enabled detailed in-depth profiling of HIV infected cells in SIV infected macaques during chronic untreated infection [116], it demonstrated a large amount of variation both between infected, mRNA+ cells and also between tissues. Furthermore, a recent report has demonstrated the concurrent detection of spliced and unspliced RNA, nuclear DNA and Gag protein by microscopy, using an approach known as multiplex immunofluorescent

cell-based detection of DNA, RNA and Protein (MICD-DRP, [117]). While the latter study focused on in vitro infection, future work will determine how both of these approaches can be applied to detect HIV-infected cells in ART-treated individuals.

Conclusions

We propose that the detection of the transcription and translation-competent cellular reservoirs provides a unique, complementary, approach to identify and probe the cells contributing to HIV persistence at a single cell level. While not all cells identified as transcription and translation-competent cellular reservoirs will harbor replication-competent virus, we propose that such cells, particularly those which express multiple HIV mRNAs, express HIV protein and downregulate CD4, are likely to be enriched for replication-competent virus. We base this speculation on the requirement for the functionality of multiple genes to bring about this phenotype, including *gag*, *tat*, *rev*, *env*, and *nef*. Thus, we suggest that these approaches close the gap between alternative reservoir measurements and provide a closer estimate of HIV reservoir size. Finally, we summarize recent evidence supporting the concept that even if such transcription/translation-competent proviruses are not replication-competent, understanding and/or removing this cellular reservoir will be important for the development of cure strategies.

Abbreviations
ART: anti-retroviral therapy; bDNA: branched DNA; CA-RNA: cell associated-RNA; CTL: cytotoxic T lymphocytes; FAST: fiber-optic array scanning technology; (F)ISH: (fluorescence) in situ hybridization; HRP: horse radish peroxidase; IUPM: infectious units per million; LRA: latency-reversing agent; TAR: trans-acting response element; Q-VOA: quantitative viral outgrowth assay; RT-PCR: reverse transcriptase-PCR; RRE: rev responsive element; SUSHI: simultaneous ultrasensitive subpopulation staining/hybridization in situ.

Authors' contributions
AEB performed the literature review and wrote the manuscript, with contributions from UO and DEK, who edited the manuscript. All authors read and approved the final manuscript.

Author details
[1] CR-CHUM, Université de Montréal, Montréal, QC, Canada. [2] Scripps CHAVI-ID, La Jolla, CA, USA. [3] Department of Pathology and Laboratory Medicine, Division of Transfusion Medicine and Therapeutic Pathology, University of Pennsylvania, Philadelphia, PA, USA.

Acknowledgements
We thank Mathieu Dubé for the critical reading of this manuscript and assistance with figure preparation.

Competing interests
The authors declare that they have no competing interests.

Funding
AEB is the recipient of a CIHR Postdoctoral Fellowship (Award No. 152536); DEK is supported by a FRQS Research Scholar Award (# 31035), CIHR #377124, NHLBI RO1-HL-092565 and UM1-AI-100663. UO receives support from NIAID R01-AI-120011 and UM1-AI-126617.

References

1. Chun TW, Finzi D, Margolick J, Chadwick K, Schwartz D, Siliciano RF. In vivo fate of HIV-1-infected T cells: quantitative analysis of the transition to stable latency. Nat Med. 1995;1:1284–90.
2. Chun TW, Carruth L, Finzi D, Shen X, DiGiuseppe JA, Taylor H, et al. Quantification of latent tissue reservoirs and total body viral load in HIV-1 infection. Nature. 1997;387:183–8.
3. Chun TW, Stuyver L, Mizell SB, Ehler LA, Mican JA, Baseler M, et al. Presence of an inducible HIV-1 latent reservoir during highly active antiretroviral therapy. Proc Natl Acad Sci USA. 1997;94:13193–7.
4. Finzi D, Hermankova M, Pierson T, Carruth LM, Buck C, Chaisson RE, et al. Identification of a reservoir for HIV-1 in patients on highly active antiretroviral therapy. Science. 1997;278:1295–300.
5. Wong JK, Hezareh M, Günthard HF, Havlir DV, Ignacio CC, Spina CA, et al. Recovery of replication-competent HIV despite prolonged suppression of plasma viremia. Science. 1997;278:1291–5.
6. Bruner KM, Hosmane NN, Siliciano RF. Towards an HIV-1 cure: measuring the latent reservoir. Trends Microbiol. 2015;23:192–203.
7. Rasmussen TA, Lewin SR. Shocking HIV out of hiding: where are we with clinical trials of latency reversing agents? Curr Opin HIV AIDS. 2016;11:394–401.
8. Imamichi H, Natarajan V, Adelsberger JW, Rehm CA, Lempicki RA, Das B, et al. Lifespan of effector memory CD4+ T cells determined by replication-incompetent integrated HIV-1 provirus. AIDS. 2014;28:1091–9.
9. Imamichi H, Dewar RL, Adelsberger JW, Rehm CA, O'Doherty U, Paxinos EE, et al. Defective HIV-1 proviruses produce novel protein-coding RNA species in HIV-infected patients on combination antiretroviral therapy. Proc Natl Acad Sci USA. 2016;113:8783–8.
10. Vandergeeten C, Fromentin R, Merlini E, Lawani MB, DaFonseca S, Bakeman W, et al. Cross-clade ultrasensitive PCR-based assays to measure HIV persistence in large-cohort studies. J Virol. 2014;88:12385–96.
11. Ho Y-C, Shan L, Hosmane NN, Wang J, Laskey SB, Rosenbloom DIS, et al. Replication-competent noninduced proviruses in the latent reservoir increase barrier to HIV-1 cure. Cell. 2013;155:540–51.
12. Bruner KM, Murray AJ, Pollack RA, Soliman MG, Laskey SB, Capoferri AA, et al. Defective proviruses rapidly accumulate during acute HIV-1 infection. Nat Publ Group. 2016;22:1043–9.
13. Siliciano JD, Kajdas J, Finzi D, Quinn TC, Chadwick K, Margolick JB, et al. Long-term follow-up studies confirm the stability of the latent reservoir for HIV-1 in resting CD4+ T cells. Nat Med. 2003;9:727–8.
14. Laird GM, Eisele EE, Rabi SA, Lai J, Chioma S, Blankson JN, et al. Rapid quantification of the latent reservoir for HIV-1 using a viral outgrowth assay. PLoS Pathog. 2013;9:e1003398.
15. Bullen CK, Laird GM, Durand CM, Siliciano JD, Siliciano RF. New ex vivo approaches distinguish effective and ineffective single agents for reversing HIV-1 latency in vivo. Nat Med. 2014;20:425–9.
16. Sanyal A, Mailliard RB, Rinaldo CR, Ratner D, Ding M, Chen Y, et al. Novel assay reveals a large, inducible, replication-competent HIV-1 reservoir in resting CD4+ T cells. Nat Med. 2017;73:5858–6099.
17. Deeks SGHIV. Shock and kill. Nature. 2012;487:439–40.
18. Margolis DM, Garcia JV, Hazuda DJ, Haynes BF. Latency reversal and viral clearance to cure HIV-1. Science. 2016;353:aaf6517–7.
19. Lederman MM, Cannon PM, Currier JS, June CH, Kiem HP, Kuritzkes DR, et al. A cure for HIV infection: "not in my lifetime" or "just around the corner"? PAI. 2016;1:154–64.
20. Churchill MJ, Deeks SG, Margolis DM, Siliciano RF, Swanstrom R. HIV reservoirs: what, where and how to target them. Nat Rev Microbiol. 2016;14:55–60.
21. Siliciano RF, Greene WC. HIV latency. Cold Spring Harbor Perspect Med. 2011;1:a007096–6.
22. Murray JM, Zaunders JJ, McBride KL, Xu Y, Bailey M, Suzuki K, et al. HIV DNA subspecies persist in both activated and resting memory CD4+ T cells during antiretroviral therapy. J Virol. 2014;88:3516–26.
23. Karn J, Stoltzfus CM. Transcriptional and posttranscriptional regulation of HIV-1 gene expression. Cold Spring Harbor Perspect Med. 2012;2:a006916.
24. Kim S-Y, Byrn R, Groopman J, Baltimore D. Temporal aspects of DNA and RNA synthesis during human immunodeficiency virus infection: evidence for differential gene expression. J Virol. 1989;63:3708–13.
25. Rojas-Araya B, Ohlmann T, Soto-Rifo R. Translational control of the HIV unspliced genomic RNA. Viruses. 2015;7:4326–51.
26. Van Lint C, Bouchat S, Marcello A. HIV-1 transcription and latency: an update. Retrovirology. 2013;10:67.
27. Mohammadi P, di Iulio J, Muñoz M, Martinez R, Bartha I, Cavassini M, et al. Dynamics of HIV latency and reactivation in a primary CD4+ T cell model. PLoS Pathog. 2014;10:e1004156.
28. Pace MJ, Graf EH, Agosto LM, Mexas AM, Male F, Brady T, et al. Directly infected resting CD4+ T cells can produce HIV Gag without spreading infection in a model of HIV latency. PLoS Pathog. 2012;8:e1002818.
29. Pace MJ, Agosto L, Graf EH, O'Doherty U. HIV reservoirs and latency models. Virology. 2011;411:344–54.
30. Schnittman SM, Greenhouse JJ, Lane HC, Pierce PF, Fauci AS. Frequent detection of HIV-1-specific mRNAs in infected individuals suggests ongoing active viral expression in all stages of disease. AIDS Res Hum Retrovir. 1991;7:361–7.
31. Graziosi C, Pantaleo G, Butini L, Demarest JF, Saag MS, Shaw GM, et al. Kinetics of human immunodeficiency virus type 1 (HIV-1) DNA and RNA synthesis during primary HIV-1 infection. Proc Natl Acad Sci USA. 1993;90:6405–9.
32. Fischer M, Joos B, Niederöst B, Kaiser P, Hafner R, von Wyl V, et al. Biphasic decay kinetics suggest progressive slowing in turnover of latently HIV-1 infected cells during antiretroviral therapy. Retrovirology. 2008;5:107.
33. Kaiser P, Joos B, Niederöst B, Weber R, Günthard HF, Fischer M. Productive human immunodeficiency virus type 1 infection in peripheral blood predominantly takes place in CD4/CD8 double-negative T lymphocytes. J Virol. 2007;81:9693–706.
34. Pasternak AO, DeMaster LK, Kootstra NA, Reiss P, O'Doherty U, Berkhout B. Minor contribution of chimeric host-HIV readthrough transcripts to the level of HIV cell-associated gag RNA. J Virol. 2015;90:1148–51.
35. Pasternak AO, Berkhout B. What do we measure when we measure cell-associated HIV RNA. Retrovirology. 2018;15(1). https://doi.org/10.1186/s12977-018-0397-2.
36. Pasternak AO, Lukashov VV. Ben Berkhout. Cell-associated HIV RNA: a dynamic biomarker of viral persistence. Retrovirology. 2013;10:41.
37. Pantaleo G, Graziosi C, Demarest JF, Butini L, Montroni M, Fox CH, et al. HIV infection is active and progressive in lymphoid tissue during the clinically latent stage of disease. Nature. 1993;362:355–8.
38. Haase AT, Henry K, Zupancic M, Sedgewick G, Faust RA, Melroe H, et al. Quantitative image analysis of HIV-1 infection in lymphoid tissue. Science. 1996;274:985–9.
39. Brenchley JM, Vinton C, Tabb B, Hao XP, Connick E, Paiardini M, et al. Differential infection patterns of CD4+ T cells and lymphoid tissue viral burden distinguish progressive and nonprogressive lentiviral infections. Blood. 2012;120:4172–81.

40. Li Q, Skinner PJ, Ha S-J, Duan L, Mattila TL, Hage A, et al. Visualizing antigen-specific and infected cells in situ predicts outcomes in early viral infection. Science. 2009;323:1726–9.

41. Patterson BK, Till M, Otto P, Goolsby C, Furtado MR, McBride LJ, et al. Detection of HIV-1 DNA and messenger RNA in individual cells by PCR-driven in situ hybridization and flow cytometry. Science. 1993;260:976–9.

42. Patterson BK, Mosiman VL, Cantarero L, Furtado M, Bhattacharya M, Goolsby C. Detection of HIV-RNA-positive monocytes in peripheral blood of HIV-positive patients by simultaneous flow cytometric analysis of intracellular HIV RNA and cellular immunophenotype. Cytometry. 1998;31:265–74.

43. Patterson BK, Czerniewski MA, Pottage J, Agnoli M, Kessler H, Landay A. Monitoring HIV-1 treatment in immune-cell subsets with ultrasensitive fluorescence-in situ hybridisation. Lancet. 1999;353:211–2.

44. Chargin A, Yin F, Song M, Subramaniam S, Knutson G, Patterson BK. Identification and characterization of HIV-1 latent viral reservoirs in peripheral blood. J Clin Microbiol. 2015;53:60–6.

45. Wang F, Flanagan J, Su N, Wang L-C, Bui S, Nielson A, et al. RNAscope: a novel in situ RNA analysis platform for formalin-fixed, paraffin-embedded tissues. J Mol Diagn. 2012;14:22–9.

46. Player AN, Shen LP, Kenny D, Antao VP, Kolberg JA. Single-copy gene detection using branched DNA (bDNA) in situ hybridization. J Histochem Cytochem. 2001;49:603–12.

47. Deleage C, Wietgrefe SW, Del Prete G, Morcock DR, Hao XP, Anderson JL, et al. Defining HIV and SIV reservoirs in lymphoid tissues. PAI. 2016;1:39–68.

48. Deleage C, Turkbey B, Estes JD. Imaging lymphoid tissues in nonhuman primates to understand SIV pathogenesis and persistence. Curr Opin Virol. 2016;19:77–84.

49. Estes JD, Kityo C, Ssali F, Swainson L, Makamdop KN, Del Prete GQ, et al. Defining total-body AIDS-virus burden with implications for curative strategies. Nat Med. 2017;23:1271–6.

50. Porichis F, Hart MG, Griesbeck M, Everett HL, Hassan M, Baxter AE, et al. High-throughput detection of miRNAs and gene-specific mRNA at the single-cell level by flow cytometry. Nat Commun. 2014;5:5641.

51. Prasad VR, Kalpana GV. FISHing out the hidden enemy: advances in detecting and measuring latent HIV-infected cells. MBio. 2017;8:e01433–17.

52. Martrus G, Niehrs A, Cornelis R, Rechtien A, García-Beltran W, Lütgehetmann M, et al. Kinetics of HIV-1 latency reversal quantified on the single-cell level using a novel flow-based technique. J Virol. 2016;90:9018–28.

53. Baxter AE, Niessl J, Fromentin R, Richard J, Porichis F, Charlebois R, et al. Single-cell characterization of viral translation-competent reservoirs in HIV-infected individuals. Cell Host Microbe. 2016;20:368–80.

54. Baxter AE, Niessl J, Fromentin R, Richard J, Porichis F, Massanella M, et al. Multiparametric characterization of rare HIV-infected cells using an RNA-flow FISH technique. Nat Protoc. 2017;12:2029–49.

55. Grau-Expósito J, Serra-Peinado C, Miguel L, Navarro J, Curran A, Burgos J, et al. A novel single-cell FISH-flow assay identifies effector memory CD4(+) T cells as a major niche for HIV-1 transcription in HIV-infected patients. MBio. 2017;8:e00876–17.

56. Kearney MF, Wiegand A, Shao W, Coffin JM, Mellors JW, Lederman MM, et al. Origin of rebound plasma HIV includes cells with identical proviruses that are transcriptionally active before stopping of antiretroviral therapy. J Virol. 2015;90:1369–76.

57. Barton K, Hiener B, Winckelmann A, Rasmussen TA, Shao W, Byth K, et al. Broad activation of latent HIV-1 in vivo. Nat Commun. 2016;7:12731.

58. Pollack RA, Jones RB, Pertea M, Bruner KM, Martin AR, Thomas AS, et al. Defective HIV-1 proviruses are expressed and can be recognized by cytotoxic T lymphocytes, which shape the proviral landscape. Cell Host Microbe. 2017;21:494–4.

59. Imamichi H, Smith M, Rehm CA, Catalfamo M, Lane HC. Evidence of production of HIV-1 proteins from "defective" HIV-1 proviruses in vivo: implication for persistent immune activation and HIV-1 pathogenesis. IAS Conference Abstract, Paris; 2017.

60. Briggs JAG, Simon MN, Gross I, Kräusslich H-G, Fuller SD, Vogt VM, et al. The stoichiometry of gag protein in HIV-1. Nat Struct Mol Biol. 2004;11:672–5.

61. Graf EH, Pace MJ, Peterson BA, Lynch LJ, Chukwulebe SB, Mexas AM, et al. Gag-positive reservoir cells are susceptible to HIV-specific cytotoxic T lymphocyte mediated clearance in vitro and can be detected in vivo. PLoS ONE. 2013;8:e71879.

62. DeMaster LK, Liu X, VanBelzen DJ, Trinité B, Zheng L, Agosto LM, et al. A subset of CD4/CD8 double negative T cells expresses HIV proteins in patients on ART. J Virol. 2015;90:2165–79.

63. Garcia JV, Miller AD. Serine phosphorylation-independent downregulation of cell-surface CD4 by nef. Nature. 1991;350:508–11.

64. Willey RL, Maldarelli F, Martin MA, Strebel K. Human immunodeficiency virus type 1 Vpu protein induces rapid degradation of CD4. J Virol. 1992;66:7193–200.

65. Aiken C, Konner J, Landau NR, Lenburg ME, Trono D. Nef induces CD4 endocytosis: requirement for a critical dileucine motif in the membrane-proximal CD4 cytoplasmic domain. Cell. 1994;76:853–64.

66. Geleziunas R, Bour S, Wainberg MA. Correlation between high level gp160 expression and reduced CD4 biosynthesis in clonal derivatives of human immunodeficiency virus type 1-infected U-937 cells. J Gen Virol. 1994;75(Pt 4):857–65.

67. Rhee SS, Marsh JW. Human immunodeficiency virus type 1 Nef-induced down-modulation of CD4 is due to rapid internalization and degradation of surface CD4. J Virol. 1994;68:5156–63.

68. Chen BK, Gandhi RT, Baltimore D. CD4 down-modulation during infection of human T cells with human immunodeficiency virus type 1 involves independent activities of vpu, env, and nef. J Virol. 1996;70:6044–53.

69. Krivacic RT, Ladanyi A, Curry DN, Hsieh HB, Kuhn P, Bergsrud DE, et al. A rare-cell detector for cancer. Proc Natl Acad Sci USA. 2004;101:10501–4.

70. Hsieh HB, Marrinucci D, Bethel K, Curry DN, Humphrey M, Krivacic RT, et al. High speed detection of circulating tumor cells. Biosens Bioelectron. 2006;21:1893–9.

71. Liu X, Hsieh HB, Campana D, Bruce RH. A new method for high speed, sensitive detection of minimal residual disease. Cytom Part A. 2012;81:169–75.

72. Perreau M, Savoye A-L, De Crignis E, Corpataux J-M, Cubas R, Haddad EK, et al. Follicular helper T cells serve as the major CD4 T cell compartment for HIV-1 infection, replication, and production. J Exp Med. 2013;210:143–56. http://jem.rupress.org/content/210/1/143.full.

73. Banga R, Procopio FA, Noto A, Pollakis G, Cavassini M, Ohmiti K, et al. PD-1+ and follicular helper T cells are responsible for persistent HIV transcription in treated aviremic individuals. Nat Med. 2016;22:754–61.

74. Pallikkuth S, Sharkey M, Babic DZ, Gupta S, Stone GW, Fischl MA, et al. Peripheral T follicular helper cells are the major HIV reservoir within central memory CD4 T cells in peripheral blood from chronic HIV infected individuals on cART. J Virol. 2015;90:JVI.02883–15–45.

75. Fromentin R, Bakeman W, Lawani MB, Khoury G, Hartogensis W, DaFonseca S, et al. CD4+ T cells expressing PD-1, TIGIT and LAG-3 contribute to HIV persistence during ART. PLoS Pathog. 2016;12:e1005761.

76. Eriksson S, Graf EH, Dahl V, Strain MC, Yukl SA, Lysenko ES, et al. Comparative analysis of measures of viral reservoirs in HIV-1 eradication studies. PLoS Pathog. 2013;9:e1003174.

77. Patterson BK, McCallister S, Schutz M, Siegel JN, Shults K, Flener Z, et al. Persistence of intracellular HIV-1 mRNA correlates with HIV-1-specific immune responses in infected subjects on stable HAART. AIDS. 2001;15:1635–41.

78. Soriano-Sarabia N, Bateson RE, Dahl NP, Crooks AM, Kuruc JD, Margolis DM, et al. Quantitation of replication-competent HIV-1 in populations of resting CD4+ T cells. J Virol. 2014;88:14070–7.

79. Hiener B, Horsburgh BA, Eden J-S, Barton K, Schlub TE, Lee E, et al. Identification of genetically intact HIV-1 proviruses in specific CD4(+) T cells from effectively treated participants. Cell Rep. 2017;21:813–22.

80. Hurst J, Hoffmann M, Pace M, Williams JP, Thornhill J, Hamlyn E, et al. Immunological biomarkers predict HIV-1 viral rebound after treatment interruption. Nat Commun. 2015;6:8495.

81. Spina CA, Anderson J, Archin NM, Bosque A, Chan J, Famiglietti M, et al. An In-depth comparison of latent HIV-1 reactivation in multiple cell model systems and resting CD4+ T cells from aviremic patients. PLoS Pathog. 2013;9:e1003834.

82. Kiselinova M, De Spiegelaere W, Buzon MJ, Malatinkova E, Lichterfeld M, Vandekerckhove L. Integrated and total HIV-1 DNA predict ex vivo viral outgrowth. PLoS Pathog. 2016;12:e1005472–17.

83. Henrich TJ, Deeks SG, Pillai SK. Measuring the size of the latent human immunodeficiency virus reservoir: the present and future of evaluating eradication strategies. J Infect Dis. 2017;215:S134–41.

84. Procopio FA, Fromentin R, Kulpa DA, Brehm JH, Bebin A-G, Strain MC, et al. A novel assay to measure the magnitude of the inducible viral reservoir in HIV-infected individuals. EBioMedicine. 2015;2:872–81.

85. Virgin HW, Wherry EJ, Ahmed R. Redefining chronic viral infection. Cell. 2009;138:30–50.

86. Letvin NL, Walker BD. Immunopathogenesis and immunotherapy in AIDS virus infections. Nat Med. 2003;9:861–6.

87. Day CL, Kaufmann DE, Kiepiela P, Brown JA, Moodley ES, Reddy S, et al. PD-1 expression on HIV-specific T cells is associated with T-cell exhaustion and disease progression. Nature. 2006;443:350–4.

88. Kaufmann DE, Kavanagh DG, Pereyra F, Zaunders JJ, Mackey EW, Miura T, et al. Upregulation of CTLA-4 by HIV-specific CD4+ T cells correlates with disease progression and defines a reversible immune dysfunction. Nat Immunol. 2007;8:1246–54.

89. Dsouza M, Fontenot AP, Mack DG, Lozupone C, Dillon S, Meditz A, et al. Programmed death 1 expression on HIV-specific CD4+ T cells is driven by viral replication and associated with T cell dysfunction. J Immunol. 2007;179:1979–87.

90. Wherry EJ, Kurachi M. Molecular and cellular insights into T cell exhaustion. Nat Rev Immunol. 2015;15:486–99.

91. Maldarelli F, Palmer S, King MS, Wiegand A, Polis MA, Mican JM, et al. ART suppresses plasma HIV-1 RNA to a stable set point predicted by pretherapy viremia. PLoS Pathog. 2007;3:e46.

92. Palmer S, Maldarelli F, Wiegand A, Bernstein B, Hanna GJ, Brun SC, et al. Low-level viremia persists for at least 7 years in patients on suppressive antiretroviral therapy. Proc Natl Acad Sci USA. 2008;105:3879–84.

93. Brenchley JM, Price DA, Schacker TW, Asher TE, Silvestri G, Rao S, et al. Microbial translocation is a cause of systemic immune activation in chronic HIV infection. Nat Med. 2006;12:1365–71.

94. Sandler NG, Douek DC. Microbial translocation in HIV infection: causes, consequences and treatment opportunities. Nat Rev Microbiol. 2012;10:655–66.

95. Klatt NR, Chomont N, Douek DC, Deeks SG. Immune activation and HIV persistence: implications for curative approaches to HIV infection. Immunol Rev. 2013;254:326–42.

96. Mexas AM, Graf EH, Pace MJ, Yu JJ, Papasavvas E, Azzoni L, et al. Concurrent measures of total and integrated HIV DNA monitor reservoirs and ongoing replication in eradication trials. AIDS. 2012;26:2295–306.

97. Azzoni L, Foulkes AS, Papasavvas E, Mexas AM, Lynn KM, Mounzer K, et al. Pegylated Interferon alfa-2a monotherapy results in suppression of HIV type 1 replication and decreased cell-associated HIV DNA integration. J Infect Dis. 2013;207:213–22.

98. Winckelmann AA, Munk-Petersen LV, Rasmussen TA, Melchjorsen J, Hjelholt TJ, Montefiori DC, et al. Administration of a toll-like receptor 9 agonist decreases the proviral reservoir in virologically suppressed HIV-infected patients. PLoS ONE. 2013;8:e62074.

99. Leth S, Schleimann MH, Nissen SK, Højen JF, Olesen R, Graversen ME, et al. Combined effect of Vacc-4x, recombinant human granulocyte macrophage colony-stimulating factor vaccination, and romidepsin on the HIV-1 reservoir (REDUC): a single-arm, phase 1B/2A trial. Lancet HIV. 2016;3:e463–72.

100. Collaboration Antiretroviral Therapy Cohort. Life expectancy of individuals on combination antiretroviral therapy in high-income countries: a collaborative analysis of 14 cohort studies. Lancet. 2008;372:293–9.

101. Deeks SG, Phillips AN. HIV infection, antiretroviral treatment, ageing, and non-AIDS related morbidity. BMJ. 2009;338:a3172.

102. Lederman MM, Funderburg NT, Sekaly R-P, NR NR, Hunt PW. Residual immune dysregulation syndrome in treated HIV infection. Adv Immunol. 2013;119:51–83.

103. Chomont N, El-Far M, Ancuta P, Trautmann L, Procopio FA, Yassine-Diab B, et al. HIV reservoir size and persistence are driven by T cell survival and homeostatic proliferation. Nat Med. 2009;15:893–900.

104. Pinzone MR, Graf E, Lynch L, McLaughlin B, Hecht FM, Connors M, et al. Monitoring integration over time supports a role for cytotoxic T lymphocytes and ongoing replication as determinants of reservoir size. J Virol. 2016;90:10436–45.

105. Yue Y, Wang N, Han Y, Zhu T, Xie J, Qiu Z, et al. A higher CD4/CD8 ratio correlates with an ultralow cell-associated HIV-1 DNA level in chronically infected patients on antiretroviral therapy: a case control study. BMC Infect Dis. 2017;17:771.

106. Gibellini L, Pecorini S, De Biasi S, Bianchini E, Digaetano M, Pinti M, et al. HIV-DNA content in different CD4+ T-cell subsets correlates with CD4+ cell: CD8+ cell ratio or length of efficient treatment. AIDS. 2017;31:1387–92.

107. Laird GM, Bullen CK, Rosenbloom DIS, Martin AR, Hill AL, Durand CM, et al. Ex vivo analysis identifies effective HIV-1 latency–reversing drug combinations. J Clin Invest. 2015;125:1901–12.

108. Søgaard OS, Graversen ME, Leth S, Olesen R, Brinkmann CR, Nissen SK, et al. The Depsipeptide romidepsin reverses HIV-1 latency in vivo. PLoS Pathog. 2015;11:e1005142.

109. DeChristopher BA, Loy BA, Marsden MD, Schrier AJ, Zack JA, Wender PA. Designed, synthetically accessible bryostatin analogues potently induce activation of latent HIV reservoirs in vitro. Nat Chem. 2012;4:705–10.

110. Jiang G, Mendes EA, Kaiser P, Sankaran-Walters S, Tang Y, Weber MG, et al. Reactivation of HIV latency by a newly modified Ingenol derivative via protein kinase Cδ-NF-κB signaling. AIDS. 2014;28:1555–66.

111. Descours B, Petitjean G, López-Zaragoza J-L, Bruel T, Raffel R, Psomas C, et al. CD32a is a marker of a CD4 T-cell HIV reservoir harbouring replication-competent proviruses. Nature. 2017;543:564–7.

112. Sattentau QJ, Stevenson M. Macrophages and HIV-1: an unhealthy constellation. Cell Host Microbe. 2016;19:304–10.

113. Honeycutt JB, Thayer WO, Baker CE, Ribeiro RM, Lada SM, Cao Y, et al. HIV persistence in tissue macrophages of humanized myeloid-only mice during antiretroviral therapy. Nat Med. 2017;23:638–43.

114. Araínga M, Edagwa B, Mosley RL, Poluektova LY, Gorantla S, Gendelman HE. A mature macrophage is a principal HIV-1 cellular reservoir in humanized mice after treatment with long acting antiretroviral therapy. Retrovirology. 2017;14:17.

115. Jambo KC, Banda DH, Kankwatira AM, Sukumar N, Allain TJ, Heyderman RS, et al. Small alveolar macrophages are infected preferentially by HIV and exhibit impaired phagocytic function. Mucosal Immunol. 2014;7:1116–26.

116. Bolton DL, McGinnis K, Finak G, Chattopadhyay P, Gottardo R, Roederer M. Combined single-cell quantitation of host and SIV genes and proteins ex vivo reveals host-pathogen interactions in individual cells. PLoS Pathog. 2017;13:e1006445.

117. Puray-Chavez M, Tedbury PR, Huber AD, Ukah OB, Yapo V, Liu D, et al. Multiplex single-cell visualization of nucleic acids and protein during HIV infection. Nat Commun. 2017;8:1882.

7

Development of broadly neutralizing antibodies in HIV-1 infected elite neutralizers

Elise Landais[1,2,3] and Penny L. Moore[4,5,6]*

Abstract

Broadly neutralizing antibodies (bNAbs), able to prevent viral entry by diverse global viruses, are a major focus of HIV vaccine design, with data from animal studies confirming their ability to prevent HIV infection. However, traditional vaccine approaches have failed to elicit these types of antibodies. During chronic HIV infection, a subset of individuals develops bNAbs, some of which are extremely broad and potent. This review describes the immunological and virological factors leading to the development of bNAbs in such "elite neutralizers". The features, targets and developmental pathways of bNAbs from their precursors have been defined through extraordinarily detailed within-donor studies. These have enabled the identification of epitope-specific commonalities in bNAb precursors, their intermediates and Env escape patterns, providing a template for vaccine discovery. The unusual features of bNAbs, such as high levels of somatic hypermutation, and precursors with unusually short or long antigen-binding loops, present significant challenges in vaccine design. However, the use of new technologies has led to the isolation of more than 200 bNAbs, including some with genetic profiles more representative of the normal immunoglobulin repertoire, suggesting alternate and shorter pathways to breadth. The insights from these studies have been harnessed for the development of optimized immunogens, novel vaccine regimens and improved delivery schedules, which are providing encouraging data that an HIV vaccine may soon be a realistic possibility.

Background

The design of a preventative HIV vaccine is one of the major current public health challenges. Despite the global successes of antiretroviral therapy, rates of new infections, especially in sub-Saharan Africa, show little sign of abating, and indeed in some areas as many as half of young women are HIV infected [1]. Despite a massive effort, no vaccine has thus far been able to elicit protective neutralizing antibodies. However, extraordinary progress has been made in understanding the immune response to HIV infection and in defining viral targets. We now have a detailed understanding of the obstacles we face in eliciting protective antibodies, and this has enabled the design of new immunogens and vaccine strategies, many of which are based on studies of infection, and will enter clinical trials in the next months and years.

The major focus for HIV vaccine design is the elicitation of broadly neutralizing antibodies (bNAbs), capable of preventing entry by diverse viruses by binding to conserved regions on the HIV envelope glycoprotein trimer, which is the sole entry complex for HIV. This focus on bNAbs is based on the narrow window between HIV infection and the establishment of latency, ideally requiring antibodies to block viral entry. In contrast, although CTL responses have been shown to contribute to HIV control and slow disease progression [2–4], these responses are unlikely to protect from infection. Compelling evidence from animal studies shows that passive administration of bNAbs into non-human primates provides complete protection from mucosal challenge [5]. Non-broadly neutralizing antibodies, though capable of Fc effector functions such as antibody dependent cellular cytotoxicity, do not protect as well [6–8], further supporting a focus on neutralization. These findings, which are currently being further tested in the first human clinical trials of bNAbs as prophylaxis, suggest that such

*Correspondence: pennym@nicd.ac.za
[4] Centre for HIV and STIs, National Institute for Communicable Diseases of the National Health Laboratory Service, Johannesburg, South Africa
Full list of author information is available at the end of the article

antibodies, if elicited at sufficiently high titers by vaccination, would be protective.

However, eliciting such bNAbs is fraught with difficulties. The Env protein, which consists of three gp120 and three gp41 molecules, has formidable defenses that hinder bNAb development [9]. The trimer is conformationally dynamic, extremely sequence variable, particularly in the antibody accessible regions of the envelope, sparsely arrayed on viral particles [10] and massively glycosylated, with glycans so tightly packed that they occlude much of the underlying protein surface [11]. Immunological decoys in the form of non-functional envelope proteins such as gp41 stumps, monomeric forms of gp120 and non-native protomers (such as uncleaved trimers) that expose non-neutralizing epitopes normally buried in the trimer, add a further layer of complexity [12].

Despite these barriers, infected individuals mount a vigorous neutralizing response though these initial responses are almost entirely strain-specific, targeting highly variable regions of Env [13–17]. However, over 2–3 years of infection, many people develop some degree of cross-reactivity [18], and a small subset of HIV infected individuals mount extremely potent and broad responses. These "elite neutralizers", which are the focus of this review, have been the subject of intense study, in the hope that they provide a template for HIV vaccine design. Extensive functional (binding and neutralization) and structural (electron microscope, crystallography and glycobiology) characterization of these antibodies, and their precursors, has shed light on the complex molecular mechanisms by which they achieved breadth. Our increased understanding of the unusual features of bNAbs, and the failure of traditional vaccine strategies, have led the field to consider next-generation vaccine regimens which are based on the deep understanding of the host and viral factors leading the development of such antibodies. In this review, we provide a summary of these studies, and define some gaps that need to be addressed to develop an effective HIV vaccine.

HIV targets and how these are accessed by bNAbs

One of the major reasons to study elite neutralizers has been the opportunity to define the targets of bNAbs on the HIV envelope. Epitope mapping was initially conducted using polyclonal plasma [19–21] (Fig. 1), but the development of new technologies has enabled efficient isolation of monoclonal antibodies, allowing much finer mapping of epitopes. Hundreds of bNAbs have now been isolated by amplification, sequencing and cloning of immunoglobulin gene transcripts from single B-cells identified by functional screening of micro-cultures and/or antigen-specific sorting. These data show that much of the Env can be targeted by bNAbs, with six distinct target regions identified on the HIV-1 envelope, almost all of which involve glycans. These are the V2-glycan site, the V3-glycan super-epitope, the membrane proximal external region (MPER), the CD4 binding site (CD4bs) and the gp120-gp41 interface, including the fusion peptide [22–24]. Most recently, antibodies targeting the so-called "silent face" have completed coverage of the Env glycoprotein [25]. However, plasma mapping studies suggest that further epitopes or sub-epitopes may remain to be identified. Novel approaches which do not rely on our knowledge of existing epitopes, such as the recently described use of cryo-electron microscopy of antibody-trimer complexes to map the specificities of plasma responses [26], will be informative in defining

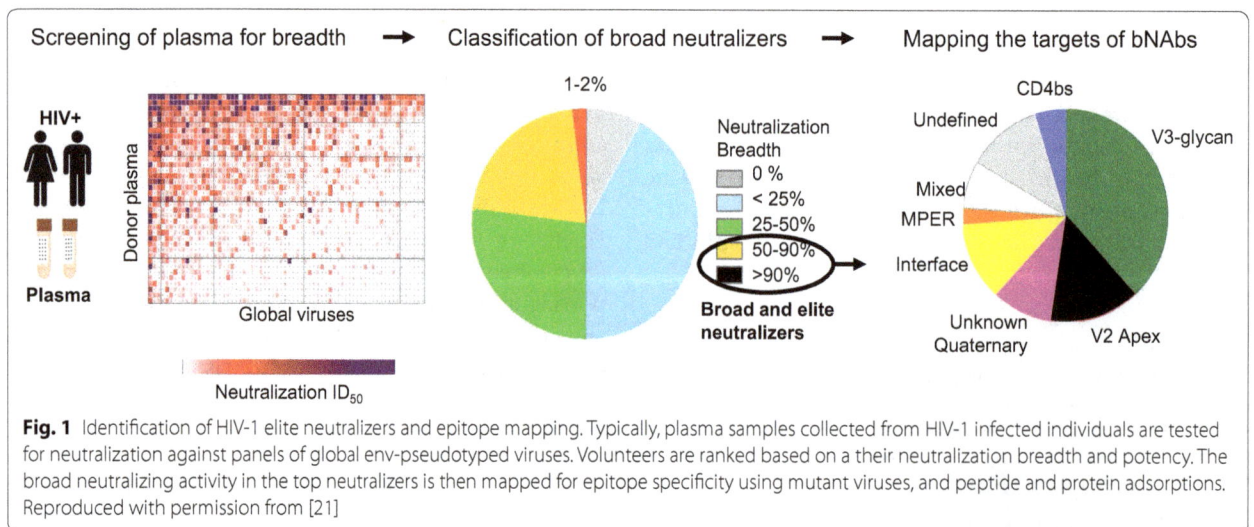

Fig. 1 Identification of HIV-1 elite neutralizers and epitope mapping. Typically, plasma samples collected from HIV-1 infected individuals are tested for neutralization against panels of global env-pseudotyped viruses. Volunteers are ranked based on a their neutralization breadth and potency. The broad neutralizing activity in the top neutralizers is then mapped for epitope specificity using mutant viruses, and peptide and protein adsorptions. Reproduced with permission from [21]

additional targets and designing more specific baits for B cell isolation.

For some bNAb epitopes, there is a degree of promiscuity with which an epitope can be recognized [9, 27]. For example, the V3-glycan supersite is relatively accessible to antibodies, perhaps explaining the prevalence of these bNAbs in infection (Fig. 1). BNAbs to this epitope show variable angles of approach centered around a series of conserved glycans at N301 and N332, but incorporating more variable elements in V1, V3 and V4 [28–31]. Similarly, bNAbs targeting the gp120/gp41 interface have diverse footprints delineating different sub-epitopes [22, 32–35]. However, other epitopes can only be accessed through very constrained angles of approach, forcing the immune system to utilize unusual structural features to access these. The stringent requirements for accessing these epitopes are reflected in the features of bNAb precursors, many of which have unusual features that are rare in the human immunoglobulin repertoire. The best examples of this are the VRC01-like CD4bs bNAbs that are characterized by conserved genetic and structural features which enable a common angle of approach [36–38]. This includes short antigen binding loops, required to avoid steric clashes with hypervariable regions and glycans [39]. In contrast, V2-directed bNAbs require a long anionic CDRH3 to penetrate the glycans protecting the apex of the trimer [40–43]. MPER bNAbs also use long variable loops and often develop membrane binding in order to access their epitopes [44, 45]. However, long loops and hydrophobic surfaces are associated with autoreactivity, such that these precursors are frequently deleted through tolerance mechanisms [43, 46–52]. Defining commonalities among bNAb precursors is the basis of "germline targeting" vaccine strategies, that are being pursued by several groups [39–41, 53–56]. Ongoing studies of immunoglobulin repertoires in diverse populations will provide insights into the possibility of reliably eliciting such bNAbs.

One feature that is common to bNAbs to several epitopes is an unusually high level of somatic hypermutation (SHM). Mutations are acquired in the complementarity determining regions of the antibodies which generally form the paratope, but also in the framework regions of antibodies which are normally more conserved [57]. Although the role of these mutations in conferring breadth is evident in studies of their ontogeny from precursors that are strain-specific [47, 58, 59], many of these mutations are "neutral", conferring no benefit in terms of breadth, and simply a consequence of prolonged maturation in the context of chronic infection [60, 61]. The isolation of less mutated antibodies, described below, may therefore fill an important gap in the field. Much SHM is associated with the need to accommodate the Env glycan shield, either through direct contact and/or by avoiding glycans. Glycan adaptation often involves insertion/deletion events [29] which are rarely observed in the B-cell repertoire as they are less likely to be productive. Recognition of glycans is itself a limitation, as glycans are typically tolerogenic and are considered "self" epitopes by the immune system. Although some degree of poly- or autoreactivity has been reported for CD4bs (PCIN63, VRC01, 12A21) and to a lesser extent, V3-glycan directed bNAb lineages, this is particularly associated with MPER bNAbs (4E10, 2F5 DH511) [62]. Notably, engineering bNAbs to achieve enhanced breadth and potency sometimes results in enhanced polyreactivity, suggesting that maturation towards breadth is balanced by the need to avoid polyreactivity in the maturation of these lineages [63, 64]. Together, these features suggest complex developmental pathways that pose challenges to traditional vaccine strategies.

Factors associated with the development of breadth

Longitudinal studies of the kinetics of plasma breadth have shown that bNAbs develop incrementally, often taking 2–3 years to emerge [19, 21]. This prolonged process suggests that extensive evolution of antibody responses is needed. Indeed, breadth has been associated with high viral loads, duration of infection, viral diversity and low CD4 T cell counts [19, 21, 65–68]. Furthermore, high overall plasma IgG levels and anti-Env IgG binding titers correlate with breadth, suggesting donors with breadth may access a more diverse repertoire of anti-Env Ab responses [21]. These findings emphasize the high levels of antigenic stimulation required to drive the extensive SHM often seen in bNAbs. However, there is also evidence that more specific viral attributes contribute to the development of breadth, with infection with subtype C viruses associated with enhanced breadth, and a bias to V2-glycan directed responses compared to the CD4bs responses more commonly observed in subtype B infected individuals [21, 65]. Another key factor associated with bNAb development is the level of circulating T follicular helper cells and germinal center (GC) function, which likely supports the SHM required for continued maturation [69, 70]. Recent data also showed that HIV-specific Fc effector function early in infection predicts the development of bNAbs, suggesting that intrinsic immune factors within the GC provide a mechanistic link between the Fc and Fab of HIV-specific antibodies [71]. Conversely, low levels of T regulatory cells, possibly enabling survival of B-cell intermediates with potential for autoreactivity, were also associated with development of bNAbs [72].

Superinfection has also been associated with broader antibody responses in some cohorts [73, 74], but not others [75]. This is an appealing observation for vaccine design, suggesting the possibility that superinfection boosts responses primed by the initial infecting virus, analogous to heterologous prime boost vaccines. However, a detailed comparison of the kinetics and targets of plasma antibodies in four superinfected donors suggested that superinfection was associated with de novo responses to both viral variants, and did not drive neutralization breadth (Sheward, Moore and Williamson, in press). This is further supported by the isolation of monoclonal antibodies (mAbs) from two superinfected donors, CAP256 and QA013. In CAP256, who developed extraordinarily potent bNAbs [76], these were directed only at the superinfecting virus [47]. Similarly, mAbs isolated from donor QA013 neutralized either primary infecting or superinfecting viruses, with none cross-neutralizing both. Furthermore, bNAbs in QA013 were largely attributable to mAbs targeting the superinfecting virus, with the mAbs that arose to the primary infecting virus only making a minor contribution to plasma breadth [77]. This suggests that HIV superinfection may enhance breadth through additive responses to each individual virus, consistent with the small effect seen in cohort studies [73], rather than through the boosting of memory responses, a distinction that is important for HIV vaccine design.

Pediatric bNAb donors: a unique group of elite neutralizers

A group particularly interesting for HIV vaccine design is pediatric donors who appear to be enriched for "elite neutralizers". BNAbs in HIV-infected children arise early in the course of infection, often during the first 2 years of life, and become more broad and potent than in adults, with 70% of children developing bNAbs that are equivalent to the top 20% of adults [78–80]. Chronically infected children frequently have an unusual phenotype of consistently high viral loads but normal CD4 counts, which may be highly conducive to the development of breadth [78]. Mapping studies show that bNAbs in children largely target previously defined epitopes, including the V2-glycan, V3-glycan, CD4bs and gp120-gp41 interface [81]. Remarkably, however, three quarters of children had antibodies targeting as many as four distinct bNAb epitopes with breadth mediated by a combination of these specificities. This polyclonality, which is also sometimes seen in adults [20, 21, 82–85], may be more pronounced in chronically infected children due to persistently high viral loads in this group, which is strongly linked to the development of neutralization breadth in adults [21, 65, 86–88]. The extraordinary breadth in

these donors may suggest fundamental differences in their development (described in more detail below). This is supported by the isolation of mAb BF520.1 that targets the V3-glycan, like many adult bNAbs, but does so despite low levels of SHM, and in the absence of insertions/deletions that characterise bNAbs to this epitope [80]. The polyclonal nature of pediatric bNAbs may suggest that the immunoglobulin repertoire in children is more diverse than that of adults, or that maternal antibodies may shape the maturation of bNAbs, as has been observed in passive antibody administration in adults [89, 90]. Lastly, studies of GCs in children will shed light into whether these are functionally distinct from those of adults. Several recent studies suggest that children may be fundamentally better at generating antibody responses in vaccination and infection [78, 79, 91–94], which may be valuable for HIV vaccine design. Additional studies will therefore be important in providing insights into whether HIV infection, and therefore vaccination, may induce unique antibody responses in pediatric donors.

Deciphering molecular pathways towards neutralization breadth

A major focus has been the need to define the cellular and molecular mechanisms leading to the development of bNAbs. The "rational design" vaccine approach critically relies on the identification and characterization of B-cell precursors and key relevant Ab intermediates as well as the Env variants responsible for the elicitation and maturation of these bNAbs. Recent advances in next-generation sequencing (NGS) technologies have been key for such studies, allowing unprecedented analysis of the memory B-cell repertoire and of the viral envelope diversity within individuals [95]. This has enabled comprehensive, multidimensional studies deciphering the molecular interplay between the virus and B-cell response over the course of infection (Fig. 2).

To date, bNAb maturation has been studied for 14 lineages isolated from 13 HIV-infected donors (Table 1). The developmental pathways of very potent and broad CD4bs (VRC01, N49P7, N60P25.1) and MPER (10E8 and DH511) bNAbs were evaluated using chronic samples from four donors and provided key insights into their maturation. In addition, longitudinal sampling from HIV-infected donors enabled seven virus antibody co-evolution studies for bNAb lineages targeting the CD4bs (CH103 and CH235 from donor CH505, and PCIN63 from donor PC63), the V2 apex (CAP256-VRC26 from donor CAP256 and PCT64 from donor PC64) and the V3-glycan high mannose patch (PCDN from donor PC76, DH270 from donor CH848 and PCIN39 from donor PC39). Such studies of the longitudinal development of bNAbs were a unique opportunity, especially as

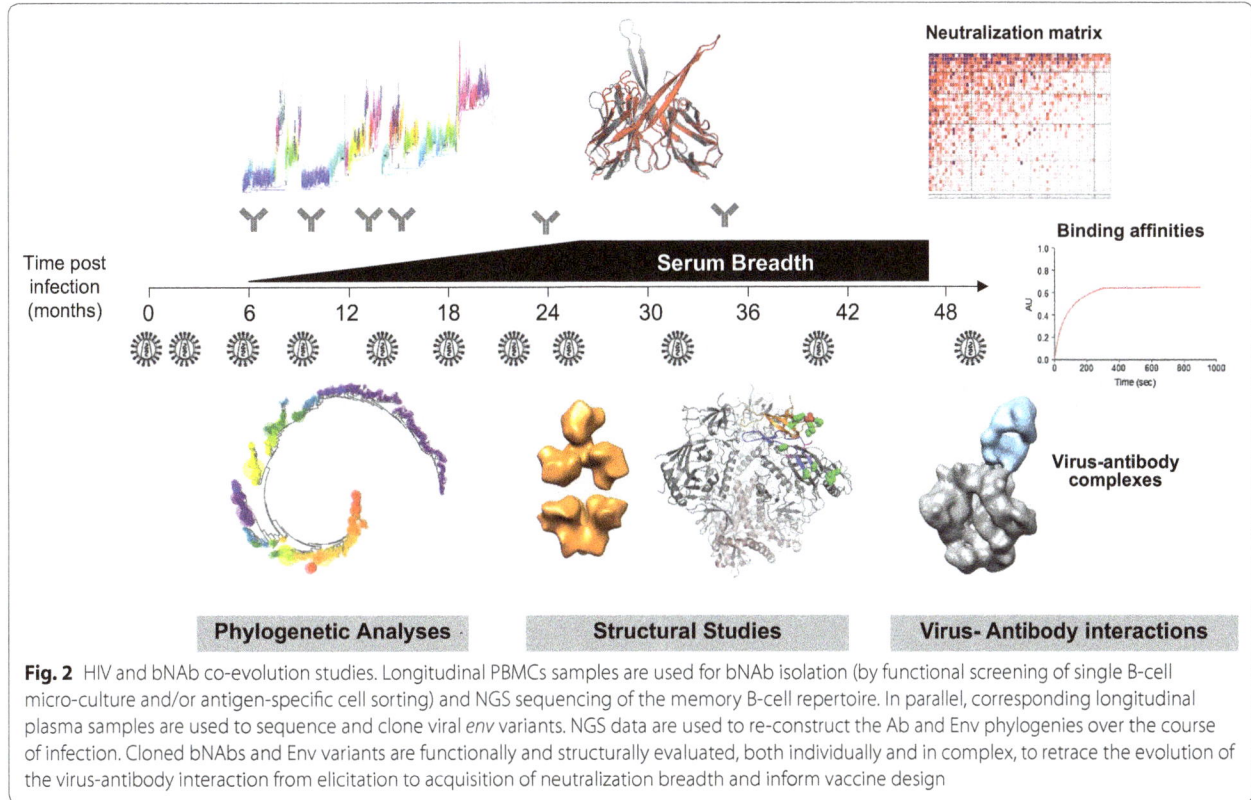

Fig. 2 HIV and bNAb co-evolution studies. Longitudinal PBMCs samples are used for bNAb isolation (by functional screening of single B-cell micro-culture and/or antigen-specific cell sorting) and NGS sequencing of the memory B-cell repertoire. In parallel, corresponding longitudinal plasma samples are used to sequence and clone viral *env* variants. NGS data are used to re-construct the Ab and Env phylogenies over the course of infection. Cloned bNAbs and Env variants are functionally and structurally evaluated, both individually and in complex, to retrace the evolution of the virus-antibody interaction from elicitation to acquisition of neutralization breadth and inform vaccine design

clinical guidelines have moved towards early treatment of HIV infection, and were extremely valuable for the HIV vaccine effort. These longitudinal mAb studies built on previous plasma studies [19, 66] to better define the timing of breadth and identified bNAb precursors between 3 and 16 months post-infection, with maturation towards breadth taking 1–2 years, depending on the level of breadth and associated SHM achieved by the lineage.

A key aspect for vaccine design has been the use of longitudinal memory B-cell NGS to accurately infer the sequence of the unmutated common ancestor (UCA) for several bNAb lineages. The accuracy of this inference is highly dependent on the availability of early, less mutated bnAb lineage sequences. In some cases, these UCAs can bind (CH235, CH103, PCT64) and even neutralize early Env variants (CH103, CAP256-VRC26 and PCT64) [47, 58, 96–98]. However, in others, no binding of precursor B-cells was detectable (PCDN, PCIN39, DH270, PCIN63). This observation led to the hypothesis that some of these bNAbs may have matured from responses to other pathogens, however it is also possible that affinity undetectable in existing assays might have been sufficient to induce BCR signaling and initiate clonal expansion in vivo [99]. Moreover, this low affinity, mainly due to the sub-optimal epitope presentation on the Env protein, can be overcome by synthetic minimal

epitope molecules such as CD4bs mimics eOD-GT8 and 426c (VRC01) [54, 100, 101], short V3-glycopeptides (DH270) [102, 103] and V2-apex scaffolds [40, 41], providing opportunities for immunogen design.

Activation of the naïve B-cell precursor induces a rapid expansion and diversification of the mAb lineage, which is typically followed by a contraction phase that is likely due to rapid viral escape preventing further maturation [59]. Memory B-cell repertoire analyses have revealed subsequent multi-limb maturation as the early antibody intermediates undergo different fates, depending on whether they can still recognize emerging new viral variants [47, 59]. Some branches display limited maturation ("dead-end" sub-lineages) due to a failure to recognize emerging viral variants [96]. Other branches continue to accumulate SHM in distinct parallel pathways through continual adaptation to new variants in the autologous virus population [47, 59, 96]. However, continued maturation is not always associated with neutralization breadth. Bhiman et al. [96] described highly mutated "off-track" CAP256-VRC26 mAbs, which have more than 20% SHM but limited neutralization breadth. Similar observations have been made in other bNAb lineages [58, 104, 105], and as mAb isolation methodologies are specifically designed to recover bNAbs, the proportion of bNAb lineages that are off-track is unknown.

Table 1 Studies of the maturation of broadly neutralizing antibodies

Epitope	Donor	Sampling	Ab lineage	Breadth Median IC50	VH-gene SHM (%nt)	VL-gene	CDR3 length	Indels	Poly/ autoreactivity	Viral subtype	Viral sequencing	UCA binds/ neutralizes T/F	References
CD4bs	NIH45	Chronic	VRC01	89%; 0.3 µg/mL	VH1-2 32%	VK3-20	H:14aa L:5 aa	Yes Del CDRL1	+	B	No		[36, 38]
	DRVI01	Chronic	DRVIA7	<10%	VH1-2 19%	VK1-5	H:13 aa L:5 aa	No		B	Yes		[120]
	CH505	Longitudinal	CH103	55%; 4.54 µg/mL	VH4-59 14%	VL3-1	H:15 aa L:10 aa	Yes Del CDRL1	++	C	Yes	Neutralization	[58]
	CH505	Longitudinal	CH235	90%; 0.6 µg/mL	VH1-46 28%	VK3-15	H:15aa L:8 aa	No	++	C	Yes	Weak binding	[108, 119]
	N60	Chronic	N60P25.1	73%	VH1-2 33%	VK1-5	H:13aa L:5 aa	No		B	No		[125]
	N49	Chronic	N49P7	98%; 0.1 µg/mL	VH1-2 33%	VL2-11	H:19aa L:5 aa	Yes Del CDRL1		B	No		[125]
	PC063	Longitudinal	PCIN63	80%; 0.24 µg/mL	VH1-2 15%	VK1-5	H:15 aa L:5 aa	No	Variable	C	Yes	No binding	Landais et al. (unpublished)
V2-glycan	CAP256	Longitudinal	VRC26-CAP256	63%; 0.003 µg/mL	VH3-30 12%	VL1-51	H:36 aa L:13 aa	No	–	C	Yes	Neutralization	[47, 96]
	PC064	Longitudinal	PCT64	37%; 0.42 µg/mL	VH3-15 13%	VK3-20	H:25aa L:8 aa	No	±	A	Yes	Binding of 293S-expressed Env	[97, 98]
V3-glycan	PC076	Longitudinal	PCDN	47%; 0.53 µg/mL	VH4-34 16%	VK3-20	H:22 aa L:8aa	No	±	C	Yes	No binding	[59]
	PC039	Longitudinal	PCN39	45%; 0.03 µg/mL	VH4-34 16%	VK3-20	H:22 aa L:10aa	Yes Ins CDRH1	++	C	Yes	No binding	Murrell, Landais et al. (unpublished)
	BF520	Longitudinal (Infant)	BF520.1	58%; 1.95 µg/mL	VH1-2 7%	VK3-15	H:20 aa L:7aa	No		A	Yes	Cell surface binding	[80]
	CH848	Longitudinal	DH270	55%; 0.08 µg/mL	VH1-2 13%	VL2-23	H:20aa L:9 aa	No	±	C	Yes	Weak binding	[102]
MPER	N152	Chronic	10E8	98%; 0.35 µg/mL	VH3-15 21%	VL3-19	H:22 aa L:11 aa	No	–	B	No		[149]
	CHO210	Chronic	DH511	99%; 1.04 µg/mL	VH3-15 18%	VK1-39	H:22 aa L:11 aa	No	++	C	No		[150]

Structural studies carried out in parallel to the repertoire analyses have also provided critical insights into the molecular basis of affinity maturation (reviewed in [106]). The detailed molecular mechanisms allowing neutralization breadth via epitope focusing and by adaptation to the glycan shield (through direct contact or by reducing steric clashes) have been better defined, and exploited for immunogen design (see below). Overall, the low affinity of bNAb precursors for cognate antigens is associated with lower thermodynamic stability, particularly of CDR loops, and SHM leads to epitope focusing [107], improved shape complementarity and increased buried surface area at the interface with the antigen, by conformational re-organization and stabilization of the paratope [47, 97]. Within bNAb lineages, these changes can occur independently within different sublineages maturing to acquire breadth [46, 47, 58, 96, 104, 105]. These varying pathways to breadth strongly demonstrate the plasticity of the immune system, which, even within one antibody lineage, can find multiple structural and genetic solutions to the same immunological problem.

The role of viral variants in selecting bNAbs

These multiple pathways to bNAb maturation also highlight the power of the selective pressure exerted by emerging Env variants. A common finding from co-evolution studies is that of Env diversity as a key driver of breadth, with the emergence of cross-neutralization within bNAb lineages associated with a burst of viral diversity [47, 58, 97]. This early viral diversification is the result of selective pressure by early (strain-specific) precursors within the bNAb lineage [96], or by unrelated "helper" or "cooperating" neutralizing antibodies that target an overlapping epitope and drive viral mutations within the bNAb epitope [102, 108–110]. Maturing bNAb lineages are thus constantly exposed to a large variety of Env "immunotypes", varying not only in amino acid sequence [96], but also in conformation and glycosylation profile [97]. These viral mutants are recognized by bNAb intermediates capable of tolerating emerging "immunotypes" within epitopes, and these continue to be selected during the next round of affinity maturation [96]. This constant exposure of the immune system to viral variants and glycoform heterogeneity selects those antibody sub-lineages able to tolerate viral diversity and indirectly drives the maturation of bNAbs [96]. The rate of viral escape also seems to be key. Within the CAP256-VRC26 lineage, constrained virus escape was associated with reduced infectivity and altered entry kinetics [111]. This observation is consistent with the likelihood that bNAb epitopes are conserved for functional reasons, with escape likely requiring compensatory mutations [97, 110], and suggests that slower viral escape supports

the development of bNAbs through prolonged exposure to antigen [96, 97, 110, 111]. This hypothesis is further supported by the demonstration in vaccine studies that extended antigen availability enhances germinal center activity and resulting neutralizing Ab responses [112, 113].

BNAb development thus depends on a sustained feedback loop, in which Env diversity and high antigen levels lead to increased diversity in the Ab response. This i) increases the chances of stimulating relevant precursors, and ii) results in maturing bNAb lineages being exposed to multiple related antigens, generated as the virus explores multiple escape pathways within a restricted landscape, eventually leading to neutralization breadth. This supports a strategy of using sequential Envs from elite neutralizers as templates for immunogen design, which has recently shown promise in animal vaccination studies, albeit in the artificial context of mice engineered to express bNAb precursors [114].

Can common patterns in bNAb development be exploited for immunogen design?

Although co-evolutionary studies provide fascinating insights into the immune system, their utility as models for vaccine design is based on the notion that there are inter-donor commonalities amenable to vaccine design. As more studies emerge, such common patterns are becoming evident, both in terms of antibody precursors and the viral variants that select them.

The exquisite structural homogeneity with which VRC01-class bNAb precursors bind to the HIV Env CD4bs has been exploited in the design of germline-targeting immunogens (eOD-GT8 and 426c) [54, 100, 101]. These could elicit narrowly neutralizing antibody responses with VRC01-like characteristics, namely VH1-2 gene usage, a 5 amino acid CDRL3 and a short/flexible CDRL1, in mouse models [53, 115–117]. As additional studies of V2 and V3-glycan directed bNAbs define common features in their precursors and in the viral envelopes bound by them, germline targeting is being expanded to other epitopes [40, 41, 55, 114, 118].

Similarly, comparison of the viral diversification that leads to breadth is identifying convergent envelope features, which could be harnessed for vaccine design. For example, in two V2-glycan bNAb donors, there is striking similarity in the viral variants associated with maturation of breadth [96, 97]. In both these donors, localized diversity at the same key V2 epitope residues, specifically residues 166 and 169, selected SHM that drove bNAb maturation toward breadth [96, 97]. Similarly, studies of CD4bs directed antibodies in several donors have highlighted the role of variation in loop D and in the V5 glycans in shaping breadth [58, 108, 119], whereas for

V3-glycan bNAbs, shifting glycans at positions 332, 335 and 301, and mutations within the V3 GDIR motif are common escape mechanisms between donors [59, 102]. While these studies support the idea of rational vaccine design and provide the first real hope that common pathways may exist, systematic structural and functional evaluation of longitudinal bNAb/Env autologous complexes and a deeper understanding of Env conformational plasticity, will provide insight into how these interactions drive bNAb lineage maturation towards breadth.

Are the unusual features of bNAbs an insurmountable hurdle for vaccine design?

The high level of SHM typically exhibited by bNAbs is seen as a major hurdle for vaccination. This is especially true of bNAbs targeting the CD4bs. Indeed, despite the detection of VRC01-class Ab precursors in the naïve repertoire of a majority of healthy individuals [101], bNAbs directed to the CD4bs rarely develop in infected individuals and typically only after several (> 5) years of infection. Although about two-thirds of the SHM seen in CD4bs directed bNAb VRC01 conferred no benefit in terms of neutralization breadth [60], adaptation to the glycan surrounding the CD4bs, such as position N276, appears to be a major hurdle for CD4bs VH1-2 antibody lineages to overcome. This was clearly demonstrated through the study of the DRIVA7 lineage which, despite being encoded by a VH1-2*02 gene, encoding the critical 5 amino acid CDRL3 associated with VRC01-class bNAbs, and acquiring critical mutations in the CDRH1, CDRH3 and FRH3, failed to achieve the light chain maturation necessary to adapt to HIV Env loop D and V5 glycans [120].

There are however some examples that suggest that there may be shortcuts to the development of breadth, providing a more feasible template for vaccine design. One such example is the CD4bs lineage from donor PC63, which has equivalent breadth and potency to VRC01, but substantially less SHM (13.7% compared to 31.6% of VH1-2 nucleotides) [121]. Notably, the SHM that appears in this lineage is highly focused at positions previously shown to be key CD4bs epitope contacts or glycan adaptation residues, suggesting that the viral variants in this donor might represent an ideal series of immunogens to drive the inclusion of "useful" SHM in CD4bs lineages, and avoiding the selection of redundant mutations that do not contribute to breadth.

In addition to the pediatric V3 glycan mAb BF520.1 described above [77], lower levels of SHM have also been described for adult bNAbs targeting the V3-glycan supersite. These include the PCDN [59], DH270 [102] and PCIN39 [122] bNAb lineages, further suggesting that shorter maturation pathways more compatible with

vaccination can be achieved for this epitope. Furthermore, three of these V3-glycan lineages also achieved breadth without insertion/deletions (indels) in CDR loops, seen as another major roadblock for vaccination. Interestingly, in the fourth example, CDRH1 insertions of different lengths occurred independently in several branches of the PCIN39 lineage. Together, these studies suggest (i) that indels may not necessarily be required for V3-glycan bNAbs (ii) that indels may be less rare than anticipated, and that given the right selection, Ab lineages with insertions could be elicited by vaccination. Thus, despite substantial genetic and structural heterogeneity, the V3-glycan supersite remains an attractive vaccine target.

For bNAbs to the V2-glycan epitope, the long CDRH3s characteristic of this class of bNAbs arise during naïve rearrangement rather than during maturation [47], and are extremely rare in the naïve repertoire [49]. Nonetheless, such specificities, once triggered can rapidly mature towards breadth with moderate levels of SHM [47]. Furthermore, V2-glycan bNAbs PCT64, VRC38 and CH01 bear slightly shorter CDRH3 loops of ~ 25 amino acids, which are much more common in the naïve repertoire. Although bNAbs with shorter CDRH3s showed significantly lower breadth than the PG9, PGDM1400 and CAP256-VRC26 bNAbs that have longer CDRH3s, this reduced breadth is potentially off-set in a vaccine scenario by higher precursor frequency [82, 123]. This balance between breadth and more "normal" genetic features of antibodies raises the question of whether the focus on elite neutralizers may have resulted in missed opportunities. With the exception of germline targeting immunogens, most vaccines aim to elicit polyclonal responses to multiple epitopes, a scenario similar to that of most HIV infected individuals, who develop some cross-reactivity [18], often targeting multiple epitopes [20, 21, 82–85]. It is therefore possible that a renewed focus on more "elicitable" antibodies, with features more representative of the overall repertoire (e.g. few insertions or deletions, lower levels of SHM and average length CDRH3 s) may be valuable in honing vaccine candidates.

Can studies of failed bNAb lineages tell us what the roadblocks are?

In addition to studies of more moderate neutralizers, studies of failed bNAb lineages may also be informative. Although most individuals mount robust neutralizing responses, the low proportion of individuals who develop breadth, and the fact that in some broad neutralizers, bNAbs represent a minority of the overall response [124, 125] suggests that the roadblocks impeding the development of breadth are profound. Analysis of the developmental pathway of Ab lineages failing to develop breadth would also shed light on the molecular events limiting the acquisition of neutralization breadth [126]. Defining both favorable and unfavorable maturation pathways may also allow a better evaluation of the responses elicited by immunization to determine whether they are on the "right" track.

Leveraging studies of infection for vaccine design: What are the gaps?

Overall, the data reviewed here suggest a model based on the stochastic recruitment of rare, low-affinity precursor B cells, often with unusual features, by Env variants that may be equally unusual, followed by the survival of randomly generated intermediates with low affinity for emerging viral escape variants. Many of the factors associated with breadth (described above), effectively act by increasing the chances of successful bNAb generation. The main goal of vaccine design is to similarly increase the odds, by optimizing immunogens and adjuvants and by defining novel vaccine regimens and delivery schedules (Fig. 3 and Table 2).

Several solutions are already being explored for the optimization of immunogens, such as the development of high-affinity germline targeting immunogens [39–41, 53–56, 103, 127]. Soluble stabilized Env trimers with key structural features are also a major focus in the field, to select critical antibody intermediates capable

of binding the functionally relevant Env native conformation (reviewed in [128]). While the design of soluble trimers has greatly advanced the field, less is known about envelope signatures that impact the thermodynamics of natural viral trimers, perhaps affecting binding/ neutralization by early bnAb intermediates. Understanding the stabilized conformation compared to membrane anchored spikes [98] and whether some degree of flexibility is necessary for productive interactions within developing bNAb lineages will be informative. Finally, variation in glycosylation also likely impacts trimer properties, and extending recent advances in glycobiology [11, 129, 130] will provide additional insights into controlling the glycan shield for acquisition of breadth [131, 132].

The rationale for further trimer stabilization is, in part, to reduce elicitation of "distracting", mostly V3 directed, strain-specific responses, which might outcompete the bNAb lineages during affinity maturation [133]. However, during infection bNAbs develop in a highly competitive environment, and immunization studies showed that autologous neutralizing titers were not enhanced by reduction of V3 responses [113, 134]. Additionally, two elegant studies recently showed that most GCs retain substantial clonal diversity during affinity maturation of complex antigens [135, 136]. The effect of interclonal competition as a limiting factor for bNAb elicitation is thus not clear. Much of what we know about the GC

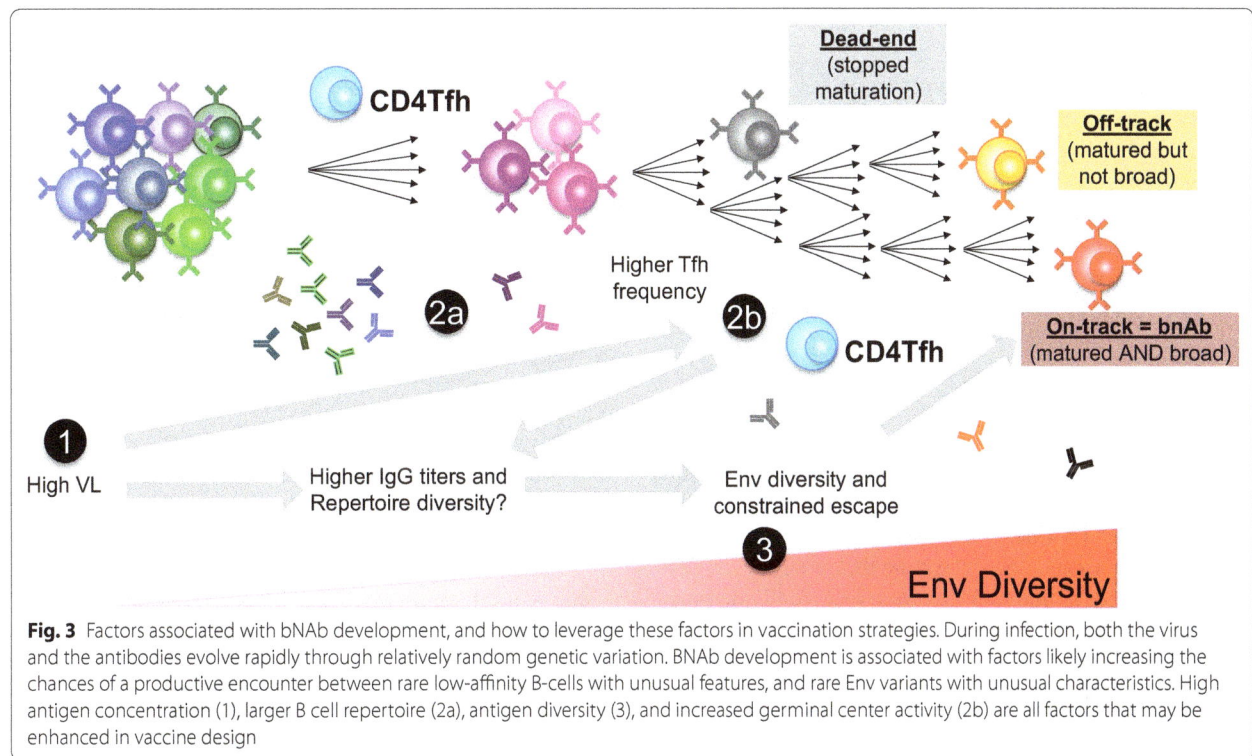

Fig. 3 Factors associated with bNAb development, and how to leverage these factors in vaccination strategies. During infection, both the virus and the antibodies evolve rapidly through relatively random genetic variation. BNAb development is associated with factors likely increasing the chances of a productive encounter between rare low-affinity B-cells with unusual features, and rare Env variants with unusual characteristics. High antigen concentration (1), larger B cell repertoire (2a), antigen diversity (3), and increased germinal center activity (2b) are all factors that may be enhanced in vaccine design

Table 2 Translating insights from studies of infection into novel immunization strategies

		Mechanism in infection	Immunization
1	High viral load	Recruitment of larger B and T cell repertoires by increasing chances of activating lower affinity precursors due to higher antigen concentration	Germline-targeting immunogen design based on UCA features → high affinity prime
			Adjuvants to boost innate immune responses
2a	High anti-Env IgG Titers and helper lineages of neutralizing antibodies	More diverse repertoire increases chance of productive bNAb UCA encountering antigen	Adjuvants to ensure high Ab titers and posibly greater diversity
		May restrict/slow down viral escape	Sustained delivery to ensure prolonged availability of Ags
			Adjuvants to boost innate immune responses
2b	High frequency of Tfh	May increase chances of activating lower affinity intermediates with unusual features, thereby sustaining affinity maturation and leading to higher SHM levels	Formulation should include T-cell epitopes
			Adjuvants to boost innate immune responses and GC reaction
3	Burst of viral diversity	Increased chances of activating/maturing low affinity intermediates with unusual features. Sustained affinity maturation and associated high levels of SHM	Immunogen design incorporating incremental diversity. Autologous versus heterologous boosts to avoid "dead-end" pathways
			Contemporaneous delivery of "variants" to quickly select relevant intermediates and positive selection

Numbering relates to Fig. 3

reaction comes from studies mimicking an acute infection with non-variable model antigens, and B-cell affinity maturation and differentiation in chronic GCs are incompletely defined (Reviewed in [137–139]). Specifically, the accumulation of higher levels of SHM and its effect on self-reactivity [140], and the impact of antigenic drift associated with HIV infection on the formation of memory subsets need to be better understood. Ongoing studies aiming to directly sample GC B cells and T follicular helper and regulatory cells during infection, as has recently been done in immunization [112], will be important.

Translating viral studies from elite neutralizers to vaccine design is another active area of research. Though incorporating some antigen diversity seems crucial, vaccine regimens cannot match the Env diversity seen during infection. How much diversity is required is not known. Several studies suggest that sequential delivery of a mix of Env immunogens may be preferable over a repeated cocktail immunization for the elicitation of bNAb responses [141, 142]. This contrasts by GC modeling studies [143] and with findings from studies of elite neutralizers, where a burst of viral diversity typically precedes acquisition of breadth [47, 58, 59]. Furthermore, the association of bNAbs with slower viral escape, and the existence of antibody "dead-ends", suggests that too much variation between prime and boost Envs may terminate a nascent lineage. While animal data suggests that a lineage of autologous Env may specifically drive the maturation of a particular lineage [55, 115, 144], whether this will be a generalizable response in vaccine recipients will require human trials.

A further challenge is how to drive maturing lineages to accommodate glycans, particularly where a given glycan, such as that at residue 276, is incompatible with binding with bNAb precursors, but globally conserved on viruses. One approach has been the creation of "glycan holes" in Env immunogens. These bare Env regions are immunodominant in vaccine studies [145, 146], however the potential of these neutralizing responses to mature to recognize or tolerate glycans is unclear. During infection, breadth is not determined by the overall autologous neutralizing response ([14, 19] Sheward, Moore and Williamson, in press). This highlights the remaining challenges in driving "glycan-hole" directed vaccine responses towards breadth. Finally, the need for sustained exposure to high concentrations of antigens, as in infected donors with high viral loads, has led to strategies incorporating subcutaneous and extended administration with promising improvements in nAb titers [113, 147, 148].

In summary, the identification of elite neutralizers, and the unprecedented detail in which these donors have been studied, has provided crucial immunological and virological insights into the development of bNAbs. The translation of these landmark studies into innovative vaccine strategies that seek to bypass the stringent limitations imposed by rare bNAb precursors, and drive these towards breadth is generating promising data in animal studies. Ongoing and planned experimental medicine trials in humans will take the HIV vaccine field into a hugely exciting era. For the first time in 30 years of an HIV pandemic that has devastated communities, these studies provide hope that an HIV vaccine may be achieved, but also provided immunological lessons that are being harnessed for the design of vaccines against other highly mutable, complex pathogens.

Authors' contributions
PLM and EL wrote this manuscript and prepared the figures. Both authors read and approved the final manuscript.

Author details
[1] International AIDS Vaccine Initiative Neutralizing Antibody Center, The Scripps Research Institute, La Jolla, CA 92037, USA. [2] Department of Immunology and Microbiology, The Scripps Research Institute, La Jolla, CA 92037, USA. [3] International AIDS Vaccine Initiative, New York, NY 10004, USA. [4] Centre for HIV and STIs, National Institute for Communicable Diseases of the National Health Laboratory Service, Johannesburg, South Africa. [5] Faculty of Health Sciences, University of the Witwatersrand, Johannesburg, South Africa. [6] Centre for the AIDS Programme of Research in South Africa (CAPRISA), University of KwaZulu-Natal, Durban, South Africa.

Acknowledgements
PLM and EL would like to thank members of our laboratories, and many collaborators and students who have contributed to this review through useful discussions.

Competing interests
The authors declare that they have no competing interests.

Funding
EL is supported by the International AIDS Vaccine Initiative. IAVI's work is made possible by generous support from many donors including: the Bill & Melinda Gates Foundation; the Ministry of Foreign Affairs of Denmark; Irish Aid; the Ministry of Finance of Japan in partnership with The World Bank; the Ministry of Foreign Affairs of the Netherlands; the Norwegian Agency for Development Cooperation (NORAD); the United Kingdom Department for International Development (DFID), and the United States Agency for International Development (USAID). The full list of IAVI donors is available at www.iavi.org. The contents are the responsibility of the International AIDS Vaccine Initiative and do not necessarily reflect the views of USAID or the United States Government. PLM is supported by the South African Research Chairs Initiative of the Department of Science and Technology and National Research Foundation of South Africa, the National Institutes for Health through a U01 grant (AI116086-01), the SA Medical Research Council SHIP program and Centre for the AIDS Program of Research (CAPRISA). Related research is conducted as part of the DST-NRF Centre of Excellence in HIV Prevention, which is supported by the Department of Science and Technology and the National Research Foundation. This collaboration was supported the generous support of the American people through USAID.

References

1. Abdool Karim Q, et al. Effectiveness and safety of tenofovir gel, an antiretroviral microbicide, for the prevention of HIV infection in women. Science. 2010;329(5996):1168–74.
2. Ackerman ME, et al. Polyfunctional HIV-specific antibody responses are associated with spontaneous HIV control. PLoS Pathog. 2016;12(1):e1005315.
3. Forthal DN, et al. FcgammaRIIa genotype predicts progression of HIV infection. J Immunol. 2007;179(11):7916–23.
4. Lambotte O, et al. Heterogeneous neutralizing antibody and antibody-dependent cell cytotoxicity responses in HIV-1 elite controllers. AIDS. 2009;23(8):897–906.
5. Walker LM, Burton DR. Passive immunotherapy of viral infections: 'super-antibodies' enter the fray. Nat Rev Immunol. 2018;18(5):297–308.
6. Hessell AJ, et al. Effective, low-titer antibody protection against low-dose repeated mucosal SHIV challenge in macaques. Nat Med. 2009;15(8):951–4.
7. Burton DR, et al. Limited or no protection by weakly or nonneutralizing antibodies against vaginal SHIV challenge of macaques compared with a strongly neutralizing antibody. Proc Natl Acad Sci USA. 2011;108(27):11181–6.
8. Dugast AS, et al. Lack of protection following passive transfer of polyclonal highly functional low-dose non-neutralizing antibodies. PLoS ONE. 2014;9(5):e97229.
9. Ward AB, Wilson IA. Insights into the trimeric HIV-1 envelope glycoprotein structure. Trends Biochem Sci. 2015;40(2):101–7.
10. Zhu P, et al. Electron tomography analysis of envelope glycoprotein trimers on HIV and simian immunodeficiency virus virions. Proc Natl Acad Sci USA. 2003;100(26):15812–7.
11. Behrens AJ, et al. Composition and antigenic effects of individual glycan sites of a trimeric HIV-1 envelope glycoprotein. Cell Rep. 2016;14(11):2695–706.
12. Moore PL, et al. Nature of nonfunctional envelope proteins on the surface of human immunodeficiency virus type 1. J Virol. 2006;80(5):2515–28.
13. Frost SD, et al. Neutralizing antibody responses drive the evolution of human immunodeficiency virus type 1 envelope during recent HIV infection. Proc Natl Acad Sci USA. 2005;102(51):18514–9.
14. Gray ES, et al. Neutralizing antibody responses in acute human immunodeficiency virus type 1 subtype C infection. J Virol. 2007;81(12):6187–96.
15. Li B, et al. Evidence for potent autologous neutralizing antibody titers and compact envelopes in early infection with subtype C human immunodeficiency virus type 1. J Virol. 2006;80(11):5211–8.
16. Richman DD, et al. Rapid evolution of the neutralizing antibody response to HIV type 1 infection. Proc Natl Acad Sci USA. 2003;100(7):4144–9.
17. Wei X, et al. Antibody neutralization and escape by HIV-1. Nature. 2003;422(6929):307–12.
18. Hraber P, et al. Prevalence of broadly neutralizing antibody responses during chronic HIV-1 infection. AIDS. 2014;28(2):163–9.
19. Gray ES, et al. HIV-1 neutralization breadth develops incrementally over 4 years and is associated with CD4+ T cell decline and high viral load during acute infection. J Virol. 2011;85(10):4828–40.
20. Tomaras GD, et al. Polyclonal B cell responses to conserved neutralization epitopes in a subset of HIV-1-infected individuals. J Virol. 2011;85(21):11502–19.
21. Landais E, et al. Broadly neutralizing antibody responses in a large longitudinal sub-Saharan HIV primary infection cohort. PLoS Pathog. 2016;12(1):e1005369.
22. Kong R, et al. Fusion peptide of HIV-1 as a site of vulnerability to neutralizing antibody. Science. 2016;352(6287):828–33.
23. Wibmer CK, Moore PL, Morris L. HIV broadly neutralizing antibody targets. Curr Opin HIV AIDS. 2015;10:135.
24. van Gils MJ, et al. An HIV-1 antibody from an elite neutralizer implicates the fusion peptide as a site of vulnerability. Nat Microbiol. 2016;2:16199.
25. Zhou T, et al. A neutralizing antibody recognizing primarily N-linked glycan targets the silent face of the HIV envelope. Immunity. 2018;48(3):500e6–513e6.

26. Bianchi M, Turner HL, Nogal B, Cottrell CA, Oyen D, Pauthner M, Bastidas R, Nedellec R, McCoy LE, Wilson IA, Burton DR, Ward AB, Hangartner L. 2018;49(2):288-300.e8. https://doi.org/10.1016/j.immuni.2018.07.009.

27. Burton DR, Hangartner L. Broadly neutralizing antibodies to HIV and their role in vaccine design. Annu Rev Immunol. 2016;34:635–59.

28. Doores KJ, et al. Two classes of broadly neutralizing antibodies within a single lineage directed to the high-mannose patch of HIV Envelope. J Virol. 2014;89(2):1105–18.

29. Walker LM, et al. Broad neutralization coverage of HIV by multiple highly potent antibodies. Nature. 2011;477(7365):466–70.

30. Garces F, et al. Structural evolution of glycan recognition by a family of potent HIV antibodies. Cell. 2014;159(1):69–79.

31. Sok D, et al. Promiscuous glycan site recognition by antibodies to the high-mannose patch of gp120 broadens neutralization of HIV. Sci Transl Med. 2014;6(236):236ra63.

32. Blattner C, et al. Structural delineation of a quaternary, cleavage-dependent epitope at the gp41-gp120 interface on intact HIV-1 Env trimers. Immunity. 2014;40(5):669–80.

33. Huang J, et al. Broad and potent HIV-1 neutralization by a human antibody that binds the gp41-gp120 interface. Nature. 2014;515(7525):138–42.

34. Scharf L, et al. Antibody 8ANC195 reveals a site of broad vulnerability on the HIV-1 envelope spike. Cell Rep. 2014;7(3):785–95.

35. Wibmer CK, et al. Structure and recognition of a novel HIV-1 gp120-gp41 interface antibody that caused MPER exposure through viral escape. PLoS Pathog. 2017;13(1):e1006074.

36. Wu X, et al. Focused evolution of HIV-1 neutralizing antibodies revealed by structures and deep sequencing. Science. 2011;333(6049):1593–602.

37. Scheid JF, et al. Sequence and structural convergence of broad and potent HIV antibodies that mimic CD4 binding. Science. 2011;333(6049):1633–7.

38. Zhou T, et al. Multidonor analysis reveals structural elements, genetic determinants, and maturation pathway for HIV-1 neutralization by VRC01-class antibodies. Immunity. 2013;39(2):245–58.

39. Jardine J, et al. Rational HIV immunogen design to target specific germline B cell receptors. Science. 2013;340(6133):711–6.

40. Andrabi R, et al. Identification of common features in prototype broadly neutralizing antibodies to HIV envelope V2 apex to facilitate vaccine design. Immunity. 2015;43(5):959–73.

41. Gorman J, et al. Structures of HIV-1 Env V1V2 with broadly neutralizing antibodies reveal commonalities that enable vaccine design. Nat Struct Mol Biol. 2016;23(1):81–90.

42. Moore PL, et al. Ontogeny-based immunogens for the induction of V2-directed HIV broadly neutralizing antibodies. Immunol Rev. 2017;275(1):217–29.

43. Walker LM, et al. Broad and potent neutralizing antibodies from an African donor reveal a new HIV-1 vaccine target. Science. 2009;326(5950):285–9.

44. Muster T, et al. A conserved neutralizing epitope on gp41 of human immunodeficiency virus type 1. J Virol. 1993;67(11):6642–7.

45. Zwick MB, et al. Anti-human immunodeficiency virus type 1 (HIV-1) antibodies 2F5 and 4E10 require surprisingly few crucial residues in the membrane-proximal external region of glycoprotein gp41 to neutralize HIV-1. J Virol. 2005;79(2):1252–61.

46. Bonsignori M, et al. Analysis of a clonal lineage of HIV-1 envelope V2/V3 conformational epitope-specific broadly neutralizing antibodies and their inferred unmutated common ancestors. J Virol. 2011;85(19):9998–10009.

47. Doria-Rose NA, et al. Developmental pathway for potent V1V2-directed HIV-neutralizing antibodies. Nature. 2014;509(7498):55–62.

48. Sok D, et al. Recombinant HIV envelope trimer selects for quaternary-dependent antibodies targeting the trimer apex. Proc Natl Acad Sci USA. 2014;111(49):17624–9.

49. Briney BS, et al. Frequency and genetic characterization of V(DD) J recombinants in the human peripheral blood antibody repertoire. Immunology. 2012;137(1):56–64.

50. Briney BS, Willis JR, Crowe JE Jr. Location and length distribution of somatic hypermutation-associated DNA insertions and deletions reveals regions of antibody structural plasticity. Genes Immun. 2012;13(7):523–9.

51. Verkoczy L, et al. Role of immune mechanisms in induction of HIV-1 broadly neutralizing antibodies. Curr Opin Immunol. 2011;23(3):383–90.

52. Doyle-Cooper C, et al. Immune tolerance negatively regulates B cells in knock-in mice expressing broadly neutralizing HIV antibody 4E10. J Immunol. 2013;191(6):3186–91.

53. Dosenovic P, et al. Immunization for HIV-1 broadly neutralizing antibodies in human Ig knockin mice. Cell. 2015;161(7):1505–15.

54. McGuire AT, et al. Engineering HIV envelope protein to activate germline B cell receptors of broadly neutralizing anti-CD4 binding site antibodies. J Exp Med. 2013;210(4):655–63.

55. Steichen JM, et al. HIV vaccine design to target germline precursors of glycan-dependent broadly neutralizing antibodies. Immunity. 2016;45(3):483–96.

56. Medina-Ramirez M, et al. Design and crystal structure of a native-like HIV-1 envelope trimer that engages multiple broadly neutralizing antibody precursors in vivo. J Exp Med. 2017;214(9):2573–90.

57. Klein F, et al. Somatic mutations of the immunoglobulin framework are generally required for broad and potent HIV-1 neutralization. Cell. 2013;153(1):126–38.

58. Liao HX, et al. Co-evolution of a broadly neutralizing HIV-1 antibody and founder virus. Nature. 2013;496(7446):469–76.

59. MacLeod DT, et al. Early antibody lineage diversification and independent limb maturation lead to broad HIV-1 neutralization targeting the Env high-mannose patch. Immunity. 2016;44(5):1215–26.

60. Jardine JG, et al. Minimally mutated HIV-1 broadly neutralizing antibodies to guide reductionist vaccine design. PLoS Pathog. 2016;12(8):e1005815.

61. Georgiev IS, et al. Antibodies VRC01 and 10E8 neutralize HIV-1 with high breadth and potency even with Ig-framework regions substantially reverted to germline. J Immunol. 2014;192(3):1100–6.

62. Haynes BF, et al. HIV-host interactions: implications for vaccine design. Cell Host Microbe. 2016;19(3):292–303.

63. Rudicell RS, et al. Enhanced potency of a broadly neutralizing HIV-1 antibody in vitro improves protection against lentiviral infection in vivo. J Virol. 2014;88(21):12669–82.

64. Burton DR, Mascola JR. Antibody responses to envelope glycoproteins in HIV-1 infection. Nat Immunol. 2015;16(6):571–6.

65. Rusert P, et al. Determinants of HIV-1 broadly neutralizing antibody induction. Nat Med. 2016;22(11):1260–7.

66. Sather DN, et al. Factors associated with the development of cross-reactive neutralizing antibodies during human immunodeficiency virus type 1 infection. J Virol. 2009;83(2):757–69.

67. Piantadosi A, et al. Breadth of neutralizing antibody response to human immunodeficiency virus type 1 is affected by factors early in infection but does not influence disease progression. J Virol. 2009;83(19):10269–74.

68. Smith SA, et al. Diversification in the HIV-1 envelope hyper-variable domains V2, V4, and V5 and higher probability of transmitted/founder envelope glycosylation favor the development of heterologous neutralization breadth. PLoS Pathog. 2016;12(11):e1005989.

69. Locci M, et al. Human circulating PD-1 + CXCR3-CXCR5+ memory Tfh cells are highly functional and correlate with broadly neutralizing HIV antibody responses. Immunity. 2013;39(4):758–69.

70. Cohen K, et al. Early preservation of CXCR5 + PD-1+ helper T cells and B cell activation predict the breadth of neutralizing antibody responses in chronic HIV-1 infection. J Virol. 2014;88(22):13310–21.

71. Richardson SI, et al. HIV-specific Fc effector function early in infection predicts the development of broadly neutralizing antibodies. PLoS Pathog. 2018;14(4):e1006987.

72. Moody MA, et al. Immune perturbations in HIV-1-infected individuals who make broadly neutralizing antibodies. Sci Immunol. 2016;1(1):aag0851.

73. Cortez V, et al. HIV-1 superinfection in women broadens and strengthens the neutralizing antibody response. PLoS Pathog. 2012;8(3):e1002611.

74. Powell RL, Kinge T, Nyambi PN. Infection by discordant strains of HIV-1 markedly enhances the neutralizing antibody response against heterologous virus. J Virol. 2010;84(18):9415–26.

75. Cornelissen M, et al. The neutralizing antibody response in an individual with triple HIV-1 infection remains directed at the first infecting subtype. AIDS Res Hum Retroviruses. 2016;32(10–11):1135–42.

76. Moore PL, et al. Potent and broad neutralization of HIV-1 subtype C by plasma antibodies targeting a quaternary epitope including residues in the V2 loop. J Virol. 2011;85(7):3128–41.

77. Williams KL, et al. Superinfection drives HIV neutralizing antibody responses from several B cell lineages that contribute to a polyclonal repertoire. Cell Rep. 2018;23(3):682–91.

78. Muenchhoff M, et al. Nonprogressing HIV-infected children share fundamental immunological features of nonpathogenic SIV infection. Sci Transl Med. 2016;8(358):358ra125.

79. Goo L, et al. Early development of broadly neutralizing antibodies in HIV-1-infected infants. Nat Med. 2014;20(6):655–8.

80. Simonich CA, et al. HIV-1 neutralizing antibodies with limited hypermutation from an infant. Cell. 2016;166(1):77–87.

81. Ditse Z, et al. HIV-1 subtype C infected children with exceptional neutralization breadth exhibit polyclonal responses targeting known epitopes. J Virol. 2018;92(17):e00878–18.

82. Bonsignori M, et al. Two distinct broadly neutralizing antibody specificities of different clonal lineages in a single HIV-1-infected donor: implications for vaccine design. J Virol. 2012;86(8):4688–92.

83. Wibmer K, et al. Viral Escape from HIV-1 Neutralizing Antibodies Drives Increased Plasma Neutralization Breadth through Sequential Recognition of Multiple Epitopes and Immunotypes. PLoS Pathog. 2013;9(10):e1003738.

84. Walker LM, et al. A limited number of antibody specificities mediate broad and potent serum neutralization in selected HIV-1 infected individuals. PLoS Pathog. 2010;6(8):e1001028.

85. Scheid JF, et al. Broad diversity of neutralizing antibodies isolated from memory B cells in HIV-infected individuals. Nature. 2009;458(7238):636–40.

86. Derdeyn CA, Moore PL, Morris L. Development of broadly neutralizing antibodies from autologous neutralizing antibody responses in HIV infection. Curr Opin HIV AIDS. 2014;9(3):210–6.

87. Gray ES, et al. The neutralization breadth of HIV-1 develops incrementally over four years and is associated with CD4+ T cell decline and high viral load during acute infection. J Virol. 2011;85(10):4828–40.

88. Moore PL, Williamson C, Morris L. Virological features associated with the development of broadly neutralizing antibodies to HIV-1. Trends Microbiol. 2015;23(4):204–11.

89. Schoofs T, et al. HIV-1 therapy with monoclonal antibody 3BNC117 elicits host immune responses against HIV-1. Science. 2016;352(6288):997–1001.

90. Ng CT, et al. Passive neutralizing antibody controls SHIV viremia and enhances B cell responses in infant macaques. Nat Med. 2010;16(10):1117–9.

91. Fouda GG, et al. Infant HIV type 1 gp120 vaccination elicits robust and durable anti-V1V2 immunoglobulin G responses and only rare envelope-specific immunoglobulin A responses. J Infect Dis. 2015;211(4):508–17.

92. Goulder PJ, Lewin SR, Leitman EM. Paediatric HIV infection: the potential for cure. Nat Rev Immunol. 2016;16(4):259–71.

93. McGuire EP, et al. HIV-exposed infants vaccinated with an MF59/recombinant gp120 vaccine have higher-magnitude anti-V1V2 IgG responses than adults immunized with the same vaccine. J Virol. 2018;92(1):e017070.

94. Roider JM, Muenchhoff M, Goulder PJ. Immune activation and paediatric HIV-1 disease outcome. Curr Opin HIV AIDS. 2016;11(2):146–55.

95. Laird Smith M, et al. Rapid sequencing of complete env genes from primary HIV-1 samples. Virus Evol. 2016;2(2):vew018.

96. Bhiman JN, et al. Viral variants that initiate and drive maturation of V1V2-directed HIV-1 broadly neutralizing antibodies. Nat Med. 2015;21(11):1332–6.

97. Landais E, et al. HIV envelope glycoform heterogeneity and localized diversity govern the initiation and maturation of a V2 apex broadly neutralizing antibody lineage. Immunity. 2017;47(5):990e9–1003e9.

98. Rantalainen K, et al. Co-evolution of HIV envelope and apex-targeting neutralizing antibody lineage provides benchmarks for vaccine design. Cell Rep. 2018;23(11):3249–61.

99. Jonsson P, et al. Remarkably low affinity of CD4/peptide-major histocompatibility complex class II protein interactions. Proc Natl Acad Sci USA. 2016;113(20):5682–7.

100. Jardine JG, et al. HIV-1 VACCINES. Priming a broadly neutralizing antibody response to HIV-1 using a germline-targeting immunogen. Science. 2015;349(6244):156–61.

101. Jardine JG, et al. HIV-1 broadly neutralizing antibody precursor B cells revealed by germline-targeting immunogen. Science. 2016;351(6280):1458–63.

102. Bonsignori M, et al. Staged induction of HIV-1 glycan-dependent broadly neutralizing antibodies. Sci Transl Med. 2017;9(381):7514.

103. Fera D, et al. HIV envelope V3 region mimic embodies key features of a broadly neutralizing antibody lineage epitope. Nat Commun. 2018;9(1):1111.

104. Sok D, et al. A recombinant HIV envelope trimer selects for quaternary dependent antibodies targeting the trimer apex. AIDS Res Hum Retroviruses. 2014;30(Suppl 1):A7–8.

105. Sok D, et al. The effects of somatic hypermutation on neutralization and binding in the PGT121 family of broadly neutralizing HIV antibodies. PLoS Pathog. 2013;9(11):e1003754.

106. Mishra AK, Mariuzza RA. Insights into the structural basis of antibody affinity maturation from next-generation sequencing. Front Immunol. 2018;9:117.

107. Zhou T, et al. Structural repertoire of HIV-1-neutralizing antibodies targeting the CD4 supersite in 14 donors. Cell. 2015;161(6):1280–92.

108. Gao F, et al. Cooperation of B cell lineages in induction of HIV-1-broadly neutralizing antibodies. Cell. 2014;158(3):481–91.

109. Moore PL, et al. Evolution of an HIV glycan-dependent broadly neutralizing antibody epitope through immune escape. Nat Med. 2012;18(11):1688–92.

110. Anthony C, et al. Co-operation between strain-specific and broadly neutralizing responses limited viral escape, and prolonged exposure of the broadly neutralizing epitope. J Virol. 2017;91(18):e00828–7.

111. Reh L, et al. Phenotypic deficits in the HIV-1 envelope are associated with the maturation of a V2-directed broadly neutralizing antibody lineage. PLoS Pathog. 2018;14(1):e1006825.

112. Havenar-Daughton C, et al. Direct probing of germinal center responses reveals immunological features and bottlenecks for neutralizing antibody responses to HIV Env trimer. Cell Rep. 2016;17(9):2195–209.

113. Pauthner M, et al. Elicitation of robust tier 2 neutralizing antibody responses in nonhuman primates by HIV envelope trimer immunization using optimized approaches. Immunity. 2017;46(6):1073e6–1088e6.

114. Escolano A, et al. Sequential immunization elicits broadly neutralizing anti-HIV-1 antibodies in Ig knockin mice. Cell. 2016;166(6):1445e12–1458e12.

115. Briney B, et al. Tailored immunogens direct affinity maturation toward HIV neutralizing antibodies. Cell. 2016;166(6):1459e11–1470e11.

116. Sok D, et al. Priming HIV-1 broadly neutralizing antibody precursors in human Ig loci transgenic mice. Science. 2016;353(6307):1557–60.

117. Tian M, et al. Induction of HIV neutralizing antibody lineages in mice with diverse precursor repertoires. Cell. 2016;166(6):1471e18–1484e18.

118. Alam SM, et al. Mimicry of an HIV broadly neutralizing antibody epitope with a synthetic glycopeptide. Sci Transl Med. 2017;9(381):eaai7521.

119. Bonsignori M, et al. Maturation pathway from germline to broad HIV-1 neutralizer of a CD4-mimic antibody. Cell. 2016;165(2):449–63.

120. Kong L, et al. Key gp120 glycans pose roadblocks to the rapid development of VRC01-class antibodies in an HIV-1-infected Chinese Donor. Immunity. 2016;44(4):939–50.

121. Landais E. Broadly neutralizing antibody development: lessons from the protocol C cohort. Keystone Symposia HIV Vaccines (2017)

122. Ver LS, Choi N, Murrell M, Murrell B, Briney B, Eren K, Wrin T, The IAVI Protocol C Investigators & the IAVI African HIV Research Network, Burton DR, Wilson IA, Landais E, Poignard P. Env escape to high-mannose patch targeting broadly neutralizing antibodies involves the V1-loop and the Co-receptor binding site. Keystone Symposia HIV Vaccines (2017)

123. Cale EM, et al. Virus-like particles identify an HIV V1V2 apex-binding neutralizing antibody that lacks a protruding loop. Immunity. 2017;46(5):777e10–791e10.

124. Huang J, et al. Identification of a CD4-binding-site antibody to HIV that evolved near-pan neutralization breadth. Immunity. 2016;45(5):1108–21.

125. Sajadi MM, et al. Identification of near-pan-neutralizing antibodies against HIV-1 by deconvolution of plasma humoral responses. Cell. 2018;173(7):1783–95.

126. Wibmer CK, et al. Structure of an N276-dependent HIV-1 neutralizing antibody targeting a rare V5 glycan hole adjacent to the CD4 binding site. J Virol. 2016;90(22):10220–35.

127. Abbott RK, et al. Precursor frequency and affinity determine B cell competitive fitness in germinal centers, tested with germline-targeting HIV vaccine immunogens. Immunity. 2018;48(1):133e6–146e6.

128. Sanders RW, Moore JP. Native-like Env trimers as a platform for HIV-1 vaccine design. Immunol Rev. 2017;275(1):161–82.

129. Panico M, et al. Mapping the complete glycoproteome of virion-derived HIV-1 gp120 provides insights into broadly neutralizing antibody binding. Sci Rep. 2016;6:32956.

130. Cao L, et al. Global site-specific N-glycosylation analysis of HIV envelope glycoprotein. Nat Commun. 2017;8:14954.

131. Andrabi R, et al. Glycans function as anchors for antibodies and help drive HIV broadly neutralizing antibody development. Immunity. 2017;47(5):1004.

132. Crooks ET, et al. Glycoengineering HIV-1 Env creates 'supercharged' and 'hybrid' glycans to increase neutralizing antibody potency, breadth and saturation. PLoS Pathog. 2018;14(5):e1007024.

133. McGuire AT, et al. HIV antibodies. Antigen modification regulates competition of broad and narrow neutralizing HIV antibodies. Science. 2014;346(6215):1380–3.

134. de Taeye SW, et al. Immunogenicity of stabilized HIV-1 envelope trimers with reduced exposure of non-neutralizing epitopes. Cell. 2015;163(7):1702–15.

135. Tas JM, et al. Visualizing antibody affinity maturation in germinal centers. Science. 2016;351(6277):1048–54.

136. Kuraoka M, et al. Complex antigens drive permissive clonal selection in germinal centers. Immunity. 2016;44(3):542–52.

137. Mesin L, Ersching J, Victora GD. Germinal center B cell dynamics. Immunity. 2016;45(3):471–82.

138. Bannard O, Cyster JG. Germinal centers: programmed for affinity maturation and antibody diversification. Curr Opin Immunol. 2017;45:21–30.

139. De Silva NS, Klein U. Dynamics of B cells in germinal centres. Nat Rev Immunol. 2015;15(3):137–48.

140. Brink R, Phan TG. Self-reactive B cells in the germinal center reaction. Annu Rev Immunol. 2018;36:339–57.

141. Wang S, et al. Manipulating the selection forces during affinity maturation to generate cross-reactive HIV antibodies. Cell. 2015;160(4):785–97.

142. Luo Y, et al. Sequential Immunizations with heterosubtypic virus-like particles elicit cross protection against divergent influenza A viruses in mice. Sci Rep. 2018;8(1):4577.

143. Shaffer JS, et al. Optimal immunization cocktails can promote induction of broadly neutralizing Abs against highly mutable pathogens. Proc Natl Acad Sci USA. 2016;113(45):E7039–48.

144. Williams WB, et al. Initiation of HIV neutralizing B cell lineages with sequential envelope immunizations. Nat Commun. 2017;8(1):1732.

145. McCoy LE, et al. Holes in the glycan shield of the native HIV envelope are a target of trimer-elicited neutralizing antibodies. Cell Rep. 2016;16(9):2327–38.

146. Crooks ET, et al. Vaccine-elicited tier 2 HIV-1 neutralizing antibodies bind to quaternary epitopes involving glycan-deficient patches proximal to the CD4 binding site. PLoS Pathog. 2015;11(5):e1004932.

147. Cirelli KM, Crotty S. Germinal center enhancement by extended antigen availability. Curr Opin Immunol. 2017;47:64–9.

148. Tam HH, et al. Sustained antigen availability during germinal center initiation enhances antibody responses to vaccination. Proc Natl Acad Sci USA. 2016;113(43):E6639–48.

149. Soto C, et al. Developmental pathway of the MPER-directed HIV-1-neutralizing antibody 10E8. PLoS ONE. 2016;11(6):e0157409.

150. Williams LD, et al. Potent and broad HIV-neutralizing antibodies in memory B cells and plasma. Sci Immunol. 2017;2(7):eaal2200.

8

The invariant arginine within the chromatin-binding motif regulates both nucleolar localization and chromatin binding of Foamy virus Gag

Joris Paris[1†], Joëlle Tobaly-Tapiero[1†], Marie-Lou Giron[1], Julien Burlaud-Gaillard[2,3], Florence Buseyne[4,5], Philippe Roingeard[2,3], Pascale Lesage[1], Alessia Zamborlini[1,6*‡] and Ali Saïb[1*‡]

Abstract

Background: Nuclear localization of Gag is a property shared by many retroviruses and retrotransposons. The importance of this stage for retroviral replication is still unknown, but studies on the Rous Sarcoma virus indicate that Gag might select the viral RNA genome for packaging in the nucleus. In the case of Foamy viruses, genome encapsidation is mediated by Gag C-terminal domain (CTD), which harbors three clusters of glycine and arginine residues named GR boxes (GRI-III). In this study we investigated how PFV Gag subnuclear distribution might be regulated.

Results: We show that the isolated GRI and GRIII boxes act as nucleolar localization signals. In contrast, both the entire Gag CTD and the isolated GRII box, which contains the chromatin-binding motif, target the nucleolus exclusively upon mutation of the evolutionary conserved arginine residue at position 540 (R540), which is a key determinant of FV Gag chromatin tethering. We also provide evidence that Gag localizes in the nucleolus during FV replication and uncovered that the viral protein interacts with and is methylated by Protein Arginine Methyltransferase 1 (PRMT1) in a manner that depends on the R540 residue. Finally, we show that PRMT1 depletion by RNA interference induces the concentration of Gag C-terminus in nucleoli.

Conclusion: Altogether, our findings suggest that methylation by PRMT1 might finely tune the subnuclear distribution of Gag depending on the stage of the FV replication cycle. The role of this step for viral replication remains an open question.

Keywords: Foamy virus, Gag, Nuclear trafficking, Nucleolus, Chromatin-binding, Post-translational modification, Methylation, PRMT

Background

Foamy viruses (FVs), also known as spumaviruses, are complex retroviruses that belong to the *Spumaretrovirinae* subfamily of the Retroviridae. They are endemic among many animal species, particularly non-human primates (NHPs) (for a review [1]). The Prototype FV (PFV) was isolated from human-derived cell culture and later found to be a chimpanzee FV [2]. It is currently well established that humans are not natural hosts but acquire infection as a consequence of zoonotic transmission of simian FVs (SFVs) through bites of captive or wild NHPs [3, 4]. FV infection is persistent and apparently benign [1] and human-to-human transmission has never been reported. Like all retroviruses, FVs reverse transcribe their RNA genome (gRNA), which encodes the typical *gag*, *pol* and *env* genes, and integrate the resulting cDNA into the host cell chromosomes. However,

*Correspondence: alessia.zamborlini@univ-paris-diderot.fr; ali.saib@univ-paris-diderot.fr
[†]Joris Paris and Joëlle Tobaly-Tapiero are the co-first authors
[‡]Alessia Zamborlini and Ali Saïb contributed equally to this work
[1] CNRS UMR7212, Hôpital St Louis, Inserm U944, Institut Universitaire d'Hématologie, Université Paris Diderot, Sorbonne Paris Cité, Paris, France
Full list of author information is available at the end of the article

specificities in the replication strategy of FVs set them apart from orthoretroviruses. These include the fact that reverse transcription occurs during viral particle production [5, 6], and that Pol is expressed independently of Gag from a specific spliced transcript [7, 8]. The structural organization and maturation profile of FV Gag are also peculiar. FV Gag lacks the major homology region (MHR) and the Cys-His zinc-finger motifs that are hallmarks of orthoretroviral Gag proteins. Moreover, FV Gag is not processed into the matrix (MA), capsid (CA) and nucleocapsid (NC) mature products like its orthoretroviral counterparts, but rather undergoes a single cleavage event that removes a 4 kDa C-terminal peptide ([9], reviewed in [10]). This feature is shared by the Gag proteins of the *Drosophila* retrovirus Gypsy [11] and the Ty1 retrotransposon of *S. cerevisiae* [12]. Recent studies showed that PFV Gag N-terminal domain (NTD, amino acids (aa) 1–180) is entirely unrelated to its orthoretroviral counterpart [13]. They also confirmed that the NTD, which harbors the cytoplasmic targeting and retention signal (CTRS) and the self-dimerization domain, plays a role similar to orthoretroviral CA in viral capsid assembly [13]. In contrast the central conserved region of PFV Gag (aa 300–477), which is involved in the formation of higher-order multimers, shares a conformation analogous to that of orthoretroviral CA, suggesting evolution from a common ancestral protein [14]. In the absence of structural data, functional studies indicate that the C-terminal domain (CTD, aa 400–648) of FV Gag plays a role related to that of orthoretroviral NC in genome packaging [10, 15]. This domain is enriched in glycine and arginine residues that in primate FV Gag proteins are clustered in three regions named GR boxes (GRI-III) [15]. GRI binds nucleic acids in vitro and was proposed to be responsible of the incorporation of both the gRNA and Pol into virions [16–18]. The GRII box shows the highest conservation throughout evolution and is involved in the accumulation of PFV Gag in the nucleus [15]. The determinant for nuclear localization within GRII maps to a 13-aa chromatin binding sequence (CBS, aa 534–546) that recognizes the H2A/H2B core histones. This interaction tethers the pre-integration complex (PIC) to host cell chromatin prior to viral integration [19–21]. The role of GRIII in FV replication is enigmatic but likely related to that of GRI, since the two motifs can functionally complement each other [22]. Although the GR boxes were initially viewed as independent entities playing both specific and redundant functions, a recent study rather indicates that the positively charged residues within the CTD, not the GR boxes individually, mediate gRNA packaging and Pol encapsidation [23].

During FV replication Gag displays different subcellular localizations, as a result of numerous interactions with the intracellular trafficking machinery, which likely match its multiple roles throughout the viral life cycle. Our previous studies showed that, as a component of the incoming PIC, Gag drives the traffic of viral particles towards the microtubule-organizing center (MTOC) where uncoating occurs [24–26]. Upon nuclear envelope breakdown, Gag associates with host cell chromosomes and critically contributes to the selection of the integration sites [19–21, 27]. At a later stage, newly synthesized Gag molecules have been shown to oligomerize in the nucleus and, next, reach the cytoplasm by engaging the CRM1 (Chromosomal Maintenance 1, also known as Exportin 1)-dependent pathway through a nuclear export signal (NES) [28], as reported for Rous Sarcoma Virus (RSV) (see below, [29]). Currently, how newly synthesized Gag crosses the intact nuclear membrane is unknown [20].

Evidence that Gag proteins shuttle between the nucleus and the cytoplasm has been reported for other retroviruses, including RSV, feline immunodeficiency virus (FIV), Human Immunodeficiency Virus (HIV), mouse mammary tumor virus (MMTV), Mazon-Pfizer monkey virus (MPMV) and murine leukemia virus (MLV) ([30] and references therein), and the Tf1 retrotransposon [31]. Gag or the isolated NCs of MMTV, RSV, FIV, HIV and MLV have also been detected in the nucleolus ([30] and references therein), a distinct subnuclear compartment that forms around the gene clusters encoding rRNAs and represents the site of ribosomes biogenesis. Although in most instances the significance of Gag nucleocytoplasmic trafficking for virus replication is elusive, RSV Gag was shown to oligomerize in the nucleus, in an RNA- and NC-dependent manner [29]. The observation that nuclear trafficking of RSV Gag is required for efficient genome encapsidation [32, 33] and that binding to a synthetic oligonucleotide mimicking the packaging signal favours the association between Gag and the nuclear export factor CRM1 in vitro [34], led to propose a model according to which RSV Gag selects the viral gRNA for packaging in the nucleus.

To deepen our understanding of the nuclear trafficking of PFV Gag, we studied the localization of the C-terminal GR boxes and established that the isolated GRI and GRIII boxes are nucleolar localization signals (NoLSs). We also found that Gag localizes at least temporarily in the nucleolus during PFV replication. Next, we investigated the mechanisms that regulate this process, and identified the evolutionary conserved arginine residue at position 540 (R540) within the GRII box as a critical factor determining whether Gag localizes in the nucleolus or is tethered to chromatin. We also established that PFV Gag interacts with and is modified by PRMT1 (Protein Arginine Methyltransferase 1) and PRMT5. Interestingly, we found that PFV Gag harboring the R540A substitution is unable to interact with PRMT1 and lost the asymmetric dimethylarginine (ADMA) mark, while retaining binding to and modification by PRMT5. Finally, we observed that siRNA-mediated depletion of PRMT1 leads to nucleolar accumulation of the C-terminus of PFV Gag fused to GFP. On the basis of these results, we hypothesize that PRMT1-mediated methylation, which requires the invariant R540 residue, could regulate the subnuclear distribution of PFV Gag antagonizing nucleolar accumulation in favor of chromosome binding.

Results

The GRI and GRIII boxes of PFV Gag are nucleolar localization signals

The GR boxes within PFV Gag CTD are short sequences enriched in arginine residues, which is a hallmark of NoLSs [35] (Fig. 1a and Additional file 1: S1A). To determine if these motifs could localize proteins to the nucleolus, we cloned each GR box in frame with the *EGFP* gene. The cellular distribution of the resulting GFP-fusion proteins was studied in HeLa cells that were stained for nucleolin, one of the most abundant proteins of the nucleolus [36]. We found that GFP-GRI was concentrated in nucleolin-positive foci, GFP-GRII displayed a diffuse nuclear staining, while GFP-GRIII was both enriched in nucleolin-positive foci and distributed throughout the nucleoplasm and the cytoplasm (Fig. 1b). GFP-GRI staining also partially overlapped with DsRed fused to the NoLS of the HIV Rev protein (DsRed-RevNoLS) (Fig. 1c), which localizes in both the Dense Fibrillar Component (DFC) and the Granular Component (GC) nucleolar compartments where the early events in rRNA transcription and processing and maturation of pre-ribosomal subunits occur, respectively [37]. In agreement with this observation, GFP-GRI co-localized with fibrillarin and nucleophosmin/B23, which specifically mark the DFC and the GC, respectively (Fig. 1c). Furthermore, an overlap between GFP-GRI and the Upstream Binding Factor (UBF) located in the Fibrillar Center (FC) was observed (Fig. 1c). Ultrastructural analysis by immunoelectron microscopy confirmed the presence of GFP-GRI and GFP-RevNoLS in the DFC and GC (Additional file 1: Fig S1B). We further observed that DsRed-GRI and GFP-GRIII co-localized when expressed in the same cell, confirming that the GRI and the GRIII box target the same subnuclear compartment (Additional file 1: Fig. S1C). A co-localization was observed between DsRed-PFV-GRI

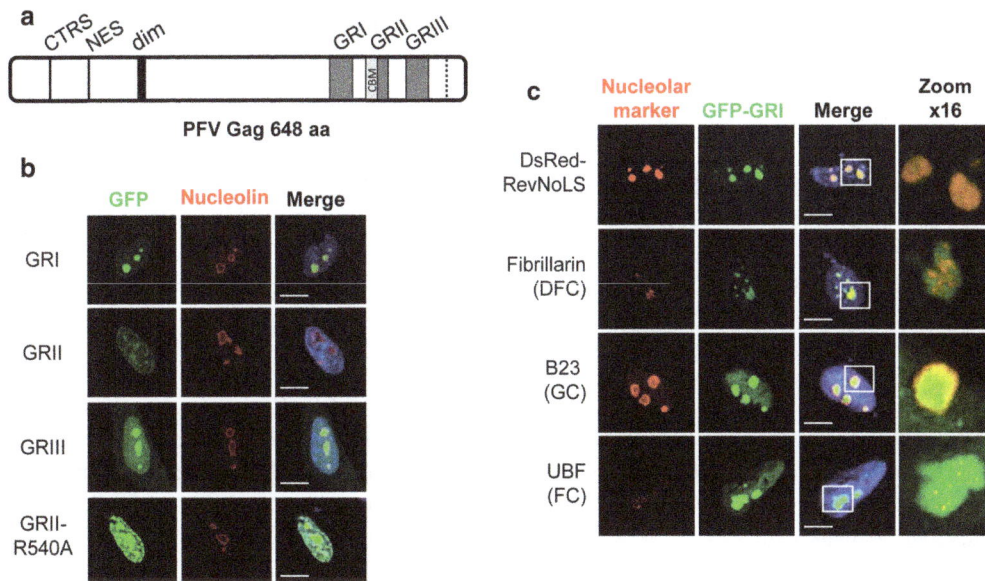

Fig. 1 GRI and GRIII boxes of PFV Gag are Nucleolar Localization Signals. **a** Scheme of PFV Gag protein where the primary protease-cleavage site at residue 621 is indicated by a dotted line. Some characterized motifs are shown. CTRS: cytoplasmic targeting and retention signal (aa 43–60); NES: nuclear export signal (aa 95–112); dim: dimerization domain (aa 130–160); GRI, GRII and GRIII: glycine-arginine rich box I (aa 485–511), II (aa 534–557) and III (aa 586–618); CBM, chromatin-binding motif (aa 536–544). **b** The subcellular localization of GRI, GRII, GRII$_{R540A}$ or GRIII expressed as GFP-fusion proteins in fixed HeLa cells was analyzed 24 h post-transfection by immunofluorescence and confocal microscopy. Nucleoli were immune-stained with an anti-nucleolin antibody (ab 22758, Abcam, 1:800) and nuclei were stained with DAPI (blue). **c** The localization of GFP-GRI expressed in HeLa cells relative to the NoLS of HIV-1 Rev protein (aa 35–51) in fusion with DsRed or specific markers of the nucleolar subcompartments was studied as in B. Cells were stained with antibodies against fibrillarin (c13c3, Cell signaling, 1:200), B23 (sc6013_R, Santa Cruz, 1:200) or UBF (H300, Santa Cruz, 1:200) to visualize the dense fibrillar component (DFC), the granular component (GC) and the fibrillar center (FC), respectively. The right column (zoom × 16) corresponds to the enlarged images from the boxed areas. Scale bar represents 10 µm

and GFP fused to either the GRI or the GRIII box of the Equine Foamy virus (EFV), the most distantly related FV (Additional file 1: Fig. S1C). Altogether these results indicate that the GRI and GRIII boxes of FV Gag proteins are NoLSs able to induce the nucleolar localization of a heterologous protein, and that this function is conserved among primate and non-primate FVs.

FV Gag transits through the nucleolus during viral replication

Having shown that GRI and GRIII are NoLSs, we asked whether FV Gag transits through the nucleolus during PFV life cycle. The fact that PFV Gag has never been detected in the nucleolus of infected cells suggests that either this process is highly dynamic and/or that only a small fraction of the protein resides in the nucleolus at steady state. To address this question, we adopted a "capture" assay similar to that used to demonstrate nucleolar trafficking of HIV Rev [38]. To this end, we established U373MG cells stably expressing a chimeric protein named Gag-TRAP-GFP, which consists of the N-terminal region of Gag (aa 1–200) including the dimerization domain [13, 39], fused with the NoLS of HIV Rev and GFP (Fig. 2a). We reasoned that if FV Gag transits through the nucleolus, it would interact with Gag-TRAP-GFP and be consequently retained at this site. As expected, Gag-TRAP-GFP accumulates in the nucleolus (Fig. 2b). We also confirmed that Gag-TRAP-GFP co-precipitates with full-length PFV Gag (Additional file 2: Fig. S2). Next, U373MG cells stably expressing Gag-TRAP-GFP, or the appropriate controls (GFP, Gag$_{1-200}$-GFP or RevNoLS-GFP), were infected with PFV. Seventy-two hours later, Gag distribution was analyzed by immunofluorescence and confocal microscopy with an antibody directed against the C-terminal half of Gag. In control cells, Gag (red staining) localized in the cytoplasm and/or in the nucleus, but was not detected in the nucleolus (Fig. 2b), while in Gag-TRAP-GFP-expressing cells, Gag was diffused in the nucleoplasm and co-localized with the chimeric protein in the nucleolus. The infectivity of viruses released in the cell culture supernatant was quantified in parallel using FAG-indicator cells [39]. Viruses produced from cells expressing RevNoLS-GFP or Gag$_{1-200}$-GFP were not significantly less infectious compared to those produced from GFP-expressing cells, used for normalization (96% ± 14 and 91% ± 3 compared to 100 ± 15, respectively) (Fig. 2c). Expression of Gag-TRAP-GFP resulted in a reduction of infectivity of about 25% (75% ± 13 and 73% ± 11 for independent duplicate samples) (Fig. 2c). Statistical analysis shows that such decrease in infectivity is statistically significant when compared to the GFP, but not to the Gag$_{1-200}$-GFP, sample (Fig. 2c).

Since we could not exclude that the interaction between Gag and Gag-TRAP-GFP occurs outside the nucleolus and that the Rev NoLS within the chimeric protein subsequently targets the complex to this subcellular site, we analyzed Gag localization in PFV-infected U937MG cells treated with leptomycine B (LMB), a specific inhibitor of CRM1-mediated nuclear export, and/or exposed to hypoxia, a setting that was previously shown to slow down protein trafficking [40]. Under these conditions, Gag (green staining) co-localized with nucleolin in about 3–10% of PFV-infected cells (Fig. 2d). Altogether these results indicate that Gag transits through the nucleolus during PFV replication.

The evolutionary conserved R540 residue is critical for both nucleolar localization and chromosome tethering of PFV Gag

Our observations showing that Gag localizes at least temporarily in the nucleolus during PFV infection, raise the question of how this process is regulated. Given that GRI and GRIII, but not GRII, are NoLSs (Fig. 1b), we decided first to study the subcellular distribution of GFP fused to PFV Gag CTD encompassing the three GR boxes (aa 477–625). The resulting GFP-GRs fusion protein was diffused throughout the nucleoplasm and excluded from the nucleoli (Fig. 3a, left panel), a localization pattern reminiscent of that of GFP-GRII (Fig. 1b). This observation suggested that the GRII box might antagonize the nucleolar-targeting function of GRI and/or GRIII. In support of this hypothesis, deletion of either the entire GRII box or the chromatin-binding motif (CBM, aa 536–544) in the context of GFP-GRs induced an accumulation of the corresponding mutants in the nucleolus (Fig. 3a, left panel). To map further the determinants of GRII that influence nucleolar-targeting, we aligned the sequences of the GRII box from several FV isolates and found that PFV CBM residues Y537 and R540 are strictly conserved, while R542 is only present in Gag from some primate FVs, EFV and in CoeEFV, an endogenous foamy virus-like element in the Coelacanth genome [41] (Table 1). Each of these residues was mutated within the GFP-GRs construct to address their contribution to nucleolar targeting. GFP-GRsR542A displayed a WT distribution in HeLa cells (Fig. 3a, left panel). GFP-GRsY537A localized in the nucleoplasm in most instances, but was detected also in the nucleolus in about a third of the transfected cells (Fig. 3a, left panel). In contrast, GFP-GRs where R540 is mutated to A, K or F accumulated in nucleoli in the whole population of transfected cells (Fig. 3a, left panel and Fig. 3b). These observations are consistent with the finding that GFP-GRII harboring the R540A mutation co-localizes with nucleolin (Fig. 1b). Finally, we found that GFP fused to the C-terminal region of EFV

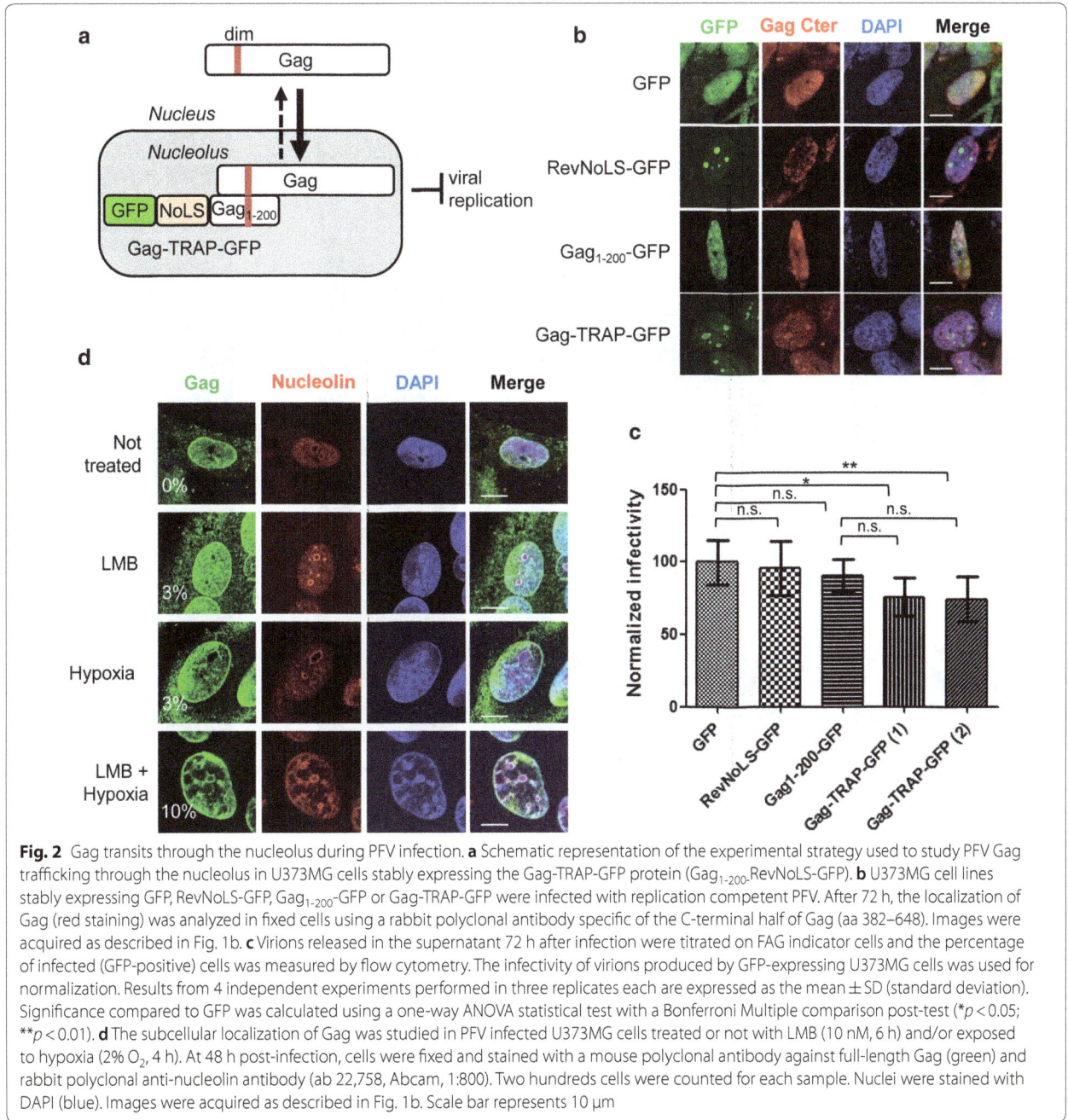

Fig. 2 Gag transits through the nucleolus during PFV infection. **a** Schematic representation of the experimental strategy used to study PFV Gag trafficking through the nucleolus in U373MG cells stably expressing the Gag-TRAP-GFP protein (Gag$_{1-200}$-RevNoLS-GFP). **b** U373MG cell lines stably expressing GFP, RevNoLS-GFP, Gag$_{1-200}$-GFP or Gag-TRAP-GFP were infected with replication competent PFV. After 72 h, the localization of Gag (red staining) was analyzed in fixed cells using a rabbit polyclonal antibody specific of the C-terminal half of Gag (aa 382–648). Images were acquired as described in Fig. 1b. **c** Virions released in the supernatant 72 h after infection were titrated on FAG indicator cells and the percentage of infected (GFP-positive) cells was measured by flow cytometry. The infectivity of virions produced by GFP-expressing U373MG cells was used for normalization. Results from 4 independent experiments performed in three replicates each are expressed as the mean ± SD (standard deviation). Significance compared to GFP was calculated using a one-way ANOVA statistical test with a Bonferroni Multiple comparison post-test (*$p < 0.05$; **$p < 0.01$). **d** The subcellular localization of Gag was studied in PFV infected U373MG cells treated or not with LMB (10 nM, 6 h) and/or exposed to hypoxia (2% O_2, 4 h). At 48 h post-infection, cells were fixed and stained with a mouse polyclonal antibody against full-length Gag (green) and rabbit polyclonal anti-nucleolin antibody (ab 22,758, Abcam, 1:800). Two hundreds cells were counted for each sample. Nuclei were stained with DAPI (blue). Images were acquired as described in Fig. 1b. Scale bar represents 10 μm

Gag (EFV GFP-GRs) was distributed in the nucleoplasm (Additional file 1: Fig. S1D). Upon alanine substitution of R472, which is equivalent of PFV Gag R540, EFV GFP-GRs accumulated in the nucleolus (Additional file 1: Fig. S1D).

We next studied the influence of R540 on full-length PFV Gag localization. PFV Gag expressed as GFP-fusion protein in HeLa cells was predominantly diffused in the cytoplasm of interphasic cells, and was excluded from the nucleolus (Fig. 3c, left panel). Upon deletion of the CBM or mutation of R540 to A, GFP-Gag accumulated in the nucleolus in a fraction of transfected HeLa cells (about 7 and 10%, respectively) (Fig. 3c, left panel). These results contrasted with the finding that GFP-GRsR540A was detected in the nucleolus in all the transfected cells (Fig. 3a, left panel). We hypothesized that this discrepancy might result at least in part from the presence of N-terminal sequences within Gag favoring its accumulation in the cytoplasm and/or antagonizing its nuclear/nucleolar localization. To

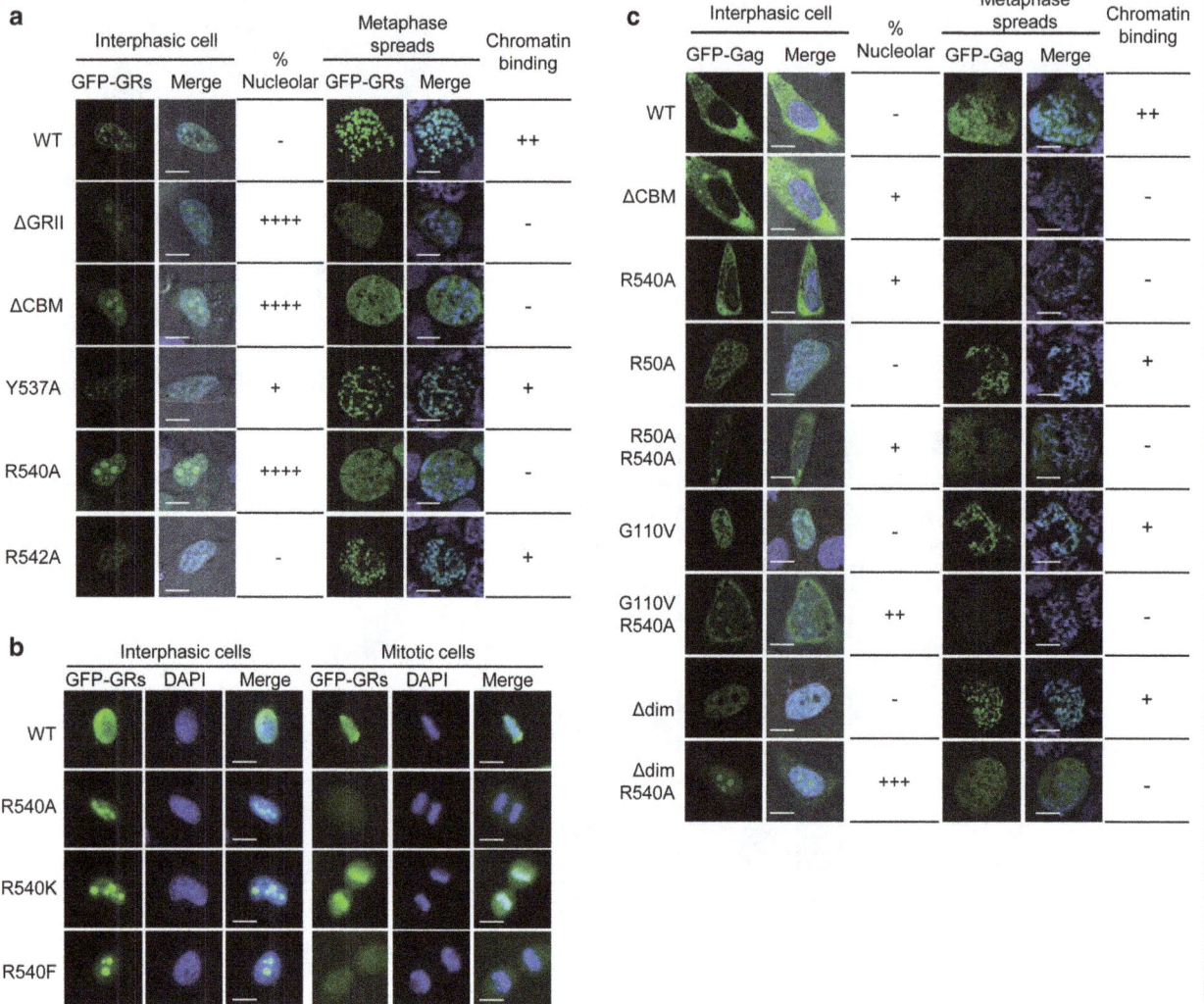

Fig. 3 The invariant R540 residue in PFV Gag regulates nucleolar localization and binding to mitotic chromosomes. Living HeLa cells expressing the indicated GFP-GRs (**a**) or GFP-Gag (**c**) constructs and stained with Hoechst 33342 were observed on a confocal microscope 24 h after transfection (left panels). Merged images correspond to GFP, nucleic acid staining and differential interference contrast to visualize the cell shape. The "% nucleolar" column indicates the percentage of transfected cells displaying GFP staining in the nucleolus (−, < 1%; +, 1–25%; ++, 26–50%; +++, 51–75%; ++++, 76–100%). To study the interaction of GFP-fusion proteins with chromatin (right panels), cells ectopically expressing indicated proteins were arrested in metaphase by treatment with colcemid (0.1 µg/mL, 2 h) and chromosome spreads counterstained with DAPI. Images were acquired as described in Fig. 1b. The chromatin binding column indicates whether the GFP-fusion protein was exclusively localized onto chromosomes (++), both on chromosomes and throughout the cell (+), or was distributed throughout the cell and did not associate with chromosomes (−). Representative images from two independent experiments are shown. Between 100 and 120 cells were analyzed for each condition. Scale bars represent 10 µm. **b** HeLa cells expressing the indicated GFP-GRs were stained with DAPI. Images were acquired as described in Fig. 1b. Scale bars represent 10 µm

address this point, we mutated three well-characterized functional domains in GFP-Gag or GFP-GagR540A, namely the CTRS (mutation R50A) [42], the NES (mutation G110 V) [28] and the dimerization domain (Δdim, deletion of aa 130–160) [39] (Fig. 1a). In agreement with these published studies, GFP-Gag bearing the R50A or G110V or Δdim mutation accumulated in the nucleus (Fig. 3c, left panel). When any of these mutations was combined with the R540A substitution, the resulting GFP-Gag variants were distributed in the cytoplasm and the nucleoplasm and also accumulated in the nucleolus, to a variable extent (Fig. 3c, left panel).

Having previously shown that deletion of the CBM impairs FV Gag binding to mitotic chromosomes [19], we also addressed the involvement of the conserved residues

Table 1 Sequence alignment of Gag CBM from different FV strains. Residues that are conserved in > 50 and 100% of the sequences are colored blue and red, respectively. The alignment was obtained using ESPript (http://espript.ibcp.fr) [58]

Primates	PFV	536GYNLRPRTY
	SFVmac	537GYNLRPRTY
	SFVagm	524GYDLRPRTY
	SFVgor	533GYNLRPRTY
	SFVora	519GYNLRPNTF
	SFVspm	518GYNLRQQIN
Non Primates	FFV	415GYNFRRNPQ
	BFV	444RYPLRPNPQ
	EFV	468RYFFRPRPS
Endogenous FV	CoeEFV	404RYDLRPRHD
Consensus >50		gYnlRprty

within the GRII box in the interaction of FV Gag with chromatin. Gag variants where Y537 or R542 are changed to A retained the ability to interact with mitotic chromosomes (Fig. 3a, c, right panel). Notably, mutation of R540 to A was sufficient to abolish binding of either the CTD or full length Gag expressed as GFP-fusion proteins to chromatin (Fig. 3a, c, right panel). The results obtained in metaphase spreads were confirmed by the observation of fixed cells expressing GFP-GRs R540A that undergo mitosis, as judged by DNA staining (Fig. 3b). Similarly, we never observed an association between mitotic chromosomes and GFP-GRs bearing the R540F mutation, which mimics constitutive methylation (Fig. 3b). Finally, we found that GFP-GRs carrying the R540 K change painted the chromosomes of mitotic cells (Fig. 3b), indicating that a positive charge at position 540 is sufficient to ensure interaction of Gag with the H2A/H2B core histones [19, 21]. Altogether our findings indicate that the phylogenetically conserved R540 residue of PFV Gag is critical to regulate the subnuclear distribution of the protein: i.e. its nucleolar localization *versus* mitotic chromosomes binding.

R540 is required for both PRMT1 binding and ADMA modification of PFV Gag

To further understand the regulation of PFV Gag subnuclear distribution by R540, we asked whether this residue might be targeted by post-translational modifications, particularly methylation. To address this point, we tested whether Gag could interact with any of the nine Protein Arginine Methyltransferases identified in human cells (PRMT1 to PRMT9) [43]. We performed co-immunoprecipitation assays on 293T cells expressing WT Gag and each PRMT protein fused to GFP and observed that Gag binds to GFP-PRMT1 and GFP-PRMT5, but no other

GFP-PRMTs (Additional file 3: Fig. S3A). These interactions were confirmed by performing the reciprocal experiment (Fig. 4a and Additional file 3: S3B). Interestingly, we found that the R540A Gag mutant lost the ability to interact with GFP-PRMT1 (Fig. 4a, IP GFP), but still co-precipitated with GFP-PRMT5 (Additional file 3: Fig. S3B, IP GFP). The R540A change also abolished the interaction between Gag CTD (comprising the three GR boxes) and endogenous PRMT1 (Fig. 4b, IP PRMT1). Therefore, R540 is specifically required for Gag binding to PRMT1. It is worth to mention that Gag CTD bearing the R540A substitution is unable to interact with the H2A histone (Fig. 4b, IP HA), which likely explains the impaired binding to mitotic chromosomes (Fig. 3).

PRMT1 is the primary methyltransferase that deposits the asymmetric dimethylarginine (ADMA) mark, whereas PRMT5 performs the symmetric dimethylarginine (SDMA) modification. In GFP-PRMT1-expressing cells WT Gag, but not the R540A mutant, can be precipitated with an antibody specific for the ADMA modification (Fig. 4a, IP ADMA). Similarly, WTHA-GRs, but not the R540A mutant, was enriched on beads coated with the anti-ADMA antibody (Fig. 4b). In contrast, both WT Gag and the R540A mutant co-precipitated with an anti-SDMA antibody, when expressed together with GFP-PRMT5 (Additional file 3: Fig. S3B).

Since mutation of R540 also leads to the accumulation of Gag in nucleoli, we finally asked whether PRMT1 might influence the subcellular distribution of the viral protein. To this purpose, we studied the localization of GFP-GRs in HeLa cells previously transfected with siRNA targeting PRMT1 or the appropriate scrambled control. As shown in Fig. 4c, GFP-GRs is distributed throughout the nucleoplasm of control cells, while accumulates in nucleoli upon siRNA-mediated knockdown of PRMT1. Altogether these results indicate that PRMT1-dependent methylation of PFV Gag C-terminal region requires the invariant R540 residue and is necessary to prevent Gag accumulation in nucleoli.

Discussion
It is well established that incoming FV Gag tethers the PIC to host cell chromatin contributing to integration site selection [19–21]. We also showed that PFV Gag harbors a NES, which integrity is required for the completion of the late stages of viral replication [28]. These observations suggest that Gag transits through the nucleus at a step following its translation although the mechanisms underlying its ability to cross the nuclear membrane are still unclear [20]. To get further insights in the role of Gag nuclear trafficking for FV replication, we investigated the localization of the C-terminal GR boxes and found that GRI and GRIII act as NoLSs able

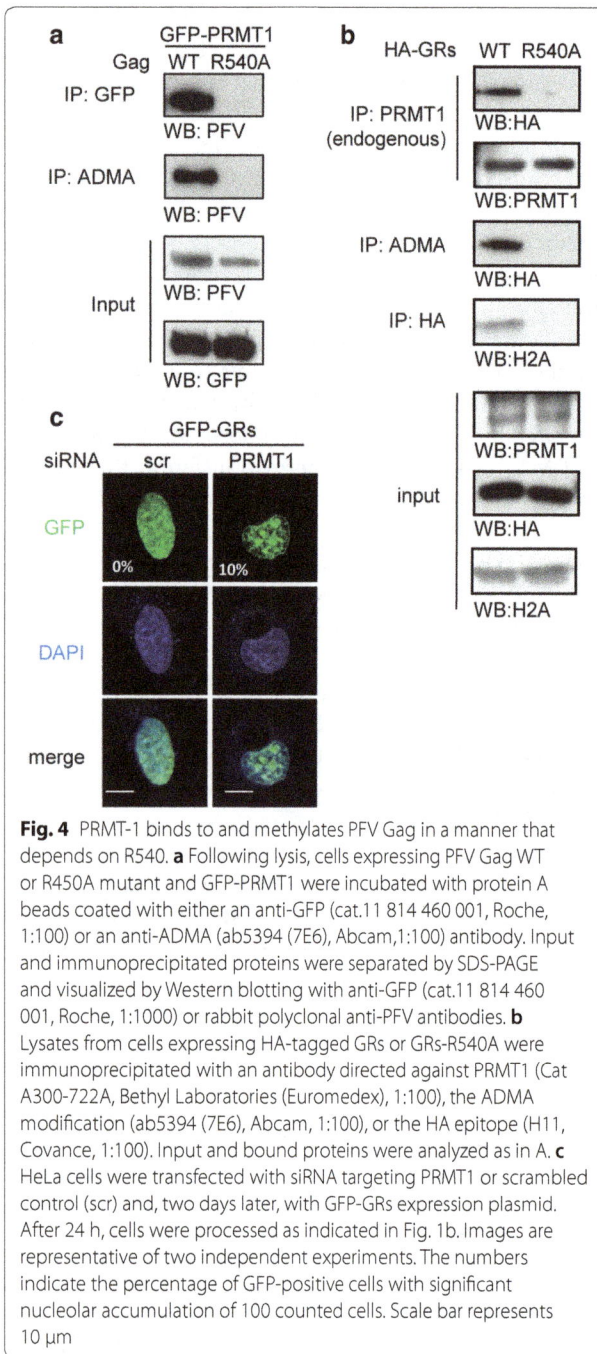

Fig. 4 PRMT-1 binds to and methylates PFV Gag in a manner that depends on R540. **a** Following lysis, cells expressing PFV Gag WT or R450A mutant and GFP-PRMT1 were incubated with protein A beads coated with either an anti-GFP (cat.11 814 460 001, Roche, 1:100) or an anti-ADMA (ab5394 (7E6), Abcam,1:100) antibody. Input and immunoprecipitated proteins were separated by SDS-PAGE and visualized by Western blotting with anti-GFP (cat.11 814 460 001, Roche, 1:1000) or rabbit polyclonal anti-PFV antibodies. **b** Lysates from cells expressing HA-tagged GRs or GRs-R540A were immunoprecipitated with an antibody directed against PRMT1 (Cat A300-722A, Bethyl Laboratories (Euromedex), 1:100), the ADMA modification (ab5394 (7E6), Abcam, 1:100), or the HA epitope (H11, Covance, 1:100). Input and bound proteins were analyzed as in A. **c** HeLa cells were transfected with siRNA targeting PRMT1 or scrambled control (scr) and, two days later, with GFP-GRs expression plasmid. After 24 h, cells were processed as indicated in Fig. 1b. Images are representative of two independent experiments. The numbers indicate the percentage of GFP-positive cells with significant nucleolar accumulation of 100 counted cells. Scale bar represents 10 μm

we visualized Gag in the nucleolus of PFV-infected cells exposed to conditions that slow down protein trafficking (hypoxia and/or LMB treatment), indicating that nucleolar accumulation occurs during the viral cycle and is not a mere artifact of Gag-TRAP-GFP expression. Our findings complement previous reports that Gag and/or the isolated NC proteins from several retroviruses display nuclear/nucleolar distribution, when expressed either as individual proteins or during viral infection (reviewed in [30]). The importance of this nuclear/nucleolar stage for retroviral replication is still unknown. Notably, the observation that many proteins of RNA viruses involved in genome packaging and viral particle assembly localize to nucleoli [44, 45] suggests that these nuclear bodies could be sites where viral ribonucleoprotein complexes form to facilitate viral RNA export and packaging [46].

Another major finding of our work is that neither full-length Gag nor an N-terminal truncation mutant encompassing the three GR boxes accumulates in nucleoli unless the entire GRII box or the CBS is deleted, leading us to assume that this region might hold determinant(s) antagonizing nucleolar targeting. We mapped this determinant to the invariant R540 residue, which mutation is sufficient to induce nucleolar targeting of the isolated GRII box or Gag CTD. Of note, localization of full-length Gag harboring the R540A mutation in nucleoli required concomitant inactivation of N-terminal motifs such as the CTRS, the NES or the dimerization domain, conditions that favor nuclear accumulation of the viral protein. Consistent with this observation, Müllers et al. [20] reported that PFV Gag displays nucleolar staining when fused to a heterologous NLS and upon simultaneous deletion of the GRII box. Similarly, Lochmann et al. [46] described nucleolar localization of RSV Gag after having enhanced its concentration in the nucleus by inhibition of CRM1-dependent nuclear export or mutation of its NES.

Having previously shown that the CBM mediates tethering of PFV Gag to chromatin [19], we assessed the implication of R540 in this process. Our data show that substitution of R540 to A prevents Gag from binding to mitotic chromosomes and interacting with the H2A histone. This finding is in agreement with the recent results of Lesbats et al. [21] demonstrating that R540 acts as an anchor motif interacting with the acidic patch on the surface of the H2A/H2B heterodimer. The role of R540 in modulating chromatin binding is further supported by the observation that insertion of the WT chromatin-binding sequence (CBS, aa 534–546) of PFV Gag, but not the corresponding R540A mutant, restores the interaction between a mutant version of MLV p12 and mitotic chromosomes [47]. Notably, we found that Gag CTD bearing the R540 K mutation associates to chromatin in

to target a heterologous protein (GFP) to the nucleolus. This observation underscores once more the functional link between these two motifs [22]. We also provide evidence that PFV Gag accumulates to nucleoli in a context of infection using two complementary approaches. First, we demonstrated that Gag binds to and, at least partially, colocalizes with a Gag-TRAP-GFP decoy constitutively localized in the nucleolus of PFV-infected cells. Second, cells undergoing unperturbed mitosis, indicating that a positive charge at position 540 is necessary and sufficient to ensure tethering of PFV Gag on chromatin, but not to antagonize nucleolar accumulation.

Finally we set to investigate how R540 regulates the subnuclear localization of PFV Gag. Post-translational modification of R by methylation has been shown to modulate the function and/or localization of several viral proteins. Studies on HIV NC revealed that mutation of R residues within the NoLSs, which are targeted by PRMT6-mediated methylation, impairs both nucleolar localization [46] and reverse transcription initiation [48]. Methylation is also proposed to control both the nucleolar distribution and the transactivation activity of the HIV Tat protein [49, 50]. In the case of HIV Rev mutation of methylated R residues or expression of catalytically inactive PRMT6 diminishes both binding to and nuclear export of RRE-containing transcripts [51]. Least but not last, methylation of R residues influences histone binding of KSHV (Kaposi Sarcoma-associated Herpesvirus) LANA (Latency-associated Nuclear Antigen) protein [52]. Based on these reports, we asked whether PFV Gag is methylated and whether this post-translational modification might influence its subnuclear distribution. In our work we show for the first time that PFV Gag interacts with and is methylated by both PRMT1 and PRMT5. We also established that Gag R540A mutant retains the ability to interact with PRMT5 and, surprisingly, displays enhanced SDMA modification compared to WT Gag. Why mutation of the R540 residue would facilitate deposition of SDMA marks by PRMT5 and at which sites this modification occurs are currently unanswered questions. Importantly, substitution of R540 with A abolished both Gag association with, and modification by, PRMT1. In addition, PFV Gag C-terminus fused to GFP (GFP-GRs) is enriched in nucleoli when PRMT1 expression is reduced by RNA interference, mimicking the phenotype of the R540 mutation. These data are consistent with a model according to which PRMT1-mediated modification of PFV Gag antagonize its nucleolar accumulation. Although we do not provide direct evidence of PRMT1-mediated methylation of R540, it is tempting to speculate that reversible modification of this amino acid might contribute to finely tune the distinct functions of Gag at different stages of the replication cycle. Nevertheless, finding that Gag mutants where R540 is mutated to A or F, which mimics constitutive methylation [53, 54], have a similar phenotype argues that methylation at this site is neither required for localization in nucleoli nor for tethering to chromatin. Another possibility is that PRMT1 controls Gag subnuclear localization by mediating ADMA modification of other residues within its R-rich C-terminal region, which await identification. PFV Gag was already known to be phosphorylated on

multiple sites [5, 9]. Recent studies established that phosphorylation of T225 occurs exclusively in virions and propose that this modification is required for the interaction between PFV Gag and Polo-like kinases, ultimately leading to efficient integration [55].

When we assessed the impact of nucleolar retention of Gag on PFV replication we found that virions produced from Gag-TRAP-GFP-expressing cells display only a moderate decrease of infectivity, which is not statistically significant as compared to the infectivity of virions released from cells expressing Gag_{1-200}-GFP, leaving the question of the role of PRMT1-dependent methylation and/or nucleolar accumulation of Gag during PFV replication open for further investigations. Given that a virus harboring the R540Q mutation within the CBM has an altered integration profile [21], it would also be interesting to address the role of Gag methylation for integration site selection.

Conclusion

In closing, our work underscores that Gag localizes in the nucleolus during PFV replication. This step is likely regulated by PRMT1-mediated methylation of Gag that depends on the invariant R540 residue. Further studies will be required to define the functional significance of the nucleolar step for FV replication as well as the consequences of PFV Gag methylation in regard to the regulation of its complex nuclear transport and integration site selection.

Methods
Cells and culture conditions
HeLa, 293T and U373MG cells were cultured in DMEM supplemented with 10% Fetal Calf serum (FBS). BHK-U3GFP indicator FAG (Fluorescence Activated GFP) cells were cultured in DMEM supplemented with 5% FBS and 500 µg/mL G418 (Gibco). Leptomycin B (LMB) (Sigma) was added to culture medium to a final concentration of 10 nM for 4 h. Hypoxic conditions (2% O_2, 5%CO_2 and 93% N_2) were induced by a continuous flow of nitrogen using a Forma Series II Water Jacket CO2 incubator (model: 3131; Thermo Scientific).

Plasmid constructions
Fusion of individual GR boxes (GRI: aa 485–511, GRII: aa 534-557, GRIII: aa 586–618) or RevNoLS (aa 35–51) to GFP or RFP was obtained by inserting annealed complementary oligonucleotides of appropriate sequence into pEGFP-C1 or pDsRed-C1. GFP-GRs (GRs: aa 477–625) and GFP-Gag were constructed by insertion of PCR products obtained using the pcziGag as template, into pEGFP-C1 (Clontech) between HindIII and BamHI sites. HA-GRs expression plasmids were generated by replacing GFP by the HA sequence. pHFVGag$\Delta_{131-162}$ [39] served as

template to generate GFP-GagΔdim (deletion of PFV Gag aa 130–160). Mutants were generated using QuickChange site-directed mutagenesis Kit according to the manufacturer's specifications (Stratagene). Fragments spanning Gag$_{1-200}$, RevNoLS or Gag$_{1-200}$ fused to RevNoLS, were inserted into pEGFP-N1, and the resulting plasmids were used as template to amplify the coding sequences to be inserted in pMSCVneo at the EcoRI and HpaI sites. Plasmids encoding GFP-tagged human PRMTs proteins were kindly provided by Mark Bedford [56].

Establishment of cell lines stably expressing Gag-TRAP-GFP
U373MG stable cell lines were established using the Murine Stem Cell Virus (MSCV)-based retroviral vector system. Recombinant retroviral vectors were generated by transfection of 293T cells with the pMSCV-neo vector encoding Gag$_{1-200}$-RevNoLS-GFP (Gag-TRAP-GFP), Gag$_{1-200}$-GFP, RevNoLS-GFP or GFP, and the packaging plasmids expressing MLV Gag-Pol and the Vesicular Stomatitis Virus envelope G glycoprotein (VSV-G) using the calcium phosphate precipitation method. Cell-free supernatants were collected 48 h post-transfection and used to transduce U373MG cells. GFP expression was analyzed 48 h post-transduction by flow cytometry. After cell sorting, GFP-positive cells were propagated in culture medium supplemented with G418 (500 µg/mL).

Immunocytochemistry
Indirect immunofluorescence imaging on fixed-cells or mitotic chromosome spreads was described elsewhere [19]. In brief, samples were incubated with the appropriate primary antibodies (4 °C, overnight) and fluorescent-labeled secondary antibody (30 min, room temperature). Nuclei were stained with 4,6-diamidino-2-phenylindole (DAPI). Images were acquired with a laser-scanning confocal microscope (LSM510 Meta; Carl Zeiss) equipped with an Axiovert 200 M inverted microscope, using a Plan Apo 63_/1.4-N oil immersion objective.

Co-immunoprecipitation assay and Western blotting
Cell pellets were lysed in 0.4 M NaCl, 1 mM MgCl$_2$, 10% sucrose, 0.5 mM DTT, 10 mM PIPES pH 6.8, 0.5% NP-40 supplemented with Protease Inhibitor Cocktail (Roche) (30 min on ice), and subsequently centrifuged (12,000g, 5 min at 4 °C). Immunoprecipitation and Western-blot were performed as previously described [28].

Immuno-electron microscopy
Transfected 293T cells were prepared as described [57]. After extensive washing, the grids were incubated with an anti-GFP monoclonal antibody (90 min,

RT), followed by an anti-rabbit antibody conjugated to 15 nm-gold particles (British Biocell International, Cardiff, UK) (90 min, RT). Ultrathin sections were stained with 5% uranyl acetate 5% lead citrate, placed on EM grids coated with collodion membrane and observed with a Jeol 1010 transmission electron microscope (Tokyo, Japan).

RNA interference
HeLa Cells were transiently transfected with ON-TARGETplus Human SMARTpool siRNA targeting PRMT-1 (Dharmacon #3276) or the scrambled control (10 nM) using the Lipofectamine RNAiMax reagent according to the manufacturer's instructions (Life Technologies). After 48 h, cells were transfected with the GFP-GRs expressor and, following further 24 h incubation, were fixed and analyzed by confocal microscopy.

Statistic testing
Graphical representation and statistical analyses were performed using the GraphPad Prism software (GraphPad Software, San Diego, CA, USA). Differences were tested for statistical significance using ne-way ANOVA statistical test with a Bonferroni Multiple comparison post-test.

Additional files

Additional file 1: Figure S1. Nucleolar targeting is a conserved feature of EFV GRI and GRIII boxes and is antagonized by R472 within GRII. **A)** Amino acid sequences of the GR boxes of PFV and EFV and the NoLS of HIV-1 Rev protein (aa 35–51). **B)** Electron microscopy images of HeLa cells expressing GFP, GFP-GRI or GFP-RevNoLS and stained with an anti-GFP antibody (ab6556, Abcam, 1:200) and a secondary antibody coupled to 15 nm gold particles (goat anti-rabbit 15 nm Gold, BBI International, 1: 60). **C)** PFV GRI fused to DsRed and PFV GRIII, EFV GRI (aa 395–427) or GRIII (aa 492–524) fused to GFP were expressed in HeLa cells. Their localization was analyzed 24 h later as described in Fig. 1b. Nuclei are stained with DAPI. **D)** The C-terminal region (GRs) of EFV Gag fused to GFP and bearing the R472A mutation or not, was expressed in HeLa cells, and its localization was studied as described in Fig. 1b. Nuclei are stained with DAPI. Scale bar represents 10 µm.

Additional file 2: Figure S2. Gag-TRAP-GFP interacts with PFV Gag. Lysates of 293T cells ectopically expressing PFV Gag and Gag-TRAP-GFP construct (Gag$_{1-200}$-RevNoLS-GFP) or the corresponding controls (GFP, Gag$_{1-200}$-GFP or RevNoLS-GFP) were immunoprecipitated on protein A beads coated with an anti-GFP antibody (cat.11 814 460 001, Roche, 1:100). Input and bound proteins were analyzed as in Fig. 4a.

Additional file 3: Figure S3. Both WT and R540A mutant Gag bind to PRMT5. **A)** Lysates from 293T cells expressing PFV Gag and each human PRMT variant in fusion with GFP were immunoprecipitated with protein A beads coated with anti-PFV antibodies. Input and bound proteins were analyzed as in Fig. 4a. **B)** Cells expressing WT or R450A mutant PFV Gag and GFP-PRMT5 were lysed and incubated with beads coated with anti-GFP (cat.11 814 460 001, Roche, 1:100) or anti-SDMA (SYM10, 07-412, Millipore, 1:100) antibodies. Input and immunoprecipitated proteins were treated as in Fig. 4a.

Authors' contributions
AS, JP, JTT conceived and designed the experiments; JP, JG, JTT, MLG, and PR performed the experimental work; AS, AZ, FB, JP, JTT, MLG, PL analyzed the data; JTT, AS and AZ wrote the manuscript. All authors read and approved the final manuscript.

Author details
[1] CNRS UMR7212, Hôpital St Louis, Inserm U944, Institut Universitaire d'Hématologie, Université Paris Diderot, Sorbonne Paris Cité, Paris, France. [2] Plateforme IBiSA de Microscopie Electronique, Université François Rabelais and CHRU de Tours, Tours, France. [3] INSERM U1259, Université François Rabelais and CHRU de Tours, Tours, France. [4] Institut Pasteur, Unité d'Epidémiologie et Physiopathologie des Virus Oncogènes, Paris, France. [5] CNRS UMR3569, Insitut Pasteur, Paris, France. [6] CNRS UMR7212, Hôpital St Louis, Inserm U944, Institut Universitaire d'Hématologie, Université Paris Diderot, Sorbonne Paris Cité, Laboratoire PVM, Conservatoire National des Arts et Métiers (Cnam), Paris, France.

Acknowledgements
We thank Axel Rethwilm and Dirk Lindemann for FV reagents; Mark Bedford for GFP-PRMTs plasmids; Christelle Doliger, Sophie Duchez and Niclas Setterblad at the Imaging, Cell selection and Genomics Department of the Institut Universitaire d'Hématologie for confocal microscopy; Claudine Pique for critical reading of the manuscript.

Competing interests
The authors declare that they have no competing interests.

Funding
This study was supported by CNRS, INSERM, Université Paris Diderot Sorbonne Paris Cité, CNAM and ANR (ANR-12-BSV3-0016 to AS, ANR-15-CE15-0008 to AS and FB).

References
1. Murray SM, Linial ML. Foamy virus infection in primates. J Med Primatol. 2006;35:225–35.
2. Heneine W, Schweizer M, Sandstrom P, Folks T. Human infection with foamy viruses. Curr Top Microbiol Immunol. 2003;277:181–96.
3. Gessain A, Rua R, Betsem E, Turpin J, Mahieux R. HTLV-3/4 and simian foamy retroviruses in humans: discovery, epidemiology, cross-species transmission and molecular virology. Virology. 2013;435:187–99.
4. Khan AS. Simian foamy virus infection in humans: prevalence and management. Expert Rev Anti-Infect Ther. 2009;7:569–80.
5. Moebes A, Enssle J, Bieniasz PD, Heinkelein M, Lindemann D, Bock M, et al. Human foamy virus reverse transcription that occurs late in the viral replication cycle. J Virol. 1997;71:7305–11.
6. Yu SF, Baldwin DN, Gwynn SR, Yendapalli S, Linial ML. Human foamy virus replication: a pathway distinct from that of retroviruses and hepadnaviruses. Science. 1996;271:1579–82.
7. Löchelt M, Flügel RM. The human foamy virus pol gene is expressed as a Pro-Pol polyprotein and not as a Gag-Pol fusion protein. J Virol. 1996;70:1033–40.
8. Enssle J, Jordan I, Mauer B, Rethwilm A. Foamy virus reverse transcriptase is expressed independently from the Gag protein. Proc Natl Acad Sci USA. 1996;93:4137–41.
9. Giron ML, Colas S, Wybier J, Rozain F, Emanoil-Ravier R. Expression and maturation of human foamy virus Gag precursor polypeptides. J Virol. 1997;71:1635–9.
10. Müllers E. The foamy virus Gag proteins: what makes them different? Viruses. 2013;5:1023–41.
11. Gabus C, Ivanyi-Nagy R, Depollier J, Bucheton A, Pelisson A, Darlix J-L. Characterization of a nucleocapsid-like region and of two distinct primer tRNALys,2 binding sites in the endogenous retrovirus Gypsy. Nucleic Acids Res. 2006;34:5764–77.
12. Merkulov GV, Swiderek KM, Brachmann CB, Boeke JD. A critical proteolytic cleavage site near the C-terminus of the yeast retrotransposon Ty1 GAG protein. J Virol. 1996;70:5548–56.
13. Goldstone DC, Flower TG, Ball NJ, Sanz-Ramos M, Yap MW, Ogrodowicz RW, et al. A unique spumavirus Gag N-terminal domain with functional properties of orthoretroviral matrix and capsid. PLoS Pathog. 2013;9:e1003376.
14. Ball NJ, Nicastro G, Dutta M, Pollard DJ, Goldstone DC, Sanz-Ramos M, et al. Structure of a Spumaretrovirus Gag central domain reveals an ancient retroviral capsid. Krausslich H-G, editor. PLOS Pathog. 2016;12:e1005981.
15. Schliephake AW, Rethwilm A. Nuclear localization of foamy virus Gag precursor protein. J Virol. 1994;68:4946–54.
16. Lee E-G, Linial ML. The C terminus of foamy retrovirus Gag contains determinants for encapsidation of Pol protein into virions. J Virol. 2008;82:10803–10.
17. Stenbak CR, Linial ML. Role of the C terminus of foamy virus Gag in RNA packaging and Pol expression. J Virol. 2004;78:9423–30.
18. Yu SF, Edelmann K, Strong RK, Moebes A, Rethwilm A, Linial ML. The carboxyl terminus of the human foamy virus Gag protein contains separable nucleic acid binding and nuclear transport domains. J Virol. 1996;70:8255–62.
19. Tobaly-Tapiero J, Bittoun P, Lehmann-Che J, Delelis O, Giron ML, de The H, et al. Chromatin tethering of incoming foamy virus by the structural Gag protein. Traffic. 2008/07/17. 2008;9:1717–27.
20. Mullers E, Stirnnagel K, Kaulfuss S, Lindemann D. Prototype foamy virus Gag nuclear localization: a novel pathway among retroviruses. J Virol. 2011;85:9276–85.
21. Lesbats P, Serrao E, Maskell DP, Pye VE, O'Reilly N, Lindemann D, et al. Structural basis for spumavirus GAG tethering to chromatin. Proc Natl Acad Sci. 2017;114:5509–14.
22. Müllers E, Uhlig T, Stirnnagel K, Fiebig U, Zentgraf H, Lindemann D. Novel functions of prototype foamy virus Gag glycine- arginine-rich boxes in reverse transcription and particle morphogenesis. J Virol. 2011;85:1452–63.
23. Hamann MV, Müllers E, Reh J, Stanke N, Effantin G, Weissenhorn W, et al. The cooperative function of arginine residues in the prototype foamy virus Gag C-terminus mediates viral and cellular RNA encapsidation. Retrovirology. 2014;11:87.
24. Petit C, Giron ML, Tobaly-Tapiero J, Bittoun P, Real EE, Jacob Y, et al. Targeting of incoming retroviral Gag to the centrosome involves a direct interaction with the dynein light chain 8. J Cell Sci. 2003;116:3433–42.
25. Lehmann-Che J, Renault N, Lou Giron M, Roingeard P, Clave E, Tobaly-Tapiero J, et al. Centrosomal latency of incoming foamy viruses in resting cells. PLoS Pathog. 2007;3:e74.
26. Saïb A, Schmid M, Périès J, De Thé H, Puvion-dutilleul F, Pe J. Nuclear targeting of incoming human foamy virus Gag proteins involves a centriolar step. J Virol. 1997;71:1155–61.
27. Hocum JD, Linde I, Rae DT, Collins CP, Matern LK, Trobridge GD. Retargeted foamy virus vectors integrate less frequently near proto-oncogenes. Sci Rep. 2016;6:36610.
28. Renault N, Tobaly-Tapiero J, Paris J, Giron M-L, Coiffic A, Roingeard P, et al. A nuclear export signal within the structural Gag protein is required for prototype foamy virus replication. Retrovirology. 2011;8:6.
29. Kenney SP, Lochmann TL, Schmid CL, Parent LJ. Intermolecular interactions between retroviral Gag proteins in the nucleus. J Virol. 2008;82:683–91.
30. Stake MS, Bann DV, Kaddis RJ, Parent LJ. Nuclear trafficking of retroviral RNAs and Gag proteins during late steps of replication. Viruses. 2013;5:2767–95.

31. Balasundaram D, Benedik MJ, Morphew M, Dang VD, Levin HL. Nup124p is a nuclear pore factor of Schizosaccharomyces pombe that is important for nuclear import and activity of retrotransposon Tf1. Mol Cell Biol. 1999;19:5768–84.

32. Scheifele LZ, Garbitt RA, Rhoads JD, Parent LJ. Nuclear entry and CRM1-dependent nuclear export of the Rous sarcoma virus Gag polyprotein. Proc Natl Acad Sci USA. 2002;99:3944–9.

33. Garbitt-Hirst R, Kenney SP, Parent LJ. Genetic evidence for a connection between Rous sarcoma virus gag nuclear trafficking and genomic RNA packaging. J Virol. 2009;83:6790–7.

34. Gudleski N, Flanagan JM, Ryan EP, Bewley MC, Parent LJ. Directionality of nucleocytoplasmic transport of the retroviral gag protein depends on sequential binding of karyopherins and viral RNA. Proc Natl Acad Sci USA. 2010;107:9358–63.

35. Emmott E, Hiscox JA. Nucleolar targeting: the hub of the matter. EMBO Rep. 2009;10:231–8.

36. Mongelard F, Bouvet P. Nucleolin: a multiFACeTed protein. Trends Cell Biol. 2007;17:80–6.

37. Dundr M, Leno GH, Hammarskjöld ML, Rekosh D, Helga-Maria C, Olson MO. The roles of nucleolar structure and function in the subcellular location of the HIV-1 Rev protein. J Cell Sci. 1995;108:2811–23.

38. Stauber R, Gaitanaris GA, Pavlakis GN. Analysis of Trafficking of Rev and Transdominant Rev Proteins in Living Cells Using Green Fluorescent Protein Fusions: Transdominant Rev Blocks the Export of Rev from the Nucleus to the Cytoplasm. Virology. 1995;1(449):439–49.

39. Tobaly-Tapiero J, Bittoun P, Giron ML, Neves M, Koken M, Saïb A, et al. Human foamy virus capsid formation requires an interaction domain in the N terminus of Gag. J Virol. 2001;75:4367–75.

40. Mekhail K, Khacho M, Gunaratnam L, Lee S. Oxygen sensing by H+: implications for HIF and hypoxic cell memory. Cell Cycle. 2004;3:1027–9.

41. Han GZ, Worobey M. An endogenous foamy-like viral element in the coelacanth genome. PLoS Pathog. 2012;8:1–7.

42. Eastman SW, Linial ML. Identification of a conserved residue of foamy virus Gag required for intracellular capsid assembly. Society. 2001;75:6857–64.

43. Bedford M, Clarke S. Protein arginine methylation in mammals: who, what, and why. Mol Cell. 2009;33:1–13.

44. Matthews D, Emmott E, Hiscox J. Viruses and the nucleolus. In: Olson M, editor. The nucleolus. Protein reviews, vol. 15. New York: Springer; 2011.

45. Wulan WN, Heydet D, Walker EJ, Gahan ME, Ghildyal R. Nucleocytoplasmic transport of nucleocapsid proteins of enveloped RNA viruses. Front Microbiol. 2015;6:553.

46. Lochmann TL, Bann DV, Ryan EP, Beyer AR, Mao A, Cochrane A, et al. NC-mediated nucleolar localization of retroviral gag proteins. Virus Res. 2013;171:304–18.

47. Schneider WM, Brzezinski JD, Aiyer S, Malani N, Gyuricza M, Bushman FD, et al. Viral DNA tethering domains complement replication-defective mutations in the p12 protein of MuLV Gag. Proc Natl Acad Sci. 2013;110:9487–92.

48. Invernizzi CF, Xie B, Frankel FA, Feldhammer M, Roy BB, Richard S, et al. Arginine methylation of the HIV-1 nucleocapsid protein results in its diminished function. AIDS. 2007;21:795–805.

49. Fulcher AJ, Sivakumaran H, Jin H, Rawle DJ, Harrich D, Jans DA. The protein arginine methyltransferase PRMT6 inhibits HIV-1 Tat nucleolar retention. Biochim Biophys Acta - Mol Cell Res. 2016;1863:254–62.

50. Xie B, Invernizzi CF, Richard S, Wainberg MA. Arginine methylation of the human immunodeficiency virus type 1 tat protein by PRMT6 negatively affects tat interactions with both cyclin T1 and the TAt transactivation region. J Virol. 2007;81:4226–34.

51. Invernizzi CF, Xie B, Richard S, Wainberg MA. PRMT6 diminishes HIV-1 rev binding to and export of viral RNA. Retrovirology. 2006;3:93.

52. Campbell M, Chang P-C, Huerta S, Izumiya C, Davis R, Tepper CG, et al. Protein arginine methyltransferase 1-directed methylation of Kaposi Sarcoma-associated Herpesvirus Latency-associated nuclear antigen. J Biol Chem. 2012;287:5806–18.

53. Mostaqul Huq MD, Gupta P, Tsai N-P, White R, Parker MG, Wei L-N. Suppression of receptor interacting protein 140 repressive activity by protein arginine methylation. EMBO J. 2006;25:5094–104.

54. Lott K, Mukhopadhyay S, Li J, Wang J, Yao J, Sun Y, et al. Arginine methylation of DRBD18 differentially impacts its opposing effects on the trypanosome transcriptome. Nucleic Acids Res. 2015;43:5501–23.

55. Zurnic I, Hütter S, Rzeha U, Stanke N, Reh J, Müllers E, et al. Interactions of Prototype Foamy Virus Capsids with Host Cell Polo-Like Kinases Are Important for Efficient Viral DNA Integration. Emerman M, editor. PLOS Pathog. 2016;12:e1005860.

56. Herrmann F, Lee J, Bedford MT, Fackelmayer FO. Dynamics of human protein arginine methyltransferase 1(PRMT1) in vivo. J Biol Chem. 2005;280:38005–10.

57. Ferraris P, Blanchard E, Roingeard P. Ultrastructural and biochemical analyses of hepatitis C virus-associated host cell membranes. J Gen Virol. 2010;91:2230–7.

58. Robert X, Gouet P. Deciphering key features in protein structures with the new ENDscript server. Nucleic Acids Res. 2014;42:W320–4.

9

The role of integration and clonal expansion in HIV infection: live long and prosper

Elizabeth M. Anderson⊙ and Frank Maldarelli[*]

Abstract

Integration of viral DNA into the host genome is a central event in the replication cycle and the pathogenesis of retroviruses, including HIV. Although most cells infected with HIV are rapidly eliminated in vivo, HIV also infects long-lived cells that persist during combination antiretroviral therapy (cART). Cells with replication competent HIV proviruses form a reservoir that persists despite cART and such reservoirs are at the center of efforts to eradicate or control infection without cART. The mechanisms of persistence of these chronically infected long-lived cells is uncertain, but recent research has demonstrated that the presence of the HIV provirus has enduring effects on infected cells. Cells with integrated proviruses may persist for many years, undergo clonal expansion, and produce replication competent HIV. Even proviruses with defective genomes can produce HIV RNA and may contribute to ongoing HIV pathogenesis. New analyses of HIV infected cells suggest that over time on cART, there is a shift in the composition of the population of HIV infected cells, with the infected cells that persist over prolonged periods having proviruses integrated in genes associated with regulation of cell growth. In several cases, strong evidence indicates the presence of the provirus in specific genes may determine persistence, proliferation, or both. These data have raised the intriguing possibility that after cART is introduced, a selection process enriches for cells with proviruses integrated in genes associated with cell growth regulation. The dynamic nature of populations of cells infected with HIV during cART is not well understood, but is likely to have a profound influence on the composition of the HIV reservoir with critical consequences for HIV eradication and control strategies. As such, integration studies will shed light on understanding viral persistence and inform eradication and control strategies. Here we review the process of HIV integration, the role that integration plays in persistence, clonal expansion of the HIV reservoir, and highlight current challenges and outstanding questions for future research.

Keywords: HIV persistence, HIV reservoirs, Proviral integration, Clonal expansion

Background

Despite the success of combination antiretroviral therapy (cART) to block viral replication and halt disease progression, HIV viremia persists in the blood and anatomic compartments for years after therapy is initiated [1]. Although current therapies improve morbidity, mortality, and quality of life [2–5], long-term cART is associated with drug toxicities and persistent immune activation that contributes to morbidity and mortality, including a higher risk for non-AIDS related diseases including cardiovascular disease, cancer, kidney disease, liver disease, neurologic disease, and bone diseases [3, 6, 7]. Furthermore, if antiretroviral treatment is interrupted, viremia rebounds to near pre-therapy levels within weeks in most patients [8–10]. As a consequence, developing strategies to eradicate or control HIV without antiretroviral therapy are a high priority [11]. HIV rebounds from a reservoir of latently infected cells and consistent with this, the rebounding virus is archival in nature [12]. The source of persistent residual viremia that gives rise to rebounding virus upon treatment interruption remains largely unknown and is paramount for HIV cure initiatives.

A hallmark of retroviruses, and a key step in the HIV replication cycle that enables viral persistence, is the integration of the HIV DNA into the host genome. Integration is a multistep process that involves both viral and

*Correspondence: fmalli@mail.nih.gov
HIV Dynamics and Replication Program, NCI, NIH, Frederick, MD 21702, USA

host factors resulting in a stable and irreversible positioning of the double stranded reverse transcription product, the provirus, within the host cell. Integration does not require that the viral DNA be replication competent or even full length, and integration may proceed with highly deleted genomes. The choice of location of the retrovirus integration site within the host genome is neither entirely random nor specifically targeted. Integration preferences for various retroviruses have been identified and influence locations within the host genome where proviral integration takes place [13, 14]. Upon integration, the HIV provirus persists for the life of the cell and transcription of viral mRNA is coordinated by host cellular mechanisms. HIV primarily infects activated CD4+ T cells, a small subset of which may transition back to a resting memory state that is non-permissive for viral gene expression [15]. Although resting cells largely restrict productive HIV infection (reviewed by Zack et al. [16]), HIV can directly infect resting cells in vitro [17, 18] providing an alternative mechanism for establishing latency. In either case, a reservoir of latently infected cells may be unaffected by host immune responses and have a very long half-life [19–22].

HIV integration into long-lived cells represents an intrinsic characteristic that is central to HIV persistence and therefore a major barrier to an HIV cure or control strategy. During cART, lymphocyte populations undergo substantial change as ongoing HIV transmission is blocked, and a degree of immune restoration occurs. The population of HIV infected cells is molded over time since these cells may persist, be lost, or undergo clonal expansion. Understanding immune and viral mechanisms responsible for persistence is essential to characterizing the population of infected cells harboring replication-competent HIV that remain on therapy for prolonged periods and are a primary objective of control and eradication.

The only HIV reservoir that gives rise to rebounding virus, making a cure unachievable as of yet, is the reservoir of replication competent proviruses. Although over 95% of all integrated proviruses are defective or deleted, a small fraction of inducible replication competent proviruses persist for years on cART [23]. Still, defective and deleted proviruses are capable of producing viral proteins which can be targeted by the immune system and may contribute to persistent immune activation and long-term HIV pathogenesis [24, 25]. The majority of replication competent HIV proviruses persist in resting CD4+ T cells of a memory phenotype [21]. Since HIV gene expression is dependent on host transcription factors that are present only during cellular activation, HIV transcription is nearly silenced in resting CD4+ T cells. This results in a stably integrated yet transcriptionally silent provirus that will persist for the life of the cell, and can be reactivated to produce infectious virus. Resting CD4+ memory T cells have a very long half-life [19] and even after years on cART, resting CD4+ memory T cells can maintain themselves in a quiescent state or through periodic cell division without reactivation of the latent virus.

The HIV reservoir is established early during primary infection and is remarkably stable with a half-life of 43–44 months [26, 27]. As a consequence, current suppressive therapies must be maintained in an individual for over 70 years to achieve complete elimination of the reservoir. Similarly, HIV DNA levels remain detectable and are stable in most patients after years on suppressive therapy [28]. HIV reservoir half-life determinations vary substantially, in part due to technical approaches. Measurements of HIV DNA vary according to the HIV proviral target measured, for example LTR compared to *gag*. Determining the number of cells with infectious HIV proviruses may vary depending on the distinct quantitative viral outgrowth assay in use [29]. Understanding the underlying mechanisms that determine the variability in reservoir half-life will shed light on how the reservoir decays and whether immune selection pressure influences the rate of decay. The intrinsic stability of the reservoir indicates that its long term maintenance is a major mechanism that supports HIV persistence. The latent reservoir can be maintained over the course of cART through periodic homeostatic proliferation and through clonal expansion of HIV infected cells, both antigen mediated and integration site driven (reviewed by Murray et al. [30]). Additionally, promotion of cell survival through antiapoptotic regulation (reviewed by Badley et al. [31]) or the integration of proviruses into certain genes may also enable cells harboring integrated proviruses to persist for prolonged periods. Targeting the mechanisms for reservoir maintenance may provide novel curative strategies to deplete the latent reservoir.

Fundamental to bridging knowledge gaps towards HIV eradication is an understanding of the establishment and maintenance of cellular reservoirs and their persistence. The dramatic example of HIV cure [32, 33], as well as accumulating reports of post treatment control without cART [34–38] suggests that viral eradication or long-term viral remission may be achievable. Further study of proviral integration and persistence will aid in the development of novel strategies towards an HIV cure. A number of reviews on integration details have been published in the last several years that summarize aspects of integration and persistence including integrase structure and enzymology [39, 40], recent methods of detecting and quantitating integration sites [41, 42], as well as studies on other retroviruses integration that have useful insights for understanding persistence of HIV infected cells [43].

Here, we review concepts and controversies regarding HIV integration and clonal expansion of infected cells in the setting of current understanding of host cell populations, and highlight unanswered questions for future research.

Dynamics of HIV infected populations
Establishing a reservoir for HIV

Characterizing HIV persistence during prolonged cART requires a fundamental understanding of infected cell populations and their dynamics in infected individuals during cART. HIV infects numerous host cell types in diverse anatomic compartments typical of cells of lymphocyte [44] and myeloid lineage [45]. Various CD4+ T cell subsets are infected, but only some are likely sources of long-term persistence. Activated cells are typically infected by HIV and frequently undergo cell death from viral induced or immune elimination. Infrequently, activated CD4+ T cells infected with HIV transition to a resting memory state that is only poorly permissive for viral gene expression if at all [20, 21, 46]. These latently infected cells have a very long half-life [19] and in the absence of any viral gene expression may evade host immune responses. New studies to address whether cells remain latent permanently and whether they may evade immune surveillance are necessary. The memory T cell pool is composed of two main compartments, central memory (T_{CM}) and effector memory (T_{EM}) T cells, which are characterized by their homing abilities and effector functions [47, 48]. An intermediate compartment has also been described and is designated as the transitional memory compartment (T_{TM}). Both T_{CM} and T_{EM} compartments persists for decades [49] however the kinetic behaviors of these populations differ [50]. T_{CM} have a high proliferative capacity and are long-lived [51]. On the other hand, T_{EM} are rapidly turned over constituting a short-lived population with an extremely low proliferative capacity [50].

Another potential contributor to the HIV reservoir is a less differentiated subset of long-lived memory T cells with a high self-renewal capacity known as stem-cell memory CD4+ T cells (T_{SCM}) [52]. T_{SCM} can be differentiated from naïve T cells via TCR stimulation in vitro supporting the idea that naïve T cells represent the precursor to T_{SCM}. T_{SCM} retain many phenotypic characteristics of naïve T cells (CD45RA+ and CCR7+) but additionally express memory T cell markers including CD95 and CD62L [52]. T_{SCM} are infected by HIV in vitro, however, only a small fraction of cells are able to support productive infection [53]. Still, prolonged survival of T_{SCM} indicate that they may become the dominating population in the reservoir after long term suppression when ongoing rounds of virus replication are halted and other memory

T cell compartments decay. Indeed, Buzon et al. found T_{SCM} infected cells contribute minimally after 1 year on suppressive therapy but their contribution increased after long term therapy [54]. These findings suggest that HIV infected T_{SCM} cells could comprise a viral niche that promotes long-term viral persistence. Furthermore, replication competent virus has been recovered from CD45+/CD62L+ memory T cells ex vivo [55]. Given the potential for T_{SCM} to survive for prolonged periods and maintain a high proliferative capacity, it is critical to determine the contribution of the T_{SCM} compartment to the HIV reservoir.

Recent reports suggest additional helper T cell populations are infectable by HIV. As described by Lichterfeld and coworkers, these additional T cell populations express sufficient CXCR4 (Th1, Th17), or CCR5 (Th2 and Th9) to be infected in vitro by X4 and R5 tropic HIV respectively [56]. Extensive cell sorting studies recovered HIV DNA from these subsets in HIV infected individuals, indicating they are infected in vivo. The longevity of these subsets remains uncertain, but they are reported to have long half-lives, and thus may represent relevant reservoirs for HIV infection.

Other cell lineages, including tissue resident cells may be infected with HIV and may represent important sources of persistence of HIV infected cells during cART [57]. Intriguingly, HIV infection occurring at the stem cell level [58–60] raises the possibility that other downstream lymphocyte lineages, including B cells, may contain HIV proviruses. Although routine analyses of B cells does not typically detect HIV proviruses, infection may be present at levels below assay limits. Collins et al. have reported the presence of such cells as well as hematopoietic stem cells (HPC) infected with HIV at low frequency [61] and have suggested HPC infection may occur in only a subset of patients [60]. Others have published conflicting reports on the presence of HIV infected HPC in vivo [62, 63]. It is essential to determine if long-lived hematopoietic stem cells also contribute to the HIV reservoir. Additional potential reservoirs for HIV infection have been reported in myeloid lineages, including brain macrophages [64–66] and astrocytes [67, 68] in the central nervous system, and podocytes in the kidney [69]. The relevance of HIV infection of these long-lived cells as reservoirs for HIV infection during long-term cART is actively under investigation.

Maintaining a reservoir of HIV infected cells during cART

Longstanding untreated infection is characterized by progressive loss of lymphocytes with a preferential decline in CD4+ cells, and consequently a decrease of CD4/CD8 ratios. As described above, not all HIV infected cells are rapidly eliminated. The proportion of all lymphocytes that are infected is relatively low (1:100–1:1000). As such, the progressive loss of CD4 cells that is characteristic of untreated HIV infection is not due to direct viral killing per se, but to associated mechanisms, such as bystander effects and activation-induced cell elimination. Long-lived infected cells are less frequent, and are revealed upon initiating cART. The frequency of HIV DNA+ cells declines within the 1–4 years on cART, but remains relatively stable thereafter within the range of 1–3 per 10,000 CD4 cells during therapy [28]. As reviewed in this Special Issue by Pinzone and O'Doherty [70], determining levels of integrated HIV DNA can shed light on how reservoirs are maintained during cART. Prior to treatment initiation, total and integrated HIV DNA levels are higher in individuals treated during chronic HIV infection and decrease to a lower extent than those treated in primary HIV infection [71–73]. Furthermore, integrated HIV DNA continues to decay after prolonged therapy in individuals treated during primary infection suggesting that enhanced immune responses in these individuals are able to clear HIV infected cells more effectively [72, 74, 75]. During this same period, CD4 cell numbers typically increase with a measure of immune restoration. Thus, the number of infected cells keep pace with the overall recovery of CD4 cells. During prolonged cART, infected cells persist, are lost, or undergo clonal expansion in the context of a dynamic (and aging) immune cell population. It is not known how the proportion of infected cells remains stable as CD4 numbers rise, but it is likely that infected cells respond to immune signals to persist and proliferate. As such, the abundance of HIV infected cells in T cell subsets during cART may be continually molded by immune forces. The factors driving the maintenance of infected cells is of critical interest in understanding persistence and have been broadly divided into homeostatic and direct immune stimulatory factors [76].

Latently HIV infected resting memory CD4+ T cells can undergo homeostatic proliferation and antigen mediated or integration site driven clonal expansion [77–80] which may maintain the reservoir during cART. T cell homeostasis is a state of equilibrium maintained through self-regulation of T cell pools. T cells present in circulation and residing in tissues provide afferent and efferent immune arms that are central to both adaptive and innate immune responses. T cell homeostasis is mediated by homeostatic cytokines that belong to the common γ chain cytokine family including IL-2, IL-4, IL-7, IL-9, IL-15, and IL-21. A strong inverse correlation between baseline CD4 count and IL-7 plasma levels has been described, but the factors associated with this correlation have not been identified [81–83]. Lymphocyte population dynamics has been directly investigated using in vivo bromodeoxyuridine (BrdU) labeling. These studies found

that the increase in IL-7 is the result of CD4 depletion, but is not the primary driver of CD4 proliferation in the context of HIV infection [84]. Conversely, IL-15 controls survival and turnover of memory CD4+ T cells. Patients with advanced HIV infection have increased type I IFN plasma levels. Ongoing exposure to homeostatic forces and type I IFN activation may be responsible for selective depletion of CD4+ T cells [85]. IL-7 increases the number of CD4+ T cells by promoting their survival and proliferation, providing a rationale for IL-7 treatment to assist immune reconstitution in the setting of HIV infection [86, 87]. However, IL-7 induces proliferation without virus reactivation indicating that homeostatic proliferation can maintain the reservoir over time [88, 89].

Antigenic stimulation driven either by specific common antigens (CMV, EBV, HPV) or nonspecific immune activators, such as bacterial cell products translocated across the leaky gut wall that is present in HIV infection, may induce generalized immune activation and could ultimately contribute to the clonal expansion of HIV infected cells. IL-2 is produced by CD4+ T cells following activation by an antigen and drives T cell proliferation [90]. It is possible that HIV infected cells can undergo clonal expansion in response to cognate or cross reacting antigens. HIV-specific CD4+ T cells are a favored target for HIV infection [91]; it is likely these HIV specific cells persist during therapy, and that low level HIV production during cART may continue to drive persistence and expansion of these specific subsets. Other antigens commonly encountered (e.g., CMV, EBV) may also represent potential sources of clonal expansion. We previously reported a cell clone that was widely anatomically distributed, but significantly enriched in cancer metastases, suggesting that these cells proliferated in response to the cancer antigen [79]. Specific T cell receptor analyses were not possible in this single example. Advances in T cell receptor characterization of individual HIV infected cell clones will be critical for understanding the role of antigen driven clonal expansion on shaping the proviral landscape. These different mechanisms can promote cellular clonal expansion to maintain or potentially increase the size of the latent reservoir of intact replication competent proviruses.

HIV infection is characterized by a state of chronic immune activation which may play a strong role in maintaining persistence and clonal expansion of HIV infected cells. Prior to cART, viremia is substantial and activated CD4+ T cells infected with HIV die rapidly with a half-life of approximately 1.5 days which can be attributed to a variety of cytopathic effects. During chronic HIV infection and in the absence of treatment, abortive infection leads to the release of inflammatory cytokines that contribute to chronic inflammation, CD4+ T cell depletion, dysregulation of T cell homeostasis and ultimately AIDS [92, 93]. Even after the introduction of cART, low level viremia persists likely as the result of the stochastic reactivation of latently infected cells [94], infected cells are slowly eliminated [26, 27], but HIV antigens continue to persist thereby potentially contributing to chronic immune activation and dysregulation [95, 96]. Previous work measuring the decay kinetics of integrated HIV DNA from individuals treated during chronic HIV infection suggest diminished immune responses could promote persistence with the inability to effectively eliminate HIV infected cells during therapy. We recently found HIV infected cells harboring proviruses that contain internal HIV genes (such as *gag*) decline at a faster rate than *gag*-lacking proviruses upon cART initiation [76]. These findings further suggest a potential role for immune pressure to shape the proviral landscape during cART. Finally, in addition to generalized systemic immune activation, HIV mediated inflammation may be anatomically restricted [97]. Understanding the forces driving persistence and clonal expansion of resident T cells in tissues will shed important light on the mechanisms of HIV persistence and pathogenesis in vivo.

Detecting reservoirs of HIV infected cells and their turnover

Recent lines of research may improve our understanding of lymphocyte kinetics, and critical advances for quantifying HIV reservoirs are essential (Reviewed in this Special Issue by Wang et al. [98]). The simplest way to determine the viral burden in various cell subsets uses standard PCR-based techniques that measure total HIV DNA but is unable to distinguish integrated from unintegrated forms of HIV DNA. The utility of measuring integrated HIV DNA to understand how reservoirs are formed and persist is reviewed in this Special Issue by Pinzone and O'Doherty [70]. To date, HIV DNA has been measured in total peripheral blood mononuclear cells (PBMCs) [99], CD4+ T cells [100], resting CD4+ T cells [101], as well as in the gut-associated lymphoid tissue (GALT) [102, 103]. Recent approaches have used a next generation platform of PCR called droplet digital PCR (ddPCR) (Reviewed in this Special Issue by Rutsaert et al. [104]). ddPCR utilizes absolute quantification rather than relative quantification based off extrapolating from a standard curve in traditional qPCR. Eliminating the error from user generated or instable standard curves enables ddPCR to be more accurate than qPCR [105]. Furthermore, PCR inhibition is limited since the bulk PCR reaction is partitioned into circa 20,000 individual reactions. ddPCR has been used to quantify total HIV DNA in vivo

from PBMCs, CD4+ T cells, T regulatory (Treg) cells, and in cells from cerebrospinal fluid [29, 106–110].

Despite these advances, total HIV DNA quantification using standard PCR-based techniques has been shown to be at least two orders of magnitude higher than latent reservoir size measurements using the quantitative viral outgrowth assay (qVOA), the gold standard technique to measure the replication competent reservoir [29]. This large discrepancy is likely due to the fact that the majority of integrated proviruses are deleted [111], therefore total HIV DNA alone cannot provide an accurate estimate of latent reservoir size. Still, HIV DNA levels remain an important biomarker for viral persistence [112] and can predict viral rebound upon treatment interruption [9, 113]. Moreover, HIV DNA levels strongly correlate with qVOA thereby providing a surrogate marker for the size of the latent reservoir using an inexpensive and less time consuming approach [29, 114]. New duplexed ddPCR strategies that quantify internal targets may improve the accuracy of amplification methods to quantify replication competent reservoirs [115].

Understanding lymphocyte dynamics and turnover is a second critical area requiring advancement. In the context of HIV infection, persistent immune activation is associated with an increase in cell proliferation and cell death. In vivo labeling can provide reliable measurements of cell turnover and proliferation. Labeling newly synthesized DNA with deuterium provides a method for directly measuring turnover in a population of cells, with the caveat that minority populations cannot be studied easily. BrdU is a thymidine analogue that is incorporated into the DNA of replicating cells and can subsequently be detected by flow cytometry with a monoclonal antibody [116]. In vivo BrdU labeling identified two populations of CD4 and CD8 T lymphocytes which can be characterized as either rapidly proliferating or slowly proliferating [117]. Activated cells have the highest proliferative rates, followed by effector and central memory, and naïve cells have the lowest proliferative rates [84]. Increased CD4+ T cell turnover is associated with higher HIV plasma RNA levels and increased CD4 depletion, suggesting that lymphocyte turnover is a direct consequence of HIV infection [117]. Additionally, immune responses also play a role in the turnover of most CD4 and CD8 memory cell subsets [84]. On the other hand, turnover of the naïve compartment can be attributed to homeostatic mechanisms rather than immune mediated activation [84]. Long term labeling with deuterated water found T cell subpopulations possess distinct half-life characteristics and that T cells died more rapidly in individuals with advanced HIV infection [118]. Continuing research to measure the turnover of cells, including HIV infected cells, in these subsets is crucial to determine the longevity of these compartments and their role in promoting long-term persistence of HIV infected cells.

Further definition of the spectrum of cell subsets infected by HIV is also essential. Novel single cell and transcriptomic studies [119–122], as well as quantitative studies of populations of CD4 and CD8 cell subsets are advancing our understanding of human immune response to pathogens, including chronic infections, and may potentially inform the status of HIV infected cells with integrated proviruses. To date, single cell methods have been useful in characterizing the fate of T cells [122]. Understanding the functionality and dynamics of T cell populations over prolonged periods as individuals age is especially germane [123–125]. Since the frequency of HIV infected cells during cART is low, functional studies of T cells infected with HIV necessitates innovative approaches that overcome technical challenges to characterizing individual infected cells.

Integration: the central event in HIV replication

The integration of the HIV provirus into the host genome is a key characteristic of retroviruses and an essential step in the HIV life cycle that enables viral persistence. Prior to integration, the virally encoded enzyme reverse transcriptase (RT) synthesizes a linear double-stranded cDNA intermediate from the viral RNA genome. This reverse transcription product is the substrate for integration and contains homologous long terminal repeat (LTR) sequences at both the 5' and 3' ends [126]. The process of integration is the product of a viral enzyme, integrase, but interactions with other viral and cellular factors are required for successful integration to take place in an in vivo setting.

Integrase structural and enzymatic studies

Integrase (IN) is a member of the transposase family of nucleotidyl transferases (E.C. 2.7.7) that catalyze the transfer of 3' OH ends of HIV DNA to a host DNA acceptor. IN has a tripartite structure consisting of an N terminal Domain (NTD), a catalytic core domain (CCD) and a C-terminal domain (CTD). NTD and CTD have important functions coordinating interactions with DNA and chromatin binding. CCD contains enzymatic activity, including a D, D, E active site motif that is found in a number of nucleotidyl transferases, which coordinates essential divalent metal cations necessary for catalysis (Fig. 1).

Understanding the structure and function of integrase has been critical to explain the establishment of the provirus and for developing integrase inhibitors. The structure of HIV integrase has been the subject of intense investigation; crystals of the catalytic portion of HIV IN have been available for years [127], but the full length enzyme has had technical issues [128, 129]. Fortunately, pivotal studies of foamy virus and maedi-visna virus integrase have greatly advanced the field [130–132] and revealed critical structural characteristics of integration [133, 134]. These studies utilized crystallographic approaches of integrase and DNA substrate co-crystals and cryo-electron microscopy (cryo-EM) approaches of integrase multimers and DNA. Structural studies combined with biochemical studies using in vitro assays of purified HIV IN enzyme and host DNA have characterized the multistep process of HIV integration (Fig. 2). HIV IN multimers are positioned at the ends of DNA product. The initial structure, denoted the intasome or stable synaptic complex, is poised to initiate the multistep integration reaction, beginning with an IN-mediated 2 nucleotide deletion at the 3' end of each viral DNA

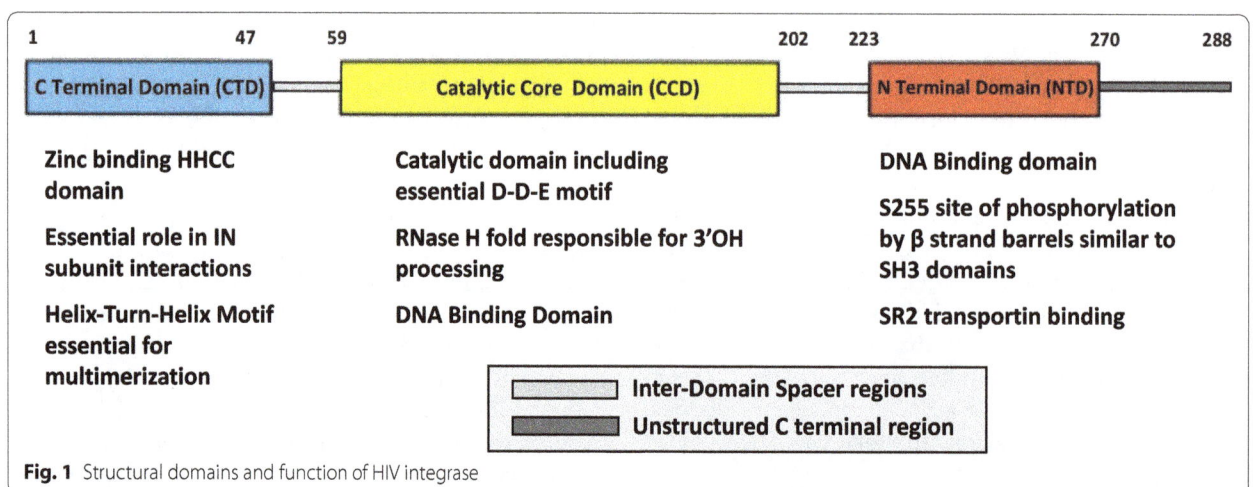

Fig. 1 Structural domains and function of HIV integrase

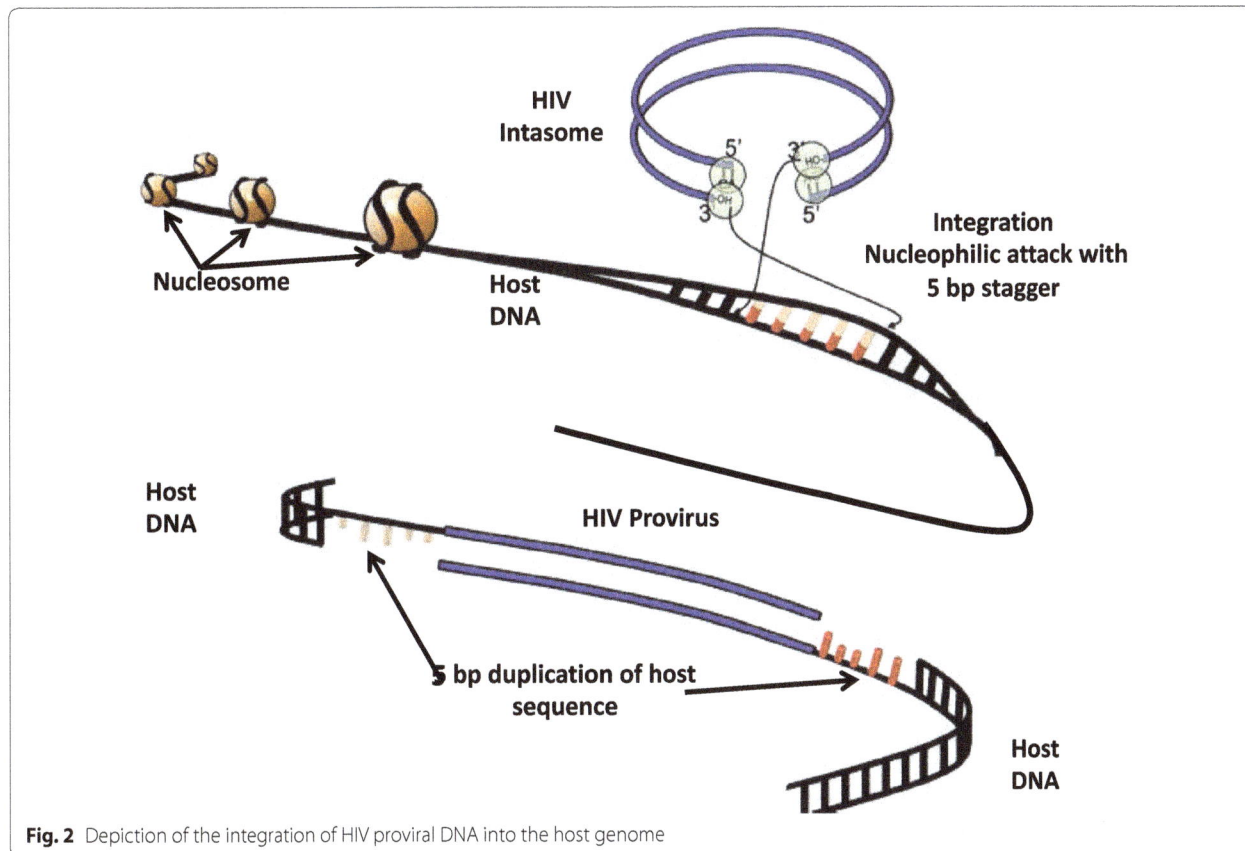

Fig. 2 Depiction of the integration of HIV proviral DNA into the host genome

molecule, creating staggered ends on the viral substrate for subsequent integration into the host DNA.

The stoichiometry of Integrase:DNA has been a subject of intense interest to discern the processes that coordinate the integration reaction. Furthermore, specific inhibitors that disrupt multimerization are currently in therapeutic development. A number of studies have suggested that IN from HIV and other retroviruses assumes a quaternary structure at the ends of the proviral DNA molecules [133]. Over the last several years, the development of cryo-EM has revolutionized the visualization of large macromolecular assemblies. Cryo-EM has permitted the visualization of HIV IN structure that has not been previously possible through traditional crystallographic approaches. Intriguing new cryo-EM studies have identified structures for HIV IN containing more than four IN molecules. The relative contributions of these higher order structures to integration and interactions with elements of the PIC remain uncertain and are topics of active investigation [135]. The development of a new class of IN inhibitors, called allosteric integrase inhibitors (ALLINIs), will be particularly useful probes in understanding the role of higher order structures in HIV IN (reviewed by Feng et al. [136]). ALLINIs bind at the IN

dimer interface resulting in aberrant IN multimerization, with a number of critical consequences for HIV replication, including the production of aberrant particles with viral ribonucleoprotein eccentrically localized in virions [136]. These defective virions have reduced reverse transcriptase activity and accelerated decay rates of viral RNA in subsequent rounds of replication [137–140]. Thus, disruption of proper IN multimerization has consequences for both early and late steps in HIV replication.

The details of binding and cutting host sequences has been extensively studied in model systems. In cryo-EM studies of maedi-visna integrase, tetramers assembled at each DNA end (with 2 nucleotides at the 3′ end of each viral DNA molecule already removed), then the CTDs bind in expanded major grooves of DNA targets effectively bending the target DNA [141]. Once bound, a target capture complex cuts the host DNA with a 5 nucleotide staggered cut yielding the strand transfer complex (Fig. 2) (for details see Lesbats et al. [142]), enabling transfer of the viral DNA to host cell DNA. The intervening 5 nucleotide gap is filled in by host DNA polymerase, and ligated by host ligase. One consequence of the 5 nucleotide staggered cutting mechanism of the host DNA by integrase is the duplication of these 5 nucleotides of host sequence directly flanking the 5′ and 3′ ends of the provirus, which provides a useful assay to confirm authentic integrations when both the 5′ and 3′ sites have been sequenced.

The extraordinary detail afforded by crystallographic and cryo-EM studies combined with an extensive understanding of IN enzymology, the role of specific domains involved in IN enzymatic activity (Fig. 1), and the effects of type I and II mutations provides a strong foundation for understanding the role of IN in HIV replication and identifying new avenues for HIV IN therapeutic development.

Determinants of integration site selection

In in vitro assays of purified integrase, integrases show little host site specificity, with the exception of weak palindromic sequences at target sites [14]. In contrast, analyses of integration site distribution in retroviral tissue culture infections and in samples from animal studies or patients reveal integration site preferences that highly influence the overall infection program. Preferences are exercised by the cellular partners that the intasome engages during the transport to the nucleus and integration. As described by Ciuffi [143], Craigie [144], and Debeyser [145, 146], these factors may be categorized as those with chaperone-like activity and those with chromatin-tethering activity. Understanding nuclear import and chromatin association is essential to understanding distribution of integration sites, as interactions with tethering and chaperone partners may have direct and indirect effects on distribution of integration sites. Cofactors for integration have been investigated for a number of retroviruses. As reviewed by Engleman [147], some retroviruses have distinct integration preferences, while others remain relatively random. Here we will review data for HIV.

Unlike many retroviruses, HIV infects non-dividing cells, requiring import of the reverse transcript into the nucleus which takes place in the context of a large multimeric pre-integration complex (PIC). PIC contents remain under study (reviewed in Suzuki & Craigie [148] and Craigie & Bushman [144]), as understanding the composition of the PIC will provide insights into requirements for initial steps in establishing the proviral state and potential targets for interruption in non-dividing cells. Viral components include HIV RT, IN, and an uncertain portion of the complement of HIV CA from the incoming core are associated with the PIC. Cellular proteins interacting with the PIC include the barrier to autointegration factor 1 (BAF1), high mobility group proteins (HMG), lamina-associated polypeptide 2α (LAP2α), lens-epithelium-derived growth factor (LEDGF/p75), and the karyopherin transportin SR2 (TRN-SR2, TNPO3). TNPO3 binds directly to the CCD and CTD of IN [149]

and may participate in shuttling the PIC to the nucleus. The size of the PIC is uncertain, but it must fit through the nuclear pore, and the process of import is essential yet remains unclear. As IN associates with the ends of the HIV DNA, the internal HIV sequence need not be full length, and can be defective or deleted, making the HIV proviral makeup in an individual highly diverse. As reverse transcription may take place in the nucleus [150], RT and associated factors may clearly be imported into the nucleus.

A number of critical outstanding questions defining the early events of infection are currently under study. These include the requirements for uncoating and transport, the composition of PIC structures, the factors required for intracellular transport and nuclear import, the coordinated involvement of cellular and nuclear cytoskeletal structures, as well as the overall kinetics and rate limiting steps of the process. A number of factors have been reported to be involved in regulating import, including nuclear membrane proteins SUN1 and SUN2 [151]. The central role for integration in HIV replication makes it an attractive target for therapy. Enzymatic inhibitors have been highly successful, allosteric inhibitors or agents that interrupt other integrase functions such as multimerization or interactions with cellular proteins have already yielded interesting candidates for further study [136, 152–154]. Critical advances in tracking single particles with elegant microscopic approaches have begun to characterize the kinetics of nuclear import [150, 155].

Once nuclear import has been accomplished the provirus can integrate into the host genome. The site of proviral integration for retroviruses is relatively nonspecific, with general preferences among the orthoretrovirinae subfamily. For HIV, integration site preferences include actively transcribed genes, gene rich regions of chromosomes, introns over exons, and generally exclude promoter regions. As introns are typically much larger than exons, the excess integrations into introns is likely due to larger overall size of introns rather than a functional constraint or preference per se. Preferences for activated genes [156] are generally mediated by cellular cofactors that bind IN [157]. As described by Ciuffi [158] and Debeyser [145, 146], these factors may be categorized as those with chaperone-like activity that are primarily involved in nuclear import, and those with chromatin-tethering activity.

Chief among the factors coordinating binding to chromatin is the transcriptional activator LEDGF/p75 [159]. Co-crystal studies identified contacts between the integrase CCD and CTD of two IN molecules and the C-terminal integrase binding domain (IBD) in LEDGF/p75 [132]. These findings suggest that LEDGF/p75 forms a bridge between the NTD domain of one IN dimer and two CCD domains of a second dimer [132, 143, 160]. The LEDGF/p75 N-terminal domain contains an AT-hook motif which mediates DNA-binding at AT-rich regions [143], and a PWWP domain that mediates binding to chromatin [161]. LEDGF/p75 knock down experiments showed no decrease in the ability of HIV DNA to integrate into the host genome, but revealed shifts the integration site distribution away from transcriptionally active and AT-rich regions [159]. In a series of domain swapping experiments, Hughes and coworkers demonstrated that replacing the AT hook and PWWP domains of LEDGF/p75 with the chromatin binding domains of proteins having euchromatin or heterochromatin binding specificities redirects integration according to the specificity of the heterologous binding domain [162]. These studies highlight the critical role of LEDGF/p75 and demonstrate approaches to manipulate integration that may be useful in the design of safer retroviral vectors [162].

Recent reports have investigated the role of nuclear architecture in integration preferences. HIV enters via nuclear pore complexes (NPCs) into regions that are typically euchromatin rich as a result of Tpr, a protein constituent of the NPC basket region that facilitates heterochromatin exclusion zones [163]. Tpr knock down results in chromatin reorganization and no exclusion of heterochromatin from NPC regions, but does not reduce HIV integration although HIV transcription is significantly impaired [159, 164]. These findings indicate that in the absence of Tpr, HIV integration continues directly after or in concert with nuclear import but into regions that are unfavorable for HIV transcription [164]. Marini et al. analyzed the topologic distribution of HIV integration sites and reported highest levels of integration in genes located near NPCs with a decreasing gradient of integration in genes at greater distance from the nuclear envelope [165]. There are a number of techniques to localize HIV proviruses within nuclei: labeling of nascent HIV DNA with 5-ethynyl-2′-deoxyuridine (EdU) and immunofluorescent detection [166], identifying integrated proviruses by immunolocalization of endonucleases that introduce specific double strand breaks in HIV [167], detecting HIV proviruses in live cells using quantum dot labeled Transcription Activator-Like Effectors (TALEs) [168], colocalizing HIV Tat with HIV LTRs of integrated proviruses in isolated live nuclei [169], and detecting HIV IN live cells using specific immunofluorescent [170]. These studies have identified HIV proviruses or HIV IN near the nuclear membrane after import. Other studies reported HIV signal at some distance from nuclear membrane [150, 166, 168], while real-time studies from Burdick et al. demonstrated slow movement away from NPCs [170].

Hope and coworkers have suggested studies to investigate the role of nuclear architecture, other HIV proteins (e.g., capsid), and cellular components in HIV integration [171]. Such studies may reveal useful insights into HIV replication and nuclear import, especially regarding how the processes of reverse transcription and nuclear import are coordinated. These approaches will require analysis of the primary targets of HIV, including lymphocytes and macrophages. While macrophages have comparatively large nuclei and are likely easier to analyze, new studies of lymphocytes are especially needed. Visualization approaches, including sensitive single cell technologies that can identify intranuclear location of HIV DNA within these nuclei are essential. Methods to simultaneously detect HIV provirus and HIV RNA transcription in infected lymphocytes have been reported [172]. Live cell studies are particularly useful to elucidate the dynamics of RNA expression from HIV proviruses [168–170].

Not all of the newly synthesized viral cDNA molecules, however, are successfully integrated into the host genome. In the nucleus, a subset of reverse transcripts comprise unintegrated episomal molecules that include 1- or 2-LTR circles and defective autointegrants [173]. Circular forms are not replicated as the cell divides, are diluted out upon cell replication, and do not contribute to ongoing replication. The longevity of such forms is a subject of debate. In tissue culture, circular LTR forms are lost several weeks after infection [174–176] but are stable in long term cultures of nondividing cells [176, 177]. In vivo they may persist for longer periods [28, 178], similar to T cell receptor excision DNA circles (TRECs) [179].

Integration in vivo: analysis of HIV integration junction sequences

Initial in vivo studies of proviral integration sites utilized inverse PCR to characterize HIV integration sites in CD4+ T cells from HIV infected individuals [180–182]. These studies confirmed what had been found from in vitro tissue culture systems with a preference for HIV DNA to integrate into transcriptionally active genes, usually within introns (range: 93–96%) [180–182]. Initial longitudinal analyses revealed that identical integration sites could persist in individuals for years during therapy. However, the methods used could not determine whether this arose through clonal expansion or simply represented long-term persistence [181]. Multiple individuals were identified as having proviral integration sites in the *BACH2* gene and all integrations were in the same orientation of the gene [181]. *BACH2* is highly expressed in B lymphocytes and plays a role in the regulation of B cell development [183]. While expression of *BACH2* has been shown in T lymphocytes in vitro [183] and in vivo [181], the function of *BACH2* in these cells remains unknown. Further, it was not understood at the time if the enrichment of integration sites in *BACH2* is the result of preferential integration or, rather, a selective advantage towards long-term persistence of cells that harbor integrants in *BACH2*.

New methods have been developed to detect and quantify HIV integration sites. Assays that can detect both the site of integration and the presence of clonal expansion represent a pivotal advance. Pioneering work from the Bangham laboratory inferred selective forces that shape the landscape of human T cell leukemia virus 1 (HTLV-1) clones in vivo [184]. A high-throughput approach was developed to identify the locations of unique HTLV-1 integration sites in the host genome [185]. This method, based on random shearing and linker-mediated PCR followed by next generation paired-end sequencing, enables simultaneous mapping and quantification of unique integration sites in HTLV-1 infected T-cells [185, 186]. Integration sites from gene therapy vectors and retroviruses, including HTLV-2 [187], murine leukemia virus (MLV) [188], and recently HIV [78], have been investigated using this approach. The abundance of specific clones can be assessed by the number of unique host break points. Identical integration sites with different lengths of host

sequence imply clonal expansion, whereas identical integration sites with identical lengths of host sequences are the product of PCR amplification (Fig. 3). A novel alternative approach to identify HIV proviral integration sites, the integration site loop amplification (ISLA) assay, was developed by Wagner and co-workers [80] (Fig. 4). ISLA utilizes linear amplification of proviral integration sites to increase their abundance, followed by loop formation using random decamers tailed with an HIV LTR U5-specific sequence [80]. This results in circularized amplicons containing HIV LTR sequence flanking the host genome at the site of integration, the HIV:host junction is then mapped using HIV LTR primers (Fig. 4). Both of these methods (reviewed in [41]) reduce bias since they do not rely on PCR amplification or restriction digestion both of which favor amplification of some integration sites.

Critically, these assays identify the integration junction sequence and the presence of clonal expansion. Yet, current approaches for integration site identification do not characterize the structure of the provirus located at the integration site. This is mainly due to the short amplicon constraints imposed by current next generation sequencing platforms. Integration site recovery has been insightful and has retrieved 10^2–10^3 integration sites from 5 to 10 million PBMCs. Initial studies revealed a number of

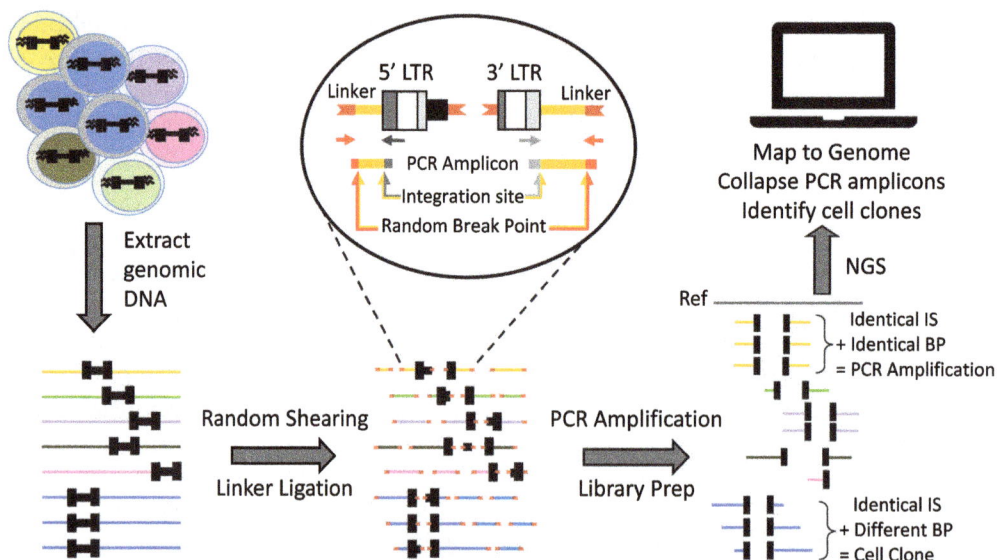

Fig. 3 Linker mediated HIV integration site assay (ISA) workflow. Total genomic DNA is first extracted then randomly sheared by Covaris sonification into 300–500 bp fragments. Sheared fragments are end repaired and a single dA overhang is added, then linkers containing a single T overhang are ligated onto the sheared ends (red). The pop out displays the PCR amplification strategy to selectively amplify integration sites. Primers that are complementary to the 5′ HIV LTR in U3 (dark grey arrow) and the 3′ HIV LTR in U5 (light grey arrow) are combined with linker specific primers (red arrows). The resulting amplicons contain linker sequence, the random breakpoint (BP), and the HIV/host junction sequence at the integration site (IS). The amplicons are then subjected to Illumina Miseq paired end sequencing. Sequences obtained are run through a stringent bioinformatics pipeline to map the location of the integrated provirus against a reference host genome and to determine the distance to breakpoint. Identical integration sites from amplicons with different break points in the host genome are the result of clonally expanded cells, whereas identical integration sites from amplicons with identical break point distances arose during PCR amplification

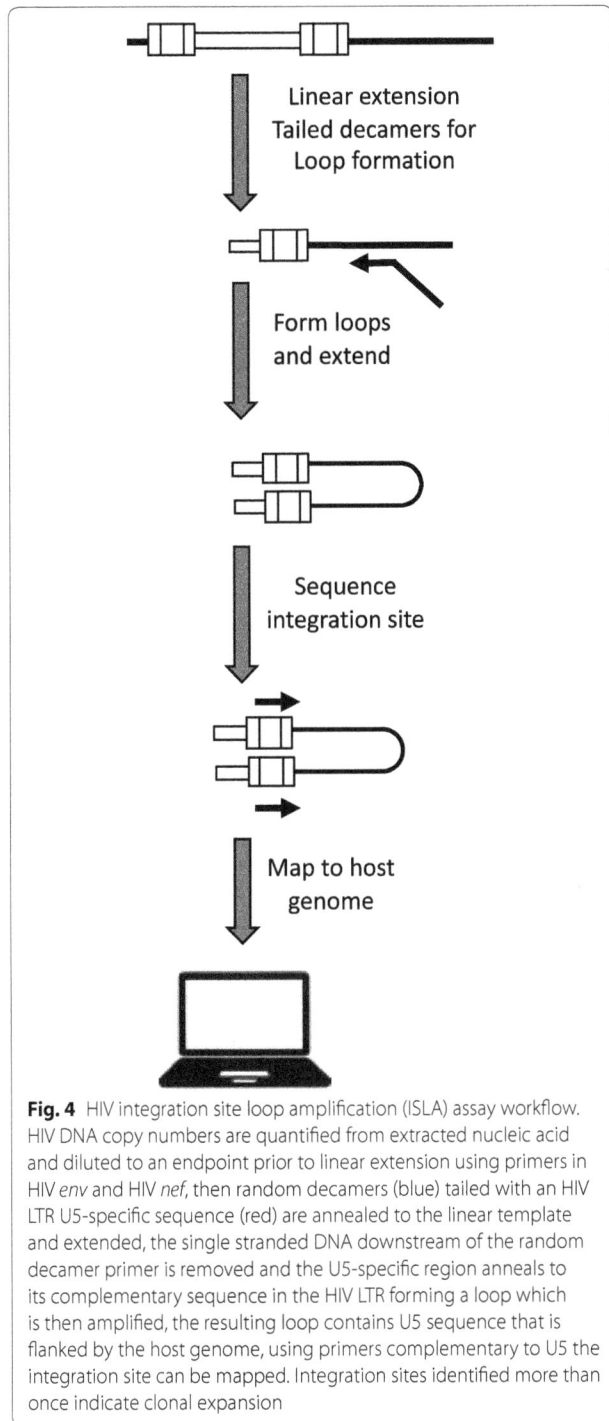

Fig. 4 HIV integration site loop amplification (ISLA) assay workflow. HIV DNA copy numbers are quantified from extracted nucleic acid and diluted to an endpoint prior to linear extension using primers in HIV *env* and HIV *nef*, then random decamers (blue) tailed with an HIV LTR U5-specific sequence (red) are annealed to the linear template and extended, the single stranded DNA downstream of the random decamer primer is removed and the U5-specific region anneals to its complementary sequence in the HIV LTR forming a loop which is then amplified, the resulting loop contains U5 sequence that is flanked by the host genome, using primers complementary to U5 the integration site can be mapped. Integration sites identified more than once indicate clonal expansion

unexpected findings: HIV infected cells present after prolonged cART are frequently clonally expanded. Overall, circa 40% of all cells harboring HIV proviruses are the product of clonal expansion. As described above, the efficiency of recovery of integrated proviruses is comparatively low, as such the actual frequency of clonal

expansion is likely to be much higher [78]. Moreover, Wagner et al. demonstrated that clonal expansion increased during antiretroviral therapy [80]. Longitudinal analyses revealed specific expanded clones were present over prolonged periods (> 10 years), demonstrating durable persistence of HIV infected cells [80].

Analysis of the distribution of integration sites using bioinformatic tools to investigate the functions of genes have revealed many proviruses were present in genes associated with cell growth [78, 80]. The cells remaining after long-term cART were infected many years prior to their sampling. Therefore, the enrichment in genes associated with cell growth raises the strong possibility that the presence of the provirus in these genes contributes to persistence, expansion, or both.

As expected, proviruses were most frequently identified in introns, and were integrated in the same or opposite direction of host transcription, similar to those detected in in vitro infections. However, proviruses in several genes, including *BACH2* and *MKL2*, were present integrated only in the same orientation as the host gene transcription. In addition, integrations into these genes were highly restricted, and identified only in a limited region of the host gene (Introns 4 and 6 for *MKL2*, Introns 4 and 5 for *BACH2*) [78]. Control experiments analyzing the distribution of HIV integration sites in acute in vitro infections of HIV demonstrated that proviruses are commonly found throughout the *MKL2* and *BACH2* genes [78]. However, the striking finding that in in vivo experiments they were only present in the same orientation as host gene transcription after prolonged cART suggested that proviruses present in intron 4 or 6 provided a direct selective advantage that contributed to persistence, and expansion [78]. Proviruses present in other parts of these genes were not detected after prolonged ART presumably because they did not have a selective advantage.

Megakaryoblastic Leukemia (MKL)/Myocardin-Like Protein 2 (MKL2) is a phosphorylation mediated transcriptional activator that modulates the transcription of many cellular early genes by regulating the transcription factor serum response factor (SRF). SRF is a reported oncogene involved in promoting proliferation of mammary and hepatocellular adenocarcinomas [189, 190]. Fusions of *MKL2* and *C11orf95* have been frequently identified in choroid lipomas, suggesting a role in growth and expansion of these neoplasms [191]. *MKL2* fusion with *RREB1* has been described in oropharyngeal sarcoma [192]. MKL2 has also been implicated in development of hippocampal neurons [193] and muscle [194, 195]. However, the precise role of MKL2 in T cell homeostasis has not been extensively studied.

The transcription regulator protein BACH2 is a member of the basic leucine zipper transcription factor family that typically associates with Maf proteins to permit the binding of a BACH2-Maf heterodimer to specific DNA promoter recognition sites (reviewed by Igarashi et al. [196]). BACH2 functions in normal B cell development [197], is frequently deleted in B cell tumors [183, 198], and reduced levels of BACH2 have been associated with poor outcome in response to chemotherapy [199]. In addition, aggressive lymphomas containing IGHCδ-BACH2 fusion protein have been identified [200]. More recently, BACH2 has been demonstrated to have critical roles in T cell homeostasis [201–203]. As reviewed by Richer et al. [204], BACH2 may participate in regulating development during T cell differentiation, especially of T-regulatory and T effector lineages. BACH2 may also contribute to maintaining cell quiescence by preventing differentiation into effector memory cells [201, 202]. It is not known how HIV integration affects BACH2 expression.

In infected cells, integrations into BACH2 were limited to introns 4 and 5, which are in the 5' untranslated region several thousand nucleotides upstream of the BACH2 start codon [78]. This suggests the possibility that transcription may be initiated from the proviral LTR promoter and not from the authentic BACH2 promoter. Indeed, Cesana et al. recently reported the detection of chimeric transcripts encoding HIV-LTR-BACH2 in a substantial number of HIV infected patients undergoing antiretroviral therapy [205]. These transcripts consists of HIV 5' untranslated sequence to the major splice donor from HIV spliced to exon 5 of BACH2. It is not yet clear whether these transcripts are initiated at +1 of HIV or represent read-through transcripts of BACH2 intron 4 [205]. These data demonstrate that chimeric host–HIV RNA is common, and increased expression of BACH2 may influence persistence and clonal expansion. Cesana et al. also demonstrated evidence of chimeric HIV transcripts with STAT5B, a transcription factor central to T cell activation, in PBMCs from a substantial number of infected individuals undergoing antiretroviral therapy [205]. Integrations into STAT5B were identified in a number of patients, but without significant orientation specificity [78]. Additional study of these specific examples of HIV integration is needed. Although integrations into these genes has been demonstrated, only limited sequence information of the HIV:host junction has been obtained and the structure of the entire proviruses in BACH2, MKL2 and STAT5B remains uncertain. The data of Cesana et al. indicate that at least the R, U5, and 5' untranslated HIV sequence to the major splice donor is present, but the remainder of the provirus structure is not known. It should be emphasized that although integrants in these genes were found in numerous HIV

infected individuals, their actual abundance in PBMC populations is quite low, on the order of 1–10 copies/million PBMC, complicating amplification and characterization of integrated proviruses.

The limits and consequences of clonal expansion remain poorly understood. Clonal expansion is detected during long-term cART, although total HIV DNA levels remain relatively constant. Thus, clonal expansions occur but do not appear to increase the abundance of virus infected cells. Control mechanisms that permit clonal expansion but restrict the number of HIV infected cells are not known. Similarly, HIV integration has not been associated, as yet, with malignant transformation of HIV infected cells. In fact, CD4+ T cell leukemia and lymphoma is distinctly uncommon in HIV infected individuals [206, 207]. It is likely that clonal amplification, even to the large abundance as we and others have identified [78, 80, 208], is insufficient for malignant transformation. Of note, clonal expansions of T cells are present in individuals infected with other human retroviruses, including both HTLV-1 and HTLV-2 [185, 187]. However, hematologic malignancies are only detected in a minority of HTLV-1 infections, suggesting that malignant transformation is likely due to additional requirements [209].

Advances in next generation sequencing approaches have enabled in depth analyses of proviral integration sites from PBMCs of HIV infected individuals on cART [78, 80, 208]. These methodologies allow quantification of multiple identical integration sites and the ability to identify clonal expansion. Since the probability of HIV integration into the exact same location in the host genome more than once is vanishingly small, clonal expansion can be defined as a population of cells derived from cell division that harbor a provirus integrated into the exact same location in the host genome. Analyses of these integration sites show clonally expanded HIV infected CD4+ T cells exist after years on therapy suggesting that clonal expansion is a major mechanism that enables HIV persistence despite the success of cART [78]. Yet, current approaches for integration site identification do not characterize the structure of the provirus located at the integration site. This is mainly due to the short amplicon constraints imposed by these sequencing platforms. Therefore, novel approaches to map integration sites and provirus structure will aid in understanding long-term HIV persistence and reservoir maintenance. Characterization of HIV integrant structures will be useful for constructing model systems in which proviruses can be specifically targeted, for instance with CRISPR/Cas, to investigate the effects of proviral integration on cell growth and differentiation. Further detailed analyses of integration site distribution in vivo will aid in the study of cellular functions in the context of HIV infection.

As integration sites are identified by various research groups, they should be compiled and made available for analyses through established public databases in order to robustly advance this key area of inquiry [210].

The role of clonal expansion in maintaining HIV persistence

Clonal expansion of HIV infected cells can persist in patients for over 10 years on suppressive cART [78, 80, 208]. Early studies found populations of virus with identical sequences emerge in the plasma of HIV infected individuals who were suppressed for years on cART suggesting that highly expanded cell clones gave rise to persistent viremia [211, 212]. The discovery of identical HIV sequences from clearly defective or APOBEC hypermutated proviruses indicated that the only way the virus could arise was through clonal expansion [213]. A mathematical model predicted that clonal expansion and contraction of latently infected cells upon sporadic antigen stimulation can generate persistent low level viremia and lead to intermittent viral blips [214]. Although experimental data is needed to confirm these findings, this model also indicates that a fraction of activated T cells can revert back to the latent state thereby providing a mechanism to continually replenish the latent reservoir [214].

The majority of HIV DNA decay occurs within the first year on cART, after which it remains relatively stable in participants treated during chronic infection [28]. Meanwhile, the reservoir of replication competent proviruses, as measured with qVOA, decays minimally [26]. Yet, the frequency of clonally expanded cells harboring integrated proviruses increase over time [80]. Therefore, the overall composition of the reservoir is dynamic and changes over time despite suppressive cART. For instance, although the majority of integrated proviruses are defective or deleted [23], some can still be transcribed and produce proteins which can be targeted by CTL for killing [24, 25]. Moreover, clonal expansion of cells harboring integrated proviruses can occur through homeostatic forces, as a consequence of the integration site, or by antigen stimulation [78, 79].

Homeostatic proliferation is a mechanism for T cell division that may play a role in maintaining the reservoir over time. Previous studies have implicated interleukin 7 (IL-7) in the homeostatic regulation of the T cell pool [215]. IL-7 is produced by non-hematopoietic cells and is involved in thymocyte development and survival [216]. During chronic infection, CD4+ T cell depletion is associated with increased levels of proliferation through elevated levels of IL-7 and ultimately larger reservoir size, indicating that IL-7 is responsible for the persistence of latently infected cells by promoting homeostatic proliferation [217]. IL-7 induced proliferation can occur without reactivation of the virus in an in vitro model of HIV latency [89] and in vivo [88]. Taken together these studies suggest T cell division of HIV infected cells permits HIV persistence in the absence of ongoing cycles of viral replication.

Integration site driven clonal expansion is believed to occur infrequently and is the result of a nearly random integration site selection process. Multiple individuals have been identified as having proviral integrations enriched in genes associated with cell growth some of which were found to be clonally expanded [78, 80]. These findings raises the possibility that the presence of the provirus within the oncogene contributes to the ability of the cell to persist or to undergo clonal expansion in an integration site driven manner. The frequency of integration site driven clonal expansion and the mechanisms that govern these cell clones are still under active investigation.

Identifying clonal populations containing replication-competent HIV proviruses is challenging because these cells are generally rare, and are present in large populations of cells containing defective proviruses. In vivo, most HIV infected cells persisting for prolonged periods on ART contain defective proviruses [23, 111]. The initial finding that many cells present after prolonged cART are the products of clonal expansion [78, 80] was thought to reflect clonal expansion of defective, but not replication competent proviruses [208]. Clonal populations harboring defective HIV can contribute to ongoing immune activation, which may enable persistence [24, 25, 111] but these populations cannot give rise to rebounding viremia upon treatment interruption and therefore do not contribute to the 'true' HIV reservoir. Initial analyses of plasma HIV during prolonged antiretroviral therapy revealed the presence of populations of identical sequences, suggesting these variants were the product of clonal expansion. Detailed analyses of one example of predominant plasma clone [79] led to identification of the integration site of the provirus responsible for the clone and that the provirus was replication competent. The provirus has a unique integration site, but is present in a region that has not been mapped to a unique location. The integrant was designated AMBI-1 (ambiguous) to reflect that the location in the human genome is ambiguous [79]. Amplification from the known integrant was determined to be replication competent in in vitro infections, and the identical virus could also be repeatedly recovered in vitro from endpoint diluted PBMC cultures. Cells harboring the AMBI-1 integrant were found to be widely anatomically distributed but enriched in cancer metastases indicating that the clone expanded in response to the cancer antigen [79]. These data demonstrated that clonally expanded populations can contain infectious HIV, and therefore represent a relevant reservoir for HIV during cART.

The finding of a clonally expanded population with infectious HIV was unexpected as HIV is frequently cytolytic and encodes an accessory protein (Vpr) which can arrest the cell cycle [218]. It is possible that cell division and virus production are compartmentalized, and do not take place concurrently. Recent studies have shown that populations of clonally expanded cells persist on cART and only a fraction of cells within the clone are transcriptionally active [219, 229]. Furthermore, upon treatment interruption, transcriptionally active cells ultimately gave rise to rebounding viremia [220]. Taken together, these studies suggest that clonally expanded cells containing replication competent proviruses comprise a portion of the true HIV reservoir and that a proportion of transcriptionally active cells within the clone contribute to low level persistent viremia and ultimately rebounding virus upon treatment interruption. A critical understanding of these populations, their HIV RNA expression levels, and mechanisms which govern their active or latent states are is crucial for targeting eradication efforts.

The frequency of clonally expanded cells that harbor replication competent proviruses, such as AMBI-1, is not known, although recent data indicate that they may be relatively common [221–223]. Unequivocal identification of such proviruses is labor intensive and technically complex, but their characterization will yield key information regarding the requirements for persistence during therapy. Such proviruses represent a substantial obstacle to HIV cure. Furthermore, the dynamics of clonal expansion of cells containing replication competent proviruses is not well described and may be shaped by immune selection pressures. Recently it was found that these clones can wax and wane or persist steadily in vivo for years [224]. The mechanisms by which these cells can proliferate without viral reactivation to maintain the reservoir despite therapy poses a major obstacle towards an HIV cure. Shock and kill strategies aimed at HIV eradication will need to reactivate quiescent cells without inducing cell replication, which could result in unintended expansion of a cellular reservoir of infected cells. A number of such agents capable of activating cells without inducing cell division are under investigation. Analysis of proviral integration sites as part of the analytic approach to HIV eradication strategies will be a useful adjunct to current reservoir studies. Current integration site assays are, as described above, not highly efficient, and sensitivity will likely need to be optimized to detect low level clonal expansion. Taken together, these findings suggests that both active CTL selection pressures and passive clonal expansion mechanisms can drive the remodeling of the HIV reservoir over time. Finally, clonal expansion provides multiple targets to decrease the probability that a cell with an intact provirus will be eliminated precluding eradication strategies.

Characterizing clonal expansion in the setting of eradication strategies

Several strategies aimed at eradicating the latent HIV reservoir have been employed. These include ART regime intensification, gene therapy, stem cell transplantation, therapeutic vaccines, and latency reversal agents (LRAs). LRAs are being used in a number of studies to potentially eliminate HIV through inducing reactivation of quiescent T cells in the hopes that these reactivated cells will undergo cell death. The original concept of purging the latent reservoir by reversing latency through activation of latently infected cells was implemented using interleukin 2 (IL-2) and T cell activators such as anti-CD3 antibodies (OKT3) [225, 226]. From these initial studies, it was clear that activation of latently infected T cells could be achieved and may enable purging of the reservoir, however, other compounds to reverse latency with reduced toxicity were needed.

Characterizing clonal expansion in the setting of eradication strategies such as 'shock and kill' sheds critical new light on the true structure of the HIV reservoir and whether that structure has been altered with treatment. The majority of current LRA strategies have utilized histone deacetylase inhibitors (HDACi). Even though some LRA strategies have successfully reversed latency in patients undergoing suppressed cART, measured by increased HIV transcription and virion production, no strategy has led to a decrease in the frequency of latently infected cells to date (reviewed by Bashiri et al. [227]). The inability of current LRA strategies to reduce the latent reservoir size can be attributed to insufficient host immune responses after latency reversal, an insufficient magnitude of latency reversal, or both. Therefore, new strategies that have higher specificity and potency to efficiently reverse latency may be needed in combination with therapies aimed at boosting the host immune response to sufficiently clear virus producing cells [228].

It is possible that LRA treatment can instead promote clonal expansion and thereby increase the reservoir size preventing elimination. IL-7 therapy has been administered to HIV-infected individuals to induce an increase in naïve and memory T-cell numbers [86, 87]. Yet, in vitro and in vivo studies predict that IL-7 administration would lead to an expansion of T-cells including HIV infected T-cells and thereby have a potential to increase the HIV reservoir without reactivating the virus [88, 89]. Characterization of individual HIV integration sites will identify which integrants were reactivated, eliminated, or expanded during latency reversal.

Conclusions

Integration is a critical and, as yet, irreversible step in HIV replication that enables the persistence of HIV in a reservoir of long-lived cells despite suppressive antiretroviral therapy. The reservoir of infected cells harboring inducible full length replication competent proviruses is a major barrier to an HIV cure. Understanding the mechanisms of reservoir maintenance may provide novel targets for therapeutic interventions. Clonal expansion of HIV infected cells is a key mechanism for maintenance of the reservoir.

Current assays to measure and characterize integration sites are costly, time consuming, and labor intensive. Therefore, novel assays to measure clonal expansion are of key interest. Alternatively, sequences can be obtained from individual HIV proviruses through endpoint dilution and PCR amplification [229]. While it is impossible to determine whether two proviruses are identical without comparing individual full length sequences, which are prohibitively expensive to generate at present, a surrogate to predict clonal expansion can be calculated with the clonal prediction score [230]. This metric considers the length of the amplicon and the intra-patient genetic diversity to determine the likelihood that individual identical sequences are the result of clonal expansion. This tool, while not definitive, may provide a measure to assess clonal expansion in the absence of intensive integration site analyses.

Methods to characterize the provirus sequence and structure as it is integrated into particular locations in the host genome need further development. For example, the generation of full length HIV genome amplicons that cross into the host at the HIV-host junction could provide insights into the abundance of replication competent proviruses in clonal populations, as well as the biological relevance of enriched integration sites. Extensive sequence data will enable phylogenetic analyses to elucidate timing of proviral integration as well as estimates of total population sizes within the host. Detailed assessments of intact versus defective and deleted proviruses can characterize the composition of HIV reservoirs over time and linking these data to the integration site may reveal novel immune selective pressures that eliminate or favor certain proviral structures over time.

Distinguishing how proviral structure influences transcription and RNA splicing within individual host genes may reveal alternative splice variants and their biological function in HIV persistence. For instance, it has been shown that HIV and lentiviral vectors may induce aberrant RNA splicing mechanisms resulting in the production of chimeric transcripts containing HIV sequence fused to cellular exon sequences [231–233]. Furthermore, it has been shown that lentiviral vectors with active LTRs can induce neoplastic transformation through the activation of cancer-related genes via promoter insertion [234]. In addition, chimeric HIV/*BACH2* transcripts were found in several individuals (34%) with HIV integrations in the *BACH2* gene, indicating that expression of these transcripts could favor the persistence of those cells [205]. Likewise studying the three-dimensional (3D) chromatin structure of integrated proviruses may provide insights into mechanisms influencing the location of integration as well as the 3D interactions between integrated proviruses and host genes.

Finally, elucidating the timing of clonal expansion may provide novel strategies to limit the size of the reservoir in HIV infected individuals. For instance, the extent of clonal expansion prior to the initiation of treatment and the effects of early treatment on the pool of infected, clonally expanded cells is of great interest. Understanding whether antiretroviral treatment permits clonal expansion or rather reveals the infected cell clones that were present prior to and upon treatment initiation is pivotal. Such studies require the development of deeper and more comprehensive integration site mapping techniques and the examination of unique cohorts of individuals identified during acute HIV infection. Characterizing clonal expansion in the setting of immune recovery is needed to determine whether the increase in CD4 cell number over time during therapy is reflected in clonally expanded populations. Gaining a deeper understanding of clonal expansion of HIV infected cells as a mechanism of HIV persistence despite cART will provide needed strategies for reservoir elimination and ultimately HIV eradication.

Abbreviations

cART: combination antiretroviral therapy; PBMC: peripheral blood mononuclear cell; GALT: gut-associated lymphoid tissue; CTL: cytotoxic T lymphocyte; APOBEC: apolipoprotein B mRNA editing enzyme; ddPCR: droplet digital PCR; qVOA: quantitative viral outgrowth assay; BrdU: bromodeoxyuridine; IN: HIV integrase; CA: HIV capsid; RT: reverse transcriptase; LTR: long terminal repeat; PIC: pre-integration complex; ALLINIs: allosteric integrase inhibitors; BAF1: barrier to autointegration factor 1; HMG: high mobility group; LAP2α: lamina-associated polypeptide 2α; TNPO3: karopherin transportin SR2; LEDGF/p75: lens epithelial-derived growth factor; TREC: T cell receptor excision DNA circles; ISLA: integration site loop amplification; ISA: integration site assay; AMBI-1: ambiguous integrant 1; *MKL2*: megakaryoblastic leukemia/myocardin-like protein 2; SRF: serum response factor; *STAT5B*: signal transducer and activator of transcription 5B; *BACH2*: BTB domain and CNC homolog 2.

Authors' contributions
EMA and FM wrote the review. All authors read and approved the final manuscript.

Acknowledgements
Not applicable.

Competing interests
The authors declare they have no competing interests.

Funding
This work was supported by Federal funds from the National Cancer Institute, an NIH Bench to Bedside award (FM), and by funds from the National Cancer Institute under Contract No HSSN261200800001E.

References

1. Palmer S, Maldarelli F, Wiegand A, Bernstein B, Hanna GJ, Brun SC, Kempf DJ, Mellors JW, Coffin JM, King MS. Low-level viremia persists for at least 7 years in patients on suppressive antiretroviral therapy. Proc Natl Acad Sci USA. 2008;105(10):3879–84.
2. Palella FJ Jr, Delaney KM, Moorman AC, Loveless MO, Fuhrer J, Satten GA, Aschman DJ, Holmberg SD. Declining morbidity and mortality among patients with advanced human immunodeficiency virus infection. HIV outpatient study investigators. N Engl J Med. 1998;338(13):853–60.
3. Palella FJ Jr, Baker RK, Moorman AC, Chmiel JS, Wood KC, Brooks JT, Holmberg SD, Investigators HIVOS. Mortality in the highly active antiretroviral therapy era: changing causes of death and disease in the HIV outpatient study. J Acquir Immune Defic Syndr. 2006;43(1):27–34.
4. d'Arminio Monforte A, Sabin CA, Phillips A, Sterne J, May M, Justice A, Dabis F, Grabar S, Ledergerber B, Gill J, Reiss P, Egger M, Antiretroviral Therapy Cohort C. The changing incidence of AIDS events in patients receiving highly active antiretroviral therapy. Arch Intern Med. 2005;165(4):416–23.
5. Mocroft A, Vella S, Benfield TL, Chiesi A, Miller V, Gargalianos P, d'Arminio Monforte A, Yust I, Bruun JN, Phillips AN, Lundgren JD. Changing patterns of mortality across Europe in patients infected with HIV-1. EuroSIDA Study Group. Lancet. 1998;352(9142):1725–30.
6. Antiretroviral Therapy Cohort C. Causes of death in HIV-1-infected patients treated with antiretroviral therapy, 1996-2006: collaborative analysis of 13 HIV cohort studies. Clin Infect Dis. 2010;50(10):1387–96.
7. Weber R, Ruppik M, Rickenbach M, Spoerri A, Furrer H, Battegay M, Cavassini M, Calmy A, Bernasconi E, Schmid P, Flepp M, Kowalska J, Ledergerber B, Swiss HIVCS. Decreasing mortality and changing patterns of causes of death in the Swiss HIV Cohort Study. HIV Med. 2013;14(4):195–207.
8. Wyl V, Gianella S, Fischer M, Niederoest B, Kuster H, Battegay M, Bernasconi E, Cavassini M, Rauch A, Hirschel B, Vernazza P, Weber R, Joos B, Gunthard HF, Swiss HIVCS-S. Early antiretroviral therapy during primary HIV-1 infection results in a transient reduction of the viral setpoint upon treatment interruption. PLoS ONE. 2011;6(11):e27463.
9. Yerly S, Gunthard HF, Fagard C, Joos B, Perneger TV, Hirschel B, Perrin L, Swiss HIVCS. Proviral HIV-DNA predicts viral rebound and viral setpoint after structured treatment interruptions. AIDS. 2004;18(14):1951–3.
10. Davey RT Jr, Bhat N, Yoder C, Chun TW, Metcalf JA, Dewar R, Natarajan V, Lempicki RA, Adelsberger JW, Miller KD, Kovacs JA, Polis MA, Walker RE, Falloon J, Masur H, Gee D, Baseler M, Dimitrov DS, Fauci AS, Lane HC. HIV-1 and T cell dynamics after interruption of highly active antiretroviral therapy (HAART) in patients with a history of sustained viral suppression. Proc Natl Acad Sci USA. 1999;96(26):15109–14.
11. IAS, Deeks SG, Autran B, Berkhout B, Benkirane M, Cairns S, Chomont N, Chun TW, Churchill M, Di Mascio M, Katlama C, Lafeuillade A, Landay A, Lederman M, Lewin SR, Maldarelli F, Margolis D, Markowitz M, Martinez-Picado J, Mullins JI, Mellors J, Moreno S, O'Doherty U, Palmer S, Penicaud MC, Peterlin M, Poli G, Routy JP, Rouzioux C, Silvestri G, Stevenson M, Telenti A, Van Lint C, Verdin E, Woolfrey A, Zaia J, Barre-Sinoussi F. Towards an HIV cure: a global scientific strategy. Nat Rev Immunol. 2012;12(8):607–14.
12. Joos B, Fischer M, Kuster H, Pillai SK, Wong JK, Boni J, Hirschel B, Weber R, Trkola A, Gunthard HF, Swiss HIVCS. HIV rebounds from latently infected cells, rather than from continuing low-level replication. Proc Natl Acad Sci USA. 2008;105(43):16725–30.
13. Serrao E, Ballandras-Colas A, Cherepanov P, Maertens GN, Engelman AN. Key determinants of target DNA recognition by retroviral intasomes. Retrovirology. 2015;12:39.
14. Wu X, Li Y, Crise B, Burgess SM, Munroe DJ. Weak palindromic consensus sequences are a common feature found at the integration target sites of many retroviruses. J Virol. 2005;79(8):5211–4.
15. Shan L, Deng K, Gao H, Xing S, Capoferri AA, Durand CM, Rabi SA, Laird GM, Kim M, Hosmane NN, Yang HC, Zhang H, Margolick JB, Li L, Cai W, Ke R, Flavell RA, Siliciano JD, Siliciano RF. Transcriptional reprogramming during effector-to-memory transition renders CD4(+) T cells permissive for latent HIV-1 infection. Immunity. 2017;47(4):766–75 e3.
16. Zack JA, Kim SG, Vatakis DN. HIV restriction in quiescent CD4(+) T cells. Retrovirology. 2013;10:37.
17. Pace MJ, Graf EH, Agosto LM, Mexas AM, Male F, Brady T, Bushman FD, O'Doherty U. Directly infected resting CD4+ T cells can produce HIV Gag without spreading infection in a model of HIV latency. PLoS Pathog. 2012;8(7):e1002818.
18. Chavez L, Calvanese V, Verdin E. HIV latency is established directly and early in both resting and activated primary CD4 T cells. PLoS Pathog. 2015;11(6):e1004955.
19. Finzi D, Blankson J, Siliciano JD, Margolick JB, Chadwick K, Pierson T, Smith K, Lisziewicz J, Lori F, Flexner C, Quinn TC, Chaisson RE, Rosenberg E, Walker B, Gange S, Gallant J, Siliciano RF. Latent infection of CD4+ T cells provides a mechanism for lifelong persistence of HIV-1, even in patients on effective combination therapy. Nat Med. 1999;5(5):512–7.
20. Chun TW, Engel D, Berrey MM, Shea T, Corey L, Fauci AS. Early establishment of a pool of latently infected, resting CD4(+) T cells during primary HIV-1 infection. Proc Natl Acad Sci USA. 1998;95(15):8869–73.
21. Finzi D, Hermankova M, Pierson T, Carruth LM, Buck C, Chaisson RE, Quinn TC, Chadwick K, Margolick J, Brookmeyer R, Gallant J, Markowitz M, Ho DD, Richman DD, Siliciano RF. Identification of a reservoir for HIV-1 in patients on highly active antiretroviral therapy. Science. 1997;278(5341):1295–300.
22. Wong JK, Hezareh M, Gunthard HF, Havlir DV, Ignacio CC, Spina CA, Richman DD. Recovery of replication-competent HIV despite prolonged suppression of plasma viremia. Science. 1997;278(5341):1291–5.
23. Ho YC, Shan L, Hosmane NN, Wang J, Laskey SB, Rosenbloom DI, Lai J, Blankson JN, Siliciano JD, Siliciano RF. Replication-competent noninduced proviruses in the latent reservoir increase barrier to HIV-1 cure. Cell. 2013;155(3):540–51.
24. Imamichi H, Dewar RL, Adelsberger JW, Rehm CA, O'Doherty U, Paxinos EE, Fauci AS, Lane HC. Defective HIV-1 proviruses produce novel protein-coding RNA species in HIV-infected patients on combination antiretroviral therapy. Proc Natl Acad Sci USA. 2016;113(31):8783–8.
25. Pollack RA, Jones RB, Pertea M, Bruner KM, Martin AR, Thomas AS, Capoferri AA, Beg SA, Huang SH, Karandish S, Hao H, Halper-Stromberg E, Yong PC, Kovacs C, Benko E, Siliciano RF, Ho YC. Defective HIV-1 proviruses are expressed and can be recognized by cytotoxic T lymphocytes, which shape the proviral landscape. Cell Host Microbe. 2017;21(4):494–506 e4.
26. Siliciano JD, Kajdas J, Finzi D, Quinn TC, Chadwick K, Margolick JB, Kovacs C, Gange SJ, Siliciano RF. Long-term follow-up studies confirm the stability of the latent reservoir for HIV-1 in resting CD4+ T cells. Nat Med. 2003;9(6):727–8.
27. Crooks AM, Bateson R, Cope AB, Dahl NP, Griggs MK, Kuruc JD, Gay CL, Eron JJ, Margolis DM, Bosch RJ, Archin NM. Precise quantitation of the

latent HIV-1 reservoir: implications for eradication strategies. J Infect Dis. 2015;212(9):1361–5.

28. Besson GJ, Lalama CM, Bosch RJ, Gandhi RT, Bedison MA, Aga E, Riddler SA, McMahon DK, Hong F, Mellors JW. HIV-1 DNA decay dynamics in blood during more than a decade of suppressive antiretroviral therapy. Clin Infect Dis. 2014;59(9):1312–21.

29. Eriksson S, Graf EH, Dahl V, Strain MC, Yukl SA, Lysenko ES, Bosch RJ, Lai J, Chioma S, Emad F, Abdel-Mohsen M, Hoh R, Hecht F, Hunt P, Somsouk M, Wong J, Johnston R, Siliciano RF, Richman DD, O'Doherty U, Palmer S, Deeks SG, Siliciano JD. Comparative analysis of measures of viral reservoirs in HIV-1 eradication studies. PLoS Pathog. 2013;9(2):e1003174.

30. Murray AJ, Kwon KJ, Farber DL, Siliciano RF. The latent reservoir for HIV-1: how immunologic memory and clonal expansion contribute to HIV-1 persistence. J Immunol. 2016;197(2):407–17.

31. Badley AD, Sainski A, Wightman F, Lewin SR. Altering cell death pathways as an approach to cure HIV infection. Cell Death Dis. 2013;4:e718.

32. Hutter G, Nowak D, Mossner M, Ganepola S, Mussig A, Allers K, Schneider T, Hofmann J, Kucherer C, Blau O, Blau IW, Hofmann WK, Thiel E. Long-term control of HIV by CCR5 Delta32/Delta32 stem-cell transplantation. N Engl J Med. 2009;360(7):692–8.

33. Yukl SA, Boritz E, Busch M, Bentsen C, Chun TW, Douek D, Eisele E, Haase A, Ho YC, Hutter G, Justement JS, Keating S, Lee TH, Li P, Murray D, Palmer S, Pilcher C, Pillai S, Price RW, Rothenberger M, Schacker T, Siliciano J, Siliciano RF, Sinclair E, Strain M, Wong J, Richman D, Deeks SG. Challenges in detecting HIV persistence during potentially curative interventions: a study of the Berlin patient. PLoS Pathog. 2013;9(5):e1003347.

34. Frange P, Faye A, Avettand-Fenoel V, Bellaton E, Descamps D, Angin M, David A, Caillat-Zucman S, Peytavin G, Dollfus C, Le Chenadec J, Warszawski J, Rouzioux C, Saez-Cirion A, Cohort AE-CP, the AEPVsg. HIV-1 virological remission lasting more than 12 years after interruption of early antiretroviral therapy in a perinatally infected teenager enrolled in the French ANRS EPF-CO10 paediatric cohort: a case report. Lancet HIV. 2016;3(1):e49–54.

35. Maggiolo F, Di Filippo E, Comi L, Callegaro A. Post treatment controllers after treatment interruption in chronically HIV infected patients. AIDS. 2018;32(5): 623-28.

36. Saez-Cirion A, Bacchus C, Hocquelou x L, Avettand-Fenoel V, Girault I, Lecroux C, Potard V, Versmisse P, Melard A, Prazuck T, Descours B, Guergnon J, Viard JP, Boufassa F, Lambotte O, Goujard C, Meyer L, Costagliola D, Venet A, Pancino G, Autran B, Rouzioux C, Group AVS. Post-treatment HIV-1 controllers with a long-term virological remission after the interruption of early initiated antiretroviral therapy ANRS VISCONTI Study. PLoS Pathog. 2013;9(3):e1003211.

37. Stohr W, Fidler S, McClure M, Weber J, Cooper D, Ramjee G, Kaleebu P, Tambussi G, Schechter M, Babiker A, Phillips RE, Porter K, Frater J. Duration of HIV-1 viral suppression on cessation of antiretroviral therapy in primary infection correlates with time on therapy. PLoS ONE. 2013;8(10):e78287.

38. Violari A, Cotton M, Kuhn L, Schramm D, Paximadis M, Loubser S, Shalekoff S, de Costa Dias B, Otwombe A, Liberty A, McIntyre J, Babiker A, Gibb D, Tiemessen C. Viral and host characteristics of a child with perinatal HIV-1 following a prolonged period after ART cessation in the CHER trial. In 9th IAS conference on HIV science; Paris, France; 2017.

39. Craigie R, Bushman FD. HIV DNA integration. Cold Spring Harb Perspect Med. 2012;2(7):a006890.

40. Hazuda DJ. HIV integrase as a target for antiretroviral therapy. Curr Opin HIV AIDS. 2012;7(5):383–9.

41. Maldarelli F. HIV-infected cells are frequently clonally expanded after prolonged antiretroviral therapy: implications for HIV persistence. J Virus Erad. 2015;1(4):237–44.

42. Maldarelli F. The role of HIV integration in viral persistence: no more whistling past the proviral graveyard. J Clin Invest. 2016;126(2):438–47.

43. Engelman A, Cherepanov P. Retroviral integrase structure and DNA recombination mechanism. Microbiol Spectr. 2014;2(6):1–22.

44. Wong JK, Yukl SA. Tissue reservoirs of HIV. Curr. Opin HIV AIDS. 2016;11(4):362–70.

45. Perelson AS, Neumann AU, Markowitz M, Leonard JM, Ho DD. HIV-1 dynamics in vivo: virion clearance rate, infected cell life-span, and viral generation time. Science. 1996;271(5255):1582–6.

46. Chun TW, Stuyver L, Mizell SB, Ehler LA, Mican JA, Baseler M, Lloyd AL, Nowak MA, Fauci AS. Presence of an inducible HIV-1 latent reservoir during highly active antiretroviral therapy. Proc Natl Acad Sci USA. 1997;94(24):13193–7.

47. Fritsch RD, Shen X, Sims GP, Hathcock KS, Hodes RJ, Lipsky PE. Stepwise differentiation of CD4 memory T cells defined by expression of CCR7 and CD27. J Immunol. 2005;175(10):6489–97.

48. Sallusto F, Geginat J, Lanzavecchia A. Central memory and effector memory T cell subsets: function, generation, and maintenance. Annu Rev Immunol. 2004;22:745–63.

49. Sallusto F, Lenig D, Forster R, Lipp M, Lanzavecchia A. Two subsets of memory T lymphocytes with distinct homing potentials and effector functions. Nature. 1999;401(6754):708–12.

50. Macallan DC, Wallace D, Zhang Y, De Lara C, Worth AT, Ghattas H, Griffin GE, Beverley PC, Tough DF. Rapid turnover of effector-memory CD4(+) T cells in healthy humans. J Exp Med. 2004;200(2):255–60.

51. Riou C, Yassine-Diab B, Van Grevenynghe J, Somogyi R, Greller LD, Gagnon D, Gimmig S, Wilkinson P, Shi Y, Cameron MJ, Campos-Gonzalez R, Balderas RS, Kelvin D, Sekaly RP, Haddad EK. Convergence of TCR and cytokine signaling leads to FOXO3a phosphorylation and drives the survival of CD4+ central memory T cells. J Exp Med. 2007;204(1):79–91.

52. Gattinoni L, Lugli E, Ji Y, Pos Z, Paulos CM, Quigley MF, Almeida JR, Gostick E, Yu Z, Carpenito C, Wang E, Douek DC, Price DA, June CH, Marincola FM, Roederer M, Restifo NP. A human memory T cell subset with stem cell-like properties. Nat Med. 2011;17(10):1290–7.

53. Tabler CO, Lucera MB, Haqqani AA, McDonald DJ, Migueles SA, Connors M, Tilton JC. CD4+ memory stem cells are infected by HIV-1 in a manner regulated in part by SAMHD1 expression. J Virol. 2014;88(9):4976–86.

54. Buzon MJ, Sun H, Li C, Shaw A, Seiss K, Ouyang Z, Martin-Gayo E, Leng J, Henrich TJ, Li JZ, Pereyra F, Zurakowski R, Walker BD, Rosenberg ES, Yu XG, Lichterfeld M. HIV-1 persistence in CD4+ T cells with stem cell-like properties. Nat Med. 2014;20(2):139–42.

55. Ostrowski MA, Chun TW, Justement SJ, Motola I, Spinelli MA, Adelsberger J, Ehler LA, Mizell SB, Hallahan CW, Fauci AS. Both memory and CD45RA+/CD62L+ naive CD4(+) T cells are infected in human immunodeficiency virus type 1-infected individuals. J Virol. 1999;73(8):6430–5.

56. Sun H, Kim D, Li X, Kiselinova M, Ouyang Z, Vandekerckhove L, Shang H, Rosenberg ES, Yu XG, Lichterfeld M. Th1/17 polarization of CD4 T cells supports HIV-1 persistence during antiretroviral therapy. J Virol. 2015;89(22):11284–93.

57. Perreau M, Savoye AL, De Crignis E, Corpataux JM, Cubas R, Haddad EK, De Leval L, Graziosi C, Pantaleo G. Follicular helper T cells serve as the major CD4 T cell compartment for HIV-1 infection, replication, and production. J Exp Med. 2013;210(1):143–56.

58. Folks TM, Kessler SW, Orenstein JM, Justement JS, Jaffe ES, Fauci AS. Infection and replication of HIV-1 in purified progenitor cells of normal human bone marrow. Science. 1988;242(4880):919–22.

59. Carter CC, Onafuwa-Nuga A, McNamara LA, Riddell JT, Bixby D, Savona MR, Collins KL. HIV-1 infects multipotent progenitor cells causing cell death and establishing latent cellular reservoirs. Nat Med. 2010;16(4):446–51.

60. McNamara LA, Onafuwa-Nuga A, Sebastian NT, Riddell JT, Bixby D, Collins KL. CD133+ hematopoietic progenitor cells harbor HIV genomes in a subset of optimally treated people with long-term viral suppression. J Infect Dis. 2013;207(12):1807–16.

61. Sebastian NT, Zaikos TD, Terry V, Taschuk F, McNamara LA, Onafuwa-Nuga A, Yucha R, Signer RAJ, Riddell JI, Bixby D, Markowitz N, Morrison SJ, Collins KL. CD4 is expressed on a heterogeneous subset of hematopoietic progenitors, which persistently harbor CXCR4 and CCR5-tropic HIV proviral genomes in vivo. PLoS Pathog. 2017;13(7):e1006509.

62. Josefsson L, Eriksson S, Sinclair E, Ho T, Killian M, Epling L, Shao W, Lewis B, Bacchetti P, Loeb L, Custer J, Poole L, Hecht FM, Palmer S. Hematopoietic precursor cells isolated from patients on long-term suppressive HIV therapy did not contain HIV-1 DNA. J Infect Dis. 2012;206(1):28–34.

63. Durand CM, Ghiaur G, Siliciano JD, Rabi SA, Eisele EE, Salgado M, Shan L, Lai JF, Zhang H, Margolick J, Jones RJ, Gallant JE, Ambinder RF, Siliciano RF. HIV-1 DNA is detected in bone marrow populations containing CD4+ T cells but is not found in purified CD34+ hematopoietic progenitor cells in most patients on antiretroviral therapy. J Infect Dis. 2012;205(6):1014–8.

64. Williams KC, Corey S, Westmoreland SV, Pauley D, Knight H, deBakker C, Alvarez X, Lackner AA. Perivascular macrophages are the primary cell type productively infected by simian immunodeficiency virus in the brains of macaques: implications for the neuropathogenesis of AIDS. J Exp Med. 2001;193(8):905–15.

65. Cosenza MA, Zhao ML, Si Q, Lee SC. Human brain parenchymal microglia express CD14 and CD45 and are productively infected by HIV-1 in HIV-1 encephalitis. Brain Pathol. 2002;12(4):442–55.

66. He J, Chen Y, Farzan M, Choe H, Ohagen A, Gartner S, Busciglio J, Yang X, Hofmann W, Newman W, Mackay CR, Sodroski J, Gabuzda D. CCR3 and CCR5 are co-receptors for HIV-1 infection of microglia. Nature. 1997;385(6617):645–9.

67. Schnell G, Spudich S, Harrington P, Price RW, Swanstrom R. Compartmentalized human immunodeficiency virus type 1 originates from long-lived cells in some subjects with HIV-1-associated dementia. PLoS Pathog. 2009;5(4):e1000395.

68. Li GH, Henderson L, Nath A. Astrocytes as an HIV reservoir: mechanism of HIV infection. Curr HIV Res. 2016;14(5):373–81.

69. Canaud G, Dejucq-Rainsford N, Avettand-Fenoel V, Viard JP, Anglicheau D, Bienaime F, Muorah M, Galmiche L, Gribouval O, Noel LH, Satie AP, Martinez F, Sberro-Soussan R, Scemla A, Gubler MC, Friedlander G, Antignac C, Timsit MO, Onetti Muda A, Terzi F, Rouzioux C, Legendre C. The kidney as a reservoir for HIV-1 after renal transplantation. J Am Soc Nephrol. 2014;25(2):407–19.

70. Pinzone MR, O'Doherty U. Measuring integrated HIV DNA ex vivo and in vitro provides insights about how reservoirs are formed and maintained. Retrovirology. 2018;15(1):22.

71. Murray JM, McBride K, Boesecke C, Bailey M, Amin J, Suzuki K, Baker D, Zaunders JJ, Emery S, Cooper DA, Koelsch KK, Kelleher AD, Pint Study T. Integrated HIV DNA accumulates prior to treatment while episomal HIV DNA records ongoing transmission afterwards. AIDS. 2012;26(5):543–50.

72. Pinzone MR, Graf E, Lynch L, McLaughlin B, Hecht FM, Connors M, Migueles SA, Hwang WT, Nunnari G, O'Doherty U. Monitoring integration over time supports a role for cytotoxic T lymphocytes and ongoing replication as determinants of reservoir size. J Virol. 2016;90(23):10436–45.

73. Ananworanich J, Chomont N, Eller LA, Kroon E, Tovanabutra S, Bose M, Nau M, Fletcher JLK, Tipsuk S, Vandergeeten C, O'Connell RJ, Pinyakorn S, Michael N, Phanuphak N, Robb ML, Rv, groups RSs. HIV DNA set point is rapidly established in acute HIV infection and dramatically reduced by early ART. EBioMedicine. 2016;11:68–72.

74. Radebe M, Gounder K, Mokgoro M, Ndhlovu ZM, Mncube Z, Mkhize L, van der Stok M, Jaggernath M, Walker BD, Ndung'u T. Broad and persistent Gag-specific CD8+ T-cell responses are associated with viral control but rarely drive viral escape during primary HIV-1 infection. AIDS. 2015;29(1):23–33.

75. Trautmann L, Mbitikon-Kobo FM, Goulet JP, Peretz Y, Shi Y, Van Grevenynghe J, Procopio FA, Boulassel MR, Routy JP, Chomont N, Haddad EK, Sekaly RP. Profound metabolic, functional, and cytolytic differences characterize HIV-specific CD8 T cells in primary and chronic HIV infection. Blood. 2012;120(17):3466–77.

76. Anderson EM, Hill S, Bell J, Simonetti FR, Rehm C, Jones S, Gorelick R, Coffin J, Maldarelli F. Accumulation and persistence of deleted HIV proviruses following prolonged ART. In: International AIDS society conference on HIV science; Paris, France; 2017.

77. Boritz EA, Darko S, Swaszek L, Wolf G, Wells D, Wu X, Henry AR, Laboune F, Hu J, Ambrozak D, Hughes MS, Hoh R, Casazza JP, Vostal A, Bunis D, Nganou-Makamdop K, Lee JS, Migueles SA, Koup RA, Connors M, Moir S, Schacker T, Maldarelli F, Hughes SH, Deeks SG, Douek DC. Multiple origins of virus persistence during natural control of HIV infection. Cell. 2016;166(4):1004–15.

78. Maldarelli F, Wu X, Su L, Simonetti FR, Shao W, Hill S, Spindler J, Ferris AL, Mellors JW, Kearney MF, Coffin JM, Hughes SH. HIV latency. Specific HIV integration sites are linked to clonal expansion and persistence of infected cells. Science. 2014;345(6193):179–83.

79. Simonetti FR, Sobolewski MD, Fyne E, Shao W, Spindler J, Hattori J, Anderson EM, Watters SA, Hill S, Wu X, Wells D, Su L, Luke BT, Halvas EK, Besson G, Penrose KJ, Yang Z, Kwan RW, Van Waes C, Uldrick T, Citrin DE, Kovacs J, Polis MA, Rehm CA, Gorelick R, Piatak M, Keele BF, Kearney MF, Coffin JM, Hughes SH, Mellors JW, Maldarelli F. Clonally expanded

CD4+ T cells can produce infectious HIV-1 in vivo. Proc Natl Acad Sci USA. 2016;113(7):1883–8.

80. Wagner TA, McLaughlin S, Garg K, Cheung CY, Larsen BB, Styrchak S, Huang HC, Edlefsen PT, Mullins JI, Frenkel LM. HIV latency. Proliferation of cells with HIV integrated into cancer genes contributes to persistent infection. Science. 2014;345(6196):570–3.

81. Llano A, Barretina J, Gutierrez A, Blanco J, Cabrera C, Clotet B, Este JA. Interleukin-7 in plasma correlates with CD4 T-cell depletion and may be associated with emergence of syncytium-inducing variants in human immunodeficiency virus type 1-positive individuals. J Virol. 2001;75(21):10319–25.

82. Napolitano LA, Grant RM, Deeks SG, Schmidt D, De Rosa SC, Herzenberg LA, Herndier BG, Andersson J, McCune JM. Increased production of IL-7 accompanies HIV-1-mediated T-cell depletion: implications for T-cell homeostasis. Nat Med. 2001;7(1):73–9.

83. Fry TJ, Connick E, Falloon J, Lederman MM, Liewehr DJ, Spritzler J, Steinberg SM, Wood LV, Yarchoan R, Zuckerman J, Landay A, Mackall CL. A potential role for interleukin-7 in T-cell homeostasis. Blood. 2001;97(10):2983–90.

84. Srinivasula S, Lempicki RA, Adelsberger JW, Huang CY, Roark J, Lee PI, Rupert A, Stevens R, Sereti I, Lane HC, Di Mascio M, Kovacs JA. Differential effects of HIV viral load and CD4 count on proliferation of naive and memory CD4 and CD8 T lymphocytes. Blood. 2011;118(2):262–70.

85. Catalfamo M, Wilhelm C, Tcheung L, Proschan M, Friesen T, Park JH, Adelsberger J, Baseler M, Maldarelli F, Davey R, Roby G, Rehm C, Lane C. CD4 and CD8 T cell immune activation during chronic HIV infection: roles of homeostasis, HIV, type I IFN, and IL-7. J Immunol. 2011;186(4):2106–16.

86. Sereti I, Dunham RM, Spritzler J, Aga E, Proschan MA, Medvik K, Battaglia CA, Landay AL, Pahwa S, Fischl MA, Asmuth DM, Tenorio AR, Altman JD, Fox L, Moir S, Malaspina A, Morre M, Buffet R, Silvestri G, Lederman MM, Team AS. IL-7 administration drives T cell-cycle entry and expansion in HIV-1 infection. Blood. 2009;113(25):6304–14.

87. Levy Y, Lacabaratz C, Weiss L, Viard JP, Goujard C, Lelievre JD, Boue F, Molina JM, Rouzioux C, Avettand-Fenoel V, Croughs T, Beq S, Thiebaut R, Chene G, Morre M, Delfraissy JF. Enhanced T cell recovery in HIV-1-infected adults through IL-7 treatment. J Clin Invest. 2009;119(4):997–1007.

88. Vandergeeten C, Fromentin R, DaFonseca S, Lawani MB, Sereti I, Lederman MM, Ramgopal M, Routy JP, Sekaly RP, Chomont N. Interleukin-7 promotes HIV persistence during antiretroviral therapy. Blood. 2013;121(21):4321–9.

89. Bosque A, Famiglietti M, Weyrich AS, Goulston C, Planelles V. Homeostatic proliferation fails to efficiently reactivate HIV-1 latently infected central memory CD4+ T cells. PLoS Pathog. 2011;7(10):e1002288.

90. Boyman O, Sprent J. The role of interleukin-2 during homeostasis and activation of the immune system. Nat Rev Immunol. 2012;12(3):180–90.

91. Douek DC, Brenchley JM, Betts MR, Ambrozak DR, Hill BJ, Okamoto Y, Casazza JP, Kuruppu J, Kunstman K, Wolinsky S, Grossman Z, Dybul M, Oxenius A, Price DA, Connors M, Koup RA. HIV preferentially infects HIV-specific CD4+ T cells. Nature. 2002;417(6884):95–8.

92. Doitsh G, Cavrois M, Lassen KG, Zepeda O, Yang Z, Santiago ML, Hebbeler AM, Greene WC. Abortive HIV infection mediates CD4 T cell depletion and inflammation in human lymphoid tissue. Cell. 2010;143(5):789–801.

93. Doitsh G, Galloway NL, Geng X, Yang Z, Monroe KM, Zepeda O, Hunt PW, Hatano H, Sowinski S, Munoz-Arias I, Greene WC. Cell death by pyroptosis drives CD4 T-cell depletion in HIV-1 infection. Nature. 2014;505(7484):509–14.

94. Hill AL. Mathematical Models of HIV Latency. Curr. Topics Microbiol. Immunol. 2018;417:131–56.

95. Wang S, Hottz P, Schechter M, Rong L. Modeling the slow CD4+ T cell decline in HIV-infected individuals. PLoS Comput Biol. 2015;11(12):e1004665.

96. Klatt NR, Chomont N, Douek DC, Deeks SG. Immune activation and HIV persistence: implications for curative approaches to HIV infection. Immunol Rev. 2013;254(1):326–42.

97. Mazzuca P, Caruso A, Caccuri F. HIV-1 infection, microenvironment and endothelial cell dysfunction. New Microbiol. 2016;39(3):163–73.

98. Wang Z, Simonetti FR, Siliciano RF, Laird GM. Measuring replication competent HIV-1: advances and challenges in defining the latent reservoir. Retrovirology. 2018;15(1):21.

99. Rouzioux C, Melard A, Avettand-Fenoel V. Quantification of total HIV1-DNA in peripheral blood mononuclear cells. Methods Mol Biol. 2014;1087:261–70.

100. Chun TW, Murray D, Justement JS, Hallahan CW, Moir S, Kovacs C, Fauci AS. Relationship between residual plasma viremia and the size of HIV proviral DNA reservoirs in infected individuals receiving effective antiretroviral therapy. J Infect Dis. 2011;204(1):135–8.

101. Soriano-Sarabia N, Bateson RE, Dahl NP, Crooks AM, Kuruc JD, Margolis DM, Archin NM. Quantitation of replication-competent HIV-1 in populations of resting CD4+ T cells. J Virol. 2014;88(24):14070–7.

102. Chun TW, Nickle DC, Justement JS, Meyers JH, Roby G, Hallahan CW, Kottilil S, Moir S, Mican JM, Mullins JI, Ward DJ, Kovacs JA, Mannon PJ, Fauci AS. Persistence of HIV in gut-associated lymphoid tissue despite long-term antiretroviral therapy. J Infect Dis. 2008;197(5):714–20.

103. Hatano H, Somsouk M, Sinclair E, Harvill K, Gilman L, Cohen M, Hoh R, Hunt PW, Martin JN, Wong JK, Deeks SG, Yukl SA. Comparison of HIV DNA and RNA in gut-associated lymphoid tissue of HIV-infected controllers and noncontrollers. AIDS. 2013;27(14):2255–60.

104. Rutsaert S, Bosman K, Trypsteen W, Nijhuis M, Vandekerckhove L. Digital PCR as a tool to measure HIV persistence. Retrovirology. 2018;15(1):16.

105. Busby E, Whale AS, Ferns RB, Grant PR, Morley G, Campbell J, Foy CA, Nastouli E, Huggett JF, Garson JA. Instability of 8E5 calibration standard revealed by digital PCR risks inaccurate quantification of HIV DNA in clinical samples by qPCR. Sci Rep. 2017;7(1):1209.

106. Strain MC, Lada SM, Luong T, Rought SE, Gianella S, Terry VH, Spina CA, Woelk CH, Richman DD. Highly precise measurement of HIV DNA by droplet digital PCR. PLoS ONE. 2013;8(4):e55943.

107. Henrich TJ, Gallien S, Li JZ, Pereyra F, Kuritzkes DR. Low-level detection and quantitation of cellular HIV-1 DNA and 2-LTR circles using droplet digital PCR. J Virol Methods. 2012;186(1–2):68–72.

108. Kiselinova M, Pasternak AO, De Spiegelaere W, Vogelaers D, Berkhout B, Vandekerckhove L. Comparison of droplet digital PCR and seminested real-time PCR for quantification of cell-associated HIV-1 RNA. PLoS ONE. 2014;9(1):e85999.

109. Dunay GA, Solomatina A, Kummer S, Hufner A, Bialek JK, Eberhard JM, Tolosa E, Hauber J, Schulze Zur Wiesch J. Assessment of the HIV-1 reservoir in CD4+ regulatory T cells by a droplet digital PCR based approach. Virus Res. 2017;240:107–11.

110. de Oliveira MF, Gianella S, Letendre S, Scheffler K, Kosakovsky Pond SL, Smith DM, Strain M, Ellis RJ. Comparative analysis of cell-associated HIV DNA levels in cerebrospinal fluid and peripheral blood by droplet digital PCR. PLoS ONE. 2015;10(10):e0139510.

111. Bruner KM, Murray AJ, Pollack RA, Soliman MG, Laskey SB, Capoferri AA, Lai J, Strain MC, Lada SM, Hoh R, Ho YC, Richman DD, Deeks SG, Siliciano JD, Siliciano RF. Defective proviruses rapidly accumulate during acute HIV-1 infection. Nat Med. 2016;22(9):1043–9.

112. Avettand-Fenoel V, Hocqueloux L, Ghosn J, Cheret A, Frange P, Melard A, Viard JP, Rouzioux C. Total HIV-1 DNA, a marker of viral reservoir dynamics with clinical implications. Clin Microbiol Rev. 2016;29(4):859–80.

113. Williams JP, Hurst J, Stohr W, Robinson N, Brown H, Fisher M, Kinloch S, Cooper D, Schechter M, Tambussi G, Fidler S, Carrington M, Babiker A, Weber J, Koelsch KK, Kelleher AD, Phillips RE, Frater J, Investigators SP. HIV-1 DNA predicts disease progression and post-treatment virological control. Elife. 2014;3:e03821.

114. Kiselinova M, De Spiegelaere W, Buzon MJ, Malatinkova E, Lichterfeld M, Vandekerckhove L. Integrated and total HIV-1 DNA predict ex vivo viral outgrowth. PLoS Pathog. 2016;12(3):e1005472.

115. Bruner KM, Pollack RA, Murray AJ, Soliman MG, Laskey SB, Strain M, Richman D, Deeks S, Siliciano J, Siliciano R. Rapid accumulation of defective proviruses complicates HIV-1 reservoir measurements. In: 25th conference on retroviruses and opportunistic infections, Boston, MA; 2018.

116. Gratzner HG. Monoclonal antibody to 5-bromo- and 5-iododeoxyuridine: a new reagent for detection of DNA replication. Science. 1982;218(4571):474–5.

117. Kovacs JA, Lempicki RA, Sidorov IA, Adelsberger JW, Herpin B, Metcalf JA, Sereti I, Polis MA, Davey RT, Tavel J, Falloon J, Stevens R, Lambert L, Dewar R, Schwartzentruber DJ, Anver MR, Baseler MW, Masur H, Dimitrov DS, Lane HC. Identification of dynamically distinct subpopulations of T lymphocytes that are differentially affected by HIV. J Exp Med. 2001;194(12):1731–41.

118. Hellerstein MK, Hoh RA, Hanley MB, Cesar D, Lee D, Neese RA, McCune JM. Subpopulations of long-lived and short-lived T cells in advanced HIV-1 infection. J Clin Invest. 2003;112(6):956–66.

119. Golumbeanu M, Cristinelli S, Rato S, Munoz M, Cavassini M, Beerenwinkel N, Ciuffi A. Single-cell RNA-Seq reveals transcriptional heterogeneity in latent and reactivated HIV-infected cells. Cell Rep. 2018;23(4):942–50.

120. Ciuffi A, Rato S, Telenti A. Single-cell genomics for virology. Viruses 2016;8(5):pii:e123.

121. Kok YL, Ciuffi A, Metzner KJ. Unravelling HIV-1 latency, one cell at a time. Trends Microbiol. 2017;25(11):932–41.

122. Phetsouphanh C, Zaunders JJ, Kelleher AD. Detecting antigen-specific T cell responses: from bulk populations to single cells. Int J Mol Sci. 2015;16(8):18878–93.

123. Molony RD, Malawista A, Montgomery RR. Reduced dynamic range of antiviral innate immune responses in aging. Exp Gerontol. 2017;107:130-35.

124. Nikolich-Zugich J. The twilight of immunity: emerging concepts in aging of the immune system. Nat Immunol. 2018;19(1):10–9.

125. Pallikkuth S, de Armas L, Rinaldi S, Pahwa S. T follicular helper cells and B cell dysfunction in aging and HIV-1 infection. Front Immunol. 2017;8:1380.

126. Hu WS, Hughes SH. HIV-1 reverse transcription. Cold Spring Harb Perspect Med. 2012;2(10):pii:a006882.

127. Dyda F, Hickman AB, Jenkins TM, Engelman A, Craigie R, Davies DR. Crystal structure of the catalytic domain of HIV-1 integrase: similarity to other polynucleotidyl transferases. Science. 1994;266(5193):1981–6.

128. Jenkins TM, Hickman AB, Dyda F, Ghirlando R, Davies DR, Craigie R. Catalytic domain of human immunodeficiency virus type 1 integrase: identification of a soluble mutant by systematic replacement of hydrophobic residues. Proc Natl Acad Sci USA. 1995;92(13):6057–61.

129. Miller MD, Bor YC, Bushman F. Target DNA capture by HIV-1 integration complexes. Curr Biol. 1995;5(9):1047–56.

130. Hare S, Gupta SS, Valkov E, Engelman A, Cherepanov P. Retroviral intasome assembly and inhibition of DNA strand transfer. Nature. 2010;464(7286):232–6.

131. Valkov E, Gupta SS, Hare S, Helander A, Roversi P, McClure M, Cherepanov P. Functional and structural characterization of the integrase from the prototype foamy virus. Nucleic Acids Res. 2009;37(1):243–55.

132. Hare S, Di Nunzio F, Labeja A, Wang J, Engelman A, Cherepanov P. Structural basis for functional tetramerization of lentiviral integrase. PLoS Pathog. 2009;5(7):e1000515.

133. Li X, Krishnan L, Cherepanov P, Engelman A. Structural biology of retroviral DNA integration. Virology. 2011;411(2):194–205.

134. Cherepanov P, Maertens GN, Hare S. Structural insights into the retroviral DNA integration apparatus. Curr Opin Struct Biol. 2011;21(2):249–56.

135. Engelman AN, Cherepanov P. Retroviral intasomes arising. Curr Opin Struct Biol. 2017;47:23–9.

136. Feng L, Larue RC, Slaughter A, Kessl JJ, Kvaratskhelia M. HIV-1 integrase multimerization as a therapeutic target. Curr Top Microbiol Immunol. 2015;389:93–119.

137. Jurado KA, Wang H, Slaughter A, Feng L, Kessl JJ, Koh Y, Wang W, Ballandras-Colas A, Patel PA, Fuchs JR, Kvaratskhelia M, Engelman A. Allosteric integrase inhibitor potency is determined through the inhibition of HIV-1 particle maturation. Proc Natl Acad Sci USA. 2013;110(21):8690–5.

138. Balakrishnan M, Yant SR, Tsai L, O'Sullivan C, Bam RA, Tsai A, Niedziela-Majka A, Stray KM, Sakowicz R, Cihlar T. Non-catalytic site HIV-1 integrase inhibitors disrupt core maturation and induce a reverse transcription block in target cells. PLoS ONE. 2013;8(9):e74163.

139. Fontana J, Jurado KA, Cheng N, Ly NL, Fuchs JR, Gorelick RJ, Engelman AN, Steven AC. Distribution and redistribution of HIV-1 nucleocapsid protein in immature, mature, and integrase-inhibited virions: a role for integrase in maturation. J Virol. 2015;89(19):9765–80.

140. Madison MK, Lawson DQ, Elliott J, Ozanturk AN, Koneru PC, Townsend D, Errando M, Kvaratskhelia M, Kutluay SB. Allosteric HIV-1 integrase inhibitors lead to premature degradation of the viral RNA genome and integrase in target cells. J Virol. 2017;91(17):pii:e00821–17.

141. Ballandras-Colas A, Maskell DP, Serrao E, Locke J, Swuec P, Jonsson SR, Kotecha A, Cook NJ, Pye VE, Taylor IA, Andresdottir V, Engelman AN,

Costa A, Cherepanov P. A supramolecular assembly mediates lentiviral DNA integration. Science. 2017;355(6320):93–5.

142. Lesbats P, Engelman AN, Cherepanov P. Retroviral DNA Integration. Chem Rev. 2016;116(20):12730–57.

143. Ciuffi A, Bushman FD. Retroviral DNA integration: HIV and the role of LEDGF/p75. Trends Genet. 2006;22(7):388–95.

144. Craigie R, Bushman FD. Host factors in retroviral integration and the selection of integration target Sites. Microbiol Spectr. 2014. https://doi.org/10.1128/microbiolspec.MDNA3-0026-2014.

145. Debyser Z, Christ F, De Rijck J, Gijsbers R. Host factors for retroviral integration site selection. Trends Biochem Sci. 2015;40(2):108–16.

146. Demeulemeester J, De Rijck J, Gijsbers R, Debyser Z. Retroviral integration: site matters: mechanisms and consequences of retroviral integration site selection. BioEssays. 2015;37(11):1202–14.

147. Engelman A. The roles of cellular factors in retroviral integration. Curr Top Microbiol Immunol. 2003;281:209–38.

148. Suzuki Y, Craigie R. The road to chromatin—nuclear entry of retroviruses. Nat Rev Microbiol. 2007;5(3):187–96.

149. Tsirkone VG, Blokken J, De Wit F, Breemans J, De Houwer S, Debyser Z, Christ F, Strelkov SV. N-terminal half of transportin SR2 interacts with HIV integrase. J Biol Chem. 2017;292(23):9699–710.

150. Burdick RC, Hu WS, Pathak VK. Nuclear import of APOBEC3Fla-beled HIV-1 preintegration complexes. Proc Natl Acad Sci USA. 2013;110(49):E4780–9.

151. Luo X, Yang W, Gao G. SUN1 regulates HIV-1 nuclear import in a manner dependent on the interaction between the viral capsid and cellular cyclophilin A. J Virol. 2018;92(13):pi:e00229–18.

152. Blokken J, De Rijck J, Christ F, Debyser Z. Protein–protein and protein–chromatin interactions of LEDGF/p75 as novel drug targets. Drug Discov Today Technol. 2017;24:25–31.

153. Demeulemeester J, Blokken J, De Houwer S, Dirix L, Klaassen H, Marchand A, Chaltin P, Christ F, Debyser Z. Inhibitors of the integrase-transportin-SR2 interaction block HIV nuclear import. Retrovirology. 2018;15(1):5.

154. Desimmie BA, Schrijvers R, Demeulemeester J, Borrenberghs D, Weydert C, Thys W, Vets S, Van Remoortel B, Hofkens J, De Rijck J, Hendrix J, Bannert N, Gijsbers R, Christ F, Debyser Z. LEDGINs inhibit late stage HIV-1 replication by modulating integrase multimerization in the virions. Retrovirology. 2013;10:57.

155. Francis AC, Melikyan GB. Single HIV-1 imaging reveals progression of infection through CA-dependent steps of docking at the nuclear pore, uncoating, and nuclear transport. Cell Host Microbe. 2018;23(4):536–48 e6.

156. Schroder AR, Shinn P, Chen H, Berry C, Ecker JR, Bushman F. HIV-1 integration in the human genome favors active genes and local hotspots. Cell. 2002;110(4):521–9.

157. Kvaratskhelia M, Sharma A, Larue RC, Serrao E, Engelman A. Molecular mechanisms of retroviral integration site selection. Nucleic Acids Res. 2014;42(16):10209–25.

158. Ciuffi A. The benefits of integration. Clin Microbiol Infect. 2016;22(4):324–32.

159. Ciuffi A, Llano M, Poeschla E, Hoffmann C, Leipzig J, Shinn P, Ecker JR, Bushman F. A role for LEDGF/p75 in targeting HIV DNA integration. Nat Med. 2005;11(12):1287–9.

160. Cherepanov P, Ambrosio AL, Rahman S, Ellenberger T, Engelman A. Structural basis for the recognition between HIV-1 integrase and transcriptional coactivator p75. Proc Natl Acad Sci USA. 2005;102(48):17308–13.

161. Turlure F, Maertens G, Rahman S, Cherepanov P, Engelman A. A tripartite DNA-binding element, comprised of the nuclear localization signal and two AT-hook motifs, mediates the association of LEDGF/p75 with chromatin in vivo. Nucleic Acids Res. 2006;34(5):1653–65.

162. Ferris AL, Wu X, Hughes CM, Stewart C, Smith SJ, Milne TA, Wang GG, Shun MC, Allis CD, Engelman A, Hughes SH. Lens epithelium-derived growth factor fusion proteins redirect HIV-1 DNA integration. Proc Natl Acad Sci USA. 2010;107(7):3135–40.

163. Krull S, Dorries J, Boysen B, Reidenbach S, Magnius L, Norder H, Thyberg J, Cordes VC. Protein Tpr is required for establishing nuclear pore-associated zones of heterochromatin exclusion. EMBO J. 2010;29(10):1659–73.

164. Lelek M, Casartelli N, Pellin D, Rizzi E, Souque P, Severgnini M, Di Serio C, Fricke T, Diaz-Griffero F, Zimmer C, Charneau P, Di Nunzio F. Chromatin

organization at the nuclear pore favours HIV replication. Nat Commun. 2015;6:6483.

165. Marini B, Kertesz-Farkas A, Ali H, Lucic B, Lisek K, Manganaro L, Pongor S, Luzzati R, Recchia A, Mavilio F, Giacca M, Lusic M. Nuclear architecture dictates HIV-1 integration site selection. Nature. 2015;521(7551):227–31.

166. Stultz RD, Cenker JJ, McDonald D. Imaging HIV-1 genomic DNA from entry through productive infection. J Virol. 2017;91(9):pii:e00034–17.

167. Di Primio C, Quercioli V, Allouch A, Gijsbers R, Christ F, Debyser Z, Arosio D, Cereseto A. Single-cell imaging of HIV-1 provirus (SCIP). Proc Natl Acad Sci USA. 2013;110(14):5636–41.

168. Ma Y, Wang M, Li W, Zhang Z, Zhang X, Tan T, Zhang XE, Cui Z. Live cell imaging of single genomic loci with quantum dot-labeled TALEs. Nat Commun. 2017;8:15318.

169. Sardo L, Lin A, Khakhina S, Beckman L, Ricon L, Elbezanti W, Jaison T, Vishwasrao H, Shroff H, Janetopoulos C, Klase ZA. Real-time visualization of chromatin modification in isolated nuclei. J Cell Sci. 2017;130(17):2926–40.

170. Burdick RC, Delviks-Frankenberry KA, Chen J, Janaka SK, Sastri J, Hu WS, Pathak VK. Dynamics and regulation of nuclear import and nuclear movements of HIV-1 complexes. PLoS Pathog. 2017;13(8):e1006570.

171. Wong RW, Mamede JI, Hope TJ. Impact of nucleoporin-mediated chromatin localization and nuclear architecture on HIV integration site selection. J Virol. 2015;89(19):9702–5.

172. Puray-Chavez M, Tedbury PR, Huber AD, Ukah OB, Yapo V, Liu D, Ji J, Wolf JJ, Engelman AN, Sarafianos SG. Multiplex single-cell visualization of nucleic acids and protein during HIV infection. Nat Commun. 2017;8(1):1882.

173. Farnet CM, Haseltine WA. Circularization of human immunodeficiency virus type 1 DNA in vitro. J Virol. 1991;65(12):6942–52.

174. Pauza CD, Trivedi P, McKechnie TS, Richman DD, Graziano FM. 2-LTR circular viral DNA as a marker for human immunodeficiency virus type 1 infection in vivo. Virology. 1994;205(2):470–8.

175. Sharkey ME, Teo I, Greenough T, Sharova N, Luzuriaga K, Sullivan JL, Bucy RP, Kostrikis LG, Haase A, Veryard C, Davaro RE, Cheeseman SH, Daly JS, Bova C, Ellison RT 3rd, Mady B, Lai KK, Moyle G, Nelson M, Gazzard B, Shaunak S, Stevenson M. Persistence of episomal HIV-1 infection intermediates in patients on highly active anti-retroviral therapy. Nat Med. 2000;6(1):76–81.

176. Pierson TC, Kieffer TL, Ruff CT, Buck C, Gange SJ, Siliciano RF. Intrinsic stability of episomal circles formed during human immunodeficiency virus type 1 replication. J Virol. 2002;76(8):4138–44.

177. Koelsch KK, Liu L, Haubrich R, May S, Havlir D, Gunthard HF, Ignacio CC, Campos-Soto P, Little SJ, Shafer R, Robbins GK, D'Aquila RT, Kawano Y, Young K, Dao P, Spina CA, Richman DD, Wong JK. Dynamics of total, linear nonintegrated, and integrated HIV-1 DNA in vivo and in vitro. J Infect Dis. 2008;197(3):411–9.

178. Pace MJ, Graf EH, O'Doherty U. HIV 2-long terminal repeat circular DNA is stable in primary CD4+ T Cells. Virology. 2013;441(1):18–21.

179. Drylewicz J, Vrisekoop N, Mugwagwa T, de Boer AB, Otto SA, Hazenberg MD, Tesselaar K, de Boer RJ, Borghans JA. Reconciling longitudinal naive T-cell and TREC dynamics during HIV-1 infection. PLoS ONE. 2016;11(3):e0152513.

180. Mack KD, Jin X, Yu S, Wei R, Kapp L, Green C, Herndier B, Abbey NW, Elbaggari A, Liu Y, McGrath MS. HIV insertions within and proximal to host cell genes are a common finding in tissues containing high levels of HIV DNA and macrophage-associated p24 antigen expression. J Acquir Immune Defic Syndr. 2003;33(3):308–20.

181. Ikeda T, Shibata J, Yoshimura K, Koito A, Matsushita S. Recurrent HIV-1 integration at the BACH2 locus in resting CD4+ T cell populations during effective highly active antiretroviral therapy. J Infect Dis. 2007;195(5):716–25.

182. Han Y, Lassen K, Monie D, Sedaghat AR, Shimoji S, Liu X, Pierson TC, Margolick JB, Siliciano RF, Siliciano JD. Resting CD4+ T cells from human immunodeficiency virus type 1 (HIV-1)-infected individuals carry integrated HIV-1 genomes within actively transcribed host genes. J Virol. 2004;78(12):6122–33.

183. Sasaki S, Ito E, Toki T, Maekawa T, Kanezaki R, Umenai T, Muto A, Nagai H, Kinoshita T, Yamamoto M, Inazawa J, Taketo MM, Nakahata T, Igarashi K, Yokoyama M. Cloning and expression of human B cell-specific transcription factor BACH2 mapped to chromosome 6q15. Oncogene. 2000;19(33):3739–49.

184. Meekings KN, Leipzig J, Bushman FD, Taylor GP, Bangham CR. HTLV-1 integration into transcriptionally active genomic regions is associated with proviral expression and with HAM/TSP. PLoS Pathog. 2008;4(3):e1000027.

185. Gillet NA, Malani N, Melamed A, Gormley N, Carter R, Bentley D, Berry C, Bushman FD, Taylor GP, Bangham CR. The host genomic environment of the provirus determines the abundance of HTLV-1-infected T-cell clones. Blood. 2011;117(11):3113–22.

186. Berry CC, Gillet NA, Melamed A, Gormley N, Bangham CR, Bushman FD. Estimating abundances of retroviral insertion sites from DNA fragment length data. Bioinformatics. 2012;28(6):755–62.

187. Melamed A, Witkover AD, Laydon DJ, Brown R, Ladell K, Miners K, Rowan AG, Gormley N, Price DA, Taylor GP, Murphy EL, Bangham CR. Clonality of HTLV-2 in natural infection. PLoS Pathog. 2014;10(3):e1004006.

188. De Ravin SS, Su L, Theobald N, Choi U, Macpherson JL, Poidinger M, Symonds G, Pond SM, Ferris AL, Hughes SH, Malech HL, Wu X. Enhancers are major targets for murine leukemia virus vector integration. J Virol. 2014;88(8):4504–13.

189. Muehlich S, Hampl V, Khalid S, Singer S, Frank N, Breuhahn K, Gudermann T, Prywes R. The transcriptional coactivators megakaryoblastic leukemia 1/2 mediate the effects of loss of the tumor suppressor deleted in liver cancer 1. Oncogene. 2012;31(35):3913–23.

190. Selvaraj A, Prywes R. Megakaryoblastic leukemia-1/2, a transcriptional co-activator of serum response factor, is required for skeletal myogenic differentiation. J Biol Chem. 2003;278(43):41977–87.

191. Huang D, Sumegi J, Dal Cin P, Reith JD, Yasuda T, Nelson M, Muirhead D, Bridge JA. C11orf95-MKL2 is the resulting fusion oncogene of t(11;16)(q13;p13) in chondroid lipoma. Genes Chromosomes Cancer. 2010;49(9):810–8.

192. Siegfried A, Romary C, Escudie F, Nicaise Y, Grand D, Rochaix P, Barres B, Vergez S, Chevreau C, Coindre JM, Uro-Coste E, Le Guellec S. RREB1-MKL2 fusion in biphenotypic "oropharyngeal" sarcoma: New entity or part of the spectrum of biphenotypic sinonasal sarcomas? Genes Chromosomes Cancer. 2017.

193. O'Sullivan NC, Pickering M, Di Giacomo D, Loscher JS, Murphy KJ. Mkl transcription cofactors regulate structural plasticity in hippocampal neurons. Cereb Cortex. 2010;20(8):1915–25.

194. Parmacek MS. Myocardin-related transcription factors: critical coactivators regulating cardiovascular development and adaptation. Circ Res. 2007;100(5):633–44.

195. Cen B, Selvaraj A, Prywes R. Myocardin/MKL family of SRF coactivators: key regulators of immediate early and muscle specific gene expression. J Cell Biochem. 2004;93(1):74–82.

196. Igarashi K, Ochiai K, Itoh-Nakadai A, Muto A. Orchestration of plasma cell differentiation by Bach2 and its gene regulatory network. Immunol Rev. 2014;261(1):116–25.

197. Muto A, Hoshino H, Madisen L, Yanai N, Obinata M, Karasuyama H, Hayashi N, Nakauchi H, Yamamoto M, Groudine M, Igarashi K. Identification of Bach2 as a B-cell-specific partner for small maf proteins that negatively regulate the immunoglobulin heavy chain gene 3′ enhancer. EMBO J. 1998;17(19):5734–43.

198. Merup M, Moreno TC, Heyman M, Ronnberg K, Grander D, Detlofsson R, Rasool O, Liu Y, Soderhall S, Juliusson G, Gahrton G, Einhorn S. 6q deletions in acute lymphoblastic leukemia and non-Hodgkin's lymphomas. Blood. 1998;91(9):3397–400.

199. Swaminathan S, Huang C, Geng H, Chen Z, Harvey R, Kang H, Ng C, Titz B, Hurtz C, Sadiyah MF, Nowak D, Thoennissen GB, Rand V, Graeber TG, Koeffler HP, Carroll WL, Willman CL, Hall AG, Igarashi K, Melnick A, Muschen M. BACH2 mediates negative selection and p53-dependent tumor suppression at the pre-B cell receptor checkpoint. Nat Med. 2013;19(8):1014–22.

200. Kobayashi S, Taki T, Chinen Y, Tsutsumi Y, Ohshiro M, Kobayashi T, Matsumoto Y, Kuroda J, Horiike S, Nishida K, Taniwaki M. Identification of IGHCdelta-BACH2 fusion transcripts resulting from cryptic chromosomal rearrangements of 14q32 with 6q15 in aggressive B-cell lymphoma/leukemia. Genes Chromosomes Cancer. 2011;50(4):207–16.

201. Roychoudhuri R, Hirahara K, Mousavi K, Clever D, Klebanoff CA, Bonelli M, Sciume G, Zare H, Vahedi G, Dema B, Yu Z, Liu H, Takahashi H, Rao M, Muranski P, Crompton JG, Punkosdy G, Bedognetti D, Wang E, Hoffmann V, Rivera J, Marincola FM, Nakamura A, Sartorelli V, Kanno Y,

Gattinoni L, Muto A, Igarashi K, O'Shea JJ, Restifo NP. BACH2 represses effector programs to stabilize T(reg)-mediated immune homeostasis. Nature. 2013;498(7455):506–10.

202. Tsukumo S, Unno M, Muto A, Takeuchi A, Kometani K, Kurosaki T, Igarashi K, Saito T. Bach2 maintains T cells in a naive state by suppressing effector memory-related genes. Proc Natl Acad Sci USA. 2013;110(26):10735–40.

203. Hu G, Chen J. A genome-wide regulatory network identifies key transcription factors for memory CD8(+) T-cell development. Nat Commun. 2013;4:2830.

204. Richer MJ, Lang ML, Butler NS. T cell fates zipped up: how the Bach2 basic leucine zipper transcriptional repressor directs T cell differentiation and function. J Immunol. 2016;197(4):1009–15.

205. Cesana D, Santoni de Sio FR, Rudilosso L, Gallina P, Calabria A, Beretta S, Merelli I, Bruzzesi E, Passerini L, Nozza S, Vicenzi E, Poli G, Gregori S, Tambussi G, Montini E. HIV-1-mediated insertional activation of STAT5B and BACH2 trigger viral reservoir in T regulatory cells. Nat Commun. 2017;8(1):498.

206. Biggar RJ, Engels EA, Frisch M, Goedert JJ, Group ACMRS. Risk of T-cell lymphomas in persons with AIDS. J Acquir Immune Defic Syndr. 2001;26(4):371–6.

207. Gilardin L, Copie-Bergman C, Galicier L, Meignin V, Briere J, Timsit JF, Bouchaud O, Gaulard P, Oksenhendler E, Gerard L. Peripheral T-cell lymphoma in HIV-infected patients: a study of 17 cases in the combination antiretroviral therapy era. Br J Haematol. 2013;161(6):843–51.

208. Cohn LB, Silva IT, Oliveira TY, Rosales RA, Parrish EH, Learn GH, Hahn BH, Czartoski JL, McElrath MJ, Lehmann C, Klein F, Caskey M, Walker BD, Siliciano JD, Siliciano RF, Jankovic M, Nussenzweig MC. HIV-1 integration landscape during latent and active infection. Cell. 2015;160(3):420–32.

209. Bangham CRM, Human T. Cell leukemia virus type 1: persistence and pathogenesis. Annu Rev Immunol. 2018;36:43–71.

210. Shao W, Shan J, Kearney MF, Wu X, Maldarelli F, Mellors JW, Luke B, Coffin JM, Hughes SH. Retrovirus integration database (RID): a public database for retroviral insertion sites into host genomes. Retrovirology. 2016;13(1):47.

211. Kearney MF, Spindler J, Shao W, Yu S, Anderson EM, O'Shea A, Rehm C, Poethke C, Kovacs N, Mellors JW, Coffin JM, Maldarelli F. Lack of detectable HIV-1 molecular evolution during suppressive antiretroviral therapy. PLoS Pathog. 2014;10(3):e1004010.

212. Bailey JR, Sedaghat AR, Kieffer T, Brennan T, Lee PK, Wind-Rotolo M, Haggerty CM, Kamireddi AR, Liu Y, Lee J, Persaud D, Gallant JE, Cofrancesco J Jr, Quinn TC, Wilke CO, Ray SC, Siliciano JD, Nettles RE, Siliciano RF. Residual human immunodeficiency virus type 1 viremia in some patients on antiretroviral therapy is dominated by a small number of invariant clones rarely found in circulating CD4+ T cells. J Virol. 2006;80(13):6441–57.

213. Josefsson L, von Stockenstrom S, Faria NR, Sinclair E, Bacchetti P, Killian M, Epling L, Tan A, Ho T, Lemey P, Shao W, Hunt PW, Somsouk M, Wylie W, Douek DC, Loeb L, Custer J, Hoh R, Poole L, Deeks SG, Hecht F, Palmer S. The HIV-1 reservoir in eight patients on long-term suppressive antiretroviral therapy is stable with few genetic changes over time. Proc Natl Acad Sci USA. 2013;110(51):E4987–96.

214. Rong L, Perelson AS. Modeling latently infected cell activation: viral and latent reservoir persistence, and viral blips in HIV-infected patients on potent therapy. PLoS Comput Biol. 2009;5(10):e1000533.

215. Bradley LM, Haynes L, Swain SL. IL-7: maintaining T-cell memory and achieving homeostasis. Trends Immunol. 2005;26(3):172–6.

216. Chetoui N, Boisvert M, Gendron S, Aoudjit F. Interleukin-7 promotes the survival of human CD4+ effector/memory T cells by up-regulating Bcl-2 proteins and activating the JAK/STAT signalling pathway. Immunology. 2010;130(3):418–26.

217. Chomont N, El-Far M, Ancuta P, Trautmann L, Procopio FA, Yassine-Diab B, Boucher G, Boulassel MR, Ghattas G, Brenchley JM, Schacker TW, Hill BJ, Douek DC, Routy JP, Haddad EK, Sekaly RP. HIV reservoir size and persistence are driven by T cell survival and homeostatic proliferation. Nat Med. 2009;15(8):893–900.

218. Goh WC, Rogel ME, Kinsey CM, Michael SF, Fultz PN, Nowak MA, Hahn BH, Emerman M. HIV-1 Vpr increases viral expression by manipulation of the cell cycle: a mechanism for selection of Vpr in vivo. Nat Med. 1998;4(1):65–71.

219. Musick A, Spindler J, Keele BF, Bale MJ, Shao W, Wiegand A, Mellors J, Coffin J, Maldarelli F, Kearney M. A smalle fraction of proviruses in expanded clones express unspliced HIV RNA in vivo. In: Conference on retroviruses and opportunistic infections; Seattle, WA; 2017.

220. Kearney MF, Wiegand A, Shao W, Coffin JM, Mellors JW, Lederman M, Gandhi RT, Keele BF, Li JZ. Origin of rebound plasma HIV includes cells with identical proviruses that are transcriptionally active before stopping of antiretroviral therapy. J Virol. 2016;90(3):1369–76.

221. Lorenzi JC, Cohen YZ, Cohn LB, Kreider EF, Barton JP, Learn GH, Oliveira T, Lavine CL, Horwitz JA, Settler A, Jankovic M, Seaman MS, Chakraborty AK, Hahn BH, Caskey M, Nussenzweig MC. Paired quantitative and qualitative assessment of the replication-competent HIV-1 reservoir and comparison with integrated proviral DNA. Proc Natl Acad Sci USA. 2016;113(49):E7908–16.

222. Hosmane NN, Kwon KJ, Bruner KM, Capoferri AA, Beg S, Rosenbloom DI, Keele BF, Ho YC, Siliciano JD, Siliciano RF. Proliferation of latently infected CD4(+) T cells carrying replication-competent HIV-1: potential role in latent reservoir dynamics. J Exp Med. 2017;214(4):959–72.

223. Bui JK, Sobolewski MD, Keele BF, Spindler J, Musick A, Wiegand A, Luke BT, Shao W, Hughes SH, Coffin JM, Kearney MF, Mellors JW. Proviruses with identical sequences comprise a large fraction of the replication-competent HIV reservoir. PLoS Pathog. 2017;13(3):e1006283.

224. Wang Z, Gurule EE, Brennan TP, Gerold JM, Kwon KJ, Hosmane NN, Kumar MR, Beg SA, Capoferri AA, Ray SC, Ho YC, Hill AL, Siliciano JD, Siliciano RF. Expanded cellular clones carrying replication-competent HIV-1 persist, wax, and wane. Proc Natl Acad Sci USA. 2018;115(11):E2575–84.

225. Prins JM, Jurriaans S, van Praag RM, Blaak H, van Rij R, Schellekens PT, ten Berge IJ, Yong SL, Fox CH, Roos MT, de Wolf F, Goudsmit J, Schuitemaker H, Lange JM. Immuno-activation with anti-CD3 and recombinant human IL-2 in HIV-1-infected patients on potent antiretroviral therapy. AIDS. 1999;13(17):2405–10.

226. Kulkosky J, Nunnari G, Otero M, Calarota S, Dornadula G, Zhang H, Malin A, Sullivan J, Xu Y, DeSimone J, Babinchak T, Stern J, Cavert W, Haase A, Pomerantz RJ. Intensification and stimulation therapy for human immunodeficiency virus type 1 reservoirs in infected persons receiving virally suppressive highly active antiretroviral therapy. J Infect Dis. 2002;186(10):1403–11.

227. Bashiri K, Rezaei N, Nasi M, Cossarizza A. The role of latency reversal agents in the cure of HIV: a review of current data. Immunol Lett. 2018;196:135–9.

228. Shan L, Deng K, Shroff NS, Durand CM, Rabi SA, Yang HC, Zhang H, Margolick JB, Blankson JN, Siliciano RF. Stimulation of HIV-1-specific cytolytic T lymphocytes facilitates elimination of latent viral reservoir after virus reactivation. Immunity. 2012;36(3):491–501.

229. Wiegand A, Spindler J, Hong FF, Shao W, Ciktor J, Cillo AR, Halvas EK, Coffin JM, Mellors JW, Kearney MF. Single-cell analysis of HIV-1 transcriptional activity reveals expression of proviruses in expanded clones during ART. Proc. Natl. Acad. Sci. USA. 2017;114(18):E3659–68.

230. Laskey SB, Pohlmeyer CW, Bruner KM, Siliciano RF. Evaluating clonal expansion of HIV-infected cells: optimization of PCR strategies to predict clonality. PLoS Pathog. 2016;12(8):e1005689.

231. Cesana D, Sgualdino J, Rudilosso L, Merella S, Naldini L, Montini E. Whole transcriptome characterization of aberrant splicing events induced by lentiviral vector integrations. J Clin Invest. 2012;122(5):1667–76.

232. Moiani A, Paleari Y, Sartori D, Mezzadra R, Miccio A, Cattoglio C, Cocchiarella F, Lidonnici MR, Ferrari G, Mavilio F. Lentiviral vector integration in the human genome induces alternative splicing and generates aberrant transcripts. J Clin Invest. 2012;122(5):1653–66.

233. Sherrill-Mix S, Ocwieja KE, Bushman FD. Gene activity in primary T cells infected with HIV89.6: intron retention and induction of genomic repeats. Retrovirology. 2015;12:79.

234. Rothe M, Modlich U, Schambach A. Biosafety challenges for use of lentiviral vectors in gene therapy. Curr Gene Ther. 2013;13(6):453–68.

10

Efficacies of Cabotegravir and Bictegravir against drug-resistant HIV-1 integrase mutants

Steven J. Smith[1], Xue Zhi Zhao[2], Terrence R. Burke Jr.[2] and Stephen H. Hughes[1*]

Abstract

Background: Integrase strand transfer inhibitors (INSTIs) are the class of antiretroviral (ARV) drugs most recently approved by the FDA for the treatment of HIV-1 infections. INSTIs block the strand transfer reaction catalyzed by HIV-1 integrase (IN) and have been shown to potently inhibit infection by wild-type HIV-1. Of the three current FDA-approved INSTIs, Dolutegravir (DTG), has been the most effective, in part because treatment does not readily select for resistant mutants. However, recent studies showed that when INSTI-experienced patients are put on a DTG-salvage therapy, they have reduced response rates. Two new INSTIs, Cabotegravir (CAB) and Bictegravir (BIC), are currently in late-stage clinical trials.

Results: Both CAB and BIC had much broader antiviral profiles than RAL and EVG against the INSTI-resistant single, double, and triple HIV-1 mutants used in this study. BIC was more effective than DTG against several INSTI-resistant mutants. Overall, in terms of their ability to inhibit a broad range of INSTI-resistant IN mutants, BIC was superior to DTG, and DTG was superior to CAB. Modeling the binding of CAB, BIC, and DTG within the active site of IN suggested that the "left side" of the INSTI pharmacophore (the side away from the viral DNA) was important in determining the ability of the compound to inhibit the IN mutants we tested.

Conclusions: Of the two INSTIs in late stage clinical trials, BIC appears to be better able to inhibit the replication of a broad range of IN mutants. BIC retained potency against several of the INSTI-resistant mutants that caused a decrease in susceptibility to DTG.

Keywords: HIV-1, Integrase, Infectivity, Potency, Susceptibility, Modeling, Resistance

Background

INSTIs are the class of antiretroviral (ARV) drugs most recently approved by the FDA to treat HIV-1 infections. INSTIs target the second reaction performed by HIV-1 Integrase (IN), strand transfer (ST), in which IN catalyzes the integration of the viral DNA into the cellular genome [1, 2]. INSTIs have a centralized pharmacophore, which contains a chelating functionality that interacts with the two catalytic Mg^{2+} ions at the IN active site [3, 4]. This central pharmacophore is joined to a halogenated benzyl moiety that interacts with the penultimate base at the 3′ end of the viral DNA [5]. Thus, INSTIs interact with both the enzyme and its nucleic acid substrate. The

combination of these interactions allows the INSTIs to target and potently inhibit HIV-1 IN. Raltegravir (RAL) and Elvitegravir (EVG) are the first and second FDA-approved INSTIs, respectively. They potently inhibit WT HIV-1; however, resistant mutants can develop relatively quickly (Fig. 1). A partial list of the well-defined primary resistance mutations includes: Y143R, N155H, G140S/Q148H, T66I, and E92Q. Other mutations that confer resistance to RAL and EVG have been identified. In many cases, mutations selected by either RAL or EVG reduce the susceptibility of IN to the other INSTI, showing that RAL and EVG have overlapping resistance profiles [6–8].

In 2013, Dolutegravir (DTG) was approved by the FDA and it quickly became a preferred drug for combination antiretroviral therapy (cART) [9–12]. DTG differs from the first generation INSTIs in that its chelating motif is located on a tri-cyclic scaffold [13, 14]. In addition, the structural component that connects the central chelating

*Correspondence: hughesst@mail.nih.gov
[1] HIV Dynamics and Replication Program, National Cancer Institute-Frederick, National Institutes of Health, Frederick, MD, USA
Full list of author information is available at the end of the article

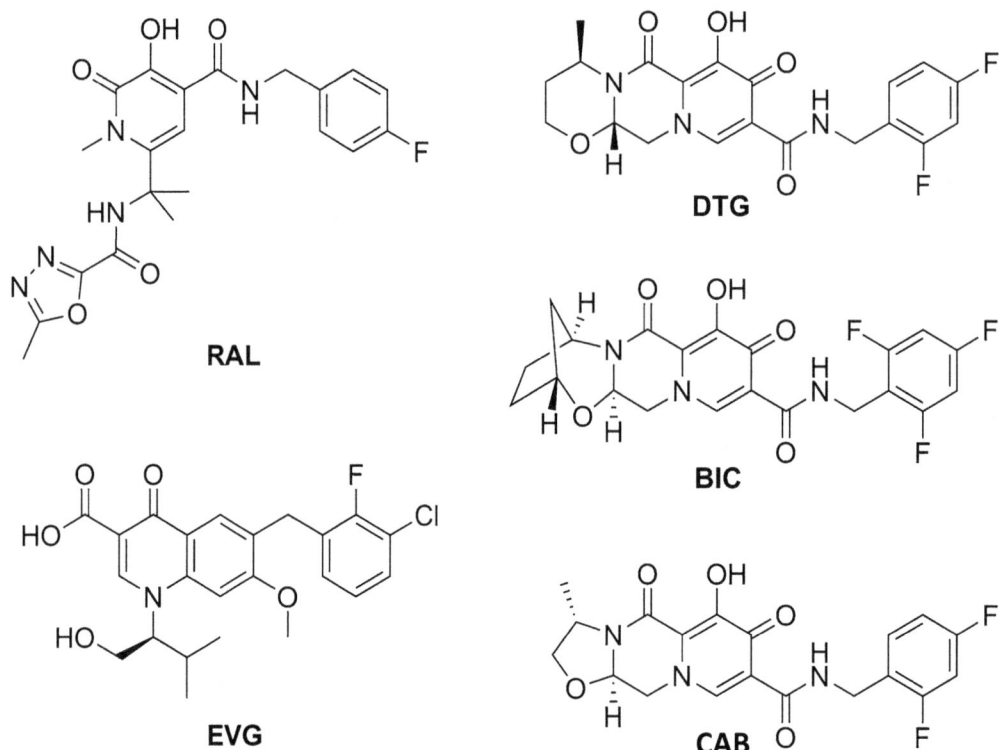

Fig. 1 Chemical structures of INSTIs. The chemical structures of RAL, EVG, DTG, BIC, and CAB are shown

moiety to the halogenated benzyl group is longer than it is in either RAL or EVG (Fig. 1) [15]. Not only do these structural differences allow DTG to be highly effective against WT HIV-1, but DTG is much more potent against IN mutants that confer resistance to the first generation INSTIs. Moreover, it has been difficult to select for DTG resistant mutants in cell culture and the treatment of HIV-1 patients using DTG has been, generally speaking, quite successful [16–21].

The usefulness of most ARV drugs is limited by the emergence of resistant mutants, and DTG will not be an exception. Recent in vitro selection studies with DTG have uncovered resistance mutations [22–24]. In clinical trials with INSTI-experienced subjects [25, 26] whose viruses had INSTI resistance mutations at the primary position Q148 plus at least one additional mutation at any of the secondary positions, L74, E138, G140, or G163, patients were put on a salvage regimen that included DTG. This change in therapy failed to lower HIV-1 below 50 copies/mL. Analysis of the virus present in the patients after the trial showed that additional mutations were selected in IN. These results showed that mutations that confer resistance to DTG can be selected in viruses that carry preexisting resistance mutations.

Recently, two new INSTIs, Cabotegravir (CAB) and Bictegravir (BIC), have been developed and these are

currently in late phase clinical trials [13, 27, 28]. BIC and CAB, which are structurally similar to DTG, (both have tri-cyclic central pharmacophores), could offer therapeutic alternatives to HIV-1 patients (Fig. 1). Here, we describe evaluation of the antiviral potency of CAB and BIC against broad panels of well-characterized INSTI-resistant single and double mutants, and against the INSTI-resistant triple mutants identified in the VIKING clinical trials. Our objective was to determine how well these new INSTIs performed compared to DTG, the current standard of care.

Results

Initial screening of CAB and BIC against primary INSTI resistant mutants

The abilities of CAB and BIC to inhibit the replication of WT HIV-1 and INSTI-resistant mutants were determined in single-round viral replication assays. We initially screened CAB and BIC against a panel of primary INSTI-resistant mutants, which included: Y143R, N155H, G140S/Q148H, T66I, E92Q, H51Y, G118R, R263K, H51Y/R263K, and E138K/E263K. Y143R, N155H, and G140S/Q148H (Fig. 2; see also Additional file 1: Table S1A) were chosen because they have been selected in patients by treatment with RAL [29–31]; the T66I and E92Q mutants were selected by treatment with EVG

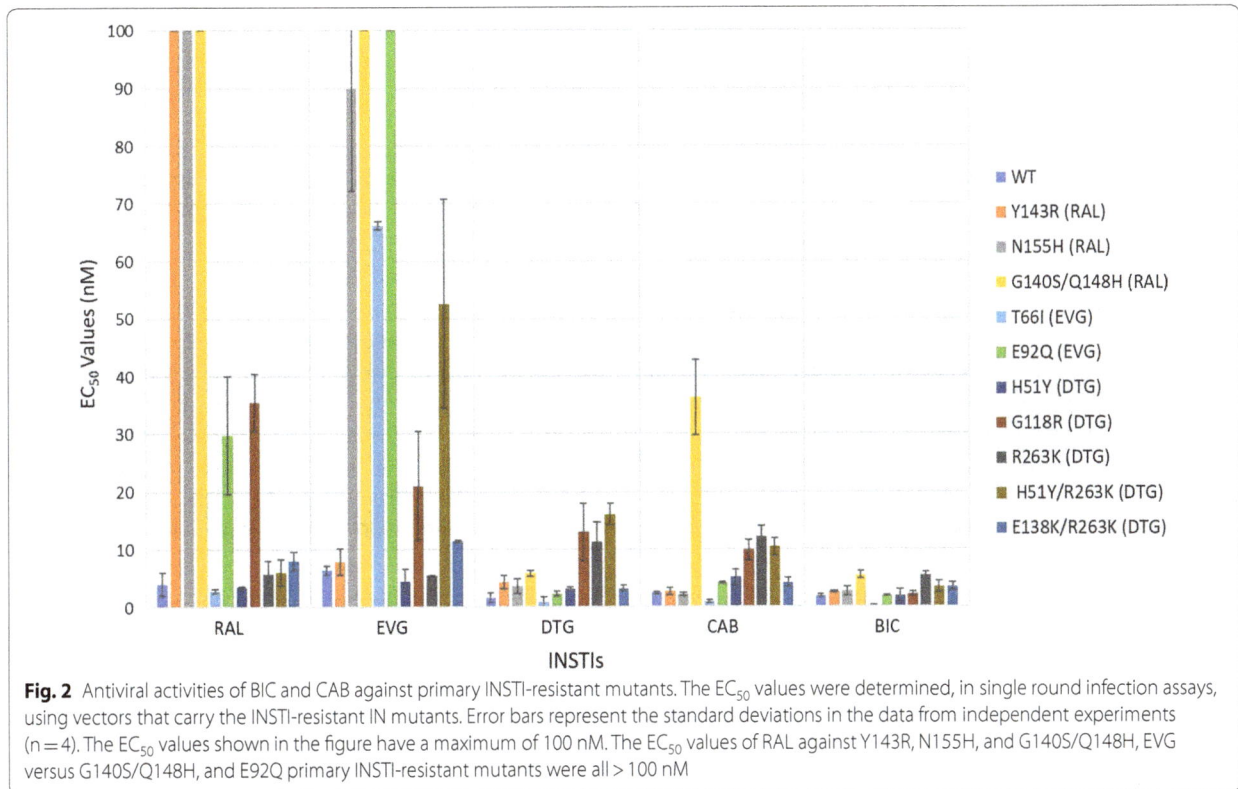

Fig. 2 Antiviral activities of BIC and CAB against primary INSTI-resistant mutants. The EC$_{50}$ values were determined, in single round infection assays, using vectors that carry the INSTI-resistant IN mutants. Error bars represent the standard deviations in the data from independent experiments (n = 4). The EC$_{50}$ values shown in the figure have a maximum of 100 nM. The EC$_{50}$ values of RAL against Y143R, N155H, and G140S/Q148H, EVG versus G140S/Q148H, and E92Q primary INSTI-resistant mutants were all > 100 nM

[32–34]. The IN mutations H51Y, G118R, R263K, H51Y/R263K, E138K/R263K mutants have been selected with DTG in cell culture [22–24]. The R263K mutation has been selected in several treatment-experienced, INSTI-naïve patients undergoing DTG therapy [16]. Both CAB and BIC potently inhibited the infection of WT HIV-1 with EC$_{50}$ values equivalent to the FDA-approved INSTIs (< 3 nM). Moreover, CAB and BIC were minimally toxic in cell culture assays with CC$_{50}$ values > 250 μM (data not shown), which is similar to the FDA-approved INSTIs. This demonstrates that these INSTIs have very favorable therapeutic indexes in cultured cells. Additionally, both CAB and BIC potently inhibited the RAL-resistant mutants Y143R and N155H; the EVG-resistant IN mutants T66I and E92Q, and the DTG-resistant IN mutant H51Y and E138K/R263K with EC$_{50}$ values < 5 nM. However, only BIC potently inhibited the well-known RAL-resistant IN double mutant G140S/Q148H and the DTG-resistant IN mutants G118R, R263K, and H51Y/R263K with EC$_{50}$ values ≤ 5 nM. The RAL-resistant IN mutant G140S/Q148H caused a substantial loss of CAB potency (36.3 ± 6.5 nM), while there was a smaller but still modest loss of potency against the DTG-resistant IN mutants G118R (12.1 ± 1.9 nM), R263K (13.4 ± 1.3 nM), and H51Y/R263K (10.4 ± 1.5 nM). These antiviral data were compared to previous screens, in which the antiviral

potencies of RAL, EVG, and DTG were measured against the same INSTI-resistant primary mutants [35, 36]. When the antiviral profiles of the second generation INSTIs, DTG, CAB and BIC were compared to the FDA-approved INSTIs for WT HIV-1 and the RAL- and EVG-resistant mutants, all of the second generation INSTIs had antiviral profiles that were obviously superior to RAL and EVG. The differences were sufficiently clear cut that the comparisons between the first and second generation INSTIs were not subjected to statistical analysis. The more important question was whether either CAB or BIC was better than DTG, in terms of their ability to inhibit the IN mutants. To make the comparison objective, the statistical significance of the EC$_{50}$ data for CAB, BIC, and DTG were analyzed using the Student's t test. The EC$_{50}$ values for WT HIV for DTG, CAB and BIC were similar, which allowed us to compare the EC$_{50}$ values for the mutants directly. In the initial screen, which included ten INSTI-resistant primary mutants, BIC was significantly better than CAB for seven of these ten primary mutants (four p values < 0.01 and three p values < 0.001; see Fig. 3 and Additional file 1: Table S1B). In addition, BIC was better than DTG against three of the primary mutants. In contrast, CAB was significantly better than DTG for one primary mutant and DTG was better than CAB for three of the primary mutants.

Antiviral activities of CAB and BIC against other common INSTI-resistant single mutants

We determined the antiviral profiles of CAB and BIC, as well as the FDA-approved INSTIs, against a second panel of additional INSTI-resistant single mutants to compare the strengths and weaknesses of the two new INSTIs and the FDA-approved INSTIs [37–39]. This panel of INSTI-resistant single mutants included: M50I, L74M, T97A, S119R, E138K, G140S, Q146L, Q146P, Q148H, Q148K, Q148R, and S153Y (Fig. 4; Additional file 1: Table S2A). BIC potently inhibited this entire panel of INSTI-resistant mutants with EC_{50} values below 5 nM, which was comparable to DTG. CAB also inhibited the majority of mutants in this panel. However, it lost some potency against the INSTI-resistant single mutants E138K (12.9 ± 1.0 nM), Q146P (10.3 ± 2.1 nM), and Q148H (6.8 ± 1.5 nM). Most of the INSTI-resistant single mutants in this panel caused significant drops in susceptibility to the first generation INSTIs, RAL and EVG, with the Q148H/K/R mutants having the greatest effect on the EC_{50} values. Based on the data obtained with the mutants in this panel, DTG was better than CAB and BIC (Fig. 3; Additional file 1: Table S2B). DTG was significantly better than CAB against six of the mutants and better than BIC against four mutants (two p values < 0.001). Conversely, BIC was better than CAB against five of these mutants.

Antiviral activities of CAB and BIC against a panel of INSTI-resistant double mutants having a primary mutation at position Q148

We next tested CAB, BIC, and the FDA-approved INSTIs against a panel of INSTI-resistant double mutants that included either one of the primary mutations at position Q148 (H/K/R), or Y143R or N155H. These primary mutations were combined with a secondary mutation at positions E138 (A/K) or G140 (A/C/S) (Fig. 5; Additional file 1: Table S3A). BIC potently inhibited ($EC_{50} < 5$ nM) the INSTI-resistant double mutants G140A/Q148H, Y143R/Q148H, Q148H/N155H, G140S/Q148K, E138A/Q148R, E138K/Q148R, and Q148R/N155H. Conversely, the INSTI-resistant double mutants G140A/Q148R (10 ± 2.5 nM), G140C/Q148R (6.4 ± 1.4 nM), G140S/Q148R (6.1 ± 1.3 nM) caused small losses in susceptibility to BIC, whereas the double mutants E138K/Q148K (59.3 ± 4.9 nM) and G140A/Q148K (137.1 ± 5.0 nM) resulted in substantial reductions in susceptibility to BIC.

However, there was a large reduction in CAB potency against most of the double mutants in the panel. The double mutants Y143R/Q148H (6.0 ± 0.4 nM), E138A/Q148R (25.6 ± 0.8 nM), E138K/Q148R (24.1 ± 0.1 nM), and G140A/Q148R (13.7 ± 2.7 nM) caused a minimal loss in susceptibility to CAB, whereas E138K/Q148K (772.1 ± 72.2 nM), G140A/Q148K (393.1 ± 51.1 nM), G140S/Q148K (87.3 ± 7.6 nM), G140C/Q148R (66.6 ± 8.1 nM), and Q148R/N155H (50.5 ± 6.5 nM) caused large reductions in susceptibility to CAB. DTG was very effective across this panel of INSTI-resistant double mutants. However, it sustained a moderate loss in potency against the INSTI-resistant double mutant E138K/Q148K (25.0 ± 2.1 nM) and significant loss in potency against the INSTI-resistant double mutant G140A/Q148K (450.7 ± 58.8 nM). The first generation INSTIs RAL and EVG exhibited considerable loss of potency against all of the mutants in this panel of INSTI-resistant double mutants. BIC was significantly better than DTG against five of these double mutants (four p values < 0.01; Fig. 3; Additional file 1: Table S3B); however, DTG was better than BIC for four of the mutants (two p values < 0.001). CAB was not significantly better than either DTG or BIC against any double mutants.

Antiviral activities of CAB and BIC against a panel of INSTI-resistant double mutants that included the primary mutations T66I and N155H and additional mutations at other positions

We determined the antiviral profiles of CAB, BIC, and the FDA-approved INSTIs against the EVG-resistant double mutant T66I/E157Q and a panel of INSTI-resistant double mutants with a primary mutation at N155H and one of the following secondary mutations: E92Q, G140S, Y143H/R, or G163R (Fig. 6; Additional file 1: Table S4A). BIC, CAB, and DTG retained potency against the INSTI-resistant double mutant T66I/E157Q and the other INSTI-resistant double mutants ($EC_{50} < 5$ nM). The first generation INSTIs, RAL and EVG, failed to potently inhibit any of these double mutants. Based on this panel of mutants, the antiviral profiles of the three second generation INSTIs were similar to each other. CAB was significantly better than BIC against two of these double mutants (one p value < 0.001; see Figs. 3 and 7 and Additional file 1: Table S4B). DTG had better activity against one of the double mutants than CAB and BIC (p value < 0.01).

(See figure on next page.)
Fig. 3 Statistical significance of the antiviral data among DTG, CAB, and BIC. The Student's t test was used to calculate the statistical significance of the differences in the antiviral activities of the INSTIs. Because of multiple comparisons, p values < 0.025 were considered statistically significant when comparing the efficacies among DTG, CAB, and BIC

Figure and Supplementary Table	p-Value < 0.025	p-Value < 0.01	p-Value < 0.001	Overall Comparison among INSTIs for Table	
Figure 2 Antiviral Data and Supplementary Table 1	BIC - DTG (R263K)	DTG – CAB (G140S/Q148H)	BIC - CAB (E92Q)	BIC > CAB	7
		BIC – CAB (G140S/Q148H)	BIC - CAB (R263K)	BIC > DTG	3
		BIC – CAB (T66I)	BIC - DTG (H51Y/R263K)	DTG > CAB	3
		DTG – CAB (E92Q)	BIC - CAB (H51Y/R263K)	DTG > BIC	0
		DTG – CAB (H51Y)		CAB > BIC	0
		BIC - DTG (H51Y)		CAB > DTG	1
		BIC - CAB (H51Y)			
		BIC - CAB (G118R)			
		CAB - DTG (H51Y/R263K)			
Figure 3 Antiviral Data and Supplementary Table 2	DTG - CAB (Q148R)	CAB - DTG (L74M)	CAB – BIC (M50I)	BIC > CAB	5
		DTG – CAB (T97A)	DTG – CAB (E138K)	BIC > DTG	0
		DTG – BIC (Q146L)	DTG – BIC (E138K)	DTG > CAB	6
		DTG – CAB (Q146P)	BIC - CAB (E138K)	DTG > BIC	4
		BIC - CAB (Q146P)	DTG – BIC (Q146P)	CAB > BIC	1
		DTG – CAB (Q148H)		CAB > DTG	1
		DTG – BIC (Q148H)			
		BIC - CAB (Q148H)			
		DTG - CAB (Q148K)			
		BIC - CAB (Q148K)			
		BIC - CAB (Q148R)			
Figure 4 Antiviral Data and Supplementary Table 3	BIC - DTG (Y143R/Q148H)	BIC - DTG (G140A/Q148H)	DTG – CAB (Y143R/Q148H)	BIC > CAB	11
	DTG – BIC (G140A/Q148R)	BIC - CAB (G140A/Q148H)	BIC - CAB (Y143R/Q148H)	BIC > DTG	5
		DTG - CAB (Q148H/N155H)	DTG – CAB (E138K/Q148K)	DTG > CAB	10
		BIC - CAB (Q148H/N155H)	DTG – BIC (E138K/Q148K)	DTG > BIC	4
		BIC - DTG (G140A/Q148K)	BIC - CAB (E138K/Q148K)	CAB > BIC	0
		BIC - CAB (G140A/Q148K)	DTG – CAB (G140S/Q148K)	CAB > DTG	0
		DTG – CAB (G140A/Q148R)	DTG – BIC (G140S/Q148K)		
		DTG – BIC (G140C/Q148R)	BIC - CAB (G140S/Q148K)		
		BIC - DTG (G140S/Q148R)	DTG - CAB (E138A/Q148R)		
		BIC - DTG (Q148R/N155H)	BIC - CAB (E138A/Q148R)		
			DTG - CAB (E138K/Q148R)		
			BIC - CAB (E138K/Q148R)		
			DTG - CAB (G140C/Q148R)		
			BIC - CAB (G140C/Q148R)		
			DTG - CAB (G140S/Q148R)		
			BIC - CAB (G140S/Q148R)		
			DTG - CAB (Q148R/N155H)		
			BIC - CAB (Q148R/N155H)		
Figure 5 Antiviral Data and Supplementary Table 4		DTG – BIC (T66I/E157Q)	CAB – BIC (T66I/E157Q)	BIC > CAB	1
		DTG - CAB (G140S/N155H)	BIC - CAB (G140S/N155H)	BIC > DTG	0
		CAB – BIC (Y143H/N155H)		DTG > CAB	1
				DTG > BIC	1
				CAB > BIC	2
				CAB > DTG	0
Figure 6 Antiviral Data and Supplementary Table 5	BIC - DTG (E138A/S147G/Q148R)	DTG - CAB (L74M/G140A/Q148R)	DTG - CAB (T97A/Y143R/Q148H)	BIC > CAB	6
		BIC - CAB (L74M/G140A/Q148R)	BIC - CAB (T97A/Y143R/Q148H)	BIC > DTG	2
		DTG - CAB (L74M/G140C/Q148R)	DTG - CAB (E138K/G140A/Q148K)	DTG > CAB	5
		BIC - DTG (L74M/G140C/Q148R)	BIC - CAB (E138K/G140A/Q148K)	DTG > BIC	1
		BIC - CAB (L74M/G140C/Q148R)	DTG - CAB (E138K/G140C/Q148R)	CAB > BIC	0
		DTG - BIC (E138K/G140C/Q148R)	BIC - CAB (E138K/G140C/Q148R)	CAB > DTG	0
			BIC - CAB (E138A/S147G/Q148R)		
Figure 7 Antiviral Data and Supplementary Table 6	BIC - CAB (T66I/T97A/E157Q)	DTG - CAB (T66I/T97A/E157Q)	DTG - CAB (T97A/Y143R/N155H)	BIC > CAB	3
		DTG - CAB (G140S/Y143R/N155H)	BIC - CAB (T97A/Y143R/N155H)	BIC > DTG	1
		BIC - CAB (G140S/Y143R/N155H)		DTG > CAB	3
		BIC - DTG (E92Q/N155H/G163R)		DTG > BIC	0
				CAB > BIC	0
				CAB > DTG	0
Figure 8 Antiviral Data and Supplementary Table 7		CAB - DTG (T97A/G140S/Q148H)	BIC - DTG (T97A/G140S/Q148H)	BIC > CAB	6
		BIC - CAB (T97A/G140S/Q148H)	DTG - CAB (E138A/G140S/Q148H)	BIC > DTG	3
		DTG - CAB (E138K/G140S/Q148H)	BIC - CAB (E138A/G140S/Q148H)	DTG > CAB	5
		DTG - CAB (G140S/Y143R/Q148H)	BIC - DTG (E138K/G140S/Q148H)	DTG > BIC	0
		BIC - CAB (G140S/Y143R/Q148H)	BIC- CAB (E138K/G140S/Q148H)	CAB > BIC	0
		DTG - CAB (G140S/Q148H/N155H)	BIC - DTG (G140S/Q148H/G163K)	CAB > DTG	1
		BIC - CAB (G140S/Q148H/N155H)	BIC -CAB (G140S/Q148H/G163K)		
		DTG - CAB (G140S/Q148H/G163K)			

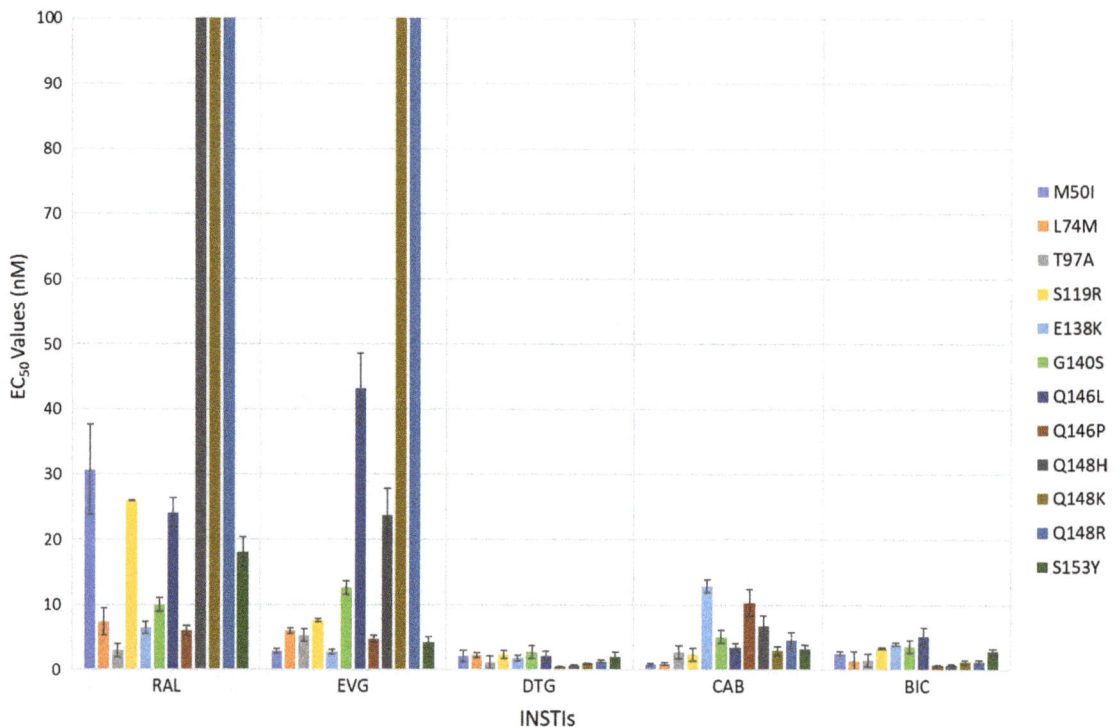

Fig. 4 Antiviral activities of BIC and CAB against common INSTI-resistant single mutants. The EC$_{50}$ values were determined using vectors that carry the INSTI-resistant IN double mutants in single round infection assays. Error bars represent the standard deviations in the data from independent experiments (n = 4). The EC$_{50}$ values shown in the figure have a maximum of 100 nM. The EC$_{50}$ values of RAL against Q148H, Q148K, and Q148R and EVG versus Q148K and Q148R INSTI-resistant mutants were all > 100 nM

Antiviral activities of CAB and BIC against a panel INSTI-resistant triple mutants that included a primary mutation (Q148H/K/R) and two additional mutations

We determined the antiviral activities of CAB, BIC, and the FDA-approved INSTIs against a panel of INSTI-resistant triple mutants that included a primary mutation at Q148 (H/K/R) with two additional mutations at primary or secondary positions. The panel of INSTI-resistant triple mutants included: T97A/Y143R/Q148H, T97A/Q148H/N155H, E138K/G140A/Q148K, L74M/G140A/Q148R, L74M/G140C/Q148R, E138K/G140C/Q148R, and E138A/S147G/Q148R (Fig. 8; Additional file 1: Table S5A). Overall, DTG and BIC showed similar antiviral profiles against these triple mutants, and in some cases, CAB also retained potency. DTG, BIC, and CAB potently inhibited (EC$_{50}$s ≤ 5 nM) the T97A/Y143R/Q148H and E138A/S147G/Q148R INSTI-resistant triple mutants. The E138K/G140C/Q148R INSTI-resistant mutant caused only a small loss of potency to DTG (5.3 ± 1.0 nM) and BIC (8.2 ± 1.1 nM). This mutant showed a significant reduction in susceptibility to CAB (134.2 ± 0.3 nM). The L74M/G140C/Q148R triple mutant was moderately susceptible to

BIC (6.1 ± 0.9 nM) and DTG (10.2 ± 1.3 nM). However, this mutant caused a massive loss in susceptibility to CAB (220.3 ± 41.2 nM). The L74M/G140A/Q148R triple mutant with a different mutation at position G140, caused a modest loss of susceptibility to both DTG (12.0 ± 2.1 nM) and BIC (11.7 ± 1.3 nM); however, this also caused a substantial loss in susceptibility to CAB (53.2 ± 14.8 nM). Finally, DTG, BIC, and CAB failed to retain potency against the E138K/G140A/Q148K INSTI-resistant triple mutant (EC$_{50}$s > 200 nM). The first generation INSTIs, RAL and EVG failed to retain potency against the entire panel of INSTI-resistant triple mutants, except for T97A/Y143R/Q148H, against which EVG showed modest inhibition, with an EC$_{50}$ value of 41.6 ± 3.0 nM. BIC had significantly higher potencies against two of the INSTI-triple mutants than DTG (one p value < 0.01, see Fig. 3 and Additional file 1: Table S5B), compared to one for DTG versus BIC against the triple mutants in this panel. Both BIC and DTG were more effective than CAB. BIC had better efficacies than CAB against six of the triple mutants (four p values < 0.001); DTG was better than CAB for five of the mutants in this panel (three p values < 0.001).

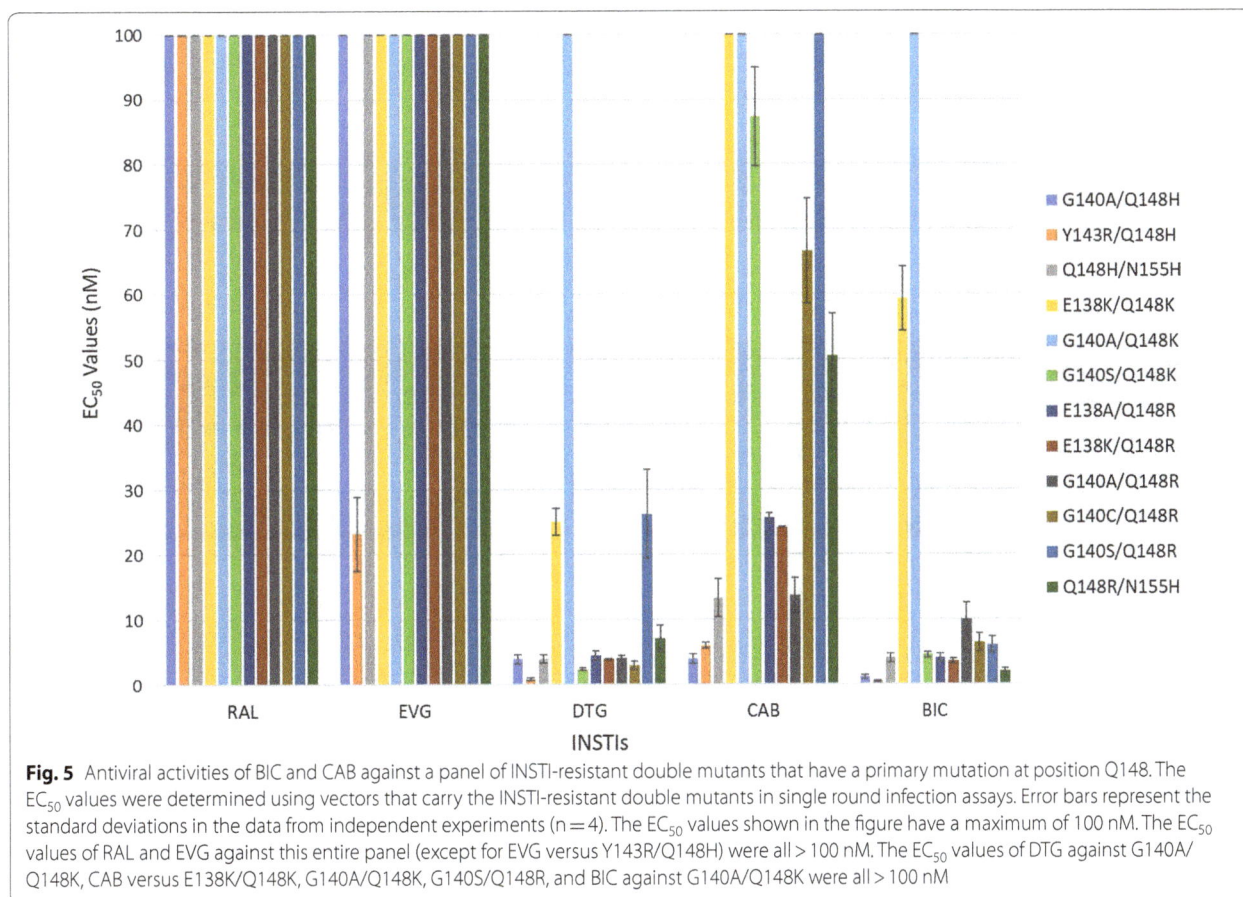

Fig. 5 Antiviral activities of BIC and CAB against a panel of INSTI-resistant double mutants that have a primary mutation at position Q148. The EC_{50} values were determined using vectors that carry the INSTI-resistant double mutants in single round infection assays. Error bars represent the standard deviations in the data from independent experiments (n = 4). The EC_{50} values shown in the figure have a maximum of 100 nM. The EC_{50} values of RAL and EVG against this entire panel (except for EVG versus Y143R/Q148H) were all > 100 nM. The EC_{50} values of DTG against G140A/Q148K, CAB versus E138K/Q148K, G140A/Q148K, G140S/Q148R, and BIC against G140A/Q148K were all > 100 nM

Antiviral activities of CAB and BIC versus a panel of INSTI-resistant triple mutants that consists of a primary mutation at T66I and N155H with additional secondary mutations

We examined CAB, BIC, and the FDA-approved INSTIs, against a panel of INSTI-triple mutants that included T66I/T97A/E157Q, T97A/Y143R/N155H, G140S/Y143R/N155H, and E92Q/N155H/G163R (Fig. 9; Additional file 1: Table S6A). The triple mutant T66I/T97A/E157Q is an EVG-resistant mutant and, as expected, this mutant showed a substantial decrease in potency to EVG (69.4 ± 11.8 nM) and a lesser loss of potency to RAL (33.5 ± 8.7 nM). In contrast, DTG (0.5 ± 0.1 nM), BIC (0.4 ± 0.2 nM), and CAB (0.8 ± 0.1 nM) retained full potency against this triple mutant. Additionally, DTG, BIC, and CAB retained high antiviral potencies against the E92Q/N155H/G163R INSTI-resistant triple mutant ($EC_{50} < 5$ nM). The G140S/Y143R/N155H triple mutant was susceptible to both DTG (2.6 ± 0.3 nM) and BIC (2.1 ± 0.1 nM), but it caused a moderate loss in potency to CAB (20.0 ± 3.5 nM). Both DTG and BIC retained significant potency against the T97A/Y143R/N155H triple mutant, 8.5 ± 1.5 nM and 8.2 ± 1.7 nM,

respectively, whereas CAB lost substantial potency (142.2 ± 8.3 nM). RAL and EVG both failed to potently inhibit the T97A/Y143R/N155H, G140S/Y143R/N155H, and E92Q/N155H/G163R INSTI-resistant triple mutants (EC_{50}s > 90 nM). Both DTG and BIC were more effective than CAB; each one had a significantly higher potency than CAB against 3 of the triple mutants in this panel (at least one p value < 0.001; see Fig. 3 and Additional file 1: Table S6B). BIC was significantly better than DTG against one of the triple mutants (p value < 0.01).

Antiviral activities of CAB and BIC against a panel of INSTI-resistant triple mutants that include the well-characterized RAL-resistant double mutant G140S/Q148H and an additional secondary mutation

We tested the antiviral potencies of CAB, BIC, and the FDA-approved INSTIs against a panel of INSTI-resistant triple mutants that included the RAL-resistant G140S/Q148H double mutations with an additional mutation: T97A, E138A/K, Y143R, N155H, or G163K (Fig. 10; Additional file 1: Table S7A). As expected, both of the first generation INSTIs, RAL and EVG, were ineffective against this panel of six INSTI-resistant triple mutants

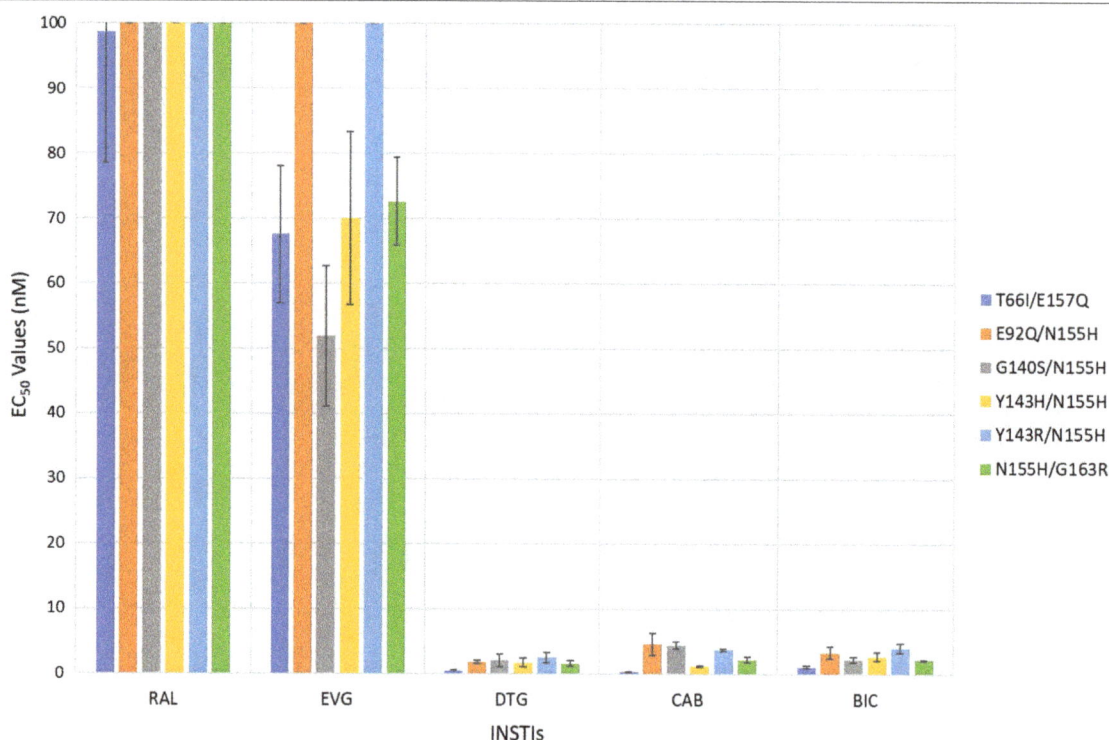

Fig. 6 Antiviral activities of BIC and CAB against a panel of INSTI-resistant double mutants that included the primary mutations T66I and N155H with additional mutations at other positions. The EC_{50} values were determined using vectors that carry the INSTI-resistant double mutants in single round infection assays. Error bars represent the standard deviations in the data from independent experiments ($n = 4$). The EC_{50} values shown in the figure have a maximum of 100 nM. The EC_{50} values of RAL against this entire panel of INSTI-resistant double mutants were all > 100 nM. The EC_{50} values of EVG against E92Q/N155H and Y143R/N155H were all > 100 nM

(EC_{50}s > 5000 nM). In addition, DTG, which potently inhibited the G140S/Q148H INSTI-resistant double mutant ($EC_{50} < 5$ nM) showed a loss of potency against the INSTI-resistant triple mutants. The E138A/G140S/Q148H, G140S/Y143R/Q148H, and G140S/Q148H/G163K triple mutants caused modest drops in potency, from 13.8 ± 4.8 nM, to 7.7 ± 2.0 nM, and 24.3 ± 1.1 nM, respectively. However, the INSTI-resistant triple mutants T97A/G140S/Q148H, E138K/G140S/Q148H, and G140S/Q148H/N155H caused substantial reductions in potency (EC_5s ≥ 55 nM). CAB was not broadly active against these INSTI-resistant triple mutants; most of the mutants caused significant drops in susceptibility to CAB. Conversely, for this panel of mutants, BIC was more effective than DTG in retaining potency. BIC showed at most a modest loss in potency against E138A/G140S/Q148H, E138K/G140S/Q148H, G140S/Y143R/Q148H, and G140S/Q148H/G163K (EC_{50}s < 10 nM. However, the INSTI-resistant triple mutant T97A/G140S/Q148H caused a larger reduction in susceptibility to BIC (29.5 ± 4.4 nM). Thus, BIC was superior to the other INSTIs in terms of its ability to retain antiviral activity against this set of triple mutants. BIC was the

superior INSTI against this panel of triple mutants, as it had significantly better potencies against five INSTI-resistant triple mutants than CAB (2 p values < 0.01 and 3 p values < 0.001, see Fig. 3 and Additional file 1: S7B) and three triple mutants than DTG (p values < 0.001). DTG was a better INSTI than CAB as it had higher efficacies against five triple mutants than CAB.

Homology modeling of the binding of BIC and CAB into the HIV-1 IN active site using PFV intasome structural data

Using the previously reported crystal structure of the PFV intasome with DTG bound at the catalytic site (PDB ID: 3S3M) [15] and the structure of the HIV-1 IN strand transfer complex (STC) solved by electron microscopy as a template (PDB ID: 5U1C) [40], homology models were prepared of BIC and CAB bound to the HIV-1 intasome (Fig. 11, panels B and C). Modeling allowed us (1) to understand better how BIC and CAB bind in the HIV-1 IN active site and (2) to identify structural features that may help (or hinder) these INSTIs in overcoming INSTI-resistant mutants. The chelating motifs of BIC and CAB aligned similarly to

Overall Comparison	BIC > CAB	39
	BIC > DTG	14
	DTG > CAB	33
	DTG > BIC	10
	CAB > BIC	3
	CAB > DTG	3
***p*-Value < 0.025**	BIC > CAB	1
	BIC > DTG	3
	DTG > CAB	1
	DTG > BIC	1
	CAB > BIC	0
	CAB > DTG	0
***p*-Value < 0.01**	BIC > CAB	17
	BIC > DTG	7
	DTG > CAB	18
	DTG > BIC	5
	CAB > BIC	1
	CAB > DTG	3
***p*-Value < 0.001**	BIC > CAB	21
	BIC > DTG	4
	DTG > CAB	14
	DTG > BIC	4
	CAB > BIC	2
	CAB > DTG	0

Fig. 7 Overall Comparison of the statistical significance of the antiviral data among DTG, CAB, and BIC. The Student's t test was used to calculate the statistical significance of the differences in the antiviral activities of the INSTIs. The p values < 0.025, < 0.01, and < 0.001 between DTG, CAB, and BIC were used to decide which INSTIs were more broadly efficacious against the mutants

flexibility of the oxazepane ring allows it to bend backwards or forwards, depending on the exact geometry of the active site, which can be modified by nearby mutations. Thus, the apparent greater conformational flexibility of the oxazepine ring could allow BIC to bind tightly to the various INSTI-resistant mutants, such as G118R and S119R, which affect the periphery of the IN active site, and limit the modifications that can be added to the "left" side of the INSTI scaffold distal to the end of the viral DNA (unpublished observations). Conversely, the oxazole ring of CAB is pointed out and away from the position occupied by the corresponding oxazine ring of DTG (Fig. 11, panel B), and its methyl group does not appear to be in a position to make an important contribution to binding, which is in good agreement with the data of Yoshinaga et al. [41], which appeared when this manuscript was in review. This could account for the fact that, although CAB and DTG adopt similar spatial orientations when bound to the IN active site, DTG is much more broadly effective against INSTI-resistant mutants (see "Discussion").

Discussion

The relatively recent development of INSTIs as potent and effective HIV-1 inhibitors permits improved treatment strategies for HIV-1 infected patients. In general, INSTIs are minimally toxic and work well in combination with other ARV drug classes [20, 42–44]. In addition, DTG appears not to readily select for resistance mutations. DTG is now widely used in therapies for the treatment of both naïve and experienced patients [11, 12, 16, 18, 19]. However, patients in advanced clinical trials that were previously on a RAL-based therapy, who switched to a DTG-based salvage therapy, have shown signs of virological failure. In some cases, additional resistance mutations were selected [25, 26]. Therefore, there is a need for new INSTIs that can overcome emerging INSTI-resistant mutants.

BIC and CAB are now in late stage clinical trials [45–48]. Based on our antiviral analysis of the ability of these new INSTIs to inhibit previously identified INSTI-resistant single, double, and triple mutants in a single round replication assay, it appears that both BIC and CAB are both more broadly effective than either of the first generation INSTIs, RAL and EVG. However, in terms of their ability to inhibit the fifty-seven INSTI-resistant mutants we tested, BIC was significantly better than DTG against fourteen out of the mutants (Fig. 7; seven featured p values < 0.01, whereas four had p values < 0.001). BIC was also better than CAB against thirty-nine of the mutants (twenty-one had p values < 0.001). Conversely, DTG was better than BIC against ten of the mutants tested (four with p values < 0.001) and better than CAB

DTG (Fig. 11, panel D), as did the halobenzyl moieties, which have π–π hydrophobic stacking interactions with the penultimate cytosine on the 3' ends of the viral DNA. However, it is the "left" side of the tricyclic ring system of BIC, which is the portion of the INSTI that is distal to the end of the viral DNA, and has an oxazepine ring which features a methylene bridge and lacks a methyl group, that appears to distinguish BIC from DTG. This cyclic modification can, in the model, adopt and maintain a different configuration from the components on the left side of DTG and CAB. Both the methyl-modified oxazine ring of DTG and the methyl-modified oxazole ring of CAB appear to be more constrained than the oxazepine ring of BIC. The greater

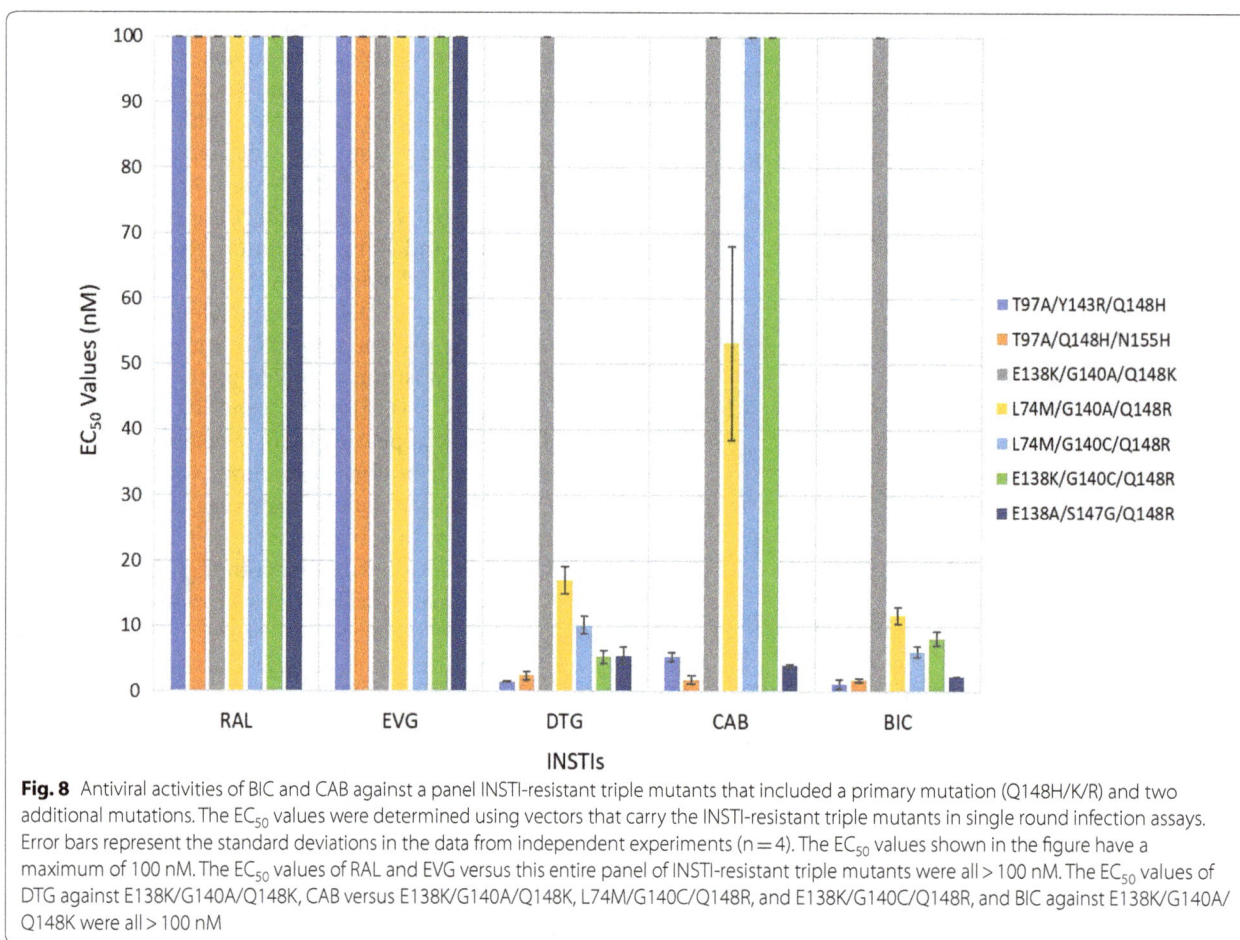

Fig. 8 Antiviral activities of BIC and CAB against a panel INSTI-resistant triple mutants that included a primary mutation (Q148H/K/R) and two additional mutations. The EC$_{50}$ values were determined using vectors that carry the INSTI-resistant triple mutants in single round infection assays. Error bars represent the standard deviations in the data from independent experiments (n = 4). The EC$_{50}$ values shown in the figure have a maximum of 100 nM. The EC$_{50}$ values of RAL and EVG versus this entire panel of INSTI-resistant triple mutants were all > 100 nM. The EC$_{50}$ values of DTG against E138K/G140A/Q148K, CAB versus E138K/G140A/Q148K, L74M/G140C/Q148R, and E138K/G140C/Q148R, and BIC against E138K/G140A/Q148K were all > 100 nM

for thirty-three of the mutants (fourteen with p values < 0.001). CAB was better than BIC and DTG for three mutants each (all three p values < 0.01 for DTG and two p values < 0.001 for BIC). Overall, our conclusions concerning the relative efficacies of the new INSTIs against mutants are in good agreement with the data of Yoshinaga et al. [41] and Neogi et al. [49], which appeared when this manuscript was in review.

Given the complexities of pharmacology, a significant difference in the behavior of a drug against a particular mutant (or mutants) may or may not translate directly into a desirable clinical outcome. However, given the problems that arise with drug resistance, it is likely that, among related compounds, those that are more broadly effective against resistant viruses will have an advantage in the clinic. In addition, in comparing the potencies of the compounds, the single round assay allows us to directly compare the efficacies of the new INSTIs against INSTI-resistant mutants in a reproducible and accurate manner. The single round assay avoids the issue of the effects of the mutations on the replication capacity, which, in turn, affects the number of viral life cycles in

assays done with replication competent viruses, and by extension, can affect the EC$_{50}$s.

Having a better understanding of how INSTIs bind to HIV-1 IN is an important part of developing more effective new drugs. However, superpositioning the available PFV and HIV IN structures has revealed differences in the PFV and HIV-1 IN active sites [15, 40]. Notably, the β4α2 loops are in different positions relative to the IN active site and there are differences in the structures and locations of the C-terminal domains (CTDs) near the IN active site. Thus, the contacts and interactions between INSTIs and the PFV intasome might not correspond exactly to the related contacts in the HIV-1 intasome. Until the structure of the HIV-1 intasome with these INSTIs bound is solved, HIV-1 IN models based on the structures of the PFV template with bound INSTIs and the available HIV-1 strand transfer (STC) structures can be used to predict how new INSTIs will bind to the HIV-1 intasome. DTG, BIC, and CAB are similar chemically and structurally. Not surprisingly, based on the model we built using the available structural information, all three compounds adopt similar configurations within

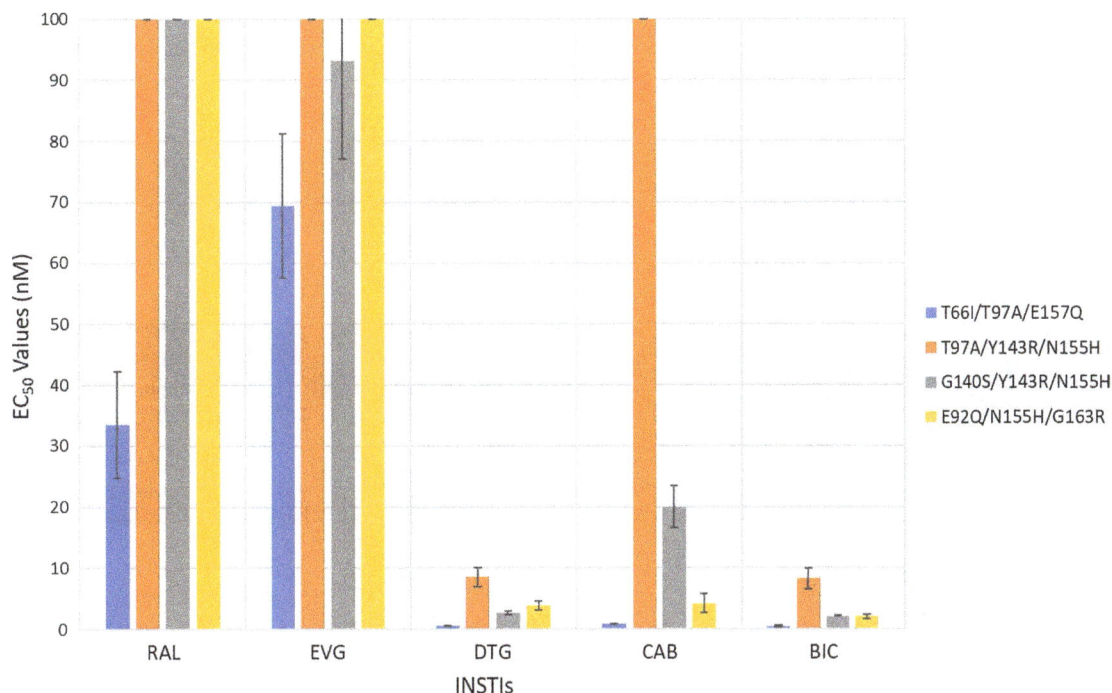

Fig. 9 Antiviral activities of BIC and CAB versus a panel of INSTI-resistant triple mutants that consists of a primary mutation at T66I and N155H with additional secondary mutations. The EC_{50} values were determined using vectors that carry the INSTI-resistant triple mutants in single round infection assays. Error bars represent the standard deviations of the data from independent experiments (n = 4). The EC_{50} value shown in the figure have a maximum of 100 nM. The EC_{50} values of RAL against T97A/Y143R/N155H, G140S/Y143R/N155H, and E92Q/N155H/G163R were all > 100 nM. The EC_{50} values of EVG versus T97A/Y143R/N155H and E92Q/N155H/G163R and CAB against T97A/Y143R/N155H were all > 100 nM

the active site of HIV-1 IN. It appears that the structural differences on the "left side" of these INSTIs, the part of the pharmacophore away from the 3′ end of the viral DNA, are largely responsible for their different resistance profiles.

Although there are similarities, as noted above, BIC is better than DTG, and DTG is better than CAB, in terms of their respective abilities to broadly inhibit the known IN mutants. We think it is likely that BIC is more broadly effective in its ability to inhibit a range of INSTI-resistant mutants, because it is better able to adjust its conformation, in response to the changes in the shape of the active site caused by the various resistance mutations. Thus, as has been proposed for the binding of non-nucleoside reverse transcriptase inhibitors (NNRTIs) to HIV-1 RT [50–53], the most broadly potent compounds are those that are able to adjust their binding mode and/or their configuration in response to changes in and around the IN active site. As briefly discussed earlier, BIC has an oxazepine ring with a methylene bridge appended to its chelating scaffold, which differs from the oxazine ring of DTG. It appears, based on the models, that the oxazepine ring of BIC is more flexible, which would allow it to be more conformationally adaptable. The introduction

of resistance mutations in residues in and around the IN active site may cause alterations in the active site geometry. These changes could potentially affect the binding of relatively rigid compounds, giving rise to resistance. The greater flexibility of the extended ring system of BIC may help it adapt to changes in the geometry in the IN active site, allowing BIC to overcome many of the known IN resistance mutations. However, the details of the binding of BIC, particularly to the INSTI-resistant forms of HIV-1 IN, will require additional high resolution structural data. Conversely, the methyl-modified oxazole ring of CAB does not appear to be in a favorable position to interact with WT IN. In addition, it does not appear to be conformationally adaptable. As a consequence, CAB may have difficulty overcoming the changes in the geometry of the active site of HIV IN caused by resistance mutants.

Generally speaking, the second generation INSTIs (DTG, BIC, and CAB) are much more proficient at inhibiting these INSTI-resistant mutants than RAL and EVG. Based on the data from our panel of mutants, DTG and BIC are more broadly effective against the mutants than CAB (Fig. 3). The potency of the second generation INSTIs can be affected by triple mutants which arise when mutations at G140 (A/C/S) and Q148 (H/R) are

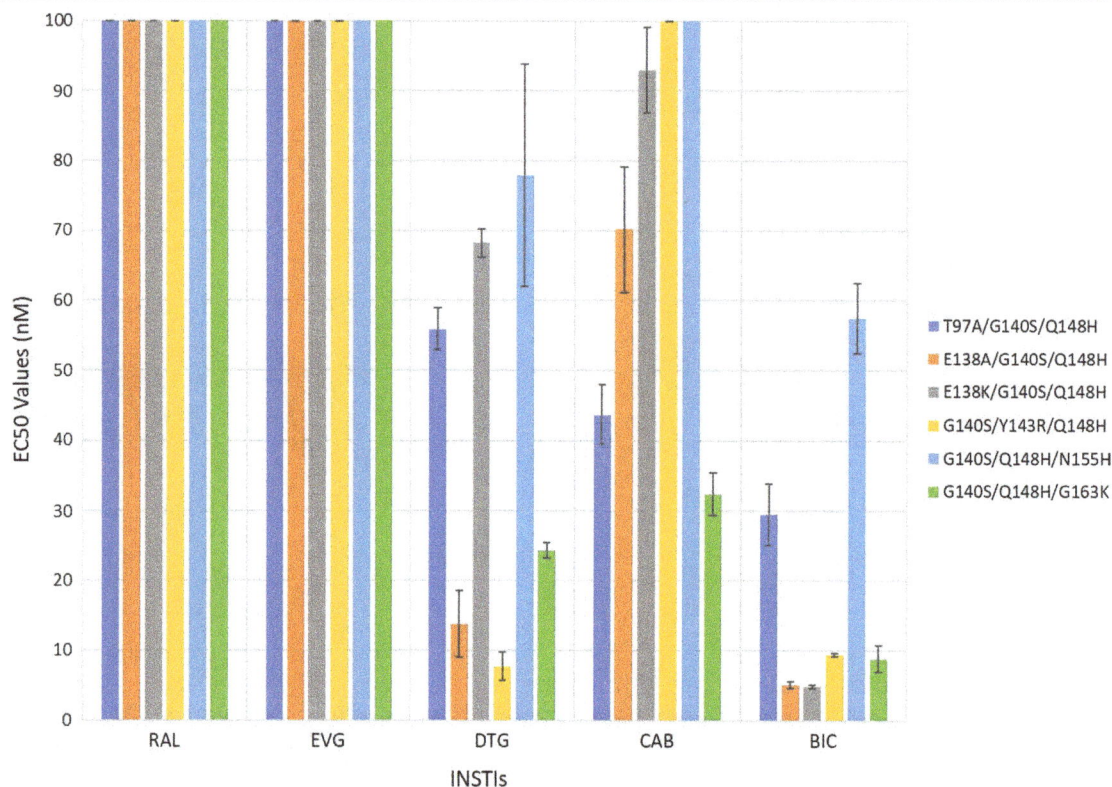

Fig. 10 Antiviral activities of CAB and BIC against a panel of INSTI-resistant triple mutants that include the well-characterized RAL-resistant double mutant G140S/Q148H plus an additional secondary mutation. The EC_{50} values were determined using vectors that carry the INSTI-resistant triple mutants in single round infection assays. Error bars represent the standard deviations in the data from independent experiments (n = 4). The EC_{50} values shown in the figure have a maximum of 100 nM. The EC_{50} values of RAL and EVG against this entire panel of INSTI-resistant triple mutants were all > 100 nM. The EC_{50} values of CAB against G140S/Y143R/Q148H and G140S/Q148H/N155H were all > 100 nM

combined with the polymorphic mutation at L74M or T97A. Although it is not entirely clear how frequently L74M and T97A occur in either B or non-B HIV-1 subtypes in INSTI-naïve patients, it is possible that, when these polymorphisms are present, that they could affect the development of resistance.

Conclusions

Based on these results, BIC appears to be a very promising INSTI. CAB has obvious disadvantages in terms of its breadth of antiviral potency relative to both BIC and DTG. However, CAB may have other advantages; it can be formulated as a long-acting compound that can be injected into patients once every 2–3 months [46, 47]. Nonetheless, based on experience with previous ARV drugs, in the long-term, resistant viruses will emerge. Thus, it is likely that at least some of the compounds that are broadly effective against the known mutants will be successful. This idea is underscored by the fact that, currently, in Washington DC, where the levels of HIV infection is still high, approximately 20% of new cases involve

a HIV strain that has at least one drug resistance mutation [54].

Methods
INSTI synthesis

Acquisition of RAL, EVG, and DTG was previously described [15, 55, 56]. BIC was obtained from Pharma-Block (Cat. No. PBLJ8958) and CAB was obtained from AbovChem LLC (Cat. No. HY-15592).

Cell-based assays

Single-round viral infectivity assays, using HIV-1 vectors that express either WT or mutant forms of IN, were used to determine antiviral potencies (EC_{50} values) of the compounds as previously described [57]. The Student's t test was used to calculate the p values used to determine statistical significance.

Vector constructs

The vector pNLNgoMIVR-ΔENV.LUC has been described previously [36]. To produce the new IN mutants used in this study, the IN open reading frame

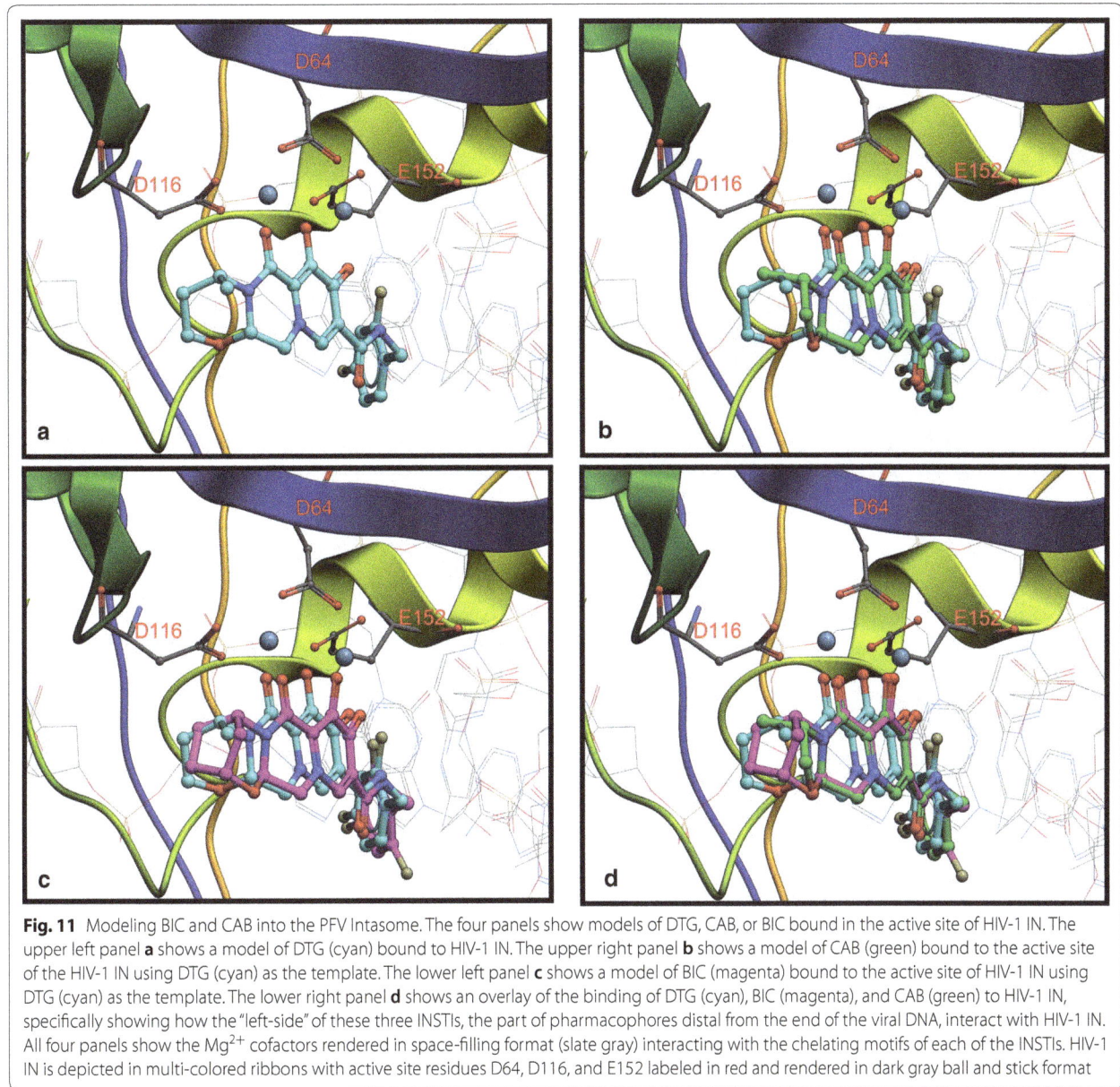

Fig. 11 Modeling BIC and CAB into the PFV Intasome. The four panels show models of DTG, CAB, or BIC bound in the active site of HIV-1 IN. The upper left panel **a** shows a model of DTG (cyan) bound to HIV-1 IN. The upper right panel **b** shows a model of CAB (green) bound to the active site of the HIV-1 IN using DTG (cyan) as the template. The lower left panel **c** shows a model of BIC (magenta) bound to the active site of HIV-1 IN using DTG (cyan) as the template. The lower right panel **d** shows an overlay of the binding of DTG (cyan), BIC (magenta), and CAB (green) to HIV-1 IN, specifically showing how the "left-side" of these three INSTIs, the part of pharmacophores distal from the end of the viral DNA, interact with HIV-1 IN. All four panels show the Mg^{2+} cofactors rendered in space-filling format (slate gray) interacting with the chelating motifs of each of the INSTIs. HIV-1 IN is depicted in multi-colored ribbons with active site residues D64, D116, and E152 labeled in red and rendered in dark gray ball and stick format

was removed from pNLNgoMIVR-ΔENV.LUC by digestion with KpnI and SalI and resulting fragment was inserted between the KpnI and SalI sites of pBluescript KS+. Using that construct as the wild-type template, we prepared the following HIV-1 IN mutants using the QuikChange II XL site directed mutagenesis kit (Agilent Technologies, Santa Clara, CA) protocol: M50I, L74M, T97A, S119R, E138K, G140S, Q146L, Q146P, Q148H, Q148K, Q148R, S153Y, T66I/E157Q, E92Q/N155H, T124A/153Y, E138A/Q148R, E138K/Q148K, E138K/ Q148R, E138K/263K, G140A/Q148H, G140A/Q148K, G140A/Q148R, G140C/Q148R, G140S/Q148K, G140S/ Q148R, G140S/N155H, Y143H/N155H, Y143R/Q148H, Y143R/N155H, Q148H/N155H, Q148R/N155H, N155H/ G163R, T66I/T97A/E157Q, L74M/G140A/Q148R, L74M/G140C/Q148R, E92Q/N155H/G163R, T97A/ G140S/Q148H, T97A/Y143R/Q148H, T97A/Y143R/ N155H, T97A/Q148H/N155H, E138A/G140S/Q148H, E138A/S147G/Q148R, E138K/G140A/Q148K, E138K/ G140C/Q148R, E138K/G140S/Q148H, G140S/Y143R/ Q148H, G140S/Y143R/N155H, G140S/Q148H/N155H, and G140S/Q148H/G163K. The following sense oligonucleotides were used with matching cognate antisense oligonucleotides (not shown) (Integrated DNA Technologies, Coralville, IA) in the mutagenesis: M50I, 5′-CAG CTAAAAGGGGAAGCCATTCATGGACAAGTAGAC

TGT-3'; T66I, 5'- ATATGGCAGCTAGATTGTATT CATTTAGAAGGAAAAGTT-3'; L74M, 5'- TTAGAA GGAAAAGTTATCATGGTAGCAGTTCATGTAGCC-3'; E92Q, 5'- GCAGAAGTAATTCCAGCACAAACA GGGCAAGAAACAGCA-3'; T97A, 5'- GCAGAGACA GGGCAAGAAGCTGCATACTTCCTCTTAAAA-3'; S119R, 5'- GTACATACAGACAATGGCCGTAATTTC ACCAGTACTACA-3'; E138A, 5'- TGGGCGGGGGATC AAGCAGGCTTTTGGCATTCCCTACAAT-3'; E138K, 5'- TGGGCGGGGATCAAGCAGAAATTTGGCATT CCCTACAAT-3'; G140A, 5'- GGGATCAAGCAGGAA TTTGCTATTCCCTACAATCCCCAA-3'; G140C, 5'- GGGATCAAGCAGGAATTTTGTATTCCCTACAAT CCCCAA-3'; G140S, 5'-GGGATCAAGCAGGAATTT TCCATTCCCTACAATCCCCAA-3'; Y143H, 5'- CAG GAATTTGGCATTCCCCATAATCCCCAAAGTCAA GGA-3'; Y143R, 5'-CAGGAATTTGGCATTCCCAGA AATCCCCAAAGTCAAGGA-3'; Q146L, 5'- GGCATT CCCTACAATCCCTTAAGTCAAGGAGTAATAGAA-3'; Q148H, 5'-TACAATCCCCAAAGTCACGGAGTA ATAGAATCT-3'; Q148K, 5'- CCCTACAATCCCCAA AGTAAAGGAGTAATAGAATCTATG-3'; Q148R, 5'- CCCTACAATCCCCAAAGTCGTGGAGTAATAGAA TCTATG-3'; S153Y, 5'- AGTCAAGGAGTAATAGAA TATATGAATAAAGAATTAAAG-3'; N155H, 5'-GGA GTAATAGAATCTATGCATAAAGAATTAAAGAAA ATT-3'; 5'-E157Q, 5'-ATAGAATCTATGAATAAACAA TTAAAGAAAATTATAGGA-3'; G163K, 5'- GAATTA AAGAAAATTATAAAACAGGTAAGAGATCAGGCT -3', G163R, 5' -GAATTAAAGAAAATTATACGTCAG GTAAGAGATCAGGCT -3'; E138K for G140S/Q148H, 5'- TGGTGGGCGGGGATCAAGCAGAAATTTTCC ATTCCCTACAATCCC-3'; S147G for E138A/Q148R, 5'- ATTCCCTACAATCCCCAAGGTCGTGGAGTAATA GAATCT-3'; E138K for G140C/Q148R, 5'- TGGGCG GGGATCAAGCAGAAATTTTGTATTCCCTACAAT-3'; E138K for G140A/Q148K, 5'- TGGGCGGGGATC AAGCAGAAATTTGCTATTCCCTACAAT-3'; E138A for G140S/Q148H, 5'- TGGGCGGGGATCAAGCAG GCATTTTCCATTCCCTACAAT-3'; Y143R for Y143R/ Q148H, 5'-CAGGAATTTGGCATTCCCAGAAAT CCCCAAAGTCACGGA-3'; Y143R for G140S/Q148H, 5'-CAGGAATTTTCCATTCCCAGAAATCCCCAA AGTCACGGA-3'; Y143R for G140S/N155H, 5'-CAG GAATTTTCCATTCCCAGAAATCCCCAAAGTCAA GGA-3'.

The following IN mutants from Fig. 2 (Additional file 1: Tables S1A and S1B), H51Y, T66I, E92Q, G118R, Y143R, N155H, R263K, H51Y/R263K, and G140S/Q148H have been described [35]. The remaining E138K/R263K double mutant was made using the previously constructed E138K mutant and the appropriate listed R263K oligonucleotides, which were used to add the second mutation.

The IN mutants from Fig. 4 (Additional file 1: Tables S2A and S2B), which includes M50I, L74M, T97A, S119R, E138K, G140S, Q146L, Q146P, Q148H, Q148K, Q148R, and S153Y, were constructed as described above using the appropriate listed oligonucleotides.

The IN mutants from Fig. 5 (Additional file 1: Tables S3A and S3B), were made as followed. The E138A/Q148R and E138K/Q148R double mutants were made using the previously generated Q148R mutant and the E138A and E138K oligonucleotides, respectively, to add the second mutation. The E138K/Q148K double mutant was constructed using the previously made E138K mutant and the appropriate Q148K oligonucleotides, which were used to add the second mutation. The G140A/Q148H and G140A/Q148K double mutants were made with the previously constructed G140A mutant and the appropriate oligonucleotides for the second mutation either Q148H or Q148K, respectively. The double mutants G140A/Q148R and G140C/Q148R were made with the previously generated Q148R mutant and the oligonucleotides for the second mutation, either G140A or G140C, respectively. The double mutants G140S/Q148K and G140S/Q148R were made using the previously generated G140S mutant and appropriate oligonucleotides for the second mutation, either Q148K or Q148R, respectively. The double mutants Q148H/N155H and Q148R/N155H were made using the previously generated N155H mutant and appropriate oligonucleotides for the second mutation, either Q148H or Q148R, respectively. The double mutant Y143R/Q148H was made using the previously generated Q148H mutant and appropriate oligonucleotides to introduce the second mutationY143R.

The IN mutants from Fig. 6 (Additional file 1: Tables S4A and S4B), were made as followed. The T66I/E157Q double mutant was made using the previously generated T66I mutant and the appropriate E157Q oligonucleotides to add the second mutation. The double mutants E92Q/N155H, G140S/N155H, Y143H/N155H, Y143R/N155H, and N155H/G163R were made using the previously generated N155H mutant and appropriate oligonucleotides for the second mutation, either E92Q, G140S, Y143H, Y143R, or G163R, respectively.

The IN mutants from Fig. 8 (Additional file 1: Tables S5A and S5B), were constructed as followed. The L74M/G140A/Q148R triple mutant was made using the previously generated G140A/Q148R double mutant and the oligonucleotides for the third mutation, L74M. The triple mutant L74M/G140C/Q148R was made with the previously generated G140C/Q148R double mutant and the oligonucleotides for the third mutation, L74M. The triple mutant T97A/Y143R/Q148H was constructed using the previously generated Y143R/Q148H double mutant and the appropriate oligonucleotides for the third mutation,

T97A. The triple mutant E138K/G140C/Q148R was made using the previously generated G140C/Q148R double mutant and the appropriate oligonucleotides to create the third mutation, E138K. The triple mutant T97A/Q148H/N155H was made using the previously constructed Q148H/N155H double mutant and the appropriate oligonucleotides for the third mutation, T97A. The triple mutant E138A/S147G/Q148R was made with the previously generated E138A/Q148R double mutant and oligonucleotides to make the third mutation, S147G. The triple mutant E138K/G140A/Q148K was made using the previously constructed double mutant G140A/Q148K double mutant and the appropriate oligonucleotides to make the third mutation, E138K.

The IN mutants from Fig. 9 (Additional file 1: Tables S6A and S6B) were made as followed. The T66I/T97A/E157Q triple mutant was made using the previously generated T66I/E157Q double mutant and the oligonucleotides for the third mutation, T97A. The E92Q/N155H/G163R triple mutant was made using the previously generated E92Q/N155H double mutant and the oligonucleotides for the third mutation, G163R. The triple mutant G140S/Y143R/N155H was made using the previously constructed G140S/N155H double mutant and the correct oligonucleotides to create the third mutation, Y143R. The triple mutant T97A/Y143R/N155H was made with the previously generated Y143R/N155H double mutant and the appropriate oligonucleotides for the third mutation, T97A.

The IN mutants from Fig. 10 (Additional file 1: Tables S7A and S7B), were constructed as followed. The triple mutants T97A/G140S/Q148H, G140S/Q148H/N155H, and G140S/Q148H/G163K were each made with the previously generated G140S/Q148H double mutant and the appropriate oligonucleotides for the third mutation, either T97A, N155H, or G163K, respectively. The triple mutant was E138A/G140S/Q148H was made using the previously constructed G140S/Q148H double mutant and oligonucleotides to make the third mutation E138A. The triple mutant E138K/G140S/Q148H was made using the previously generated G140S/Q148H double mutant and the correct oligonucleotides to make the third mutation, E138K. The triple mutant G140S/Y143R/Q148H was made using the previously constructed G140S/Q148H double mutant and the appropriate oligonucleotides to make the third mutation Y143R.

The DNA sequence of each construct was verified independently by DNA sequence determination. The mutated IN coding sequences from pBluescript KS+ were then subcloned into pNLNgoMIVR-ΔEnv.LUC (between the KpnI and SalI sites) to produce mutant HIV-1 constructs; the sequence of the final construct was checked by DNA sequencing.

Computer modeling

All modeling was conducted using MOE 2016.0802 (Chemical computing group, Montreal, Quebec, Canada). The sequences and structures of DTG bound in the PFV intasome (PDB ID: 3S3M) and HIV-1 IN (PDB ID: 5U1C) served as the structural templates to construct a HIV-1 IN model with DTG bound in the active site. First, the N-terminal portions of the NTD, CCD, and CTD domains of the PFV and HIV-1 IN were used to align the domains properly. Next the sequences and structures of HIV-1 and PFV INs were aligned so that the HIV IN sequence was matched to superpose the HIV-1 and PFV IN. The coordinates of the HIV-1 IN structure (PDB ID: 5U1C) from the aforementioned alignment were used as the IN template to construct the HIV-1 IN model. This structure was modified to fit the structural coordinates of DTG, Mg^{2+} cofactors, and the viral DNA from the PFV intasome (PDB ID: 3S3M). The model of the HIV-1 intasome with DTG bound was energy minimized using a PFROSST forcefield with relative field solvation as recommended by the manufacturer. The new HIV-1 IN model was then aligned (structure only) with the HIV-1 IN structure (PDB ID: 5U1C) from the aforementioned alignment with PFV IN (PDB ID: 3S3M) and aligned to a RMSD value of 0.82 Å. Additionally, the new HIV-1 IN model was aligned with the previously solved HIV-1 IN structure (PDB ID: 5U1C) and aligned to a RMSD value of 1.12 Å. The surface (Van der Waals) of DTG was determined to locate possible steric clashes with the active site residues in the model. To identify potential contacts with CAB and BIC, both INSTIs were docked using DTG as the template. CAB or BIC were placed using the triangle matcher method and scored with London dG with approximately 30 poses and then the putative ligand poses were further refined using the rigid receptor method in MOE and scored with the GBVI/WSA dG function. If the expected ligand poses were not created, a pharmacophore editor tool in the docking function was used to add certain features that made the appropriate docking of CAB or BIC to DTG easier to view and the resulting structures were refined in the manner described above. The poses with the best docking scores were selected based on how well the bound compounds overlay with the DTG scaffold, bound to Mg^{2+}, and how well their halogenated benzyl moiety interacted hydrophobically through π–π stacking with the penultimate cytosine on the 3' end of the bound viral DNA. Docking poses images were refined using MolSoft ICM Pro software version 3.8-5 (MolSoft LLC, San Diego, CA).

Abbreviations

INSTI's: integrase strand transfer inhibitors; ARV: antiretroviral; STC: strand transfer complex; HIV: human immunodeficiency virus; PFV: prototype foamy virus; NNRTI's: non-nucleoside reverse transcriptase inhibitors; FDA: Food and Drug Administration; EC_{50}: half maximal inhibitory concentration.

Author details

[1] HIV Dynamics and Replication Program, National Cancer Institute-Frederick, National Institutes of Health, Frederick, MD, USA. [2] Chemical Biology Laboratory, National Cancer Institute-Frederick, National Institutes of Health, Frederick, MD, USA.

Acknowledgements

The authors would like to thank Teresa Burdette for help in preparing the manuscript, Alan Kane for help with the figures, and Brian Luke for help with the statistical analysis. This research was supported by the Intramural Research Programs of the National Cancer Institute and the Intramural AIDS Targeted Antiviral Program.

Authors' contributions

SS performed the experiments. SS and SH designed the experiments. SS, XZ, TB, and SH analyzed the data. XZ and TB contributed with compounds and imaging software. SS and SH drafted the manuscript. All authors read and approved the final manuscript.

Competing interests

The authors declare that they have no competing interests.

Funding

This research was supported by the Intramural Research Programs of the National Cancer Institute.

References

1. Bushman FD, Craigie R. Activities of human immunodeficiency virus (HIV) integration protein in vitro: specific cleavage and integration of HIV DNA. Proc Natl Acad Sci USA. 1991;88:1339–43.
2. Engelman A, Mizuuchi K, Craigie R. HIV-1 DNA integration: mechanism of viral DNA cleavage and DNA strand transfer. Cell. 1991;67:1211–21.
3. Hazuda DJ, Felock P, Witmer M, Wolfe A, Stillmock K, Grobler JA, Espeseth A, Gabryelski L, Schleif W, Blau C, Miller MD. Inhibitors of strand transfer that prevent integration and inhibit HIV-1 replication in cells. Science. 2000;287:646–50.
4. Wainberg MA, Mesplede T, Raffi F. What if HIV were unable to develop resistance against a new therapeutic agent? BMC Med. 2013;11:249.
5. Hare S, Gupta SS, Valkov E, Engelman A, Cherepanov P. Retroviral intasome assembly and inhibition of DNA strand transfer. Nature. 2010;464:232–6.
6. Metifiot M, Johnson B, Smith S, Zhao XZ, Marchand C, Burke T, Hughes S, Pommier Y. MK-0536 inhibits HIV-1 integrases resistant to raltegravir. Antimicrob Agents Chemother. 2011;55:5127–33.
7. Zhao XZ, Smith SJ, Metifiot M, Johnson BC, Marchand C, Pommier Y, Hughes SH, Burke TR Jr. Bicyclic 1-hydroxy-2-oxo-1,2-dihydropyridine-3-carboxamide-containing HIV-1 integrase inhibitors having high antiviral potency against cells harboring raltegravir-resistant integrase mutants. J Med Chem. 2014;57:1573–82.
8. Zhao XZ, Smith SJ, Metifiot M, Marchand C, Boyer PL, Pommier Y, Hughes SH, Burke TR Jr. 4-amino-1-hydroxy-2-oxo-1,8-naphthyridine-containing compounds having high potency against raltegravir-resistant integrase mutants of HIV-1. J Med Chem. 2014;57:5190–202.
9. Ballantyne AD, Perry CM. Dolutegravir: first global approval. Drugs. 2013;73:1627–37.
10. Shah BM, Schafer JJ, Desimone JA Jr. Dolutegravir: a new integrase strand transfer inhibitor for the treatment of HIV. Pharmacotherapy. 2014;34:506–20.
11. Walmsley SL, Antela A, Clumeck N, Duiculescu D, Eberhard A, Gutierrez F, Hocqueloux L, Maggiolo F, Sandkovsky U, Granier C, et al. Dolutegravir plus abacavir-lamivudine for the treatment of HIV-1 infection. N Engl J Med. 2013;369:1807–18.
12. Clotet B, Feinberg J, van Lunzen J, Khuong-Josses MA, Antinori A, Dumitru I, Pokrovskiy V, Fehr J, Ortiz R, Saag M, et al. Once-daily dolutegravir versus darunavir plus ritonavir in antiretroviral-naive adults with HIV-1 infection (FLAMINGO): 48 week results from the randomised open-label phase 3b study. Lancet. 2014;383:2222–31.
13. Johns BA, Kawasuji T, Weatherhead JG, Taishi T, Temelkoff DP, Yoshida H, Akiyama T, Taoda Y, Murai H, Kiyama R, et al. Carbamoyl pyridone HIV-1 integrase inhibitors 3. A diastereomeric approach to chiral nonracemic tricyclic ring systems and the discovery of dolutegravir (S/GSK1349572) and (S/GSK1265744). J Med Chem. 2013;56:5901–16.
14. Kobayashi M, Yoshinaga T, Seki T, Wakasa-Morimoto C, Brown KW, Ferris R, Foster SA, Hazen RJ, Miki S, Suyama-Kagitani A, et al. In Vitro antiretroviral properties of S/GSK1349572, a next-generation HIV integrase inhibitor. Antimicrob Agents Chemother. 2011;55:813–21.
15. Hare S, Smith SJ, Metifiot M, Jaxa-Chamiec A, Pommier Y, Hughes SH, Cherepanov P. Structural and functional analyses of the second-generation integrase strand transfer inhibitor dolutegravir (S/GSK1349572). Mol Pharmacol. 2011;80:565–72.
16. Cahn P, Pozniak AL, Mingrone H, Shuldyakov A, Brites C, Andrade-Villanueva JF, Richmond G, Buendia CB, Fourie J, Ramgopal M, et al. Dolutegravir versus raltegravir in antiretroviral-experienced, integrase-inhibitor-naive adults with HIV: week 48 results from the randomised, double-blind, non-inferiority SAILING study. Lancet. 2013;382:700–8.
17. Min S, Sloan L, DeJesus E, Hawkins T, McCurdy L, Song I, Stroder R, Chen S, Underwood M, Fujiwara T, et al. Antiviral activity, safety, and pharmacokinetics/pharmacodynamics of dolutegravir as 10-day monotherapy in HIV-1-infected adults. AIDS. 2011;25:1737–45.
18. Raffi F, Jaeger H, Quiros-Roldan E, Albrecht H, Belonosova E, Gatell JM, Baril JG, Domingo P, Brennan C, Almond S, et al. Once-daily dolutegravir versus twice-daily raltegravir in antiretroviral-naive adults with HIV-1 infection (SPRING-2 study): 96 week results from a randomised, double-blind, non-inferiority trial. Lancet Infect Dis. 2013;13:927–35.
19. Raffi F, Rachlis A, Stellbrink HJ, Hardy WD, Torti C, Orkin C, Bloch M, Podzamczer D, Pokrovsky V, Pulido F, et al. Once-daily dolutegravir versus raltegravir in antiretroviral-naive adults with HIV-1 infection: 48 week results from the randomised, double-blind, non-inferiority SPRING-2 study. Lancet. 2013;381:735–43.
20. van Lunzen J, Maggiolo F, Arribas JR, Rakhmanova A, Yeni P, Young B, Rockstroh JK, Almond S, Song I, Brothers C, Min S. Once daily dolutegravir (S/GSK1349572) in combination therapy in antiretroviral-naive adults with HIV: planned interim 48 week results from SPRING-1, a dose-ranging, randomised, phase 2b trial. Lancet Infect Dis. 2012;12:111–8.
21. Wainberg MA, Han YS. Will drug resistance against dolutegravir in initial therapy ever occur? Front Pharmacol. 2015;6:90.
22. Quashie PK, Mesplede T, Han YS, Oliveira M, Singhroy DN, Fujiwara T, Underwood MR, Wainberg MA. Characterization of the R263K mutation in HIV-1 integrase that confers low-level resistance to the second-generation integrase strand transfer inhibitor dolutegravir. J Virol. 2012;86:2696–705.
23. Quashie PK, Mesplede T, Han YS, Veres T, Osman N, Hassounah S, Sloan RD, Xu HT, Wainberg MA. Biochemical analysis of the role of G118R-linked dolutegravir drug resistance substitutions in HIV-1 integrase. Antimicrob Agents Chemother. 2013;57:6223–35.
24. Mesplede T, Osman N, Wares M, Quashie PK, Hassounah S, Anstett K, Han Y, Singhroy DN, Wainberg MA. Addition of E138K to R263K in HIV integrase increases resistance to dolutegravir, but fails to restore activity

of the HIV integrase enzyme and viral replication capacity. J Antimicrob Chemother. 2014;69:2733–40.

25. Castagna A, Maggiolo F, Penco G, Wright D, Mills A, Grossberg R, Molina JM, Chas J, Durant J, Moreno S, et al. Dolutegravir in antiretroviral-experienced patients with raltegravir- and/or elvitegravir-resistant HIV-1: 24-week results of the phase III VIKING-3 study. J Infect Dis. 2014;210:354–62.

26. Eron JJ, Clotet B, Durant J, Katlama C, Kumar P, Lazzarin A, Poizot-Martin I, Richmond G, Soriano V, Ait-Khaled M, et al. Safety and efficacy of dolutegravir in treatment-experienced subjects with raltegravir-resistant HIV type 1 infection: 24-week results of the VIKING Study. J Infect Dis. 2013;207:740–8.

27. Yoshinaga T, Kobayashi M, Seki T, Miki S, Wakasa-Morimoto C, Suyama-Kagitani A, Kawauchi-Miki S, Taishi T, Kawasuji T, Johns BA, et al. Antiviral characteristics of GSK1265744, an HIV integrase inhibitor dosed orally or by long-acting injection. Antimicrob Agents Chemother. 2015;59:397–406.

28. Tsiang M, Jones GS, Goldsmith J, Mulato A, Hansen D, Kan E, Tsai L, Bam RA, Stepan G, Stray KM, et al. Antiviral activity of bictegravir (GS-9883), a novel potent HIV-1 integrase strand transfer inhibitor with an improved resistance profile. Antimicrob Agents Chemother. 2016;60:7086–97.

29. Cooper DA, Steigbigel RT, Gatell JM, Rockstroh JK, Katlama C, Yeni P, Lazzarin A, Clotet B, Kumar PN, Eron JE, et al. Subgroup and resistance analyses of raltegravir for resistant HIV-1 infection. N Engl J Med. 2008;359:355–65.

30. Malet I, Delelis O, Valantin MA, Montes B, Soulie C, Wirden M, Tchertanov L, Peytavin G, Reynes J, Mouscadet JF, et al. Mutations associated with failure of raltegravir treatment affect integrase sensitivity to the inhibitor in vitro. Antimicrob Agents Chemother. 2008;52:1351–8.

31. Fransen S, Gupta S, Danovich R, Hazuda D, Miller M, Witmer M, Petropoulos CJ, Huang W. Loss of raltegravir susceptibility by human immunodeficiency virus type 1 is conferred via multiple nonoverlapping genetic pathways. J Virol. 2009;83:11440–6.

32. Goethals O, Clayton R, Van Ginderen M, Vereycken I, Wagemans E, Geluykens P, Dockx K, Strijbos R, Smits V, Vos A, et al. Resistance mutations in human immunodeficiency virus type 1 integrase selected with elvitegravir confer reduced susceptibility to a wide range of integrase inhibitors. J Virol. 2008;82:10366–74.

33. Shimura K, Kodama E, Sakagami Y, Matsuzaki Y, Watanabe W, Yamataka K, Watanabe Y, Ohata Y, Doi S, Sato M, et al. Broad antiretroviral activity and resistance profile of the novel human immunodeficiency virus integrase inhibitor elvitegravir (JTK-303/GS-9137). J Virol. 2008;82:764–74.

34. Margot NA, Hluhanich RM, Jones GS, Andreatta KN, Tsiang M, McColl DJ, White KL, Miller MD. In vitro resistance selections using elvitegravir, raltegravir, and two metabolites of elvitegravir M1 and M4. Antiviral Res. 2012;93:288–96.

35. Zhao XZ, Smith SJ, Maskell DP, Metifiot M, Pye VE, Fesen K, Marchand C, Pommier Y, Cherepanov P, Hughes SH, Burke TR Jr. HIV-1 integrase strand transfer inhibitors with reduced susceptibility to drug resistant mutant integrases. ACS Chem Biol. 2016;11:1074–81.

36. Zhao XZ, Smith SJ, Maskell DP, Metifiot M, Pye VE, Fesen K, Marchand C, Pommier Y, Cherepanov P, Hughes SH, Burke TR Jr. Structure-guided optimization of HIV integrase strand transfer inhibitors. J Med Chem. 2017;60:7315–32.

37. Markowitz M, Morales-Ramirez JO, Nguyen BY, Kovacs CM, Steigbigel RT, Cooper DA, Liporace R, Schwartz R, Isaacs R, Gilde LR, et al. Antiretroviral activity, pharmacokinetics, and tolerability of MK-0518, a novel inhibitor of HIV-1 integrase, dosed as monotherapy for 10 days in treatment-naive HIV-1-infected individuals. J Acquir Immune Defic Syndr. 2006;43:509–15.

38. Metifiot M, Marchand C, Maddali K, Pommier Y. Resistance to integrase inhibitors. Viruses. 2010;2:1347–66.

39. Johnson VA, Calvez V, Gunthard HF, Paredes R, Pillay D, Shafer RW, Wensing AM, Richman DD. Update of the drug resistance mutations in HIV-1: March 2013. Top Antivir Med. 2013;21:6–14.

40. Passos DO, Li M, Yang R, Rebensburg SV, Ghirlando R, Jeon Y, Shkriabai N, Kvaratskhelia M, Craigie R, Lyumkis D. Cryo-EM structures and atomic model of the HIV-1 strand transfer complex intasome. Science. 2017;355:89–92.

41. Yoshinaga T, Seki T, Miki S, Miyamoto T, Suyama-Kagitani A, Kawauchi-Miki S, Kobayashi M, Sato A, Stewart E, Underwood M, Fujiwara T. Novel sec-ondary mutations C56S and G149A confer resistance to HIV-1 integrase strand transfer inhibitors. Antiviral Res. 2018;152:1–9.

42. Steigbigel RT, Cooper DA, Teppler H, Eron JJ, Gatell JM, Kumar PN, Rockstroh JK, Schechter M, Katlama C, Markowitz M, et al. Long-term efficacy and safety of Raltegravir combined with optimized background therapy in treatment-experienced patients with drug-resistant HIV infection: week 96 results of the BENCHMRK 1 and 2 Phase III trials. Clin Infect Dis. 2010;50:605–12.

43. Eron JJ Jr, Rockstroh JK, Reynes J, Andrade-Villanueva J, Ramalho-Madruga JV, Bekker LG, Young B, Katlama C, Gatell-Artigas JM, Arribas JR, et al. Raltegravir once daily or twice daily in previously untreated patients with HIV-1: a randomised, active-controlled, phase 3 non-inferiority trial. Lancet Infect Dis. 2011;11:907–15.

44. Sax PE, DeJesus E, Mills A, Zolopa A, Cohen C, Wohl D, Gallant JE, Liu HC, Zhong L, Yale K, et al. Co-formulated elvitegravir, cobicistat, emtricitabine, and tenofovir versus co-formulated efavirenz, emtricitabine, and tenofovir for initial treatment of HIV-1 infection: a randomised, double-blind, phase 3 trial, analysis of results after 48 weeks. Lancet. 2012;379:2439–48.

45. Gallant JE, Thompson M, DeJesus E, Voskuhl GW, Wei X, Zhang H, White K, Cheng A, Quirk E, Martin H. Antiviral activity, safety, and pharmacokinetics of bictegravir as 10-Day monotherapy in HIV-1-infected adults. J Acquir Immune Defic Syndr. 2017;75:61–6.

46. Margolis DA, Gonzalez-Garcia J, Stellbrink HJ, Eron JJ, Yazdanpanah Y, Podzamczer D, Lutz T, Angel JB, Richmond GJ, Clotet B, et al. Long-acting intramuscular cabotegravir and rilpivirine in adults with HIV-1 infection (LATTE-2): 96-week results of a randomised, open-label, phase 2b, non-inferiority trial. Lancet. 2017;390:1499–510.

47. Markowitz M, Frank I, Grant RM, Mayer KH, Elion R, Goldstein D, Fisher C, Sobieszczyk ME, Gallant JE, Van Tieu H, et al. Safety and tolerability of long-acting cabotegravir injections in HIV-uninfected men (ECLAIR): a multicentre, double-blind, randomised, placebo-controlled, phase 2a trial. Lancet HIV. 2017;4:e331–40.

48. Sax PE, DeJesus E, Crofoot G, Ward D, Benson P, Dretler R, Mills A, Brinson C, Peloquin J, Wei X, et al. Bictegravir versus dolutegravir, each with emtricitabine and tenofovir alafenamide, for initial treatment of HIV-1 infection: a randomised, double-blind, phase 2 trial. Lancet HIV. 2017;4:e154–60.

49. Neogi U, Singh K, Aralaguppe SG, Rogers LC, Njenda DT, Sarafianos SG, Hejdeman B, Sonnerborg A. Ex-vivo antiretroviral potency of newer integrase strand transfer inhibitors cabotegravir and bictegravir in HIV type 1 non-B subtypes. AIDS. 2018;32:469–76.

50. Das K, Clark AD Jr, Lewi PJ, Heeres J, De Jonge MR, Koymans LM, Vinkers HM, Daeyaert F, Ludovici DW, Kukla MJ, et al. Roles of conformational and positional adaptability in structure-based design of TMC125-R165335 (etravirine) and related non-nucleoside reverse transcriptase inhibitors that are highly potent and effective against wild-type and drug-resistant HIV-1 variants. J Med Chem. 2004;47:2550–60.

51. Das K, Lewi PJ, Hughes SH, Arnold E. Crystallography and the design of anti-AIDS drugs: conformational flexibility and positional adaptability are important in the design of non-nucleoside HIV-1 reverse transcriptase inhibitors. Prog Biophys Mol Biol. 2005;88:209–31.

52. Smith SJ, Pauly GT, Akram A, Melody K, Ambrose Z, Schneider JP, Hughes SH. Rilpivirine and doravirine have complementary efficacies against NNRTI-resistant HIV-1 mutants. J Acquir Immune Defic Syndr. 2016;72:485–91.

53. Smith SJ, Pauly GT, Akram A, Melody K, Rai G, Maloney DJ, Ambrose Z, Thomas CJ, Schneider JT, Hughes SH. Rilpivirine analogs potently inhibit drug-resistant HIV-1 mutants. Retrovirology. 2016;13:11.

54. Kassaye SG, Grossman Z, Balamane M, Johnston-White B, Liu C, Kumar P, Young M, Sneller MC, Sereti I, Dewar R, et al. Transmitted HIV drug resistance is high and longstanding in metropolitan Washington. DC. Clin Infect Dis. 2016;63:836–43.

55. Varadarajan J, McWilliams MJ, Hughes SH. Treatment with suboptimal doses of raltegravir leads to aberrant HIV-1 integrations. Proc Natl Acad Sci USA. 2013;110:14747–52.

56. Varadarajan J, McWilliams MJ, Mott BT, Thomas CJ, Smith SJ, Hughes SH. Drug resistant integrase mutants cause aberrant HIV integrations. Retrovirology. 2016;13:71.

57. Smith SJ, Hughes SH. Rapid screening of HIV reverse transcriptase and integrase inhibitors. J Vis Exp. 2014;86:51400.

11

Impact of the HIV-1 genetic background and HIV-1 population size on the evolution of raltegravir resistance

Axel Fun[1], Thomas Leitner[2], Linos Vandekerckhove[3], Martin Däumer[4], Alexander Thielen[5], Bernd Buchholz[6], Andy I. M. Hoepelman[7], Elizabeth H. Gisolf[8], Pauline J. Schipper[1], Annemarie M. J. Wensing[1,7] and Monique Nijhuis[1*]

Abstract

Background: Emergence of resistance against integrase inhibitor raltegravir in human immunodeficiency virus type 1 (HIV-1) patients is generally associated with selection of one of three signature mutations: Y143C/R, Q148K/H/R or N155H, representing three distinct resistance pathways. The mechanisms that drive selection of a specific pathway are still poorly understood. We investigated the impact of the HIV-1 genetic background and population dynamics on the emergence of raltegravir resistance. Using deep sequencing we analyzed the integrase coding sequence (CDS) in longitudinal samples from five patients who initiated raltegravir plus optimized background therapy at viral loads > 5000 copies/ml. To investigate the role of the HIV-1 genetic background we created recombinant viruses containing the viral integrase coding region from pre-raltegravir samples from two patients in whom raltegravir resistance developed through different pathways. The in vitro selections performed with these recombinant viruses were designed to mimic natural population bottlenecks.

Results: Deep sequencing analysis of the viral integrase CDS revealed that the virological response to raltegravir containing therapy inversely correlated with the relative amount of unique sequence variants that emerged suggesting diversifying selection during drug pressure. In 4/5 patients multiple signature mutations representing different resistance pathways were observed. Interestingly, the resistant population can consist of a single resistant variant that completely dominates the population but also of multiple variants from different resistance pathways that coexist in the viral population. We also found evidence for increased diversification after stronger bottlenecks. In vitro selections with low viral titers, mimicking population bottlenecks, revealed that both recombinant viruses and HXB2 reference virus were able to select mutations from different resistance pathways, although typically only one resistance pathway emerged in each individual culture.

Conclusions: The generation of a specific raltegravir resistant variant is not predisposed in the genetic background of the viral integrase CDS. Typically, in the early phases of therapy failure the sequence space is explored and multiple resistance pathways emerge and then compete for dominance which frequently results in a switch of the dominant population over time towards the fittest variant or even multiple variants of similar fitness that can coexist in the viral population.

*Correspondence: m.nijhuis@umcutrecht.nl
[1] Department of Medical Microbiology, Virology, University Medical Center Utrecht, Heidelberglaan 100, HP G04.614, 3584 CX Utrecht, The Netherlands
Full list of author information is available at the end of the article

Background

Currently, viral replication is successfully suppressed in the majority of HIV-infected patients treated with combination antiretroviral therapy (cART) [1]. However, virological failure associated with the emergence of drug resistant viruses may still limit the success of cART. The emergence of drug resistance in HIV is a direct consequence of the high error-rate of the HIV reverse transcriptase (RT) enzyme [2–4]. The frequent incorrect nucleotide incorporations result in evolution of the viral population and generate a myriad of viral variants upon which selective forces may act. The population size and replication rate are important viral parameters that contribute to the probability that resistance emerges and to how HIV-1 drug resistance evolves [5–9].

Integrase inhibitors comprise a class of antiretroviral drugs that specifically prevent the integration of the viral genome into the human genome. Raltegravir is the first representative of a class of integrase inhibitors that target the strand transfer reaction (INSTIs) of the viral DNA into the host genome which is performed by the viral enzyme integrase. Like other INSTIs, raltegravir preferentially binds and inhibits the viral DNA-integrase complex (intasome) over unbound integrase [10–12].

It was the first integrase inhibitor used in clinical practice (since 2007) but was recently registered by the FDA for once daily dosing [13] and is very well tolerated [14] due to a low toxicity profile [15]. Resistance is commonly associated with selection of one of the signature raltegravir resistance mutations Y143C/R/H, Q148H/K/R or N155H [16–18]. Mutations at each of these three amino acids represent a distinct resistance pathway and all signature mutations are associated with reductions in viral replication [17, 19, 20]. Accumulation of secondary resistance mutations is often associated with a greater loss of drug susceptibility and/or improved viral fitness [21–23]. Different mutational combinations vary greatly in their impact on raltegravir susceptibility and viral replication. In general, substitutions at amino acid position 148 confer higher levels of resistance than substitutions at amino acid Y143 or N155. The G140S plus Q148H combination is considered the most resistant variant and has little effect on viral replication. The resistance patterns observed in HIV-1 patients on a raltegravir containing regimen are very diverse and Q148H/K/R (usually with G140A/C/S and/or E138A/K) and N155H (often together with E92Q or V151I) mutations are observed more frequently than Y143 mutations [24]. The different resistance pathways are believed to be mutually exclusive and multiple primary mutations (especially 148 + 155 mutations) are generally not observed on the same viral genome [25]. Remarkably, replacement of the dominant resistant population by a viral population with a completely different resistance pattern during continuous non-suppressive INSTI therapy has been observed [26–29].

The mechanisms that drive selection and switching of resistance pathways are inadequately understood. Understanding these mechanisms is essential in view of other INSTIs that are in clinical use (elvitegravir and dolutegravir) or in clinical trial (bictegravir and cabotegravir), since their resistance profiles partially overlap with that of raltegravir [25]. For instance, raltegravir resistance mutations Q148H/K/R and N155H show a high level of cross-resistance with elvitegravir, but elvitegravir susceptibility is unaffected by Y143 mutations [30, 31], a difference that is beautifully explained by crystal structures of the intasome in presence of raltegravir or elvitegravir [11]. The VIKING studies demonstrated dolutegravir's superior resistance profile attested by sustained activity against all raltegravir resistant variants, except for viruses with a mutation at amino acid 148 in combination with at least one secondary mutation at position 138 and/or 140 [32–34]. These observations were corroborated by in vitro analysis of resistance profiles [35–37] which also uncovered two atypical INSTI resistance mutations (G118R and F121Y) that confer pan-INSTI resistance [38, 39].

We investigated the impact of the HIV-1 genetic background and population size on the evolution of raltegravir resistance and their role in determining selection of a particular resistance pathway. Using next-generation sequencing (NGS) we analyzed patient-derived viral integrase sequences from samples taken before and during raltegravir therapy failure. Frequency and dynamics analysis of the deep sequencing data was used to evaluate intra-patient evolution of resistance.

To investigate the role of the genetic background we generated recombinant viruses containing the viral integrase CDS from pre-raltegravir samples from two patients experiencing virological failure receiving raltegravir therapy. With these recombinant viruses we conducted multiple low multiplicity of infection (MOI) in vitro selections in parallel, with the advantage that all resistant variants generated are allowed to replicate and different raltegravir resistance pathways can be identified.

Results

During raltegravir resistance development, multiple resistant variants emerge that compete to become the dominant variant

We studied five patients who initiated raltegravir therapy as part of a cART regimen and subsequently demonstrated virological failure to the raltegravir containing regimen. Of note, all 5 patients were heavily pre-treated and raltegravir was part of a (partly) compromised backbone. This may partially explain the moderate virological responses and limited therapy success in these patients. Patient (Pt) 1, Pt2, Pt3 and Pt5 were infected with HIV-1 subtype B strains, Pt4 was infected with a HIV-1 CRF02_ AG strain. All patients started raltegravir therapy with viral loads > 5000 copies/ml (c/ml) of HIV-1 RNA, as measured in the last viral load test before initiation of raltegravir therapy. To investigate if the emerged resistant variants existed as minority variants before raltegravir therapy and how the resistant population evolved we analyzed longitudinal samples from these patients by NGS.

Patient 1

HIV-1 RNA initially decreased after start of raltegravir containing cART (2.2 log decrease in HIV-1 RNA), but the viral load rebounded quickly after therapy initiation (< 81 days, Fig. 1a). Population sequencing revealed presence of raltegravir resistance mutations (E138E/K + Q148Q/ K/R + N155H/H) and raltegravir was discontinued from the regimen after 124 days. NGS revealed very small populations at baseline containing Q148R and E138K (0.1% of the population, Fig. 2a), but they were not present on the same genomes (Fig. 2b). 40 days after start of raltegravir, virus with Q148R had increased to 1.7% of the population and virus with E138K + Q148K had increased to 0.5% (Fig. 2a, b). These two variants dominated the population after 90 days (red nodes, Fig. 1a) but a third resistant variant appeared, N155H which already comprised 13% of the population. In the subsequent sample (153 days after start of raltegravir, black nodes Fig. 1a) the N155H variant replaced the Q148R variant and dominated the population together with the E138K + Q148K variant. Surprisingly, 4 weeks after raltegravir discontinuation, wild-type virus had not reseeded the viral population which was consisted entirely of raltegravir resistant variants (Fig. 2).

Patient 2

Pt2 was off therapy for a few weeks due to toxicity related issues but a new five-drug regimen including raltegravir and darunavir resulted in a rapid decline of the viral load but was discontinued again because of darunavir-related toxicity (Fig. 1b). Shortly thereafter, the same regimen was restarted without darunavir resulting in a further decline of the viral load to undetectable levels. After brief virological suppression (HIV-1 RNA < 50 c/ml, a 3.0 log decrease in HIV-1 RNA), viral load rebounded and population sequencing showed gradual accumulation of raltegravir resistance mutations: initially primary resistance mutation N155H appeared followed by two secondary resistance mutations, first Q95K and later V151I. NGS revealed no major raltegravir resistance mutations at baseline or mutations at positions 143 or 148 at any time-point, not even as minority variants (Fig. 2).

Patient 3

Pt3 only showed a partial virological response to the raltegravir containing therapy (a 1.0 log decrease in HIV-1 RNA

was observed) and full suppression was never achieved. The viral load rebounded shortly after start of raltegravir containing cART (< 70 days, Fig. 1c) and the viral population contained N155H mutants. In a later time-point, 169 days after start of raltegravir, this population was replaced by a variant with primary mutation Y143R and several secondary mutations including L74M, T97A and G163E. NGS revealed only secondary mutations in the sample before raltegravir therapy, mostly as very low frequency variants (Fig. 2), including T97A and Y143C (both 0.2%). In a sample taken 28 days later, 77.5% of the population contained N155H, 15.4% had T97A and variants with Y143C were not detected anymore. In the subsequent sample 70 days after start of raltegravir therapy, N155H had increased to 88.6% and Y143C had reappeared in 11.8% of the reads. Y143C and N155H did not appear to be on the same genome (Fig. 2b). After 169 days the resistant population had shifted dramatically, with Y143R making up 99.7% of the population and complete absence of N155H. Mutations L74M, T97A and G163R appeared in nearly the entire viral population.

Patient 4

Pt4 was also a partial responder (1.1 log decrease in HIV-1 RNA) in whom virological suppression was not achieved during 48 weeks of raltegravir containing therapy. Sanger sequencing revealed only very small (< 20%) populations of Q148H/Q148R and N155H and resistant variants never dominated the population (Fig. 1d). Before raltegravir therapy, mutation Y143H was detected at low frequency (0.2%) by NGS but did not appear in any of the later samples during raltegravir treatment. In samples 8 and 81 days after start of raltegravir therapy also no significant raltegravir resistance mutations were observed (Fig. 2a). However, in the sample 123 days after raltegravir therapy initiation several primary and secondary raltegravir resistance mutations occurred. N155H was found in 14.4%, of the population, Q148H in 7.5% of which approximately half (4.1%) in combination with G140S and the remainder in combination with E157D (Fig. 2b). Q148R was present in 2.4% of the population and G163R in 2.7%.

Patient 5

In addition to a compromised backbone, this patient also had sub-therapeutic levels of raltegravir levels due to a drug–drug interaction with rifampicin (an interaction unknown at time of raltegravir prescription). Despite the suboptimal levels of raltegravir, switching to a raltegravir containing regimen quickly resulted in complete viral suppression (< 26 days, 3.3 log decrease in HIV-1 RNA) but viral load rebounded within 21 weeks (Fig. 1e). Population sequencing (sample 457 days after initiation of raltegravir) demonstrated that virus with integrase substitutions G140S + Q148H completely dominated the viral population.

a Pt 1.

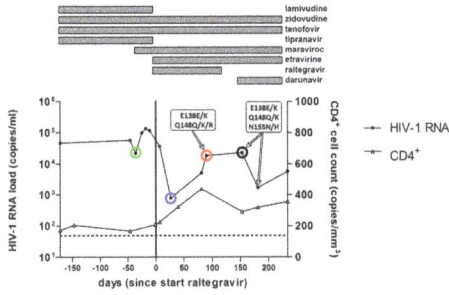

Residues E138 / Q148 / N155

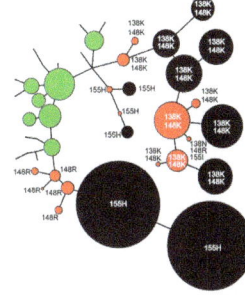

b Pt 2.

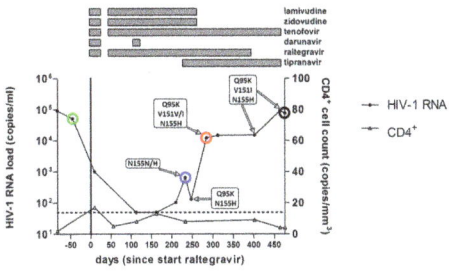

Residues V151 / N155

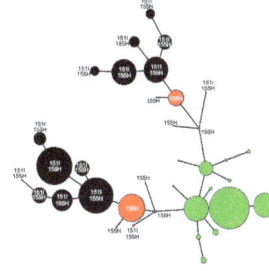

c Pt 3.

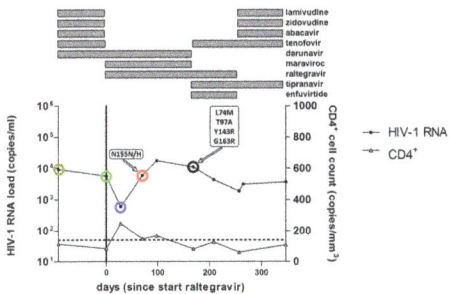

Residues Y143 / N155

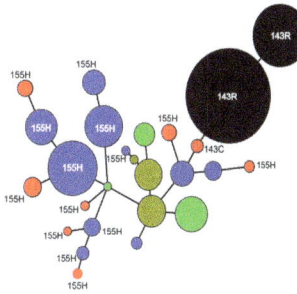

d Pt 4.

Residues Q148 / N155

e Pt 5.

Residues Y143 / Q148 / N155

(See figure on previous page.)

Fig. 1 Development of raltegravir resistance during raltegravir containing cART. Left hand panels: therapy history, HIV-1 RNA load, CD4[+] cell count and resistance mutations detected by population sequencing of five patients receiving raltegravir therapy. All viral load measurements are marked by a solid black circle. The CD4[+] cell counts are represented by open triangles. Samples analyzed by 454 deep sequencing are marked by colored circles. Resistance mutations detected by Sanger population sequencing are indicated in boxes. Only raltegravir resistance associated mutations are given. Right hand panels: evolution of resistance pathways, deep sequence analysis of the integrase core domain. Data was obtained by 454 pyrosequencing. Relevant resistance mutations are indicated at the respective nodes. Figures were generated using the nucleotide sequences and the redundancy-level for calling a variant was set at 80. No mutation information indicates wild-type amino acids. The size of each node is scaled to reflect the relative abundance and viral load at each time point and patient. Time points are indicated by color and correspond to the colored circles in the left hand panels: green is the baseline sample, blue the first sample after raltegravir therapy initiation; red is the second sample after raltegravir therapy initiation; black is the final sample after raltegravir therapy initiation. In patient 3 gold is another baseline sample predating the green sample

No major resistance mutations were detected at baseline by NGS. Interestingly, in the first sample during therapy failure (blue nodes Fig. 1e) mutations from all three major resistance pathways including double mutants with secondary mutations were observed with G140S + Q148H being the most frequently occurring double mutant (Fig. 2). In this sample the variant with mutation N155H was the dominant variant but was outcompeted in the subsequent sample (red nodes Fig. 1e) by double mutant G140S + Q148H.

Evidence for elevated diversification following extinction from drug pressure on large viral populations

To get an impression of the evolution of the viral population during raltegravir pressure we analyzed how the number of derived sequences and unique variants related to the viral load. To allow for easy comparisons, each of these measures were normalized on a 0–1 scale and plotted in the same graph (Fig. 3, left panels). In all patients, the total number of derived sequences and the number of unique variants detected correlated with the viral load

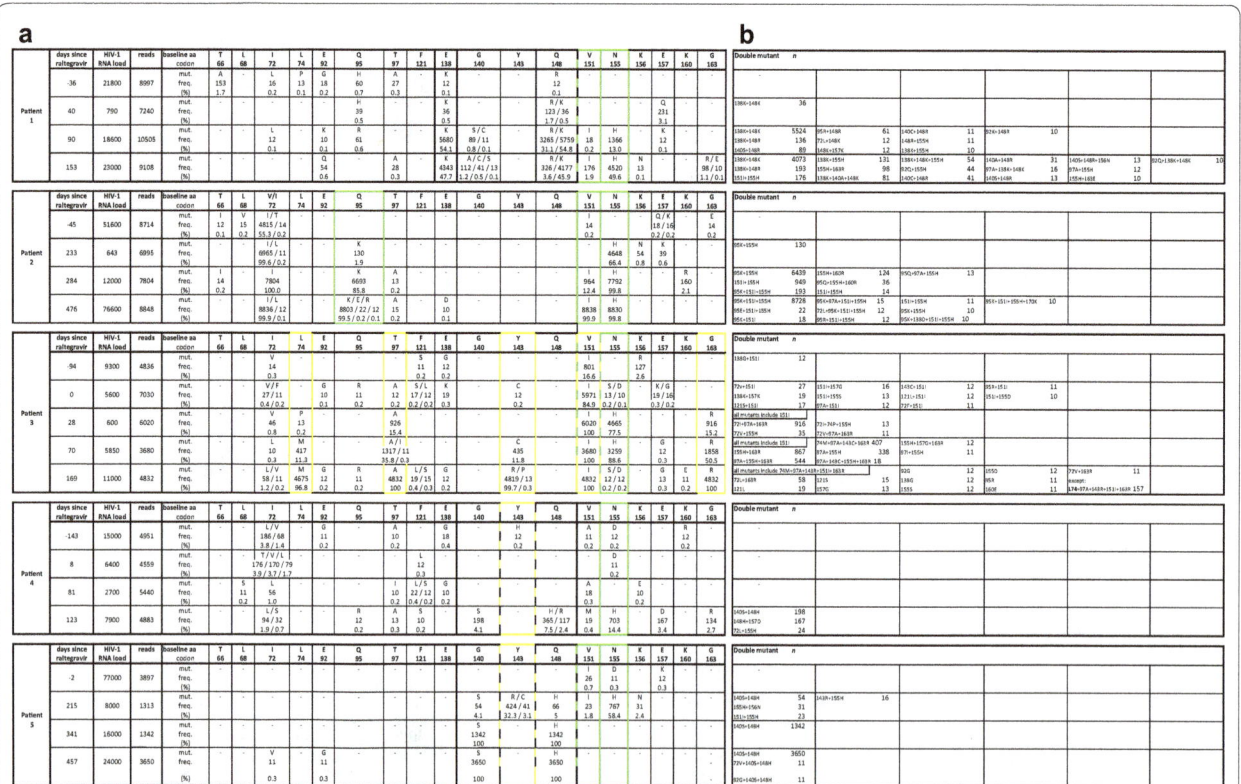

Fig. 2 Analysis of the longitudinal 454 deep sequencing data. **a** Analysis of the frequency of all non-synonymous mutations detected by deep sequencing at the 18 codons associated with raltegravir resistance. Only unique variants with a minimum of 10 reads were included in the analysis. Total number of reads and the proportion of reads containing the denoted mutations relative to the total number of reads are given. Mutations of interest are highlighted by colored boxes. Similar colored boxes are mutations that appeared to be on the same genome. Red boxes indicate mutations from the Q148 pathway, yellow boxes indicate the Y143 pathway and green boxes the N155 pathway. **b** Sequences containing multiple mutations are shown. Double mutants are sorted by frequency

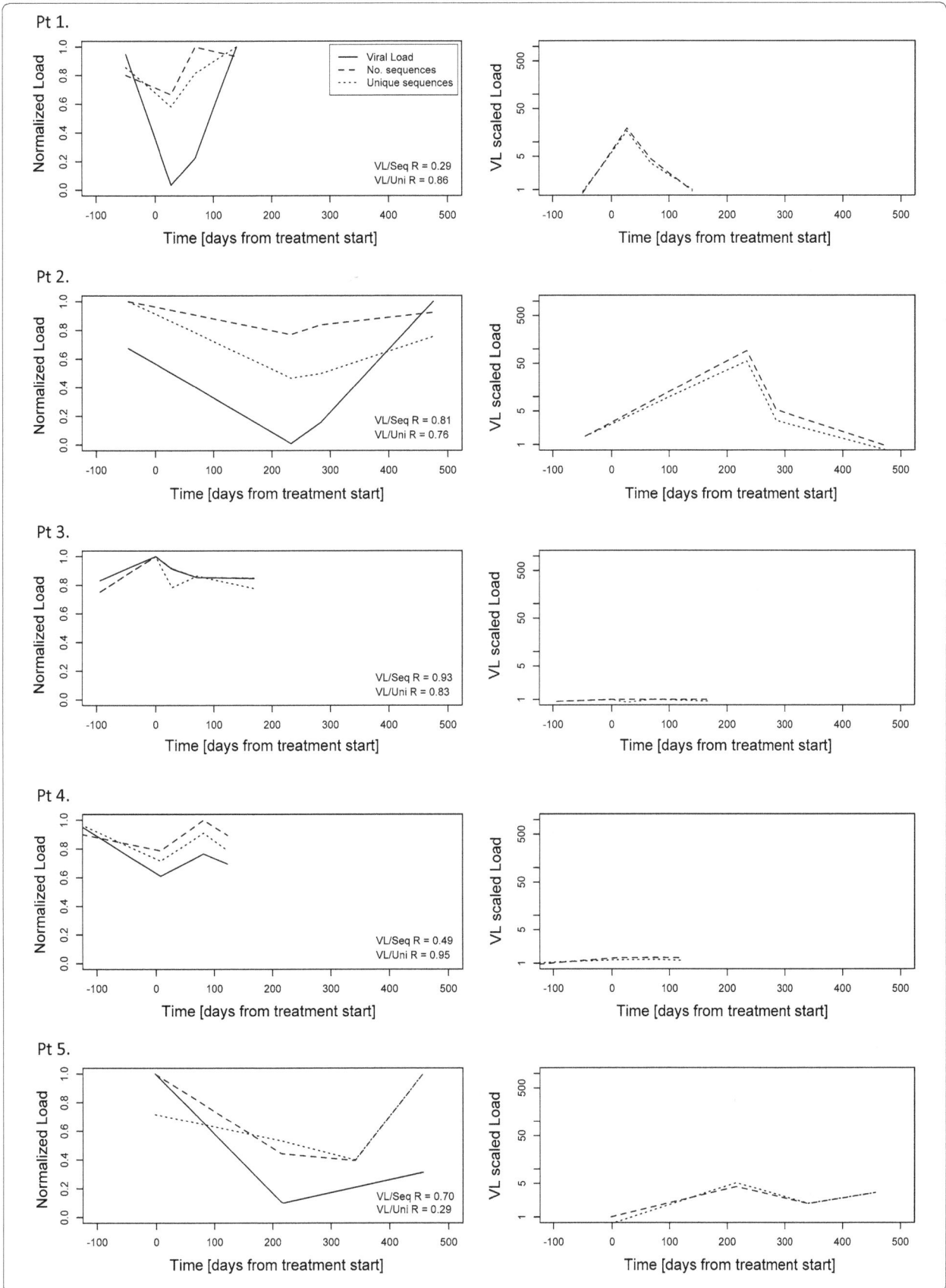

Fig. 3 Viral load versus total number of sequences and number of unique variants. Left panels: the normalized (range 0–1) viral load, number of detected sequences and unique number of variants. The correlation coefficient, R, is indicated for the comparisons to the viral load. Right panels: the relative number of derived sequences and the number of unique variants relative to the viral load. Figures were generated using the nucleotide sequences and the redundancy-level for calling a variant was set at 80

(R = 0.29–0.95). However, in a few cases either the number of sequences detected (Pt1 and Pt4) or the number of unique variants (Pt5) showed weaker correlations and thus we also investigated the population diversity relative to the viral load. Therefore, the normalized number of sequences and unique variants were divided by the normalized viral load respectively (Fig. 3, right panels). Interestingly, in patients 1, 2 and 5, the proportion of unique sequence variants appeared to increase when the viral load dropped. This suggests a sudden diversifying pressure on the viral population. In contrast, in patients 3 and 4 there appeared to be no correlation between the relative number of unique variants and the viral load which coincided with the smallest reductions in viral load during raltegravir containing cART (Fig. 1c, d). These data indicate that the stronger the bottleneck is (i.e. largest reduction in viral load), the larger the effect is on subsequent diversification. Thus, extinction due to antiretroviral treatment appears to induce diversification.

The genetic background is not paramount for the emerging INSTI resistance pathway

To investigate the role of the viral genetic background in determining the raltegravir resistance pathway we cloned the integrase coding region from pre-raltegravir therapy

samples from two patients (Pt1 and Pt2) in an HXB2 reference background. These recombinant viruses were derived from amplicons of pre-raltegravir samples with a viral load of 21,800 and 51,600 c/ml respectively, creating libraries containing thousands of patient-derived sequences for both samples.

In these patients, raltegravir resistance developed through different pathways during raltegravir therapy. In Pt1, resistance developed initially through E138K + Q148K and later a second variant emerged with N155H (Fig. 1a). In Pt2, raltegravir resistance developed initially through N155H and was complemented by two secondary mutations, Q95K and V151I, which made up nearly 100% of the viral population during prolonged therapy failure (Fig. 1b). With the recombinant viruses of these raltegravir baseline samples and HXB2 reference virus (molecular clone from pHXB2AF, therefore a single sequence input per replicate) multiple in vitro selections were performed in parallel.

All cultures were maintained for 10 serial passages to a final concentration of 1024 nM raltegravir. HXB2 virus predominantly selected mutation Q148K (in three out of the five independent cultures), N155H was selected once and in one culture only secondary resistance mutations emerged (Fig. 4). Two of the Q148K mutations were

									Integrase									
	position	68	72	74	92	121	138	140	143	148	151	155	163	230	232	233	265	280
	HXB2 aa	L	V	L	E	F	E	G	Y	Q	V	N	G	S	N	P	A	C
n = 5																		
#1	HXB2	-	-	-	-	-	-	A	-	K	-	-	-	-	-	-	-	-
#2	HXB2	-	-	M	-	Y	-	-	-	-	I	-	R	-	-	-	-	-
#3	HXB2	-	V/I	-	-	-	K	-	-	K	-	-	-	-	-	-	-	-
#4	HXB2	-	-	-	-	-	-	A	-	K	-	-	-	-	-	-	-	-
#5	HXB2	-	-	-	Q	-	-	-	-	-	I	H	-	-	-	-	-	-
n = 5	baseline aa		I												D		V	
#1 pt1 (148 pathway)		-	I	-	-	-	K	C	-	K	-	-	-	-	D	-	V	-
#2 pt1 (148 pathway)		-	I	L/M	-	-	-	-	C	-	-	H	R	S/K/R/N	D	-	V	-
#3 pt1 (148 pathway)		-	I	-	-	-	-	R	-	H	-	-	-	D	S	V	-	
#4 pt1 (148 pathway)		-	I	-	-	-	-	S	-	R	-	-	-	-	D	-	A	-
#5 pt1 (148 pathway)		-	I	-	-	-	-	S	-	H	-	-	-	-	D	-	V	-
n = 5	baseline aa		V/I												D			
#1 pt2 (155 pathway)		-	I	-	-	-	-	S	-	H	-	-	R	-	D	-	-	-
#2 pt2 (155 pathway)		-	I	-	-	-	-	S	-	H	-	-	-	-	H	-	-	Y
#4 pt2 (155 pathway)		V	I	-	-	-	-	-	-	-	-	-	-	-	D	-	-	-

Fig. 4 Raltegravir in vitro selections with patient-derived integrase recombinant viruses. Raltegravir concentration was doubled in each serial passage to a final concentration of 1024 nM of raltegravir in passage 10. All differences from the HXB2 reference sequence are given and mutations emerging during the raltegravir in vitro selections in the viral integrase coding region are indicated in red. The indicated mutations were detected by population sequencing of viral RNA in the culture supernatants from passage 10. Cultures 3 and 5 from Pt2 were discontinued due to failed virus propagation

accompanied by G140A, the third by E138K. G140S was probably not selected because it required two nucleotide changes in this HXB2 background; G140A and E138K required just one. The N155H-virus additionally acquired mutations V151I and later E92Q. Amino acid substitutions at residue 143 were not observed. In vitro selections with Pt1 recombinant virus yielded amino acid substitutions at all three major resistance positions. Again, Q148 mutations dominated (3/5 cultures). Interestingly, in the two other cultures, N155H emerged in combination with amino acid substitutions at position 143 (one with Y143C and one with Y143R, Fig. 4). The mutations selected in vitro differed remarkably from what was observed in vivo. The difference between in vivo and in vitro resistance was even more profound for Pt2. In vivo, only mutations relating to the N155H pathway were observed and no other significant mutations were detected by deep sequencing. In contrast, in vitro only mutations from the Q148 pathway were detected (Fig. 4). Cultures #1 and #2 both developed raltegravir resistance through G140S + Q148H. Culture #1 initially selected G140S + Q148R but later switched to Q148H (not shown). Two of the five cultures were not able to replicate at higher raltegravir concentrations. When an earlier passage of both cultures was sequenced, no mutations in the viral integrase were found so these cultures were discontinued. A third culture only selected an L68V substitution, but this virus did not demonstrate phenotypic resistance when tested (data not shown).

Discussion

We investigated the impact of the genetic background and viral population size on the development and evolution of raltegravir resistance in vitro and in vivo. Deep sequencing revealed presence of major raltegravir resistance mutations at baseline in 3/5 patients (patients (1, 3 and 4, Fig. 2a) at very low frequencies ($\leq$ 0.2%). Only the major resistance mutation detected before therapy in Pt3, Y143C (0.2% in 2nd sample on day 0), ultimately became the dominant variant in the resistant population although it surprisingly disappeared from the subsequent sample to reappear in the 4th sample (11.8% on day 70). In the final sample (169 days) Y143C was not detected anymore but virus with mutation Y143R completely dominated the viral population. In the majority of subtype B viruses, the Y143R substitution requires two nucleotide changes (Y143 = T$\underline{A}$C $\rightarrow$ T$\underline{G}$C = 143C $\rightarrow$ $\underline{C}$GC = 143R). So it appears that the Y143C variant detected at baseline facilitated selection of the more resistant Y143R variant [27] in this patient. In Pt 1, secondary resistance mutation E138K was detected at baseline (0.1%) and appeared to have acquired Q148K as in the subsequent sample a double mutant with E138K + Q148K was detected (0.5%)

which persevered in the population (44.7% in the final sample). This suggests that minor variants present at baseline can play a role in the development and evolution of raltegravir resistance but are not essential for the emergence of resistance [40–42], which is also seen for other drug classes [43, 44].

Remarkably, in Pt1 a variant with major mutation N155H and no apparent secondary resistance mutations emerged after and then co-existed alongside the E138K + Q148K double mutant, each comprising roughly 50% of the viral population. This suggests a fitness advantage for the N155H single mutant over the E138K + Q148K double mutant. This is unexpected considering the in vitro observations regarding resistance and replication of these mutants [17, 45, 46]. A possible explanation could be the so-called hitchhiking effect; this particular variant had a fitness advantage that was located outside the investigated region. For instance, resistance against any of the other antiretrovirals in the therapy regimen (e.g. efavirenz) could have been present in this variant but not in the other variants. While the chances that this occurs in one of the minority variants and not in any of the dominant species are small, the possibility cannot be excluded. Another possible explanation is that the variant with the N155H mutation is more fit than the E138K + Q148K mutant in the presence of raltegravir in this particular setting due to other factors (e.g. specific viral genetic background, immunological host factors, etc.).

We also observed a correlation between the number of unique sequence variants emerging and the magnitude of the virological response. Good virological response in Pts 1, 2 and 5 (> 2 log reductions in HIV-1 RNA) coincided with the number of unique sequence variants observed; the proportion of unique sequence variants increased when the viral load dropped. Pts 3 and 4 demonstrated moderate responses with viral load drops of around 1 log and showed no change in the relative frequencies of unique variants over the course of sampling. This suggests that in Pts 1, 2 and 5, treatment with raltegravir induced an elevated diversification to escape drug pressure while in Pts 3 and 4 the pressure on the population seemed to occur to a much lesser extent. This observation reminds of the explosive diversifications on a macro-evolutionary scale observed in other fields of biology after ice ages and the cataclysmic extinction of dinosaurs [47, 48]. However, regardless of treatment efficacy, i.e. both in patients with less dramatic and more severe virus load reductions, raltegravir resistance mutations developed and multiple resistance pathways were observed in 4/5 patients. The large extinction opens up previously occupied niches for new virus variants, (1) such that all new mutations are accepted and not compete for resources until the population regains a size limited by the carrying capacity of the system, or (2) most of the diversity pre-existed as a permanent, extremely low frequency pool of highly diverse viruses persisting in the shadow of more fit and high frequency variants. Once the high frequency variants are eradicated (e.g. by newly introduced drugs) a glimpse of that diversity surfaces. The larger the impact on the high frequency variants (i.e. reduction in viral load) the larger the proportion of the low frequency pool appears (i.e. number of unique variants increases when the viral load drops). Subsequently, one or two of the low frequency variants gain fitness in the new environment and become dominant, lowering the mean diversity again. The same can be argued from the point of viral escape. If the viral population doesn't have to go that low to find fit variants (in the new environment), the impact on viral load is also less severe.

The raltegravir in vitro selections in which we mimicked population bottlenecking by using a low MOI allowing all resistant variants that are generated to emerge, clearly indicate that the resistance pathway that is selected to escape raltegravir pressure is not predisposed in the genetic background of the integrase CDS. Evaluation of the combined in vivo and in vitro data indicates that stochastic selection plays a major role during the initial development of raltegravir resistance.

In conclusion, the development and evolution of raltegravir resistance can be separated in multiple phases/components: (1) minority variants present at baseline can contribute to the emergence of raltegravir resistance but this is not preordained and seems to occur arbitrarily; (2) during the viral load drop due to drug pressure a burst of new sequence variants emerges creating diversifying selection; (3) these new variants usually include multiple raltegravir resistant variants (from multiple resistance pathways) that can pass the imposed bottleneck; (4) competition of these resistant variants determines the ultimate shape of the viral population. The resistant population can be the product of a single variant that outcompetes all others and only one variant represents the population or multiple variants with a similar fitness emerge that coexist in the viral population.

Further investigation is needed to better assess the exact impact of baseline minority resistance variants and the population size on the development and evolution of raltegravir resistance and determine the clinical implications of these factors.

Conclusions

Emergence of resistance against integrase inhibitor raltegravir in HIV-1 patients is generally associated with selection of one of three distinct resistance pathways. The mechanisms that drive selection of a specific pathway

are still poorly understood. Using deep sequencing we observed an inverse correlation between the virological response and the relative amount of unique sequence variants emerging, suggesting diversifying selection during drug pressure. In 4/5 patients multiple signature mutations representing different resistance pathways were observed. In addition, in vitro selections revealed that identical viral clones were also able to select mutations from different resistance pathways indicating that raltegravir resistance is not predisposed in the genetic background of the viral integrase. Importantly, raltegravir resistance develops progressively and discontinuation during early phases of therapy failure is justified to preserve future options with second-generation INSTIs.

Methods
Genotypic analysis
Population sequencing

HIV-1 RNA was isolated using the Nuclisens Islolation kit (BioMérieux, Boxtel, The Netherlands). Briefly, 100 µl of sample was mixed with 900 µl lysisbuffer and 40 µl silica and incubated for 10 min at room temperature to allow binding of the nucleic acid to the silica particles. Unbound material was removed by several washing steps after which the RNA was eluted at 56 °C with 100 µl of 40 ng/µl poly-A RNA. The isolated viral RNA was used to reverse transcribe and amplify the viral integrase coding region in a single-step reaction using the Titan One Tube RT-PCR kit (Roche). The RT-PCR was conducted with primers 5′INoutF1 (5′-GGA ATC ATT CAA GCA CAA CCA GA-3′; 4059–4081) and 3′INoutR1 (5′-TGT ATG CAG ACC CCA ATA TGT TG-3′; 5262–5241). The amount of amplified product was further enhanced in a second PCR using the Expand High fidelity kit (Roche) with primers 5′INinF1 (5′-TAT CTG GCA TGG GTA CCA GCA C-3′; 4143–4164) and 3′INinR1 (5′-TAG TGG GAT GTG TAC TTC TGA AC-3′; 5217–5195). All PCR-amplified products were purified using the QIAquick PCR purification kit (Qiagen, Leusden, The Netherlands). Sequence analysis was performed with the BigDye Terminator v3.1 Cycle Sequencing Kit (Applied Biosystems, Foster City, CA, USA). Integrase sequences were obtained using six primers: Intseq1 (5′-ATT GGA GGA AAT GAA CAA GT-3′; 4173–4192), Intseq2 (5′-AGC AGA AGT TAT TCC AGC AG-3′; 4484–4503), INT-3 (5′-TTC GGG TTT ATT ACA G-3′; 4897–4912), INT-4 (5′-CTT GTA TTA CTA CTG C-3′; 4986–4971), Intseq-5 (5′-CTG GCT ACA TGA ACT GCT AC-3′; 4470–4452) and 3′INinR2 (5′-GCT TTC ATA GTG ATG TCT ATA AAA CC-3′; 5178–5153). Sequence editing and contig assembly were performed using SeqScape v2.6 (Applied Biosystems) with HXB2 as a reference sequence.

Next-generation sequencing and data analysis

To examine the mutation frequencies within the viral integrase by pyrosequencing, RNA was reverse transcribed and amplified in a single step in a touch-down PCR using bar-coded primers to enable 454 pyrosequencing with pooled amplicons. The integrase core domain from amino acid position 53 to amino acid 180 was analyzed. All mutations in the viral integrase at 18 different codons associated with raltegravir resistance [16, 20, 23, 45, 49–52] were evaluated and included amino acids: T66, L68, V72, L74, E92, Q95, T97, F121, E138, G140, Y143, Q148, V151, N155, K156, E157, K160 and G163.

All amplicons were purified with AMPure magnetic beads (Agencourt, Beckman Coulter, Krefeld, Germany), quality checked and quantified using an Agilent 2100 Bioanalyser (Agilent Life Sciences, Waldbronn, Germany) and picogreen using the fluorometer Fluostar Optima (BMG Labtech, Offenburg, Germany), respectively. After equimolar pooling of the amplicons, emulsion PCRs were performed. Pyrosequencing was done using primers A and B (Titanium emPCR kit Lib-L v2; Roche-454 Life Sciences, Branford, CT, USA). After bead recovery and enrichment, approximately 250,000 beads per pool were loaded on one region of a GS FLX PicoTiter plate subdivided with a four-lane gasket. Pyrosequencing was performed on a Genome Sequencer FLX (Roche-454 Life Sciences). Sequence readings from the 454 pyrosequencing run were extracted directly from the Standard-Flowgram-Files (sff). Reads were pair-wise aligned against the integrase sequence of reference strain HXB2. Multiple mutations present in a single read were assumed to originate from the same genome.

The dynamics of the sequence populations were investigated on de-aligned sets to avoid artifacts due to inconsistent alignment gap placements using statistical functions in R [53]. For the analyses of the dominant variants in the populations, the redundancy-level for calling a variant was set at 80, i.e. only variants detected at least 80 times were considered. This level resulted in a strict filter that removed all known 454-sequencing artifacts [54–56]. The resulting dominant variants were aligned using MAFFT [57] and distance matrices were estimated using the R library ape [58] under a F84 substitution model (the choice of substitution model had no effect on the subsequent analyses). The R library sna [59] was used to construct minimum spanning trees (MSTs) based on the distance matrices of patient's HIV population. Nodes were scaled according to both viral load and the relative abundance of each detected variant at time of sampling. We tracked known resistance mutations on the edges and edge lengths were drawn arbitrary in order to make the resulting graphs easy to look at.

Construction of deletion clone HXB2ΔINT

An HXB2 molecular clone (pHXB2AF) was used to construct a molecular deletion clone lacking the integrase coding region. pHXB2AF is derived from pHXB2WT [60], which expresses the full length HIV-1 sequence HXB2 (9719 bp, Genbank accession number K03455.1), with all bacterial sequences non-essential for bacterial expression and replication removed.

The NdeI site present in Gp120 (at HXB2 nt 6404) was inactivated to create a unique NdeI site at the 3′ end of the integrase CDS. Therefore pHXB2AF was digested with NcoI (Roche Diagnostics, Almere, The Netherlands) and NheI (New England Biolabs, Ipswich, MA, USA) to remove a 1586 bp fragment containing the NdeI site. PCR, using Vent$_R$ ® DNA polymerase (New England BioLabs) was performed on pHXB2AF with primers, NcoI-out (5′ CAC TAG AGC TTT TAG AGG AGC TTA AGA-3′; 5614–5640), NheI-out (5′-TTT TAT TAT TTC CAA ATT GTT CTC TTA-3′; 7296–7270) and NdeI-KO (5′-TCA G̲AT GCT AAA GCG TAT GAT ACA G-3′; 6390–6414). Primer NdeI-KO contained one silent nucleotide change (underlined) to inactivate the NdeI site in the PCR fragment. The amount of amplified product was further increased and enriched by performing a second amplification using Vent$_R$ ® DNA polymerase with primers NcoI-in (5′-GAG CTT TTA GAG GAG CTT AAG AAT GAA-3′; 5619–5645), NheI-in (5′-ATT GTT CTC TTA ATT TGC TAG CTA TCT-3′; 7281–7255) and NdeI-KO. This PCR fragment was then digested with NcoI and NheI and ligated with the digested pHXB2AF, resulting in pHXB2AFNdeIKO which was confirmed by sequence analysis of the complete fragment.

Subsequently, the integrase coding region was removed from pHXB2AFNdeIKO. Therefore pHXB2AFNdeIKO was digested with MluNI (Roche) and NdeI (New England BioLabs). The fragment between MluNI and the 5′ end of integrase was restored by performing a PCR on pHXB2AF using primers RT19 (5′-GGA CAT AAA GCT ATA GGT ACA G-3′; 2454–2472) and NgoMIV-INTlinker (5′-TAA TAT CAT ATG GAC AGC GTC G̲CC GG̲C ACT GAC TAA TTT ATC TAC TTG TTC-3′). Primer NgoMIV-INTlinker contained two silent nucleotide changes with respect to pHXB2AFNdeIKO, thereby introducing a unique NgoMIV site (underlined 4209–4214) in the PCR fragment. In addition to these nucleotide changes the primer NgoMIV-INTlinker contains a linker sequence with a unique NdeI site and an AspI site. AspI was used to prevent re-ligation of the vector and the linker. The amount of amplified product was further increased and enriched by performing a second amplification using Vent$_R$ ® DNA polymerase with primers RT19new2 (5′-GGA CCT ACA CCT GTC AAC ATA ATT GG-3′; 2484–2509) and NgoMIV-INTlinker. The

PCR fragment was then digested with MluNI and NdeI and ligated with the digested pHXB2AFNdeIKO, resulting in a molecular deletion clone lacking the integrase coding region (pHXB2AFΔINT), which was confirmed by sequencing the complete fragment.

Generation of recombinant virus

To generate recombinant viruses, the second PCR as described in the population sequencing section, was performed with a different primer pair: forward primer NgoMIV-Int2 (5'-TTA GTC AGT GCC GGC ATC AGG AAA G-3'; 4200–4224) which contains a NgoMIV restriction site (underlined) and reverse primer 3INinR2. The obtained integrase fragment and vector pHXB2AFΔINT were digested with restriction enzymes NgoMIV (New England BioLabs) and NdeI. The PCR product and vector pHXB2AFΔINT were ligated overnight at 4 °C using the Rapid Ligation System (Promega, Benelux, Leiden, The Netherlands). After ligation, plasmids were digested with AspI and subsequently transformed into competent cells. Bacteria were cultured overnight at 37 °C. Plasmid isolation was performed using the QIAgen Plasmid Mini kit (Qiagen).

Viruses were generated by transfecting 293T cells with 10 ug plasmid DNA using Lipofectamine 2000 reagent (Invitrogen) according the manufacturer's protocol. Two days after infection cell free virus was harvested and the viral infectivity ($TCID_{50}$) was determined using endpoint dilutions in MT2 cells.

Viral and cell culture

Cells

SupT1 and MT-2 cells were maintained in RPMI 1640 medium with L-glutamine (Lonza, Verviers, Belgium) supplemented with 10% FBS (FBS; Sigma-Aldrich, Zwijndrecht, The Netherlands) and 10 µg/ml gentamicin (Invitrogen, Breda, The Netherlands). 293T cells were maintained in DMEM with L-glutamine (Lonza) supplemented with 10% FBS and 10 µg/ml gentamicin.

In vitro selection experiments

The raltegravir in vitro selection experiments with two recombinant viruses that contained patient-derived integrase CDS and HIV-1 reference strain HXB2 were each performed 5 times. The in vitro selections were initiated by infecting 2×10^6 SupT1 cells at a multiplicity of infection (MOI) of 0.001. The initial raltegravir concentration was 2 nM Raltegravir. Cultures were monitored daily for cytopatic effect (CPE) and twice a week half of the medium was replaced by fresh medium supplemented with raltegravir. When full blown CPE was observed, cell free virus was harvested. The raltegravir concentration

was raised in each passage to a final concentration of 1024 nM in passage 10. After passage 10, HIV-1 RNA was isolated from all cultures for genotypic analysis. As a control, in vitro evolution experiments (10 passages) were performed with HXB2 reference strain (5 individual cultures) to monitor the evolution of the integrase CDS during culture in absence of inhibitor.

Phenotypic drug susceptibility analysis

Drug susceptibility was determined by a multiple cycle cell-killing assay [61]. MT-2 cells (4×10^4 in 200 µl RPMI 10% FBS per well) were plated in 96-well microplates. Sample virus and reference virus were inoculated for five days on a single 96-well plate in the presence of threefold dilutions of raltegravir. Both sample virus and reference virus were inoculated at multiple MOIs to adjust for any differences in viral RC. Fold change (FC) values were calculated by dividing the mean 50% inhibitory concentration (EC_{50}) for a sample virus by that of the HXB2 reference strain.

Authors' contributions

AF, LV, AW and MN designed the study. MD, BB, IH and AW collected patient information and provided samples or sequences. AF, MD, AT and PS generated the data. AF, TL, AW and MN analyzed and interpreted the data and wrote the manuscript. All authors read and approved the final manuscript.

Author details

[1] Department of Medical Microbiology, Virology, University Medical Center Utrecht, Heidelberglaan 100, HP G04.614, 3584 CX Utrecht, The Netherlands. [2] Theoretical Biology and Biophysics, Los Alamos National Laboratory, Los Alamos, NM, USA. [3] Department of General Internal Medicine and Infectious Diseases, Ghent University Hospital, Ghent, Belgium. [4] Institute of Immunology and Genetics, Kaiserslautern, Germany. [5] Max Planck Institute for Informatics, Saarbrücken, Germany. [6] Pediatric Clinic, University Medical Center Mannheim, Mannheim, Germany. [7] Department of Internal Medicine and Infectious Diseases, University Medical Center Utrecht, Utrecht, The Netherlands. [8] Department of Internal Medicine, Rijnstate Hospital, Arnhem, The Netherlands.

Acknowledgements

Raltegravir was obtained through the NIH AIDS Reagent Program, Division of AIDS, NIAID, NIH: Raltegravir (Cat # 11680) from Merck & Company, Inc.

Competing interests

The authors declare no competing financial or other interests.

Funding

This work was supported by (AF) the Dutch AIDS Fund (Project Number 2006028), (MN) the Netherlands Organization for Scientific Research (NOW VIDI Grant 91796349) and TL was supported by the National Institutes of Health (NIH Grant R01AI087520). The funders had no role in study design, collecting, analyzing or interpreting the data, or in the preparation of the manuscript.

References

1. Palella FJ Jr, Delaney KM, Moorman AC, Loveless MO, Fuhrer J, Satten GA, Aschman DJ, Holmberg SD. Declining morbidity and mortality among patients with advanced human immunodeficiency virus infection. HIV Outpatient study investigators. N Engl J Med. 1998;338:853–60.

2. Boyer JC, Bebenek K, Kunkel TA. Unequal human immunodeficiency virus type 1 reverse transcriptase error rates with RNA and DNA templates. Proc Natl Acad Sci USA. 1992;89:6919–23.

3. Ji JP, Loeb LA. Fidelity of HIV-1 reverse transcriptase copying RNA in vitro. Biochemistry. 1992;31:954–8.

4. Menendez-Arias L. Molecular basis of fidelity of DNA synthesis and nucleotide specificity of retroviral reverse transcriptases. Prog Nucleic Acid Res Mol Biol. 2002;71:91–147.

5. Bonhoeffer S, May RM, Shaw GM, Nowak MA. Virus dynamics and drug therapy. Proc Natl Acad Sci USA. 1997;94:6971–6.

6. Nowak MA, Bonhoeffer S, Shaw GM, May RM. Anti-viral drug treatment: dynamics of resistance in free virus and infected cell populations. J Theor Biol. 1997;184:203–17. https://doi.org/10.1006/jtbi.1996.0307.

7. Nijhuis M, Boucher CA, Schipper P, Leitner T, Schuurman R, Albert J. Stochastic processes strongly influence HIV-1 evolution during suboptimal protease-inhibitor therapy. Proc Natl Acad Sci USA. 1998;95:14441–6.

8. Duffy S, Shackelton LA, Holmes EC. Rates of evolutionary change in viruses: patterns and determinants. Nat Rev Genet. 2008;9:267–76. https://doi.org/10.1038/nrg2323.

9. Alexander HK, Bonhoeffer S. Pre-existence and emergence of drug resistance in a generalized model of intra-host viral dynamics. Epidemics. 2012;4:187–202. https://doi.org/10.1016/j.epidem.2012.10.001.

10. Espeseth AS, Felock P, Wolfe A, Witmer M, Grobler J, Anthony N, Egbertson M, Melamed JY, Young S, Hamill T, et al. HIV-1 integrase inhibitors that compete with the target DNA substrate define a unique strand transfer conformation for integrase. Proc Natl Acad Sci USA. 2000;97:11244–9. https://doi.org/10.1073/pnas.200139397.

11. Hare S, Gupta SS, Valkov E, Engelman A, Cherepanov P. Retroviral intasome assembly and inhibition of DNA strand transfer. Nature. 2010;464:232–6. https://doi.org/10.1038/nature08784.

12. Krishnan L, Li X, Naraharisetty HL, Hare S, Cherepanov P, Engelman A. Structure-based modeling of the functional HIV-1 intasome and its inhibition. Proc Natl Acad Sci USA. 2010;107:15910–5. https://doi.org/10.1073/pnas.1002346107.

13. ISENTRESS™ (raltegravir) for treatment of HIV (NDA 22145 S036). FDA May 31 2017. https://www.accessdata.fda.gov/drugsatfda_docs/label/2017/022145s036,203045s013,205786s004lbl.pdf.

14. Messiaen P, Wensing AM, Fun A, Nijhuis M, Brusselaers N, Vandekerckhove L. Clinical use of HIV integrase inhibitors: a systematic review and meta-analysis. PLoS ONE. 2013;8:e52562. https://doi.org/10.1371/journal.pone.0052562.

15. Rockstroh JK, DeJesus E, Lennox JL, Yazdanpanah Y, Saag MS, Wan H, Rodgers AJ, Walker ML, Miller M, DiNubile MJ, et al. Durable efficacy and safety of raltegravir versus efavirenz when combined with tenofovir/emtricitabine in treatment-naive HIV-1-infected patients: final 5-year results from STARTMRK. J Acquir Immune Defic Syndr. 2013;63:77–85. https://doi.org/10.1097/QAI.0b013e31828ace69.

16. Cooper DA, Steigbigel RT, Gatell JM, Rockstroh JK, Katlama C, Yeni P, Lazzarin A, Clotet B, Kumar PN, Eron JE, et al. Subgroup and resistance analyses of raltegravir for resistant HIV-1 infection. N Engl J Med. 2008;359:355–65.

17. Miller MD, Danovich R, Ke Y, Witmer M, Zhao J, Harvey C, Nguyen BY, Hazuda DJ: Longitudinal analysis of resistance to the HIV-1 integrase inhibitor raltegravir: results from P005 a phase 2 study in treatment experienced patients. In: XVII international HIV drug resistance workshop, Sitges, Spain. 2008.

18. Johnson VA, Brun-Vezinet F, Clotet B, Gunthard HF, Kuritzkes DR, Pillay D, Schapiro JM, Richman DD. Update of the drug resistance mutations in HIV-1: December 2010. Top HIV Med. 2010;18:156–63.

19. Fransen S, Gupta S, Danovich R, Hazuda D, Miller M, Witmer M, Petropoulos CJ, Huang W. Loss of raltegravir susceptibility by human immunodeficiency virus type 1 is conferred via multiple nonoverlapping genetic pathways. J Virol. 2009;83:11440–6.

20. Malet I, Delelis O, Valantin MA, Montes B, Soulie C, Wirden M, Tchertanov L, Peytavin G, Reynes J, Mouscadet JF, et al. Mutations associated with failure of raltegravir treatment affect integrase sensitivity to the inhibitor in vitro. Antimicrob Agents Chemother. 2008;52:1351–8.

21. Nakahara K, Wakasa-Morimoto C, Kobayashi M, Miki S, Noshi T, Seki T, Kanamori-Koyama M, Kawauchi S, Suyama A, Fujishita T, et al. Secondary mutations in viruses resistant to HIV-1 integrase inhibitors that restore viral infectivity and replication kinetics. Antivir Res. 2009;81:141–6.

22. Quercia R, Dam E, Perez-Bercoff D, Clavel F. Selective-advantage profile of human immunodeficiency virus type 1 integrase mutants explains in vivo evolution of raltegravir resistance genotypes. J Virol. 2009;83:10245–9.

23. Fun A, Van Baelen K, van Lelyveld SF, Schipper PJ, Stuyver LJ, Wensing AM, Nijhuis M. Mutation Q95K enhances N155H-mediated integrase inhibitor resistance and improves viral replication capacity. J Antimicrob Chemother. 2010;65:2300–4.

24. Blanco JL, Varghese V, Rhee SY, Gatell JM, Shafer RW. HIV-1 integrase inhibitor resistance and its clinical implications. J Infect Dis. 2011;203:1204–14.

25. Anstett K, Brenner B, Mesplede T, Wainberg MA. HIV drug resistance against strand transfer integrase inhibitors. Retrovirology. 2017;14:36. https://doi.org/10.1186/s12977-017-0360-7.

26. Malet I, Delelis O, Soulie C, Wirden M, Tchertanov L, Mottaz P, Peytavin G, Katlama C, Mouscadet JF, Calvez V, Marcelin AG. Quasispecies variant dynamics during emergence of resistance to raltegravir in HIV-1-infected patients. J Antimicrob Chemother. 2009;63:795–804.

27. Reigadas S, Anies G, Masquelier B, Calmels C, Stuyver LJ, Parissi V, Fleury H, Andreola ML. The HIV-1 integrase mutations Y143C/R are an alternative pathway for resistance to Raltegravir and impact the enzyme functions. PLoS ONE. 2010;5:e10311. https://doi.org/10.1371/journal.pone.0010311.

28. da Silva D, Van Wesenbeeck L, Breilh D, Reigadas S, Anies G, Van Baelen K, Morlat P, Neau D, Dupon M, Wittkop L, et al. HIV-1 resistance patterns to integrase inhibitors in antiretroviral-experienced patients with virological failure on raltegravir-containing regimens. J Antimicrob Chemother. 2010;65:1262–9. https://doi.org/10.1093/jac/dkq099.

29. Mukherjee R, Jensen ST, Male F, Bittinger K, Hodinka RL, Miller MD, Bushman FD. Switching between raltegravir resistance pathways analyzed by deep sequencing. AIDS. 2011;25:1951–9. https://doi.org/10.1097/QAD.0b013e32834b34de.

30. Goethals O, Vos A, Van Ginderen M, Geluykens P, Smits V, Schols D, Hertogs K, Clayton R. Primary mutations selected in vitro with raltegravir confer large fold changes in susceptibility to first-generation integrase inhibitors, but minor fold changes to inhibitors with second-generation resistance profiles. Virology. 2010;402:338–46.

31. Metifiot M, Vandegraaff N, Maddali K, Naumova A, Zhang X, Rhodes D, Marchand C, Pommier Y. Elvitegravir overcomes resistance to raltegravir induced by integrase mutation Y143. Aids. 2011;25:1175–8.

32. Castagna A, Maggiolo F, Penco G, Wright D, Mills A, Grossberg R, Molina JM, Chas J, Durant J, Moreno S, et al. Dolutegravir in antiretroviral-experienced patients with raltegravir- and/or elvitegravir-resistant HIV-1: 24-week results of the phase III VIKING-3 study. J Infect Dis. 2014;210:354–62. https://doi.org/10.1093/infdis/jiu051.

33. Akil B, Blick G, Hagins DP, Ramgopal MN, Richmond GJ, Samuel RM, Givens N, Vavro C, Song IH, Wynne B, Ait-Khaled M. Dolutegravir versus placebo in subjects harbouring HIV-1 with integrase inhibitor resistance associated substitutions: 48-week results from VIKING-4, a randomized study. Antivir Ther. 2015;20:343–8. https://doi.org/10.3851/IMP2878.

34. Hofstra LM, Nijhuis M, Mudrikova T, Fun A, Schipper P, Schneider M, Wensing A. Use of dolutegravir in two INI-experienced patients with multiclass resistance resulted in excellent virological and immunological responses. J Int AIDS Soc. 2014;17:19755. https://doi.org/10.7448/IAS.17.4.19755.

35. Seki T, Kobayashi M, Wakasa-Morimoto C, Yoshinaga T, Sato A, Fujiwara T, Underwood MR, Garvey EP, Johns BA: S/GSK1349572 is a potent next generation HIV integrase inhibitor and demonstrates a superior resistance profile substantiated with 60 integrase mutant molecular clones. In: 17th conference on retroviruses and opportunistic infections, San Francisco, CA, USA. 2010.

36. Brenner BG, Wainberg MA. Clinical benefit of dolutegravir in HIV-1 management related to the high genetic barrier to drug resistance. Virus Res. 2017;239:1–9. https://doi.org/10.1016/j.virusres.2016.07.006

37. Laskey SB, Siliciano RF. Quantitative evaluation of the antiretroviral efficacy of dolutegravir. JCI Insight. 2016;1:e90033. https://doi.org/10.1172/jci.insight.90033.

38. Malet I, Gimferrer Arriaga L, Artese A, Costa G, Parrotta L, Alcaro S, Delelis O, Tmeizeh A, Katlama C, Valantin MA, et al. New raltegravir resistance pathways induce broad cross-resistance to all currently used integrase inhibitors. J Antimicrob Chemother. 2014;69:2118–22. https://doi.org/10.1093/jac/dku095.

39. Brenner BG, Thomas R, Blanco JL, Ibanescu RI, Oliveira M, Mesplede T, Golubkov O, Roger M, Garcia F, Martinez E, Wainberg MA. Development of a G118R mutation in HIV-1 integrase following a switch to dolutegravir monotherapy leading to cross-resistance to integrase inhibitors. J Antimicrob Chemother. 2016;71:1948–53. https://doi.org/10.1093/jac/dkw071.

40. Liu J, Miller MD, Danovich RM, Vandergrift N, Cai F, Hicks CB, Hazuda DJ, Gao F. Analysis of low-frequency mutations associated with drug resistance to raltegravir before antiretroviral treatment. Antimicrob Agents Chemother. 2010;55:1114–9. https://doi.org/10.1128/AAC.01492-10.

41. Charpentier C, Laureillard D, Piketty C, Tisserand P, Batisse D, Karmochkine M, Si-Mohamed A, Weiss L. High frequency of integrase Q148R minority variants in HIV-infected patients naive of integrase inhibitors. AIDS. 2010;24:867–73. https://doi.org/10.1097/QAD.0b013e3283367796.

42. Codoner FM, Pou C, Thielen A, Garcia F, Delgado R, Dalmau D, Santos JR, Buzon MJ, Martinez-Picado J, Alvarez-Tejado M, et al. Dynamic escape of pre-existing raltegravir-resistant HIV-1 from raltegravir selection pressure. Antivir Res. 2010;88:281–6. https://doi.org/10.1016/j.antiviral.2010.09.016.

43. Johnson JA, Geretti AM. Low-frequency HIV-1 drug resistance mutations can be clinically significant but must be interpreted with caution. J Antimicrob Chemother. 2010;65:1322–6. https://doi.org/10.1093/jac/dkq139.

44. Li JZ, Paredes R, Ribaudo HJ, Svarovskaia ES, Metzner KJ, Kozal MJ, Hullsiek KH, Balduin M, Jakobsen MR, Geretti AM, et al. Low-frequency HIV-1 drug resistance mutations and risk of NNRTI-based antiretroviral treatment failure: a systematic review and pooled analysis. JAMA. 2011;305:1327–35. https://doi.org/10.1001/jama.2011.375.

45. Kobayashi M, Nakahara K, Seki T, Miki S, Kawauchi S, Suyama A, Wakasa-Morimoto C, Kodama M, Endoh T, Oosugi E, et al. Selection of diverse and clinically relevant integrase inhibitor-resistant human immunodeficiency virus type 1 mutants. Antivir Res. 2008;80:213–22.

46. Hu Z, Kuritzkes DR. Effect of raltegravir resistance mutations in HIV-1 integrase on viral fitness. J Acquir Immune Defic Syndr. 2010;55:148–55. https://doi.org/10.1097/QAI.0b013e3181e9a87a.

47. Weir JT, Haddrath O, Robertson HA, Colbourne RM, Baker AJ. Explosive ice age diversification of kiwi. Proc Natl Acad Sci USA. 2016;113:E5580–7. https://doi.org/10.1073/pnas.1603795113.

48. Halliday TJD, Goswami A. Eutherian morphological disparity across the end-Cretaceous mass extinction. Biol J Lin Soc. 2016;118:152–68.

49. Charpentier C, Karmochkine M, Laureillard D, Tisserand P, Belec L, Weiss L, Si-Mohamed A, Piketty C. Drug resistance profiles for the HIV integrase gene in patients failing raltegravir salvage therapy. HIV Med. 2008;9:765–70.

50. Goodman D, Hluhanich R, Waters J, Margot NA, Fransen S, Gupta S, Huang W, Parkin N, Borroto-Esoda K, Svarovskaia ES, et al: Integrase inhibitor resistance involves complex interactions among primary and secondary resistance mutations: a novel mutation L68V/I associates with E92Q and increases resistance. In: XVII international HIV drug resistance workshop, Sitges, Spain. 2008.

51. Markowitz M, Nguyen BY, Gotuzzo E, Mendo F, Ratanasuwan W, Kovacs C, Prada G, Morales-Ramirez JO, Crumpacker CS, Isaacs RD, et al. Rapid and durable antiretroviral effect of the HIV-1 integrase inhibitor raltegravir as part of combination therapy in treatment-naive patients with HIV-1 infection: results of a 48-week controlled study. J Acquir Immune Defic Syndr. 2007;46:125–33.

52. Sichtig N, Sierra S, Kaiser R, Daumer M, Reuter S, Schulter E, Altmann A, Fatkenheuer G, Dittmer U, Pfister H, Esser S. Evolution of raltegravir resistance during therapy. J Antimicrob Chemother. 2009;64:25–32.

53. Team RDC: R: a language and environment for statistical computing. R Foundation for Statistical Computing, Vienna, Austria. http://www.R-project.org. 2008.

54. Brodin J, Mild M, Hedskog C, Sherwood E, Leitner T, Andersson B, Albert J. PCR-induced transitions are the major source of error in cleaned ultra-deep pyrosequencing data. PLoS ONE. 2013;8:e70388. https://doi.org/10.1371/journal.pone.0070388.

55. Hedskog C, Mild M, Jernberg J, Sherwood E, Bratt G, Leitner T, Lundeberg J, Andersson B, Albert J. Dynamics of HIV-1 quasispecies during antiviral treatment dissected using ultra-deep pyrosequencing. PLoS ONE. 2010;5:e11345. https://doi.org/10.1371/journal.pone.0011345.

56. Tsibris AM, Korber B, Arnaout R, Russ C, Lo CC, Leitner T, Gaschen B, Theiler J, Paredes R, Su Z, et al. Quantitative deep sequencing reveals dynamic HIV-1 escape and large population shifts during CCR5 antagonist therapy in vivo. PLoS ONE. 2009;4:e5683. https://doi.org/10.1371/journal.pone.0005683.

57. Katoh K, Asimenos G, Toh H. Multiple alignment of DNA sequences with MAFFT. Methods Mol Biol. 2009;537:39–64. https://doi.org/10.1007/978-1-59745-251-9_3.

58. Paradis E, Claude J, Strimmer K. APE: analyses of phylogenetics and evolution in R language. Bioinformatics. 2004;20:289–90.

59. Butts SF, Owen C, Mainigi M, Senapati S, Seifer DB, Dokras A. Assisted hatching and intracytoplasmic sperm injection are not associated with improved outcomes in assisted reproduction cycles for diminished ovarian reserve: an analysis of cycles in the United States from 2004 to 2011. Fertil Steril. 2014;102(1041–1047):e1041. https://doi.org/10.1016/j.fertnstert.2014.06.043.

60. van Maarseveen NM, Huigen MC, de Jong D, Smits AM, Boucher CA, Nijhuis M. A novel real-time PCR assay to determine relative replication capacity for HIV-1 protease variants and/or reverse transcriptase variants. J Virol Methods. 2006;133:185–94. https://doi.org/10.1016/j.jviromet.2005.11.008.

61. Boucher CA, Keulen W, van Bommel T, Nijhuis M, de Jong D, de Jong MD, Schipper P, Back NK. Human immunodeficiency virus type 1 drug susceptibility determination by using recombinant viruses generated from patient sera tested in a cell-killing assay. Antimicrob Agents Chemother. 1996;40:2404–9.

12

RNA-induced epigenetic silencing inhibits HIV-1 reactivation from latency

Catalina Méndez, Scott Ledger, Kathy Petoumenos, Chantelle Ahlenstiel*[iD] and Anthony D. Kelleher

Abstract

Background: Current antiretroviral therapy is effective in controlling HIV-1 infection. However, cessation of therapy is associated with rapid return of viremia from the viral reservoir. Eradicating the HIV-1 reservoir has proven difficult with the limited success of latency reactivation strategies and reflects the complexity of HIV-1 latency. Consequently, there is a growing need for alternate strategies. Here we explore a "block and lock" approach for enforcing latency to render the provirus unable to restart transcription despite exposure to reactivation stimuli. Reactivation of transcription from latent HIV-1 proviruses can be epigenetically blocked using promoter-targeted shRNAs to prevent productive infection. We aimed to determine if independent and combined expression of shRNAs, PromA and 143, induce a repressive epigenetic profile that is sufficiently stable to protect latently infected cells from HIV-1 reactivation when treated with a range of latency reversing agents (LRAs).

Results: J-Lat 9.2 cells, a model of HIV-1 latency, expressing shRNAs PromA, 143, PromA/143 or controls were treated with LRAs to evaluate protection from HIV-1 reactivation as determined by levels of GFP expression. Cells expressing shRNA PromA, 143, or both, showed robust resistance to viral reactivation by: TNF, SAHA, SAHA/TNF, Bryostatin/TNF, DZNep, and Chaetocin. Given the physiological importance of TNF, HIV-1 reactivation was induced by TNF (5 ng/mL) and ChIP assays were performed to detect changes in expression of epigenetic markers within chromatin in both sorted GFP$^-$ and GFP$^+$ cell populations, harboring latent or reactivated proviruses, respectively. Ordinary two-way ANOVA analysis used to identify interactions between shRNAs and chromatin marks associated with repressive or active chromatin in the integrated provirus revealed significant changes in the levels of H3K27me3, AGO1 and HDAC1 in the LTR, which correlated with the extent of reduced proviral reactivation. The cell line co-expressing shPromA and sh143 consistently showed the least reactivation and greatest enrichment of chromatin compaction indicators.

Conclusion: The active maintenance of epigenetic silencing by shRNAs acting on the HIV-1 LTR impedes HIV-1 reactivation from latency. Our "block and lock" approach constitutes a novel way of enforcing HIV-1 "super latency" through a closed chromatin architecture that renders the virus resistant to a range of latency reversing agents.

Keywords: HIV-1, Latency, Reactivation, Latent reservoir, Epigenetic silencing, Transcriptional gene silencing, Transcription

Background

Human immunodeficiency virus type 1 (HIV-1) latent proviruses are not targeted by current therapeutic strategies. Antiretroviral therapy, when commenced very early in infection has shown significant reduction on the size of the reservoir but limited decay beyond 1 year of therapy [1], and cessation of therapy results in rapid recrudescence of plasma viraemia.

Viral reactivation strategies have emerged as possible approaches to eradicate the latent HIV-1 reservoir. However, the successful reactivation of latent HIV-1 ex vivo and in vivo has proven difficult [2–6]. Therefore, novel strategies that aim to permanently block HIV-1 replication warrant investigation. Importantly, eradication of the latent provirus may not be necessary if spontaneous viral reactivation can be thwarted by mechanisms such

*Correspondence: cahlenstiel@kirby.unsw.edu.au
Department of Immunovirology and Pathogenesis, Level 5, Wallace Wurth Building, The Kirby Institute for Infection and Immunity, UNSW Sydney, Kensington, Sydney, NSW 2052, Australia

as inducing or maintaining viral epigenetic silencing, also known as transcriptional gene silencing (TGS) [7, 8].

We have identified two si/shRNAs, 143 [9] and Prom A [10], as inducers of TGS, able to act individually or combined to efficiently suppress HIV-1 replication. The epigenetic mechanism, involves the induction of altered chromatin architecture associated with the recruitment of Argonaute 1 (AGO1), histone deacetylases (HDACs), histone 3 lysine 9 trimethylation (H3K9me3) and histone 3 lysine 27 trimethylation (H3K27me3). The regions targeted by these si/shRNAs in the HIV-1 5′LTR are separated by ~ 200 nt. The target si/shRNA 143 sequence is located upstream of Nuc-0 in a region rich in transcription factor (TF) binding sites, including AP-1 and COUP-TF [7]. Si/shRNA PromA sequence targets the unique NF-κB tandem binding site in the region between Nuc-0 and Nuc-1 [7, 9, 10]. An illustration of the HIV-1 LTR indicating TFs and si/shRNAs can be found in [9].

HIV-1 reactivation from latency can be triggered by signaling through various cellular pathways that induce nuclear translocation of specific TFs to the HIV-1 promoter [11–13]. We hypothesized that given the strategic location of the si/shRNAs target sites, each si/shRNA may vary in their ability to provide protection from different reactivation stimuli. Consequently, combined expression of both si/shRNAs may provide broader protection against diverse endogenous and exogenous stimuli that threaten to reactivate latent HIV-1. We reasoned that resistance to HIV-1 reactivation might originate from the continuous re-establishment of repressive epigenetic marks induced by the constant supply of each siRNA from an shRNA cassette, even during treatment with LRAs. Therefore, we evaluated the ability of these single shRNAs and their combined expression to impede HIV-1 reactivation from latency, despite treatment with various reactivation stimuli, and characterized the epigenetic profile associated with resistance to reactivation.

Methods
shRNAs and lentiviral vectors
ShRNAs were cloned into the lentiviral vectors psi-LVRU6MP or psi-LVRU6MH (GeneCopoeia, Rockville, MD), with an mCherry reporter [9]. ShRNAs: PromA (GGGACTTTCCGCTGGGGACTTCTGTGAAGCC ACAGATGGGAAGTCCCCAGCGGAAAGTCCC, targets region 350–370); 143 (GCTAGTACCAGTTGAGCC ATTCTGTGAAGCCACAGATGGGAATGGCTCAAC TGGTACTAGC, targets region 143–163); locations are based on HXB2 genomic coordinates. Specificity controls included shRNA sequences containing specific mutations in "seed regions" of target sequences of PromA and 143: M2 for PromA (GGGACTTTaaGCTGGGGACTTCTGT GAAGCCACAGATGGGAAGTCCCCACttAAAGTC

CC) [14] and 143_3M for 143 (GCTAGatCCgGTTGAG CCATTCTGTGAAGCCACAGATGGGAATGGCTC AACcGGatCTAGC,); mutations are indicated in lower case; and a scrambled control shRNA CtrL (GCTTCG CGCCGTAGTCTTA, purchased from GeneCopoeia). Lentiviral vectors were generated in HEK293 cells using PEI based transduction, as previously described [15]. Herein, the prefix "sh" before each name is used to refer to the shRNA: shPromA, shM2, sh143, sh143_3M and shControl.

Cell culture
J-Lat 9.2 cell line, a model of HIV-1 latency that expresses GFP upon reactivation of full-length provirus [16], and Jurkat E6 cells were obtained through the NIH AIDS Reagent Program, Division of AIDS, NIAID, NIH: J-Lat 9.2 (Cat. No. 9848) from Dr. Eric Verdin [16] and Jurkat E6-1 (Cat. No. 177) from Dr. Arthur Weiss [17]. Cells were grown in RPMI supplemented with 10% FCS (Gibco®, ThermoFisher Scientific, Massachusetts, USA), 8 mM GlutaMax, 5 U/mL penicillin and 50 mg/mL streptomycin (Life Technologies, ThermoFisher Scientific, Massachusetts, USA). Transduced cells were grown under selection with 400 µg/mL of Hygromycin-B (PromA), 1 µg/mL of Puromycin (143, 143_3M, M2 and Ctrl) or both (cells transduced with PromA and 143 from independent lentiviral vectors). For convenience, the name of the stably transduced shRNA is used to refer to the transduced cell line: PromA, 143, PromA/143, M2, 143_3M, Control. PromA/143 is abbreviated to A/143 only in the figures. The terms, Parental and E6, are used to refer to the untransduced J-Lat 9.2 and Jurkat E6 cell lines, respectively.

The DNA sequence of each shRNA was confirmed by sequencing of cellular DNA. Transduced cell lines were purified via sorting based on their mCherry expression after three weeks of lentiviral transduction.

Quantitation of shRNA expression
RNA was extracted from all JLat 9.2 cell lines using Monarch Total RNA Miniprep kit as per the manufacturer's instructions (NEB, Cat# 2010S). RNA was quantitated by Nanospectrometer and 1000 ng of RNA was transcribed using the miScript II RT Kit as per the manufacturer's protocol (Qiagen, Cat# 218161). cDNA was diluted as per kit instructions using nuclease free H_2O (from 20 µL to 500 µL volume). qPCR was then performed using miScript SYBR Green PCR kit (Qiagen Cat# 218073). Primer pairs used were a universal loop primer 5′-TTC TGT GAA GCC ACA GAT GGG AA-3′ and the Qiagen universal reverse primer supplied with the miScript kit. The qPCR was run on a Roche LightCycler 480 using the following cycle; initial step 95 °C 15 min, 45 cycles of

94 °C for 10 s, 58 °C for 20 s, 70 °C for 20 s. Expression was normalised to the Hs_RNU6-2_11 referencing gene (QIAGEN, #MS00033740).

Viral Quantitation
Reverse Transcriptase activity (RT-assay) in culture supernatants and Cell-associated HIV-1 gag-mRNA were quantitated as described [18, 19]. Integrated HIV-1 was detected using a nested real-time HIV-1 Alu PCR, as described [20]. Detection of latent HIV-1 and HIV-1 reactivated from latency was performed via flow cytometry on Parental and transduced J-Lat 9.2 cell lines (See Flow cytometry section).

Infection of Jurkat E6 cell lines
A total of 3×10^5 untransduced or transduced Jurkat E6 cells were seeded in 12-well plates and infected with 375 µU/mL RT activity of HIV-1$_{SF162}$. Infection proceeded for a period of 10 days, during which samples were collected for RT-assay. At day 10 cells were harvested for RNA and DNA extraction.

Drug treatments
In reactivation experiments concentrations of TNF (R&D Systems, Inc. Minneapolis, USA) ranged from 0.001 to 100 ng/mL, in 1:2 dilution series. Bryostatin (Sigma-Aldrich Co. Missouri, USA.) was used at 1, 5 and 10 ng/mL, each in combination with 5 ng/mL of TNF. Suberoylanilide Hydroxamic Acid (SAHA) (Sigma-Aldrich Co. Missouri, USA) was evaluated at concentrations of 0.001 to 100 µM, and when combined with TNF the range was adjusted to a maximum of 25 µM. Chaetocin (Sigma-Aldrich Co. Missouri, USA) was used at 0, 25, 50, 100 nM. DZNep (Sigma-Aldrich Co. Missouri, USA) was used at 0, 25, 50, 100 µM. No-drug controls contained the diluent used to dissolve each drug alone.

Reactivation experiments and flow cytometry
Treatments were added for 48 or 72 h to 50,000 cells per well in 96-well plates. Following treatment, the wells were washed once with 100 µL of cold DBPS, centrifuged at 500g at 4 °C for 1 min and resuspended in 50 µL of DPBS containing 1 µL/mL of LIVE/DEAD® Fixable Near-IR Dead cell stain for 633/635 nm to stain dead cells following manufacturer's instructions (Thermo Fisher Scientific Inc. (NSYE: TMO)), and fixed in 100 µL of 0.5% PFA. High throughput flow cytometry was performed directly from the 96-well plates using a BD LSRFortessa™ SORP cell analyser using the BD™ High Throughput Sampler Option (HTS)-LSRFortessa microplate adaptor and acquisition was performed using the following detection settings: Near-IR from the Red laser 780/60-A [642 nm], mCherry from the Yellow-Green laser 610/20-A [561 nm]

and GFP from the Blue laser 530/30-A [488 nm]. Reactivation from latency was measured only in live single-cells by negative gating of dead cells, followed by gating on mCherry$^+$ (transduced cell lines only), and then GFP$^+$ or GFP$^-$. Reactivation from HIV-1 latency was quantitated as the percentage of GFP positive cells and as the mean fluorescent intensity (MFI) of the GFP signal.

Cell sorting of mCherry$^+$/GFP$^+$ and mCherry$^+$/GFP$^-$ cells
A total of 1×10^7 transduced J-Lat 9.2 mCherry$^+$ cells per transduced cell line were resuspended in 20 mL of supplemented RPMI containing 5 ng/mL of TNF, for 48 h. After 48 h cells were washed and stained with LIVE/DEAD® Fixable Near-IR Dead cell stain. The live, Near-IR$^-$/mCherry$^+$ cells were sorted into GFP$^+$ and GFP$^-$ populations, and pellets immediately processed using the Magna ChIP™ HT96 Chromatin Immunoprecipitation Kit (Merck-Millipore, Darmstadt, Germany). Cell sorting was performed in a BD Biosciences Influx v7 cell sorter using the color channels 750/LP [640 nm] for Near-IR Live/Dead fixable dye, 610/20 [561 nm] for mCherry and 545/27 [488 nm] for GFP.

ChIP assays
Chromatin was sheared into fragments of ~200 bp using a QSonica 700 sonicator at 4 °C at 50% power, for 15 min (1 min ON, 1½ min OFF), with an internal threshold shutdown temperature of 12 °C. Immunoprecipitations (IP) were performed in duplicates from biological replicates in 96-well plates using 3 µg/mL of antibody with 10 µL of magnetic beads per IP, in a final volume of 100 µL per well, following manufacturer's instructions. Each IP contained 8×10^4 cell equivalents from sorted mCherry$^+$/GFP$^+$ HIV-1 reactivated cells or 1×10^5 cell equivalents from mCherry$^+$/GFP$^-$ HIV-1 latent cells. Each plate included No-Antibody controls per chromatin sample to correct background signal from IPs performed with antibodies of different isotypes and/or specificities.

The following antibodies were used for ChIP assays; Anti-AGO1 clone 4G7-E12 (Cat. No. MABE143), ChIPAb + Acetyl-Histone H3 (Lys9) (Cat. No. 17-658), ChIPAbTM + Trimethyl-Histone H3 (Lys9) (Cat. No. 17-625), ChIPAb + Trimethyl-Histone H3 (Lys27) (Cat No. 17-622), ChIPAbTM + HDAC1 (Cat. No. 17-10199), ChIPAb + TM Trimethyl-Histone H3 (Lys4) (Cat No. 17-614), Anti-RNA polymerase II subunit B1 (phospho CTD Ser-2) Antibody clone 3E10 (Cat No. 04-1571), and Anti-RNA polymerase II subunit B1 (phospho-CTD Ser-5) clone 3E8 (Cat No. 04-1572). All antibodies were purchased from Merck-Millipore (Darmstadt, Germany).

DNA eluted from the HIV-1 LTR region targeted by shPromA/sh143 was quantified by real time PCR as previously described [10]. Percent of Input was used to

(See figure on next page.)
Fig. 1 Protective shRNAs inhibit HIV-1$_{SF162}$ replication in Jurkat E6 cells. **a** Diagram illustrating the conduct of experiments. For simplicity, Parental and E6 untransduced cell lines are not indicated, however these cells underwent the same experimental procedures with the exception of the gating strategy for flow cytometry, as these do not express mCherry protein. **b** Upper left panel: Parental and transduced Jurkat E6 cells were infected with 375 μU/mL of HIV-1$_{SF162}$ for 10 days and RT-assays performed in duplicates at the indicated time points post-infection. Lower left panel: Cells were harvested at D10 and cell-associated HIV-1 *gag*-mRNA was quantitated in duplicates via qRT-PCR and were normalised against *GAPDH* mRNA. The dotted line at $10° = 1$, indicates the level at which transcription of *GAPDH* and HIV-1 *gag*-mRNA is equivalent. Upper right panel: Schematic of chromatin structure following siRNA treatment. Lower right: Levels of integrated HIV-1 were quantitated at D10 using a HIV-1 nested real-time Alu PCR. Second-round PCRs were performed in triplicates and are presented normalised to β-actin. Data are presented as the number of HIV-1 integrated DNA copies per 500 ng of DNA, with 500 ng equivalent to the DNA amount of 80,000 cells. Data are from one time-course performed with duplicate biological replicates and are shown as Mean ± SD

calculate the amount of immunoprecipitated DNA, and was either used as an absolute, or as a relative value normalized to the Parental cell line.

Statistical analyses

Data from HIV-1 reactivation assays were analysed using the non-parametric Kruskal–Wallis test corrected for multiple comparisons using the Dunn's test with adjusted *P* value and results are shown as mean ± SD. Data from the shRNA expression assay was analysed using the non-parametric Wilcoxon matched-pairs signed rank test with results shown as mean ± SD. ChIP data were analysed by performing an Ordinary two-way ANOVA followed by post hoc Holm Šídák multiple comparison tests (See Additional file 1: Statistical analyses, for details). $P \leq 0.05$ was the minimal threshold for determining statistical significance. The different levels of significance are represented in each plot and explained in the figure legends. Analyses were performed using Prism Version 6.0 (Graphpad Software, San Diego, CA).

In the ANOVA the dependent variable is the relative quantity of DNA that immunoprecipitated with each antibody, measured as the normalised or absolute % of Input. For AGO1, HDAC1 and epigenetic marks analyses, the % Input was normalized to the Parental control. The two independent categorical variables or factors are "cell line" and "condition". The analysis involves interaction and comparisons between the factors. The factor "cell line" refers to each of the six shRNA-transduced J-Lat 9.2 cell lines plus the corresponding Parental control. The factor "condition" refers to the transcriptional state of the HIV-1 promoter as either in latency or during reactivation treatment with TNF. We performed two types of comparisons using the standard ANOVA terminology: (1) "in-between" cell lines, in which the effect of the shRNA from each cell line is compared to the Parental cell line within the same condition (either pre or post reactivation treatment); and (2) "in-within" cell lines, in which the effect of the shRNA is compared between the two conditions within each cell line in order to compare the epigenetic changes that occur from latency to

reactivation (pre vs post treatment with TNF). In contrast, in the studies of bivalency and phosphorylation states of RNA Pol II, data were analysed using an ordinary two-way ANOVA comparing the absolute % Input of two epigenetic or chromatin-associated marks, only during HIV-1 latency. Thus, factor two now corresponds to the epigenetic- or chromatin-associated marks whose absolute levels are being compared: H3K4me3 compared to H3K27me3, and RNA Pol II pSer2 compared to RNA Pol II pSer5.

Results

TGS-inducing shRNAs protect Jurkat E6-1 cells from HIV-1$_{SF162}$ replication

To confirm the shRNAs silencing activity we performed a time-course of infection on Jurkat E6 cells (Fig. 1a, top right) and measured the levels of HIV-1 replication via RT-assays, qRT-PCR of HIV-1 *gag*-mRNA and qPCR of Alu HIV-1 integrated DNA. Suppression of viral replication by 100% matched shRNAs in this setting, is expected to translate as resistance to reactivation during latency. Previous experiments in our laboratory have demonstrated that stable expression of PromA in MOLT-4 cells provides prolonged and potent protection for over 1 year [21]. Therefore, to further challenge and possibly disrupt RNA-induced epigenetic silencing in cells expressing TGS-inducing shRNAs, we used an extremely high amount of HIV-1$_{SF162}$ virus, 1125 mU/uL per 3×10^5 cells. This also increased the likelihood of having all the cells infected with at least one provirus. Despite the high virus inoculum, on Day 10 (D10) there was at least 10-fold difference in the levels of RT activity between controls and protected cell lines (Fig. 1b, upper left panel), confirming that PromA, 143 and PromA/143 combined expressing cells were able to specifically repress HIV-1 transcription (Fig. 1b, upper right panel). A/143 showed some variation at D10, but the levels remained within the same range (> 10 μU/mL) as those of PromA and 143. Similarly, HIV-1 *gag*-mRNA expression was > 1000 times less in PromA, ~ 80 times less in 143, and > 100 times less in PromA/143, compared to the infected parental cell line (Fig. 1b, lower left panel). Also, the levels of integrated

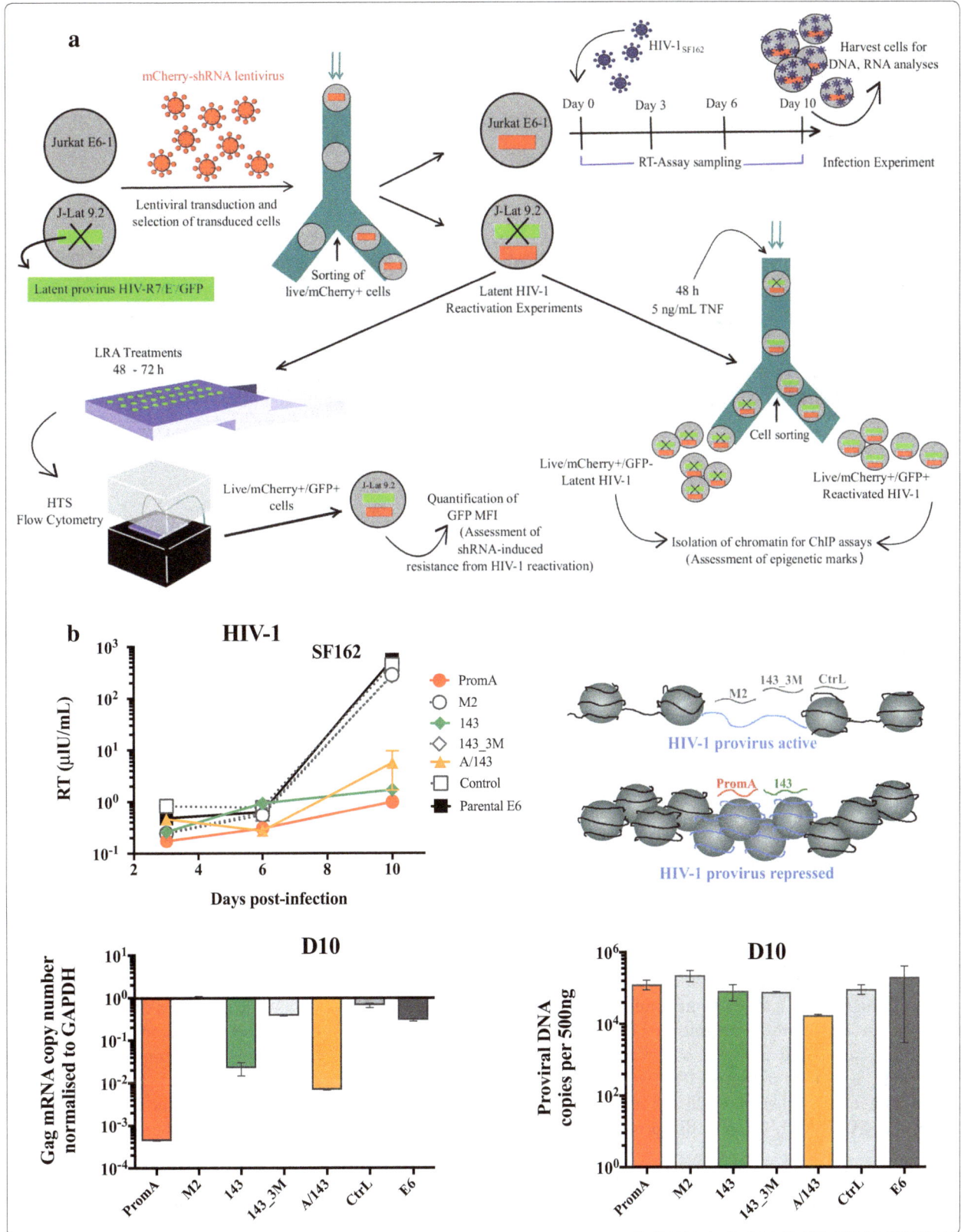

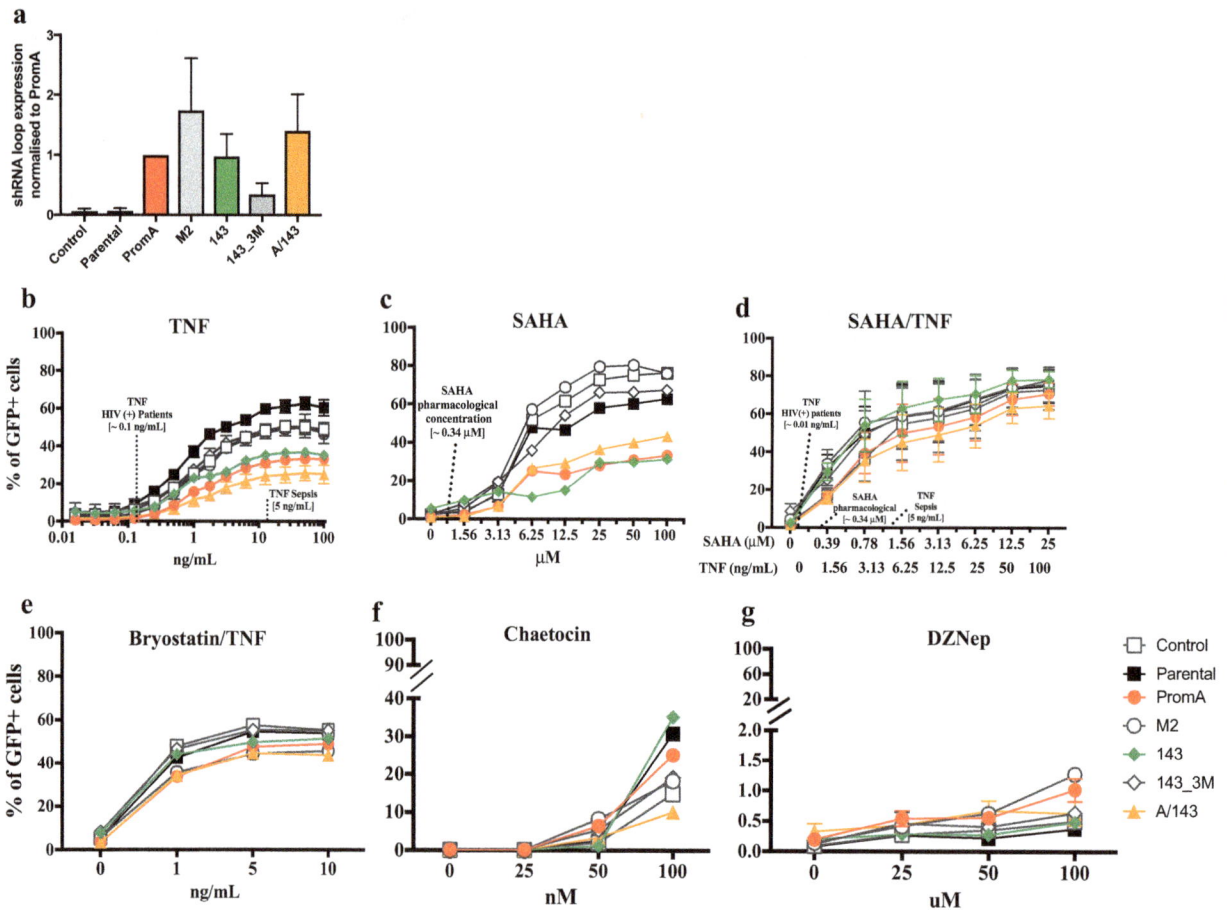

Fig. 2 Protective shRNAs inhibit reactivation of latent HIV-1. Parental and transduced J-Lat 9.2 cells were quantified for shRNA expression **a** and then treated with increasing concentrations of **b** TNF, **c** SAHA, **d** SAHA and TNF, **e** Bryostatin and TNF, **f** Chaetocin, **g** DZNep,. All treatments went for 48 h, except from Chaetocin and DZNep, which were for 72 h. Percentage of GFP + cells was measured through flow cytometry from the live (Parental) or live/mCherry + cells (transduced cell lines) and a total of 10,000 events were collected from each sample from the live cell population. The relevant concentrations of TNF and SAHA are indicated in the corresponding plots. Comparisons shown were performed against the Parental cell line using the Kruskal–Wallis Multiple comparison test, correcting for multiple comparison with Dunn's test (*$p \leq 0.05$)(Mean ± SD). Data shown is from at least one independent representative experiment performed in triplicate

HIV-1 DNA were approximately the same in all the cell lines (Fig. 1b, lower right panel). This was not unexpected because the experimental conditions were directed to infect all the cells with at least one viral particle and the shRNAs do not prevent integration of proviral DNA. These data confirmed previous observations that these constructs are able to suppress HIV-1 replication during a robust infection challenge, while 2–3 mismatches in the target shRNA sequence disabled this protective effect.

Protective shRNAs provide resistance to HIV-1 reactivation during LRA treatments

We previously showed that stable expression of shPromA, sh143 or shPromA/143 provided protection from HIV-1 reactivation when challenged with TNF,

SAHA or a combination thereof [9]. This, in addition to the strong silencing observed during the time course infection, prompted us to challenge the transduced and Parental J-Lat 9.2 cell lines with a panel of potential LRAs (Fig. 2) to assess if combined expression of the two protective shRNAs resulted in stronger or broader protection to a wider range of stimuli.

We first quantitated the levels of shRNA expression in all JLat 9.2 cell lines to determine whether each shRNA construct was expressed to the same degree. We observed similar shRNA expression across all J-Lat 9.2 cell lines, with no significant differences observed (Fig. 2a). The loop sequence was not present in the scrambled Control construct or the untransduced cell line and was therefore not detected in these cell lines.

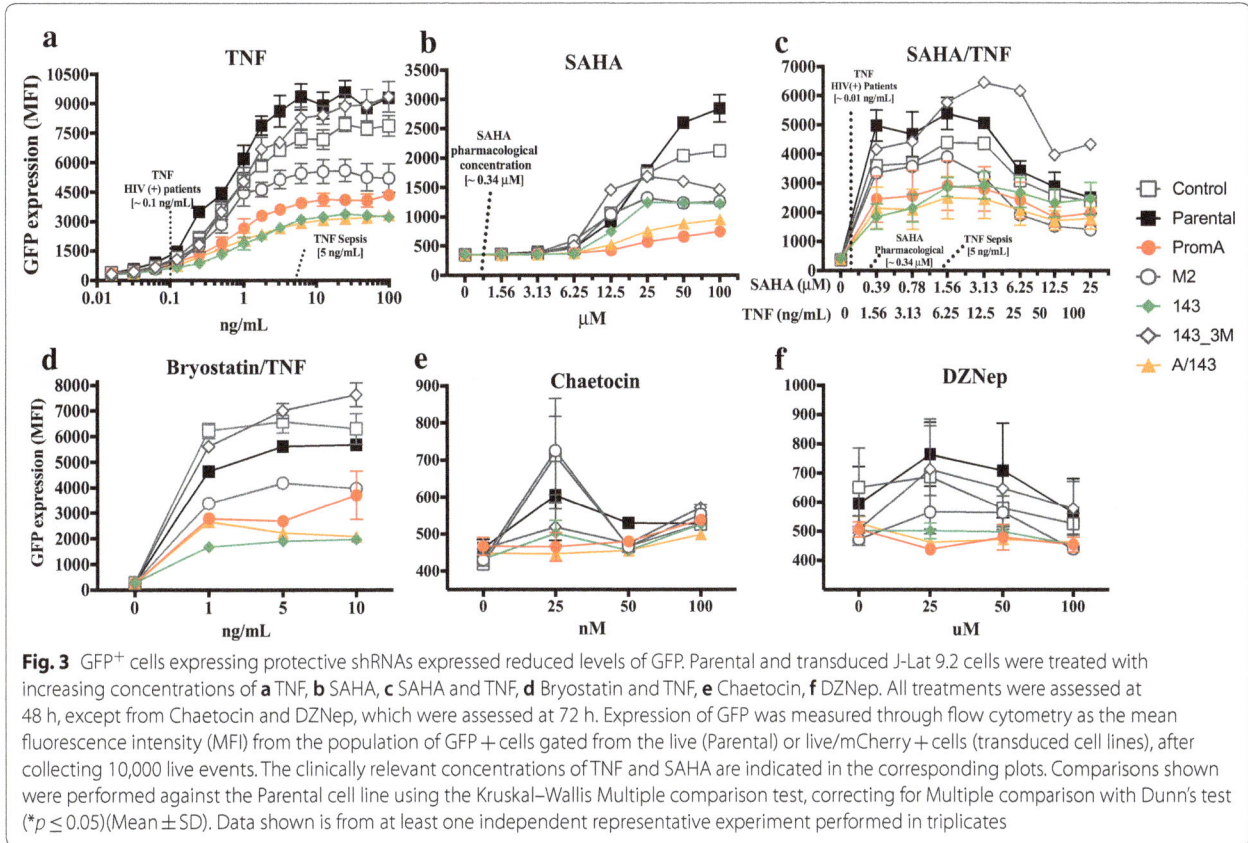

Fig. 3 GFP+ cells expressing protective shRNAs expressed reduced levels of GFP. Parental and transduced J-Lat 9.2 cells were treated with increasing concentrations of **a** TNF, **b** SAHA, **c** SAHA and TNF, **d** Bryostatin and TNF, **e** Chaetocin, **f** DZNep. All treatments were assessed at 48 h, except from Chaetocin and DZNep, which were assessed at 72 h. Expression of GFP was measured through flow cytometry as the mean fluorescence intensity (MFI) from the population of GFP + cells gated from the live (Parental) or live/mCherry + cells (transduced cell lines), after collecting 10,000 live events. The clinically relevant concentrations of TNF and SAHA are indicated in the corresponding plots. Comparisons shown were performed against the Parental cell line using the Kruskal–Wallis Multiple comparison test, correcting for Multiple comparison with Dunn's test (*$p \leq 0.05$)(Mean ± SD). Data shown is from at least one independent representative experiment performed in triplicates

After treatment with TNF the protected cells lines showed the lowest levels of GFP+ cells (Fig. 2b) and the lowest levels of GFP expression (MFI) (Fig. 3a), both compared to the parental cell line and specificity controls. This indicates decreased proviral reactivation and decreased transcriptional activity from reactivated proviruses. The highest concentration of TNF in viremic HIV-1 infected patients is 100 pg/mL(0.1 ng/mL), (27), while 5 ng/mL is the highest reported during fatal acute sepsis (37, 62). At 0.1 ng/mL the proportion of GFP+ cells in PromA and PromA/143 cells was significantly less compared to Parental (Fig. 4a, left panel), though, the overall extent of reactivation was extremely low across all cell lines and therefore not significant (Fig. 4a, lower). At 5 ng/mL of TNF, both the percentage of GFP+ cells and levels of GFP expression were significantly lower in PromA, 143 and PromA/143 ($p = 0.0005$ and $p = 0.02$, $p = 0.003$ and $p = 0.0005$, and $p < 0.0001$ both, respectively) (Fig. 4b). In addition, cell viability was slightly more affected in PromA and M2, than any of the other cell line (Fig. 5a).

We then examined the effect of SAHA, a pan-histone deacetylase inhibitor (HDACi) [22, 23] which has been extensively studied in vivo as an HIV-1 LRA [3, 4]. A concentration of ~0.335 μM has been previously used as

an in vitro equivalent of 400 mg, the protein-unbound pharmacological concentration after single dose of Vorinostat(ZOLINZA®) (63–64), also known as SAHA. At ~0.56 μM SAHA, the nearest to 0.335 μM tested, we found no significant differences in the % GFP+ cells nor in the levels of GFP expression (Figs. 2c, 3b, 4c). At higher concentrations the protected cell lines showed the lowest proportion of reactivated cells, and these cells had reduced GFP expression, with PromA and A/143 showing ~3-fold less compared to Parental (Figs. 2c, 3b). Interestingly, while 143 showed the least proportion of reactivated cells, these cells were expressing GFP at levels that paralleled those of the M2 control cell line, indicating that the sh143 induced-TGS is more susceptible to SAHA reactivation (Figs. 2c, 3b). Overall, SAHA reactivated a greater proportion of cells from the unprotected cell lines compared to TNF and the induced expression was much lower (Figs. 2c, 3b). Additionally, viability was substantially affected at higher concentrations of SAHA (Fig. 5b).

We next combined TNF with SAHA aiming to disrupt silencing via two different reactivation pathways. We decreased the dose-range of SAHA to evaluate the pharmacologically relevant concentration of ~0.335 μM in combination with a concentration of TNF that falls

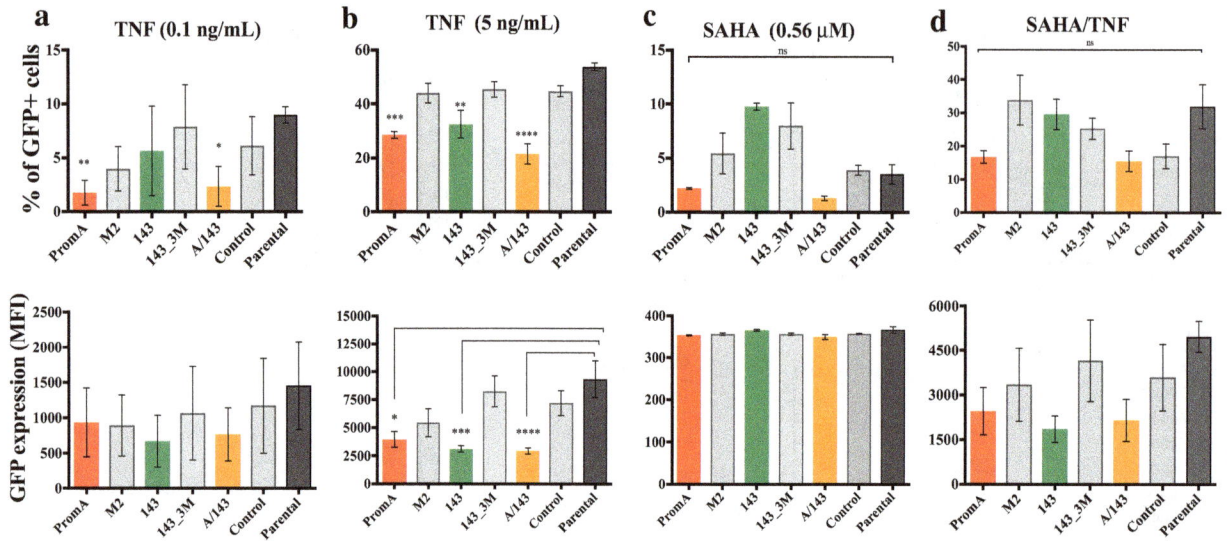

Fig. 4 Statistical significance of shRNA-induced protection at concentrations analogous to physiological levels of the LRAs. The levels of GFP expression during HIV-1 reactivation with **a**, **b** TNF, **c** SAHA, or **d** SAHA and TNF at the indicated relevant concentrations, were analysed for a significant decrease in comparison to Parental (dark-grey) by using the non-parametric Kruskal–Wallis Multiple comparison test, correcting for multiple comparisons using the Dunn's Test with adjusted *P* value. Data shown are from two independent experiments performed in triplicate (Mean ± SD). Significance levels are as follows: * = *p* values from 0.05 to 0.01, ** = *p* values from 0.009 to 0.001, *** = *p* values from 0.0009 to 0.0001 and **** = *p* values < 0.0001

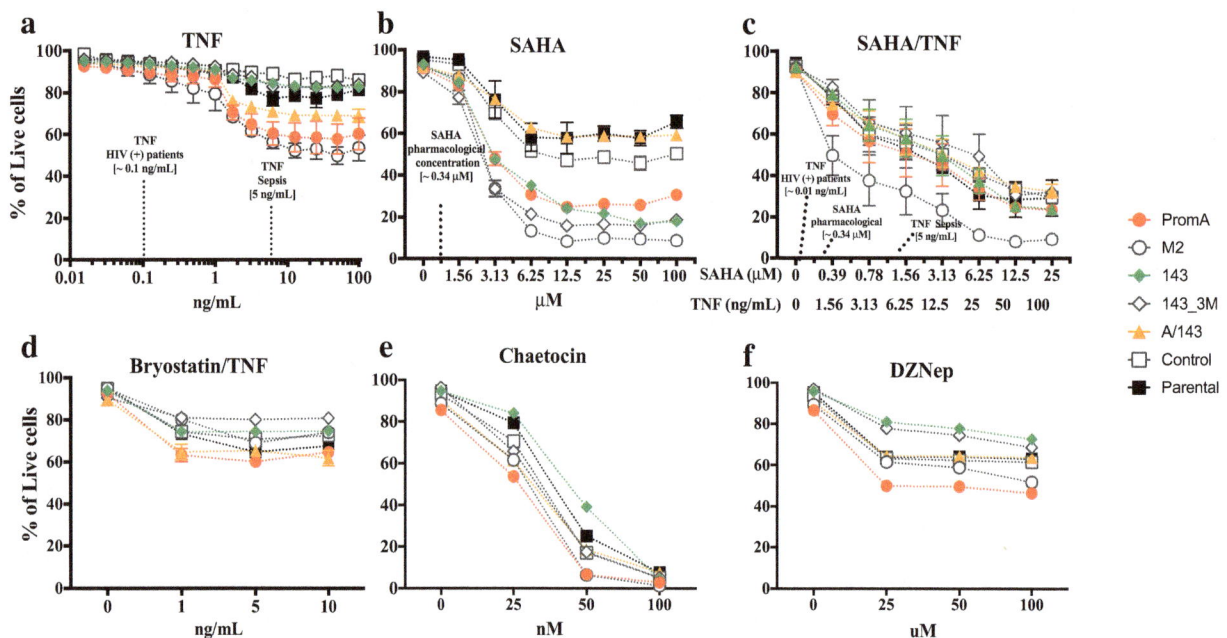

Fig. 5 Cell viability during LRA treatment. The percentage of live cells was measured via negative gating of dead cells using the LIVE/DEAD fixable dye. These live cells were further gated to measure the GFP expression levels shown in Figs. 2 and 3, 10,000 live events were collected. **a** TNF, **b** SAHA, **c** SAHA and TNF, **d** Bryostatin and TNF, **e** Chaetocin, **f** DZNep. All treatments were assessed at 48 h, except from Chaetocin and DZNep, which were assessed at 72 h. The clinically relevant concentrations of TNF and SAHA are indicated in the corresponding plots. Comparisons shown were performed against the Parental cell line using the Kruskal–Wallis Multiple comparison test, correcting for Multiple comparison with Dunn's test (**p* ≤ 0.05)(Mean ± SD). Data shown is from at least one independent representative experiment performed in triplicates

within the high range observed in the plasma of HIV-1$^+$ patients (1.5 ng/mL) [24]. Increasing concentrations of the combined treatment SAHA/TNF induced the highest percentage of GFP$^+$ cells in all the cell lines with A/143 showing the lowest (Figs. 2d, 3c, 4d), and were increasingly toxic (Fig. 5c). Although, not significant, PromA, 143 and PromA/143 showed ∼ 2 fold lower GFP expression and thus less proviral reactivation compared to Parental, up to supra physiologic concentrations of 3.13 μM for SAHA and 12.5 ng/mL for TNF (Fig. 3c). After this point, GFP expression declined in all the cell lines.

Activation of PKC pathways in conjunction with NF-kB can induce potent reactivation of latent HIV-1. Therefore, we sought to induce activation of different PKC isoforms along with the NF-κB pathway by treating the cells with increasing concentrations of Bryostatin [25] in combination with a fixed concentration of TNF (5 ng/mL). The combined treatment reactivated comparable percentages of GFP$^+$ cells in all the cell lines (Fig. 2e). However, the protected cell lines showed the lowest GFP expression levels revealing impairment of proviral transcription, while the controls revealed increased GFP expression at all concentrations tested (Figs. 2e, 3d). Cell line 143 appeared less susceptible to disruption by the combined treatment than PromA. In addition, cell viability was comparable across all cell lines (Fig. 5d).

In order to obtain insight into the epigenetic profile induced by the protective shRNAs, we investigated the effect of inhibiting the histone lysine methyltransferases (HKMTs), SUV39H1 and EZH2, using Chaetocin [26] and DZNep [27], respectively. These have been previously used to indirectly assess the epigenetic profile of latent HIV-1 [26, 27]. SUV39H1 mediates the trimethylation of lysine 9 in histone 3 (H3K9me3,) whereas EZH2 mediates the trimethylation of lysine 27 in histone 3 (H3K27me3) [28]. Both, Chaetocin and DZNep were not efficient reactivation treatments under the conditions tested. Chaetocin at its highest concentration reactivated a maximum of ∼ 40% in the Parental cell line, 143 and PromA, while A/143 showed the least percentage of reactivated cells (Fig. 2f). Expression was only detected in the specificity controls at 25 nM, while the protected cell lines did not show expression at any concentration (Fig. 3e). Chaetocin was highly toxic at its highest concentrations (Fig. 5e). DZNep was the least efficient treatment for reactivation of latent HIV-1, reactivating a maximum of ∼ 1% GFP$^+$ cells in PromA and M2 at 100 μM (Fig. 2g). GFP expression was low, but only detected for the specificity controls and the Parental cell lines with peak effect at 25 nM, while undetected in PromA, 143 and PromA/143 across the concentrations tested (Fig. 3f). Viability was mostly affected in PromA (Fig. 5f).

Altogether, the shRNAs showed a differential ability to protect the cells from HIV-1 reactivation depending on the stimuli. The data indicated that protective shRNAs inhibit HIV-1 reactivation at concentrations of LRAs considerably beyond those likely to be relevant in vivo, and that dual expression of shPromA and sh143 generally provided broader protection across a variety of stimuli.

TGS-inducing shRNAs recruit AGO1 and HDAC1, and maintain the epigenetic repressive mark H3K27me3 at the HIV-1 promoter during TNF-induced reactivation

To investigate the epigenetic changes occurring at the HIV-1 promoter during the LRA challenges, we treated all J-Lat 9.2 cell lines for 48 h with 5 ng/mL of TNF; equivalent to the highest pathological TNF concentration reported in human serum during sepsis [29]. We used this higher concentration to induce levels of GFP expression detectable via ChIP assays enabling the comparison of epigenetic marks between reactivation and latency. We performed ChIP assays on sorted live-GFP$^+$ or GFP$^-$ cells (Fig. 1a, lower right), and analysed changes in the expression of several markers of heterochromatin associated with the 5′LTR using an ordinary two-way ANOVA to compare the normalized % Input to determine whether the shRNAs modified epigenetic profiles. We use the term "latent" when referring to the sorted GFP$^-$ population in which the provirus had not been reactivated, and "reactivated" when referring to the GFP$^+$ population in which the provirus reactivated from latency following TNF treatment.

Significant interactions between the effects of the cell lines (shRNA-transduced or Parental) and the condition (latent or reactivated) were identified in the epigenetic profile of the HIV-1 LTR, for the relative presence of AGO1, HDAC1, H3K27me3, H3K9me2 and H3K9me3, but not H3K9Ac. Simple main effects analyses indicated significant differences within each of the factors, "in between" cell line and condition, for all these epigenetic related marks and proteins (Additional file 1: Table A1). These data indicate that some shRNAs modify the epigenetic profile of HIV-1 during latency, during TNF reactivation or during both. The specific interactions between cell lines and conditions were further identified (See Additional file 1: Table A2 for the Summary of P values) and are explained below.

We first evaluated the changes in the levels of repressive and activating epigenetic marks. "In between" comparisons did not find significant differences in levels of H3K27me3 between any of the transduced cell lines and Parental, during latency (Fig. 6a, left). In contrast, PromA/143 demonstrated significantly higher levels of H3K27me3 during TNF driven HIV-1 reactivation when compared to Parental (Fig. 6a, middle) ($p < 0.0001$) indicative of an overdrive mechanism maintaining closed chromatin despite the reactivation stimulus. This provides an explanation of how reactivation is limited in these circumstances. In addition, H3K27me3 levels were considerably higher in PromA/143 during reactivation compared to the levels in latency ($p < 0.0001$) (Fig. 6a, right). In contrast 143 did not show any difference in H3K27me3 levels during reactivation by TNF compared to the parental cell line (Fig. 6a, left and middle), but did show a significant increase of this mark when comparing between latency and TNF reactivation ($p = 0.004$)(Fig. 6a, right). The levels of H3K27me3 in PromA were not different to Parental during both conditions (Fig. 6a, left and middle), nor post activation compared to latency (Fig. 6a, right).

Only 143_3M had significant lower levels of H3K9me2 in comparison to Parental during HIV-1 latency ($p = 0.04$) (Fig. 6b, left) and showed a significant decrease during HIV-1 reactivation ($p = 0.01$) (Fig. 6b, middle). Intriguingly, H3K9me2 was not affected by TNF treatment in any of the other cell lines, except in the 143, in which it showed an increase compared to Parental ($p = 0.002$) (Fig. 6b, right).

We found no differences in the levels of H3K9me3, across cell lines during HIV-1 latency when compared to Parental (Fig. 6c, left). However, upon TNF stimulation M2, PromA/143 and Control cell lines completely lost this epigenetic mark from the HIV-1 promoter (Fig. 6c, middle). In fact, the levels of this mark were so low for these cell lines that the calculated relative % Input fell below the background and hence the negative values indicate a profound depletion of the epigenetic mark. When comparing the levels of H3K9me3 between HIV-1 latency and HIV-1 reactivation in each cell line, all the transduced cell lines appeared to show a decrease upon treatment with TNF, though this decrease was only significant in M2, PromA/143 and Control (Fig. 6c, right).

Consistent with the more limited interaction of H3K9me3 between the two factors, cell lines and transcriptional conditions, there were no significant differences in the levels of H3K9Ac in any of the conditions, or between latency to reactivation (Fig. 6d, Additional file 1: Table A2). This indicates that acetylation of this residue is not affected by the addition of the shRNAs during latency and that TNF treatment has the same effect on all the cell lines tested.

"In-between" multiple comparisons revealed significantly lower levels of AGO1 at the HIV-1 LTR for the specificity controls M2 ($p = 0.01$) and 143_3M ($p = 0.005$) cell lines during HIV-1 latency, when compared to Parental (Fig. 7a, left panel). These differences were not observed for PromA, 143 or PromA/143 (Fig. 7a, left panel). In contrast during reactivation, PromA, 143 and PromA/143 showed significant higher levels of AGO1 at

the HIV-1 promoter (all $p < 0.0001$), when compared to Parental (Fig. 7a, middle). "In-within" multiple comparisons determined that this increase in AGO1 during reactivation was highly significant ($p < 0.0001$) compared to levels of AGO1 during latency (Fig. 7a, right).

For HDAC1, M2, 143_3M and Control, all showed significant lower levels during latency ($p < 0.0001$, $p = 0.001$ and $p = 0.0006$, respectively), conversely, PromA, 143 and PromA/143, did not (Fig. 7b, left). HDAC1 levels of Control and M2 showed a significant increase from latency to reactivation (Fig. 7b, right) but these levels were no different to those of Parental during TNF reactivation (Fig. 7b, middle); whereas 143 and PromA/143 showed a significant increase during reactivation (both, $p < 0.0001$) (Fig. 7b, middle), and the magnitude of this increase was significant when compared to the levels during HIV-1 latency (Fig. 7b, right).

Together these data support specific recruitment of AGO1 and HDAC1, in addition to H3K27me3, to the HIV-1 LTR by shPromA, sh143 and shPromA/143 during TNF reactivation conditions and is consistent with these constructs acting specifically at the HIV-1 LTR, to maintain epigenetic repression. The protective constructs appear to induce the relative maintenance of certain repressive epigenetic marks despite the presence of drivers of reactivation (Fig. 7c). These results explain how proviral transcription was impaired in the small percentage of protected cells in which the provirus reactivated.

Maintenance of H3K27me3 is induced by protective shRNAs during reactivation with TNF

The coexistence of H3K4me3 and H3K27me3 in promoter regions is associated with poised or inducible genes (Reviewed in (30)). Their coexistence or bivalency in the HIV-1 promoter may be characteristic of inducible latent proviruses. The ordinary two-way ANOVA did not identify a significant interaction between the cell lines (shRNAs) and these epigenetic marks during latency (Additional file 1: Table A3.). Further, there were no differences in the absolute % Input of H3K4me3 between the transduced cell lines and Parental (Fig. 8a, left and middle). Only 143_3M cell line showed slightly less H3K27me3 compared to Parental cell line (Fig. 8a, middle) ($p = 0.02$).

However, post hoc Holm Šídák multiple comparisons (Additional file 1: Table A4) found significant higher levels of H3K27me3 compared to H3K4me3 within all the cell lines, during HIV-1 latency (PromA, M2, 143 and A/143: p > 0.0001; Control $p = 0.009$) (Fig. 8a, right). These data are consistent with the latent state of the provirus in J-Lat 9.2 cells, suggesting H3K27me3 is imposing a strong repressive signal while H3K4me3 allows for transcriptional activation upon stimulation.

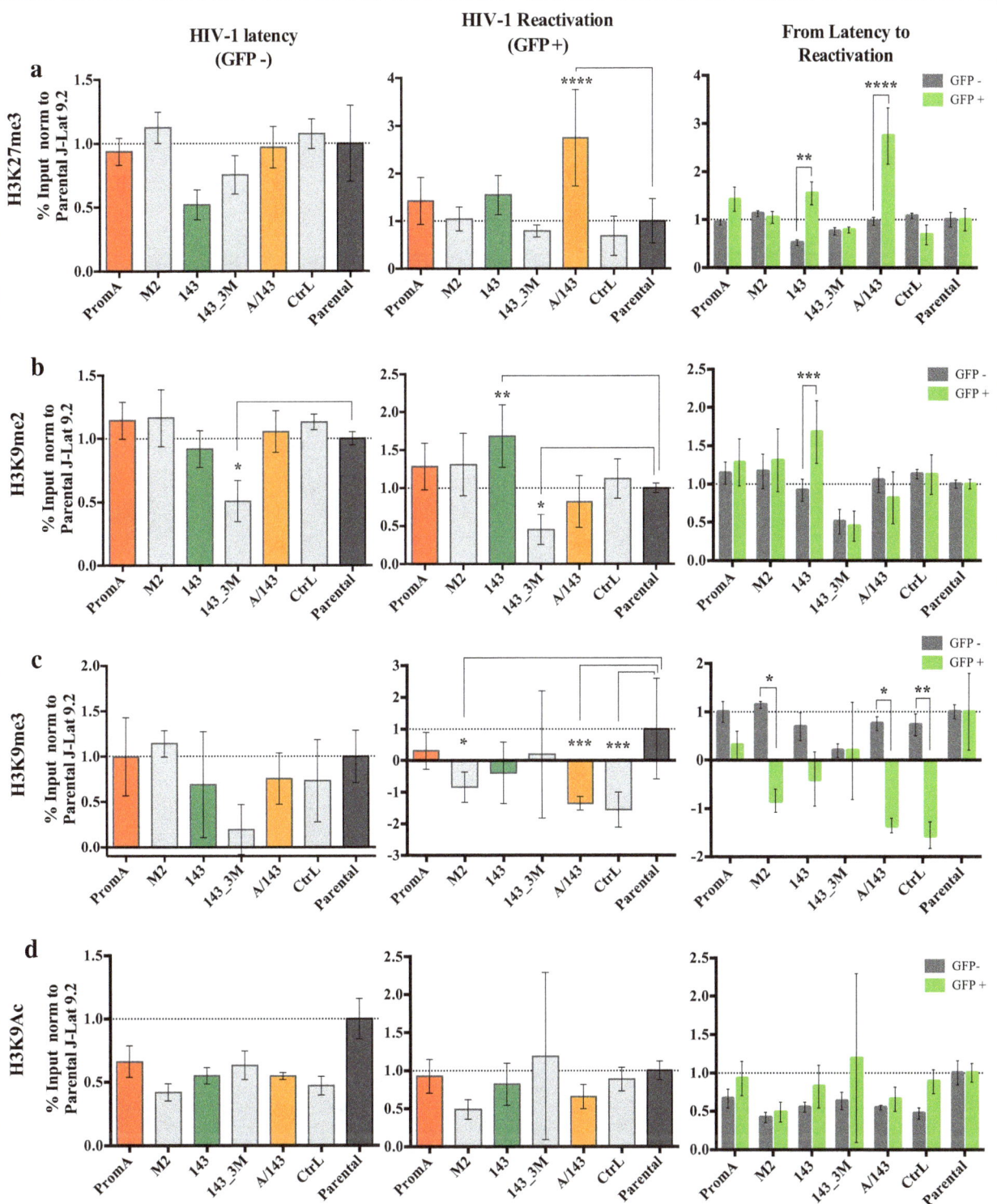

Fig. 6 TGS-inducing shRNAs affect the epigenetic profile of the HIV-1 LTR during TNF reactivation. Parental and transduced J-Lat 9.2 cell lines were stimulated for 48 h with 5 ng/mL of TNF, and ChIP assays performed on sorted live GFP- and GFP + populations. The statistical significance of immunoprecipitation levels of **a** H3K27me3, **b** H3K9me2, **c** H3K9me3, and **d** H3K9Ac, during HIV-1 latency (left panels) and HIV-1 reactivation (middle panels), was analyzed by performing "in-between" cell lines multiple comparisons against Parental (dark-grey bar). Multiple comparisons "in-within" cell lines were also performed to examine significant changes from latency to reactivation within each cell line (right panels). Data shows Mean ± SD (n = 4) from two independent ChIP assays and are presented as the % Input normalised to Parental (* = p values from 0.05 to 0.01, ** = p values from 0.009 to 0.001, *** = p values from 0.0009 to 0.0001 and **** = p values < 0.0001)

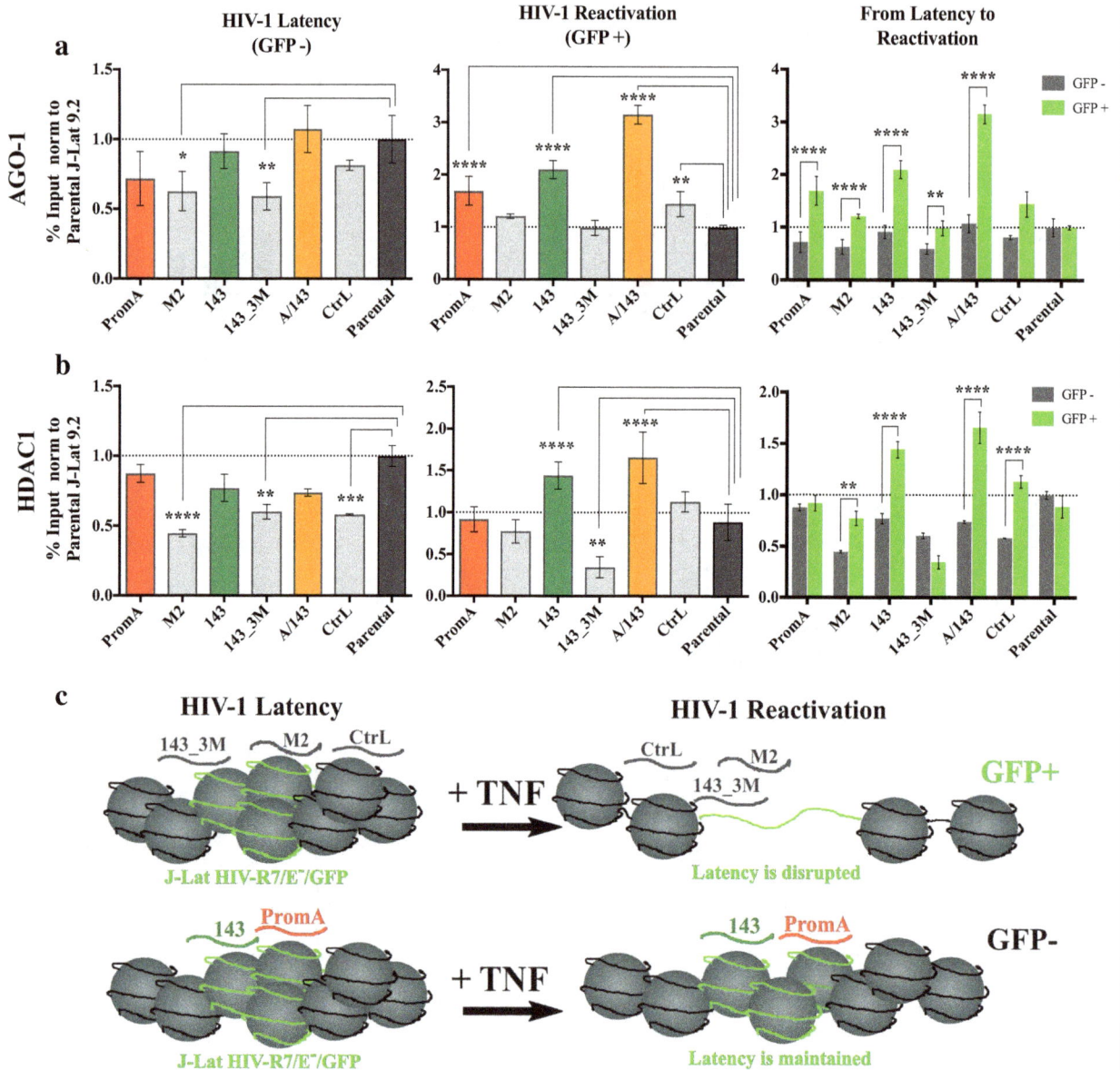

Fig. 7 Protective shRNAs recruit AGO1 and HDAC1 during HIV-1 reactivation with TNF. Parental and transduced J-Lat 9.2 cell lines were stimulated for 48 h with 5 ng/mL of TNF, and ChIP assays performed on sorted live GFP- and GFP + populations. Significance of immunoprecipitation levels of **a** AGO1 and **b** HDAC1 during HIV-1 latency (left panels) and HIV-1 reactivation (middle panels), was analysed by performing "in-between" cell lines multiple comparisons against Parental (dark-grey bar). Multiple comparisons "in- within" cell lines where also performed to examine significant changes from latency to reactivation for each cell line (right panels). Data are presented as the % Input normalised to Parental from two independent ChIP assays (Mean ± SD)(n = 4)(* = p values from 0.05 to 0.01, ** = p values from 0.009 to 0.001, *** = p values from 0.0009 to 0.0001 and **** = p values < 0.0001). **c** Upper panel: Schematic of latency disruption during HIV-1 reactivation with TNF. Lower panel: Schematic of latency maintenance by TGS-inducing si/shRNAs during treatment with TNF. ShA/143 is not explicitly illustrated because PromA/143 cell line simultaneously co-expresses each, PromA and 143, from independent lentiviral cassettes

Phosphorylation of RNA Pol II at Serine 2 of indicates the presence of an elongating polymerase a the Latent HIV-1 promoter

RNA Pol II can be processive or non-processive depending on the phosphorylation state of, Serine 5 (pSer5) and 2 (pSer2) within the Carboxyl-terminal domain (CTD).

The phosphorylation status of these residues is differentially associated with initiation and productive elongation of transcription [30, 31]. Statistical analyses identified an interaction between the cell lines and the phosphorylated species of RNA Pol II ($p = 0.02$) (Additional file 1: Table A3). The "in-within" cell line multiple comparisons

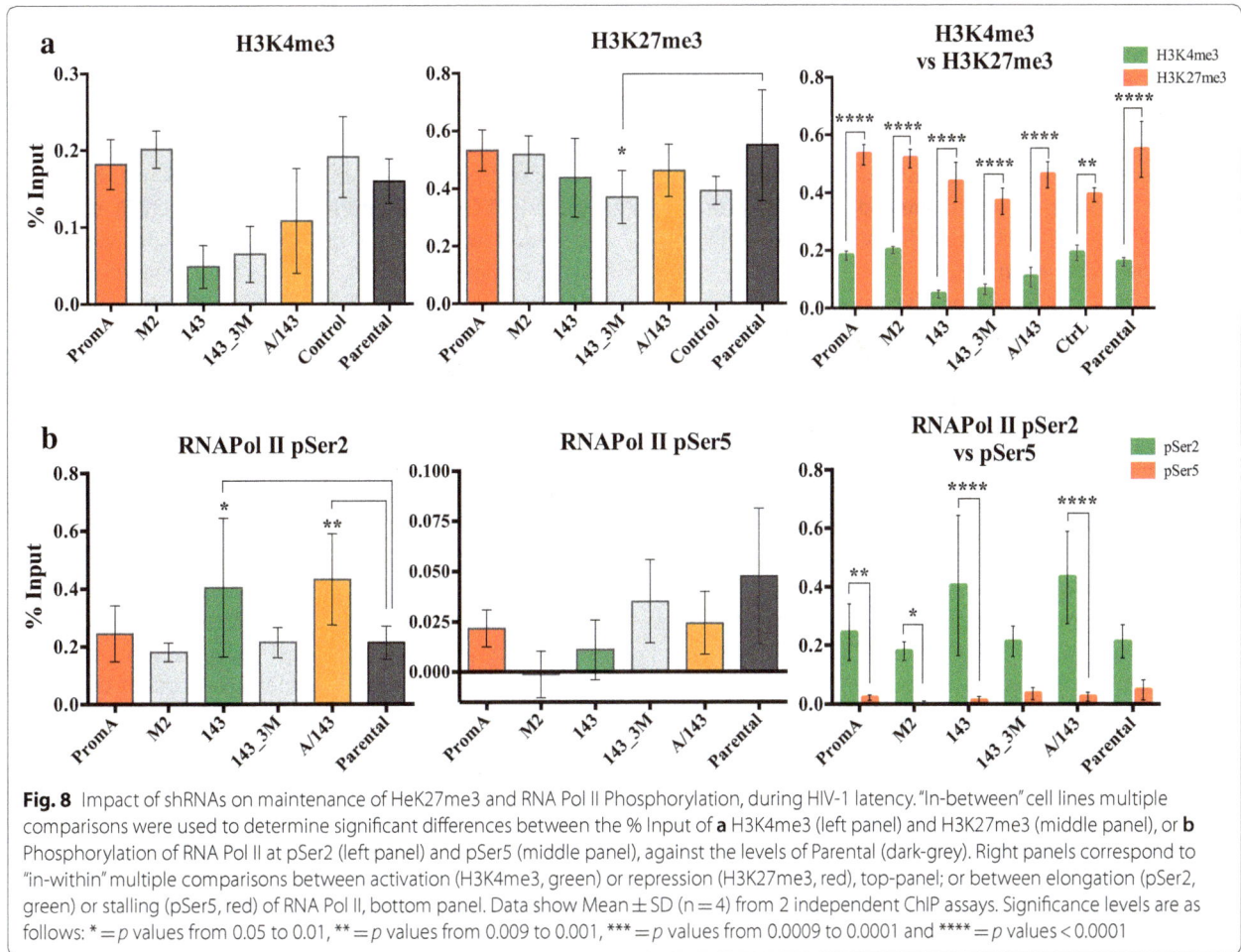

Fig. 8 Impact of shRNAs on maintenance of HeK27me3 and RNA Pol II Phosphorylation, during HIV-1 latency. "In-between" cell lines multiple comparisons were used to determine significant differences between the % Input of **a** H3K4me3 (left panel) and H3K27me3 (middle panel), or **b** Phosphorylation of RNA Pol II at pSer2 (left panel) and pSer5 (middle panel), against the levels of Parental (dark-grey). Right panels correspond to "in-within" multiple comparisons between activation (H3K4me3, green) or repression (H3K27me3, red), top-panel; or between elongation (pSer2, green) or stalling (pSer5, red) of RNA Pol II, bottom panel. Data show Mean ± SD (n = 4) from 2 independent ChIP assays. Significance levels are as follows: * = p values from 0.05 to 0.01, ** = p values from 0.009 to 0.001, *** = p values from 0.0009 to 0.0001 and **** = p values < 0.0001

determined a significant higher % Input of RNA Pol II pSer2, compared to that of pSer5, during HIV-1 latency in PromA ($p = 0.009$), 143 ($p < 0.0001$), PromA/143 ($p < 0.0001$) and M2 ($p = 0.05$) (Fig. 8b, right and Additional file 1: Table A4 top). M2 showed the lowest % Input for both marks (Fig. 8b, left and middle). *Post-Hoc* Holm Šídák "in-between" cell line comparisons (Additional file 1: Table A4, bottom) determined the levels of RNA Pol II pSer2 were significantly higher in 143 ($p = 0.03$) and in PromA/143 ($p = 0.009$), compared to Parental (Fig. 8b, left). No significant differences were identified for RNA Pol II pSer5 (Fig. 8b, middle). These data suggest the TGS mechanism induced by shRNAs PromA, 143 and A/143 possibly involves stalling of the elongating pSer2 RNA Pol II early after transcription initiation, interfering with efficient transcription elongation during reactivation stimuli.

Discussion

Despite effective antiretroviral therapy, HIV-1 provirus persists in the latent reservoir. We have proposed stabilizing HIV-1 latency via a "block and lock" strategy, namely

shRNA-induced TGS, as an alternative mechanism of controlling the reservoir. Using the J-Lat model of HIV-1 latency, we stably transfected J-Lats with constructs expressing shRNAs to induce TGS or specificity controls, challenged the induced epigenetic silencing with LRAs possessing different modes of action and assessed the resulting epigenetic profile. Here we have presented evidence that TGS-inducing shRNAs (PromA, 143 and PromA/143) provide robust resistance to reactivation by LRAs in J-Lat 9.2 cells and the impaired proviral gene expression was due to repressive epigenetic mechanisms.

Overall, the protective constructs impeded the reactivation of HIV-1 provirus from a larger population of cells compared to the reactivation events observed in the unprotected cell lines (Fig. 2). Mostly important is that the proviral transcription from the small population of cells expressing the protective constructs was in all cases below the levels measured in the control cell lines (Fig. 3).

Generally, PromA and 143 cell lines appeared more susceptible to HIV-1 reactivation by agents that activated TFs whose binding sites are adjacent to their specific targets in the HIV-1 promoter. Considering that PromA targets the NF-κB binding motifs, some interaction and susceptibility to TNF was expected. Similarly, as sh143 does not target the NF-κB binding motifs, it is not surprising that better protection was observed to TNF than that induced by shPromA, and when combined with shPromA, protection was enhanced. The effect of TNF on HIV-1 promoter during RNA-directed epigenetic silencing is modelled in Fig. 7c.

Interestingly, we observed the opposite during treatment with SAHA, where the 143-transduced cell line showed less protection than PromA. This can be explained in part by the sh143 target site mapping to a cluster of TF binding motifs, specifically AP-1/COUP-TF and NFAT [7, 9], which can provide an anchor for HDAC recruitment [7]. The combination of SAHA/TNF was able to reactivate the provirus in a larger number of protected cells (GFP$^+$ cells), consistent with the treatment affecting the target sites of PromA and 143 (Fig. 2d). However, proviral transcription remained impaired demonstrating some level of protection (GFP MFI) (Fig. 3c).

Bryostatin-1 has been tested as an LRA for HIV-1 eradication [6, 25]. It activates not only PKC-α and −δ, through which it is thought to induce reactivation of latent HIV-1 [32], but also induces PKC- ε [33], which promotes T cell survival [34, 35]. In J-Lat 9.2 cells Bryostatin-1 has induced less proviral reactivation than TNF alone [36]. Given that Bryostatin-1 and TNF act via different signaling pathways, we expected the combination of both to be a stronger challenge for our TGS-inducing constructs. Consistent with this, Bryostatin/TNF treatment reactivated comparable number of proviruses in all the cell lines (Fig. 2e), although compared to TNF alone GFP expression was not as high (Fig. 3c). Thus, there seems to be complementarity between these two activators and its combination is able to target more proviruses. Importantly, the protected cell lines showed reduced GFP expression compared to controls indicating the protective shRNAs were impairing proviral transcription (Fig. 3c). Bryostatin inhibits CDK2 through dephosphorylation of threonine 160 [37], indirectly affecting transactivation and interfering with Tat function [38, 39]. Hence, while Bryostatin-1 potentially induces reactivation of latent HIV-1 via activation of PKCs, it simultaneously impairs the HIV-1 transactivation loop by Tat, potentially explaining why the levels of GFP expression were below those of TNF alone.

Thus, PromA and 143 appear to maintain silencing despite reactivation stimuli, but may rely on subtly different epigenetic mechanisms. When both shRNAs are expressed in combination as in PromA/143, they either compensate each other or provide a more stable epigenetic landscape resulting in a more effective lock down of the HIV-1 LTR (Fig. 9).

Treatment with inhibitors of SUV39H1 and EZH2 resulted minimal viral reactivation in the controls at the conditions tested (Fig. 2f,g). Chaetocin seemed to disrupt PromA, 143 and Parental, although not A/143, but expression was barely detected indicating limited contribution of H3K9me3 in the induced-TGS in this setting (Fig. 3e). DZNep resulted in even fewer GFP$^+$ cells, but expression was evident in the controls consistent with partial involvement H3K27me3 in maintenance of proviral latency in J-Lat 9.2 (Fig. 3f). Both treatments, in particular Chaetocin, were toxic (Fig. 5e,f), which may be related to the global effect of these ubiquitous methylases in the epigenome.

During LRA treatments, none of the specificity controls were able to provide protection from HIV-1 reactivation, confirming the highly sequence specific nature of shRNA-induced TGS. In stark contrast, the dual construct (shPromA/sh143) broadened the protective effect of the single constructs, demonstrating robust protection from HIV-1 reactivation by modulators of multiple cellular and epigenetic pathways. It was therefore important to examine the epigenetic profiles that occur at the HIV-1 LTR during reactivation from transcriptional control, in the few cells in which it was disrupted. We chose TNF reactivation for these experiments as this is arguably the most powerful and physiologically relevant of activation stimuli tested. We treated the cell lines with 5 ng/mL of TNF because this concentration corresponds to the highest concentration reported in humans during acute sepsis [29], and is sufficiently high to increase the odds of detecting epigenetic changes by ChIP, during low-level proviral reactivation in protected cell lines based on the reactivation data.

The protection from TNF reactivation observed with PromA, 143 and PromA/143 was associated with the recruitment of AGO1 to the HIV-1 promoter. Although PromA had a trend towards higher levels of H3K27me3, H3K9me3 and HDAC1, these increases were not significant compared to Parental (Fig. 2b), consistent with PromA being more susceptible to TNF reactivation than 143 and PromA/143. However, given that PromA still impaired HIV-1 transcription (Fig. 3a), it also indicates that PromA may induce and maintain other epigenetic marks in addition to the previously reported increases in H3K9me2, HDAC1 [10], and H3K27me3 [9, 10].

In contrast, 143 and PromA/143 both showed a remarkable recruitment of AGO1 and HDAC1 during HIV-1 reactivation. PromA/143 had the highest retention of H3K27me3 with no variation in the levels of H3K9me2, whereas the inverse was true for 143 (Fig. 6a,b). Therefore, shPromA and sh143 induced distinct epigenetic profiles and when expressed together, the resulting epigenetic profile is further modified. Complementary to

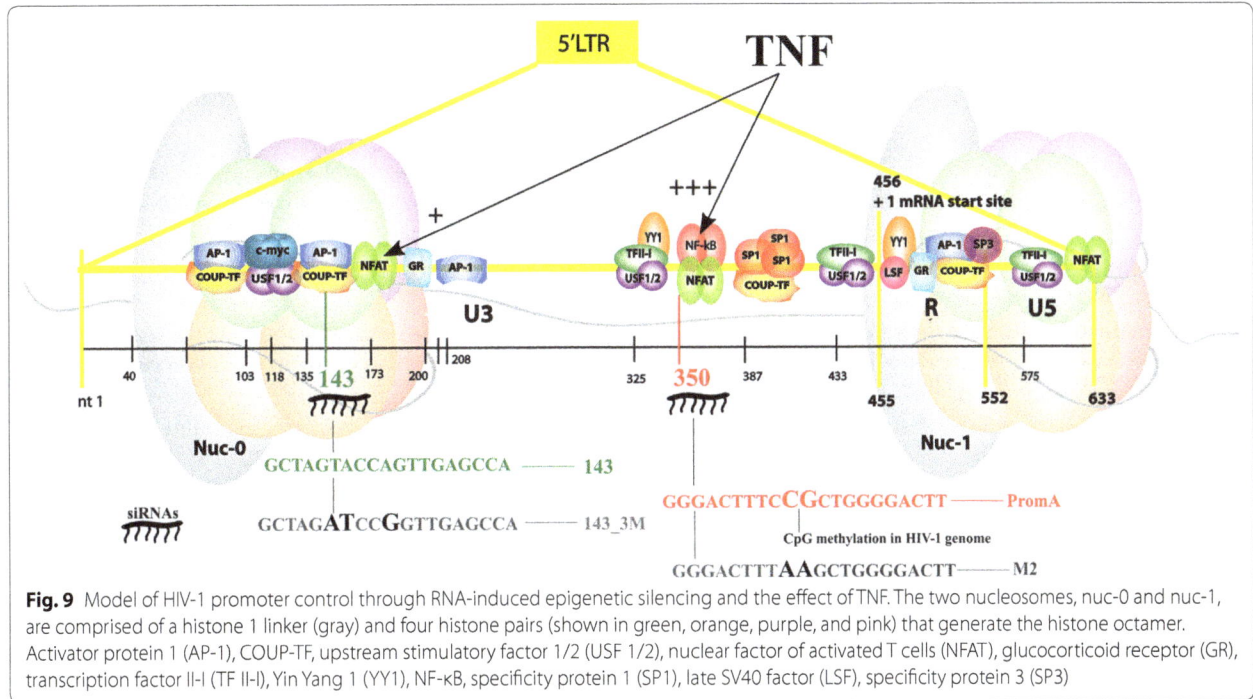

Fig. 9 Model of HIV-1 promoter control through RNA-induced epigenetic silencing and the effect of TNF. The two nucleosomes, nuc-0 and nuc-1, are comprised of a histone 1 linker (gray) and four histone pairs (shown in green, orange, purple, and pink) that generate the histone octamer. Activator protein 1 (AP-1), COUP-TF, upstream stimulatory factor 1/2 (USF 1/2), nuclear factor of activated T cells (NFAT), glucocorticoid receptor (GR), transcription factor II-I (TF II-I), Yin Yang 1 (YY1), NF-κB, specificity protein 1 (SP1), late SV40 factor (LSF), specificity protein 3 (SP3)

these data, M2 and 143_3M showed reduced levels of AGO1 and HDAC1 during latency compared to Parental, indicating the mismatch sequences may be disrupting latency. In fact, 143_3M also showed decreased levels of H3K9me2 during latency, and loss of HDAC1 recruitment after TNF stimulation, as if inducing transcriptional gene activation (TGA) rather than TGS. Further investigations may shed light on the molecular underpinning of TGA by sh/siRNAs.

The observed increase in AGO1 could be the result of TGS reinforcement compensating for TGS disruption. That is, the levels of AGO1-shRNA complexes required to re-establish TGS during exposure to TNF are higher than those required for maintenance of TGS during cell homeostasis. The increased recruitment may be due to TNF also affecting transcription of other genes, including the lentiviral vector and perhaps indirectly *AGO1*, since AGO1 interacts with RNA Pol II and binds to active promoters [40, 41]. In addition, novel transcriptional [42] and microRNA [43] targets were described for NF-κB in HeLa cells treated with TNF, pending to be fully characterized. Interestingly, most genome-wide binding by NF-κB occurs via non-canonical κB sites [44]. Hence, the possibility exists for an indirect effect on AGO1 within this regulatory network.

Quite surprisingly, H3K9Ac levels did not change. This residue does not seem to be considerably involved in the reactivation of latent HIV-1 from J-Lat 9.2 cells (Fig. 6d), though it may function as an anchor for recruitment of other epigenetic marks that affect transcription activation or elongation. In such a scenario other residues, such as H3K27Ac, may become preferentially acetylated during HIV-1 reactivation from latency. Indeed, the residues H3K4me3, H3K9Ac and H3K14Ac co-exist in promoters of paused genes that employ RNA Pol II and are stalled at initiation of transcription [45]. This pattern is found in developmental genes that require a signal to trigger transcription elongation. Further work is required to see if such patterns exist in the HIV-1 promoter in any of its states of latency.

Like H3K9Ac, the levels of H3K9me3 at the HIV-1 promoter were not different across the cell lines while latent. Only PromA showed apparent retention of this mark upon TNF treatment, while complete loss of this mark was observed in other cell lines. Values of H3K9me3 near background levels were consistent with minor reactivation observed with Chaetocin (Fig. 2e). Thus, it appears this epigenetic mark does not explain the resistance to reactivation observed in protected cell lines.

As expected, we found H3K27me3 and H3K4me3 present within the HIV-1 promoter, indicating bivalency, consistent with a latent, but inducible state of the provirus in the J-Lat 9.2 cells. Importantly, different species of phosphorylated RNA Pol II are associated with coexistence of these two epigenetics marks. For instance, paused RNA Pol II, phosphorylated at Ser5 (pSer5), is present in poised developmental genes that remain repressed as a result of PRC2 [46], and are enriched for H3K4me3 and

H3K27me3 [31]. The presence of pSer5 state of RNA Pol II is associated with genes susceptible to rapid reactivation. In contrast, phosphorylation at Serine 2 (pSer2) indicates an elongating polymerase. Therefore, we investigated the levels of different forms of phosphorylated RNA Pol II at the LTR region. We expected higher levels of pSer5 compared to pSer2 for PromA, 143 and PromA/143. However, this was not the case. Intriguingly, 143 and PromA/143 showed significantly higher levels of RNA Pol II pSer2 compared to Parental. Levels of pSer5 are known to decrease towards the 3′ end of active genes while those of pSer2 increase [30]. The higher ratio of pSer2 over pSer5 in all the cell lines suggests that the latent provirus in J-Lat 9.2 cells had already initiated transcription before becoming epigenetically silent through endogenous mechanisms. Stalling of RNA Pol II has been described in highly transcribed genes indicating that transcriptional control can occur at any instance of the process. Therefore, our data implicates a more complex mechanism, in which the shRNAs may be interacting with the transcription machinery along with other chromatin related factors to induce inhibition of transcription during the elongation process. Indeed, RNA Pol III transcribed sncRNAs have been shown to inhibit transcription of RNA Pol II transcribed genes [47, 48]. Thus our shRNAs, which are transcribed by the RNA Pol III, could potentially be directing a similar mechanism, perhaps even acting at the 3′end of the antisense HIV-1 specific long non-coding RNA [49, 50]. Importantly, the detection of epigenetic marks in the LTR may correspond partially or completely to the 3′LTR, as it is not possible to distinguish the 3′ from the 5′LTR in the ChIP assay, based on DNA fragment size and on the positioning of the nucleosomes in this region. It is therefore possible that the protective shRNAs are targeting one or both LTRs. Naturally, this means they can also target the 3′UTR of viral transcripts. However, we have previously reported limited contribution of PTGS via mRNA cleavage [9, 10], hence only translational repression on the 3′UTR of viral transcripts is possible during the time it takes for TGS to be established. PTGS is unlikely to be the main mechanism as HIV-1 rapidly develops resistance and multiplex approaches combining siRNAs targeting viral and cellular sequences are essential to control viral replication via this RNAi pathway (Reviewed in [51]).

For the ChIP assays it was important that latent HIV-1 provirus was present in most, preferably all, of the cell population, given that uninfected cells contribute to background noise. J-Lat 9.2 cells provided a practical way of measuring the epigenetics of virus reactivation and due to their clonal characteristic provided consistency in downstream laboratory techniques. Indeed, it would be interesting to investigate the epigenetic profiles of inducible latent HIV-1 proviruses directly from samples of suppressed HIV-1+ patients, however this is technically very challenging. We chose J-Lat 9.2 cells because HIV-1 latency arose spontaneously following infection of Jurkat cells with a full-length virus expressing GFP [16]. Hence, this model resembles one of the mechanisms by which latency may be naturally established in vivo, when latency is epigenetically induced in infected cells that are actively dividing rather than as a result of a transition to quiescence.

The data presented suggest that although the silencing action of two protective constructs is associated with epigenetic changes in the proviral promoter, these changes are qualitatively different indicating subtle variations in the exact underpinning mechanism of each si/shRNA. Given the broad and sustained resistance to HIV-1 reactivation, and the epigenetic profile of PromA/143, this combination shows promise as a potential lead candidate to prevent HIV-1 reactivation. The natural epigenetic profile of latent HIV-1 could be super-enforced by the action of TGS-inducing si/shRNAs and consequently become resistant to reactivation. In this way, the si/shRNAs will not only reproduce a latency-like state in actively replicating HIV-1, but will also thwart reactivation from latency, making HIV-1 less sensitive to naturally occurring reactivation stimuli.

Several studies have used CRISPR-Cas9 technology to target HIV-1 (Reviewed in [52]), including targeting cellular receptors required for HIV-1 entry [53], excising the HIV-1 genome from infected cells [54], and reactivating [55] or eradicating latent HIV-1 [56]. While promising, this approach has limitations, such as efficient targeted delivery to the required cells, choice of vector (viral or non-viral origin), adverse effects arising from the choice of vector and immune reactions, most of which are shared amongst gene therapy strategies. Additionally, resistant variants have emerged as a result of the cellular non-homologous end joining repair pathway (NHEJ) and possibly viral transcription, indicating that continuous expression of a combination of highly conserved gRNAs and Cas9 will be necessary [57].

Additionally, studies have investigated the "block and lock" approach using didehydro-cortistatin A (dCA), a Tat-mediated HIV-1 inhibitor that also induces epigenetic modifications [58].

However, this potential anti-HIV-1 therapy needs to develop a sustained response, as current data shows suppression for ~3 weeks post-treatment cessation. The "block and lock" cure strategy presented here has the advantages that HIV-1 is unlikely to develop escape mutations and si/shRNAs will be resistant to reactivation.

Authors' contributions

CM conducted all experiments, except for the shRNA expressoin assays which were performed by SL, and KP provided support in statistical analysis of ChIP data. CM, SL, CA and AK designed the experiments and wrote the paper. All authors read and approved the final manuscript.

Acknowledgements

We would like to thank Mr. Chris Brownlee, Flow Cytometry Scientist and Manager of the Flow Cytometry Facility at the Biological Resources Imaging Laboratory in UNSW and Mr. David Snowden, Technical officer at the same facility, for their advice and guidance in the use of the High Throughput Sampler for flow cytometry and for performing cell sorting for the ChIP assays. In addition, Ms Katherine Marks, from St. Vincent's Centre for Applied Medical Research, collaborated in the generation of the lentiviral particles.

Competing interests

The authors declare that they have no competing interests. CM, CA and AD hold a patent for the siRNA sequences.

Funding

This work was supported by NHMRC Project Grant APP1120812.

References

1. Koelsch KK, et al. Impact of treatment with raltegravir during primary or chronic HIV infection on RNA decay characteristics and the HIV viral reservoir. AIDS. 2011;25(17):2069–78.
2. Ho YC, et al. Replication-competent noninduced proviruses in the latent reservoir increase barrier to HIV-1 cure. Cell. 2013;155(3):540–51.
3. Cillo AR, et al. Quantification of HIV-1 latency reversal in resting CD4 + T cells from patients on suppressive antiretroviral therapy. Proc Natl Acad Sci USA. 2014;111(19):7078–83.
4. Elliott JH, et al. Activation of HIV transcription with short-course vorinostat in HIV-infected patients on suppressive antiretroviral therapy. PLoS Pathog. 2014;10(10):e1004473.
5. Bullen CK, et al. New ex vivo approaches distinguish effective and ineffective single agents for reversing HIV-1 latency in vivo. Nat Med. 2014;20(4):425–9.
6. Darcis G, et al. An in-depth comparison of latency-reversing agent combinations in various in vitro and ex vivo HIV-1 latency models identified bryostatin-1 + JQ1 and ingenol-B + JQ1 to potently reactivate viral gene expression. PLoS Pathog. 2015;11(7):e1005063.
7. Mendez C, Ahlenstiel CL, Kelleher AD. Post-transcriptional gene silencing, transcriptional gene silencing and human immunodeficiency virus. World J Virol. 2015;4(3):219–44.
8. Weinberg MS, Morris KV. Transcriptional gene silencing in humans. Nucl Acids Res. 2016;44(14):6505–17.
9. Ahlenstiel C, et al. Novel RNA duplex locks HIV-1 in a latent state via chromatin-mediated transcriptional silencing. Mol Ther Nucleic Acids. 2015;4:e261.
10. Suzuki K, et al. Closed chromatin architecture is induced by an RNA duplex targeting the HIV-1 promoter region. J Biol Chem. 2008;283(34):23353–63.
11. Nabel G, Baltimore D. An inducible transcription factor activates expression of human immunodeficiency virus in T cells. Nature. 1987;326(6114):711–3.
12. Rohr O. COUP-TF and Sp1 interact and cooperate in the transcriptional activation of the human immunodeficiency virus type 1 long terminal repeat in human microglial cells. J Biol Chem. 1997;272(49):31149–55.
13. Yang X, Chen Y, Gabuzda D. ERK MAP kinase links cytokine signals to activation of latent HIV-1 infection by stimulating a cooperative interaction of AP-1 and NF-kappaB. J Biol Chem. 1999;274(39):27981–8.
14. Suzuki K, et al. Transcriptional gene silencing of HIV-1 through promoter targeted RNA is highly specific. RNA Biol. 2011;8(6):1035–46.
15. Aggarwal A, et al. Mobilization of HIV spread by diaphanous 2 dependent filopodia in infected dendritic cells. PLoS Pathog. 2012;8(6):e1002762.
16. Jordan A, Bisgrove D, Verdin E. HIV reproducibly establishes a latent infection after acute infection of T cells in vitro. EMBO J. 2003;22(8):1868–77.
17. Weiss A, Wiskocil RL, Stobo JD. The role of T3 surface molecules in the activation of human T cells: a two-stimulus requirement for IL 2 production reflects events occurring at a pre-translational level. J Immunol. 1984;133(1):123–8.
18. Suzuki K, et al. Poly A-linked colorimetric microtiter plate assay for HIV reverse transcriptase. J Virol Methods. 1993;44(2–3):189–98.
19. Suzuki K, et al. Prolonged transcriptional silencing and CpG methylation induced by siRNAs targeted to the HIV-1 promoter region. J RNAi Gene Silencing. 2005;1(2):66–78.
20. McBride K, et al. The majority of HIV type 1 DNA in circulating CD4 + T lymphocytes is present in non-gut-homing resting memory CD4 + T cells. AIDS Res Hum Retroviruses. 2013;29(10):1330–9.
21. Yamagishi M, et al. Retroviral delivery of promoter-targeted shRNA induces long-term silencing of HIV-1 transcription. Microbes Infect. 2009;11(4):500–8.
22. Singh RK, et al. Kinetic and thermodynamic rationale for suberoylanilide hydroxamic acid being a preferential human histone deacetylase 8 inhibitor as compared to the structurally similar ligand, trichostatin A. Biochemistry. 2013;52(45):8139–49.
23. Thaler F, Mercurio C. Towards selective inhibition of histone deacetylase isoforms: what has been achieved, where we are and what will be next. ChemMedChem. 2014;9(3):523–6.
24. De Pablo-Bernal RS, et al. TNF-alpha levels in HIV-infected patients after long-term suppressive cART persist as high as in elderly, HIV-uninfected subjects. J Antimicrob Chemother. 2014;69(11):3041–6.
25. Diaz L, et al. Bryostatin activates HIV-1 latent expression in human astrocytes through a PKC and NF-kB-dependent mechanism. Sci Rep. 2015;5:12442.
26. Bernhard W, et al. The Suv39H1 methyltransferase inhibitor chaetocin causes induction of integrated HIV-1 without producing a T cell response. FEBS Lett. 2011;585(22):3549–54.
27. Friedman J, et al. Epigenetic silencing of HIV-1 by the histone H3 lysine 27 methyltransferase enhancer of Zeste 2. J Virol. 2011;85(17):9078–89.
28. Chen T, Dent SY. Chromatin modifiers and remodellers: regulators of cellular differentiation. Nat Rev Genet. 2014;15(2):93–106.
29. Damas P, et al. Tumor necrosis factor and interleukin-1 serum levels during severe sepsis in humans. Crit Care Med. 1989;17(10):975–8.
30. Kim H, et al. Gene-specific RNA polymerase II phosphorylation and the CTD code. Nat Struct Mol Biol. 2010;17(10):1279–86.
31. Ng HH, et al. Targeted recruitment of Set1 histone methylase by elongating Pol II Provides a localized mark and memory of recent transcriptional activity. Mol Cell. 2003;11(3):709–19.
32. Mehla R, et al. Bryostatin modulates latent HIV-1 infection via PKC and AMPK signaling but inhibits acute infection in a receptor independent manner. PLoS One. 2010;5(6):e11160.
33. Ekinci FJ, Shea TB. Selective activation by bryostatin-1 demonstrates unique roles for PKC epsilon in neurite extension and tau phosphorylation. Int J Dev Neurosci. 1997;15(7):867–74.
34. Bertolotto C, et al. Protein kinase C theta and epsilon promote T-cell survival by a rsk-dependent phosphorylation and inactivation of BAD. J Biol Chem. 2000;275(47):37246–50.
35. Gutierrez-Uzquiza A, et al. PKCepsilon Is an essential mediator of prostate cancer bone metastasis. Mol Cancer Res. 2015;13(9):1336–46.
36. Spina CA, et al. An in-depth comparison of latent HIV-1 reactivation in multiple cell model systems and resting CD4 + T cells from aviremic patients. PLoS Pathog. 2013;9(12):e1003834.

37. Asiedu C, et al. Inhibition of leukemic cell growth by the protein kinase C activator bryostatin 1 correlates with the dephosphorylation of cyclin-dependent kinase 2. Cancer Res. 1995;55(17):3716–20.

38. Nekhai S, et al. HIV-1 Tat-associated RNA polymerase C-terminal domain kinase, CDK2, phosphorylates CDK7 and stimulates Tat-mediated transcription. Biochem J. 2002;364(Pt 3):649–57.

39. Breuer D, et al. CDK2 regulates HIV-1 transcription by phosphorylation of CDK9 on serine 90. Retrovirology. 2012;9:94.

40. Huang V, et al. Ago1 Interacts with RNA polymerase II and binds to the promoters of actively transcribed genes in human cancer cells. PLoS Genet. 2013;9(9):e1003821.

41. Allo M, et al. Argonaute-1 binds transcriptional enhancers and controls constitutive and alternative splicing in human cells. Proc Natl Acad Sci USA. 2014;111(44):15622–9.

42. Zhou F, et al. Identification of novel NF-kappaB transcriptional targets in TNFalpha-treated HeLa and HepG2 cells. Cell Biol Int. 2017;41(5):555–69.

43. Zhou F, et al. NF-kappaB target microRNAs and their target genes in TNFalpha-stimulated HeLa cells. Biochim Biophys Acta. 2014;1839(4):344–54.

44. Xing Y, et al. Characterization of genome-wide binding of NF-kappaB in TNFalpha-stimulated HeLa cells. Gene. 2013;526(2):142–9.

45. Guenther MG, et al. A chromatin landmark and transcription initiation at most promoters in human cells. Cell. 2007;130(1):77–88.

46. Tee WW, et al. Erk1/2 activity promotes chromatin features and RNAPII phosphorylation at developmental promoters in mouse ESCs. Cell. 2014;156(4):678–90.

47. Espinoza CA, et al. B2 RNA binds directly to RNA polymerase II to repress transcript synthesis. Nat Struct Mol Biol. 2004;11(9):822–9.

48. Ponicsan SL, et al. The non-coding B2 RNA binds to the DNA cleft and active-site region of RNA polymerase II. J Mol Biol. 2013;425(19):3625–38.

49. Kobayashi-Ishihara M, et al. HIV-1-encoded antisense RNA suppresses viral replication for a prolonged period. Retrovirology. 2012;9:38.

50. Saayman S, et al. An HIV-encoded antisense long noncoding RNA epigenetically regulates viral transcription. Mol Ther. 2014;22(6):1164–75.

51. Eekels JJ, Berkhout B. Toward a durable treatment of HIV-1 infection using RNA interference. Prog Mol Biol Transl Sci. 2011;102:141–63.

52. Wang G, et al. CRISPR-Cas based antiviral strategies against HIV-1. Virus Res. 2018;244:321–32.

53. Xu L, et al. CRISPR/Cas9-mediated CCR5 ablation in human hematopoietic stem/progenitor cells confers HIV-1 resistance in vivo. Mol Ther. 2017;25(8):1782–89.

54. Kaminski R, et al. Excision of HIV-1 DNA by gene editing: a proof-of-concept in vivo study. Gene Ther. 2016;23(8–9):690–5.

55. Limsirichai P, Gaj T, Schaffer DV. CRISPR-mediated activation of latent HIV-1 expression. Mol Ther. 2016;24(3):499–507.

56. Hu W, et al. RNA-directed gene editing specifically eradicates latent and prevents new HIV-1 infection. Proc Natl Acad Sci USA. 2014;111(31):11461–6.

57. Wang Z, et al. CRISPR/Cas9-derived mutations both inhibit HIV-1 replication and accelerate viral escape. Cell Rep. 2016;15(3):481–9.

58. Kessing CF, et al. In vivo suppression of HIV rebound by didehydro-cortistatin A, a "block-and-lock" strategy for HIV-1 treatment. Cell Rep. 2017;21(3):600–11.

13

HIV-1 Tat phosphorylation on Ser-16 residue modulates HIV-1 transcription

Andrey Ivanov[1], Xionghao Lin[1], Tatiana Ammosova[1,2,3], Andrey V. Ilatovskiy[4,5], Namita Kumari[1], Hatajai Lassiter[1], Nowah Afangbedji[1], Xiaomei Niu[1], Michael G. Petukhov[4,5] and Sergei Nekhai[1,2*] ⓘD

Abstract

Background: HIV-1 transcription activator protein Tat is phosphorylated in vitro by CDK2 and DNA-PK on Ser-16 residue and by PKR on Tat Ser-46 residue. Here we analyzed Tat phosphorylation in cultured cells and its functionality.

Results: Mass spectrometry analysis showed primarily Tat Ser-16 phosphorylation in cultured cells. In vitro, CDK2/cyclin E predominantly phosphorylated Tat Ser-16 and PKR—Tat Ser-46. Alanine mutations of either Ser-16 or Ser-46 decreased overall Tat phosphorylation. Phosphorylation of Tat Ser-16 was reduced in cultured cells treated by a small molecule inhibitor of CDK2 and, to a lesser extent, an inhibitor of DNA-PK. Conditional knock-downs of CDK2 and PKR inhibited and induced one round HIV-1 replication respectively. HIV-1 proviral transcription was inhibited by Tat alanine mutants and partially restored by S16E mutation. Pseudotyped HIV-1 with Tat S16E mutation replicated well, and HIV-1 Tat S46E—poorly, but no live viruses were obtained with Tat S16A or Tat S46A mutations. TAR RNA binding was affected by Tat Ser-16 alanine mutation. Binding to cyclin T1 showed decreased binding of all Ser-16 and Ser-46 Tat mutants with S16D and Tat S46D mutiations showing the strongest effect. Molecular modelling and molecular dynamic analysis revealed significant structural changes in Tat/CDK9/cyclin T1 complex with phosphorylated Ser-16 residue, but not with phosphorylated Ser-46 residue.

Conclusion: Phosphorylation of Tat Ser-16 induces HIV-1 transcription, facilitates binding to TAR RNA and rearranges CDK9/cyclin T1/Tat complex. Thus, phosphorylation of Tat Ser-16 regulates HIV-1 transcription and may serve as target for HIV-1 therapeutics.

Background

Complete eradication of HIV-1 virus in infected individuals is hindered by the presence of latent HIV-1 provirus, which is not affected by the existing anti-HIV-1 drugs [1]. Thus, novel approaches are needed to better understand and successfully target latent HIV-1 infection. HIV-1 transcription from HIV-1 LTR depends on both host cell factors and HIV-1 transactivation Tat protein [2]. HIV-1 Tat activates viral transcription by recruiting Positive Transcription Elongation Factor b (P-TEFb) that contains CDK9/cyclin T1 to TAR RNA [2]. Inability of Tat to recruit CDK9/cyclin T1 to TAR RNA may contribute to the establishment of latency [1]. Our

earlier study showed that CDK2 phosphorylated HIV-1 Tat in vitro, although the phosphorylated residues were not clearly identified [3]. Subsequently, we found that Tat was phosphorylated in cultured cells and that the phosphorylation was significantly reduced when Ser-16 or Ser-46 residues were mutated [4]. Co-expression of Flag-tagged Tat S16A or Tat S46A mutants failed to activate integrated HIV-1 provirus with defective Tat [4]. We also showed that inhibition of CDK2 by iron chelators, 311 and ICL670, reduced Tat phosphorylation in cultured cells [5]. A recent study from Tyagi's lab showed that Tat was phosphorylated in vitro by DNA-dependent protein kinase (DNA-PK) on Ser-16 and Ser-62 residues and that alanine mutations in these sites, separately or in combination, reduced HIV-1 replication [6]. HIV-1 Tat was also shown to be phosphorylated in vitro by a double-stranded RNA activated protein kinase R (PKR) on

*Correspondence: snekhai@howard.edu
[1] Center for Sickle Cell Disease, Howard University, 1840 7th Street, N.W. HURB1, Suite 202, Washington, DC 20001, USA
Full list of author information is available at the end of the article

C-terminal residues [7, 8] and by protein kinase C (PKC) on Ser-46 [9]. PKR interacted with Tat in cultured cells [7] and phosphorylated Tat [8] or Tat-derived peptides [10] on C-terminal Ser-62, Thr-64 and Ser-68 residues. Phosphorylation of Tat by PKR enhanced Tat binding to TAR RNA and alanine mutations in Ser-62, Thr-64 and Ser-68 reduced Tat-mediated HIV-1 transcription activation [10]. In a recent study, PKR was shown to phosphorylate additional Tat residues including Thr-23, Thr-40, Ser-46, Ser-62 and Ser-68 in vitro [11]. In cultured cells, phosphorylation of Tat by PKR inhibited HIV-1 transcription by preventing the interaction of Tat with TAR RNA and reducing Tat translocation to the nucleus [11]. In addition to being phosphorylated, Tat was also shown to be methylated, acetylated and ubiquitinated (reviewed in [12]). Monoubiquitination of Tat on Lys-71 residue by Hdm2 increased Tat's ability to activate HIV-1 transcription and did not lead to its degradation [13].

Here, we analyzed Tat phosphorylation in cultured cells using high resolution mass spectrometry. We detected with high confidence phosphorylation of Ser-16 residue, and with lower confidence phosphorylation of Ser-46, Thr-77, Ser-81, Thr-82 and Ser-87 residues. Using synthetic peptides that span several potential phosphorylation sites of Tat, we showed that CDK2/cyclin E predominantly phosphorylated Tat Ser-16 and that PKR predominantly phosphorylated Tat peptide containing Ser-46. Alanine mutations of either Ser-16 or Ser-46 decreased overall Tat phosphorylation. We used small molecule inhibitors of CDK2 and DNA-PK and high resolution mass spectrometry to explore the effect of CDK2 and DNA-PK inhibition on Tat Ser-16 phosphorylation in cultured cells. We developed conditional knock-downs of CDK2 and PKR in CEM T cells and tested them for HIV-1 replication which showed induction and inhibition of one round HIV-1 replication by PKR KD and CDK2 KD, respectively. To analyze functional consequences of Ser-16 and Ser-46 phosphorylation, we analyzed transcriptional activity of HIV-1 proviral DNA containing Ser-16 and Ser-46 alanine and phosphorylation-mimicking glutamic acid mutations which showed complete inhibition of transcription by alanine mutations

and partial restoration of transcription by S16E mutation and poor restoration by S46E mutation. We also assembled pseudotyped viruses from mutant pNL4-3 Luc vectors that showed partial and weak compensation by Tat S16E and Tat S46E mutations, respectively. We were not able to assemble proviruses with Tat S16A or Tat S46A mutations. We also analyzed nuclear localization of Tat using EGFP-fused alanine and glutamic acid mutants of Ser-16 and Ser-46, which showed deficiency in nuclear localization for Tat S46E. Analysis of Tat ubiquitination showed no strong effects of Tat mutants on ubiquitination. TAR RNA binding was analyzed and found to be only affected by Tat S16A mutation. Analysis of Tat binding to cyclin T1 showed decreased binding of all mutants and Tat S16D and Tat S46D were having the strongest effect. Molecular modelling and molecular dynamic analysis revealed significant structural changes in Tat/CDK9/cyclin T1 complex with phosphorylated Ser-16, but not with phosphorylated Ser-46. Together, our results indicate Tat Ser-16 phosphorylation is an important event in HIV-1 transcription regulation and that it may facilitate binding to TAR RNA and the rearrangement of CDK9/cyclin T1/Tat complex.

Results

Analysis of HIV-1 Tat phosphorylation in cultured cells

Our previous studies showed that Tat is phosphorylated in vitro and in cultured cells [3, 4]. Alanine mutations of serine residues located within $S^{16}QPR^{19}$ and $S^{46}YGR^{49}$ sequences of HIV-1 significantly reduced Tat phosphorylation suggesting that these residues might be phosphorylated in vivo [4]. Here, we analyzed phosphorylation of HIV-1 Tat expressed in cultured cells using high resolution mass spectrometry. Flag-Tat was expressed in 293T cells which were briefly treated with 0.1 M okadaic acid prior to Tat isolation by immunoprecipitation with anti-Flag antibodies and purification on SDS PAGE (Fig. 1a). Tat was in gel digested with trypsin (see Methods) and subjected to LC-MS/MS analysis (Fig. 1b). Recovered Tat-derived peptides depicted 90% coverage of the Flag-Tat sequence and included potential phosphorylation sites (Fig. 1b). Analysis of posttranslational modifications

(See figure on next page.)
Fig. 1 Tat phosphorylation in cultured cells. **a** Purification of Flag-tagged HIV-1 Tat for mass spectrometry analysis. Flag-tagged Tat was expressed in 293T cells, immunoprecipitated from cellular lysate with anti-Flag antibodies and resolved on 10% SDS-PAGE. Peptides were in-gel digested with trypsin, eluted and subjected to MS analysis on Thermo LTQ Orbitrap XL mass spectrometer. Position of Flag-Tat is shown. **b** MS/MS analysis of Tat phosphorylation. SEQUEST search results are shown for Tat peptides identified with high, median and low confidence indicated in green, blue and red, respectively. Peptides that were not detected are shown in black. Phosphorylated serine and threonine residues are marked by asterisks. Identified phosphopeptides are shown in the table. **c–f** Phosphopeptides spectra. **c** MS/MS spectra of the Ser-16 phosphorylated Tat peptide 8–19. **d** Ser-46/Tyr-47 phosphorylated Tat peptide 41–50. **e** Ser-81 phosphorylated Tat peptide 72–89. **f** Ser-87 phosphorylated Tat peptide 72–89. The colored peaks indicate matched MS/MS fragments. Green color indicates precursor ions. Blue and red colors indicate y and b ions, respectively

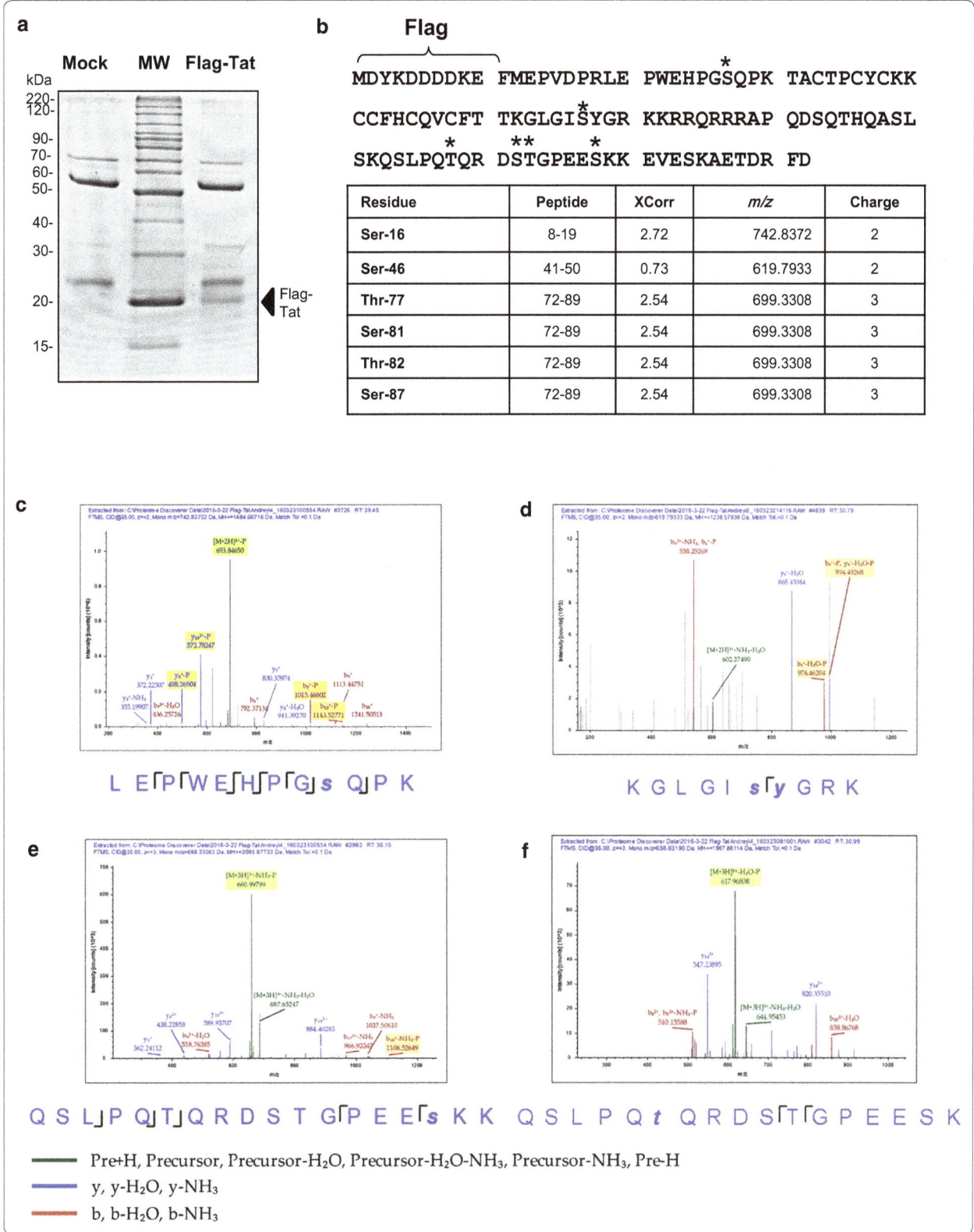

a

b

Flag

MDYKDDDDKE FMEPVDPRLE PWEHPGS*QPK TACTPCYCKK

CCFHCQVCFT TKGLGIS*YGR KKRRQRRRAP QDSQTHQASL

SKQS*LPQTQR D*S*TGPEES*KK EVESKAETDR FD

Residue	Peptide	XCorr	m/z	Charge
Ser-16	8-19	2.72	742.8372	2
Ser-46	41-50	0.73	619.7933	2
Thr-77	72-89	2.54	699.3308	3
Ser-81	72-89	2.54	699.3308	3
Thr-82	72-89	2.54	699.3308	3
Ser-87	72-89	2.54	699.3308	3

c

L E⌐P⌐WE⌐H⌐P⌐G⌐s Q⌐P K

d

K G L G I s⌐y G R K

e

f

Q S L⌐P Q⌐T⌐QR D S T G⌐P E E⌐s K K   Q S L P Q t QR D S⌐T⌐G P E E S K

— Pre+H, Precursor, Precursor-H₂O, Precursor-H₂O-NH₃, Precursor-NH₃, Pre-H
— y, y-H₂O, y-NH₃
— b, b-H₂O, b-NH₃

in Tat showed multiple phosphorylation sites on serine and threonine residues including Ser-16, Ser-46, Thr-77, Ser-81, Thr-82 and Ser-87 (Fig. 1b–f). While signal for phospho Ser-16 containing peptide was relatively high ($\sim 10^6$), signals for all other phosphorylated peptides including GLGIsyGR peptide that contains Ser-46 were significantly lower ($\sim 10^3$) (Fig. 1c–f) suggesting that Ser-16 was the major phosphorylation site and that all other sites had much lower levels of phosphorylation. Thus, mass spectrometry analysis identified the N-terminal Ser-16, Ser-46 and several C-terminal residues of Tat being phosphorylated in vivo.

CDK2 phosphorylates Tat Ser-16 in vitro

We further analyzed HIV-1 Tat phosphorylation in vitro by CDK2 and PKR using Tat peptides that span potential phosphorylation sites including Ser-16 (residues 12–29); Thr-39 and Thr-40 (residues 29–45); Ser-46 (residues 41–57); and Ser-62, Thr-64, Ser-68 and Ser-70 (residues 57–71) (Fig. 2a). Tat-derived peptides were resolved on SDS PAGE containing 6 M urea and stained with Coomassie (Fig. 2b, lower panels). Tat peptide 12–29 contains Ser-16 and also four cysteine residues that resulted in its aggregation despite the addition of 1 mM DTT and sonication. This peptide migrated as a major band at 70 kDa (Fig. 2b, lower panel, lane 1). Peptide 29–45 also aggregated and formed a smear on a Coomassie stained gel (Fig. 2b, lower panel, lane 2). Peptide 41–57 containing Ser-46 was fully soluble and migrated with the front (Fig. 2b, lower panel, lane 3). Peptide 57–71 could not be seen on a Coomassie stained gel even when loaded at high amount (20 μg) on the gel (Fig. 2b, lower panel, lane 4). Recombinant enzymes CDK2/cyclin E, CDK9/cyclin T1 and PKR were used for in vitro phosphorylation of Tat peptides. Recombinant CDK2/cyclin E primarily phosphorylated a peptide containing Ser-16 (Fig. 2b, lane 1) and to a lesser extent peptides containing Thr-39/Thr-40 and Ser-46 (Fig. 2b, lanes 3–4; see quantifications

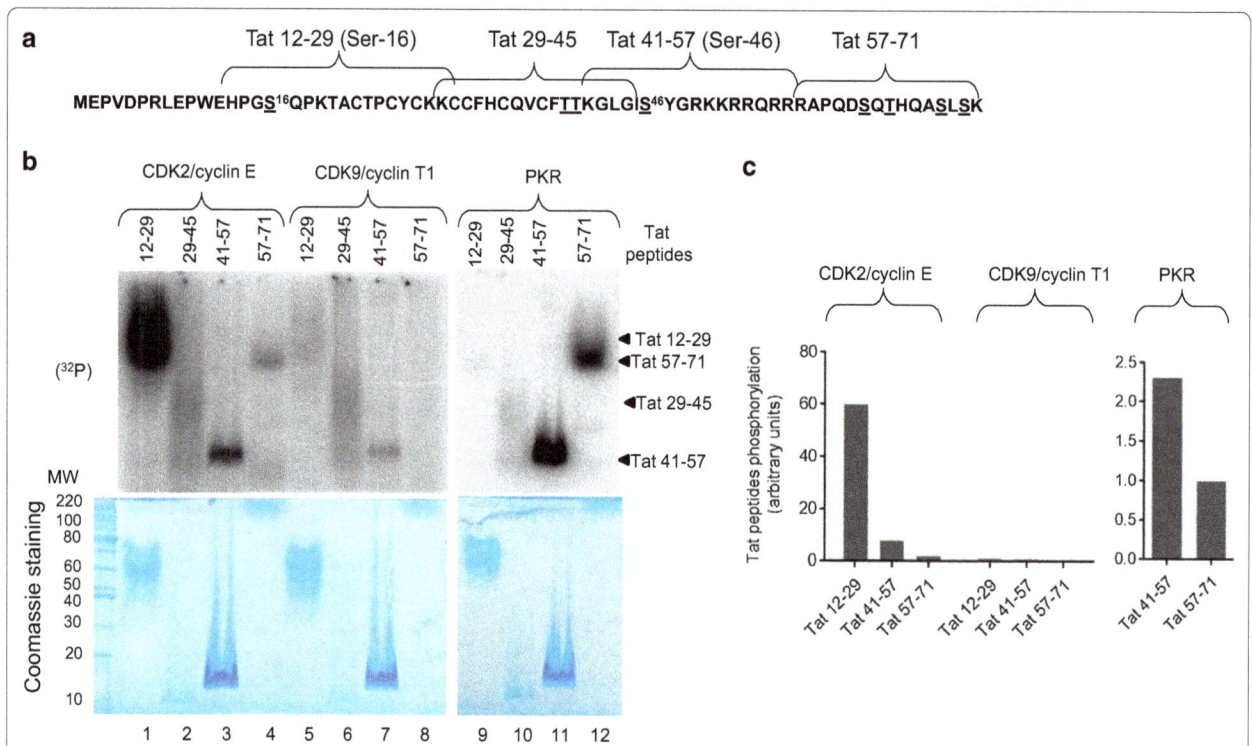

Fig. 2 CDK2 phosphorylates Tat Ser-16 and PKR phosphorylates Tat Ser-46 in vitro. **a** Sequence of Flag-tagged HIV-1 Tat indicating peptides that were used for the analysis of Tat phosphorylation in vitro. Potential phosphorylation sites are underscored. Tat Ser-16 and Ser-46 residues are further indicated with superscript numbering. Ser-16 (peptide 12–29); Thr-39 and Thr-40 (peptide 29–45); Ser-46 (peptide 41–57); and Ser-62, Thr-64, Ser-68 and Ser-70 (peptide 57–71). **b** Phosphorylation of Tat peptides in vitro. Upper panels, Tat peptides (4 μg) were phosphorylated in vitro with recombinant enzymes CDK2/cyclin E (lanes 1–4), CDK9/cyclin T1 (lanes 5–8), and PKR (lanes 9–12) with γ(^{32}P)ATP as described in Methods. Phosphorylated peptides were resolved on 12% SDS Tris-Tricine gel containing 6 M urea, stained with SimpleBlue SafeStain (Coomassie), dried and analyzed by Phospho Imager. Phosphorylated Tat peptides position indicated with arrows on the right. Lower panel, Coomassie stained gel of Tat peptides showing 20 μg of Tat peptides 12–29, 29–45 and 57–71 and 2 μg of Tat peptide 41–57 resolved on 12% SDS Tris-Tricine gel with urea and stained with SimpleBlue SafeStain (Coomassie). **c** Relative intensities of the peptides phosphorylated by CDK2/cyclin E, CDK9/cyclin T1 or PKR were quantified with OptiQuant software (Packard)

in Fig. 2c). Recombinant CDK9/cyclin T1 showed low levels of phosphorylation of peptides containing Ser-16, Thr-39/Thr-40 and Ser-46 (Fig. 2b, lanes 5 and 7; and Fig. 2c). PKR phosphorylated Tat 41–57 peptide containing Ser-46 (Fig. 2b, lane 11), and also strongly phosphorylated Tat 57–71 peptide containing C-terminal serine and threonine residues (Fig. 2b, lane 12). Quantification analysis showed that PKR primarily phosphorylated Ser-46 containing peptide (Fig. 2c).

We further verified that Tat Ser-16 containing peptide is phosphorylated by CDK2/cyclin E using Hunter peptide thin layer electrophoresis system that resolves (^{32}P) peptides. We previously utilized this technique for the analysis of CDK9 phosphorylation [14]. Tat peptides were phosphorylated by CDK2/cyclin E and PKR in vitro and resolved on Hunter peptide mapping system. Then their positions were determined by ninhydrin staining

(Fig. 3, left panels). Peptide phosphorylation detected by PhosphoImager showed that CDK2/cyclin E phosphorylated Tat 12–29 peptide containing Ser-16 (Fig. 3) and PKR phosphorylated peptide Tat 41–57 containing Ser-46 (Fig. 3). We could not detect phosphorylation of Tat 29–45 as this peptide migrates with the (^{32}P) ATP containing front. Taken together, the Tat peptides phosphorylation analysis indicated that Tat Ser-16 was the major phosphorylation site for CDK2/cyclin E and Tat Ser-46—for PKR.

Tat phosphorylation in vivo

To confirm phosphorylation of Tat in vivo, Flag-tagged WT Tat, Tat S16A and Tat S46A mutants were expressed in 293T cells. The cells were metabolically labeled with (^{32}P)-orthophosphate for 3 h and Tat was immunoprecipitated with anti-Flag antibodies (Fig. 4a). Mutation of

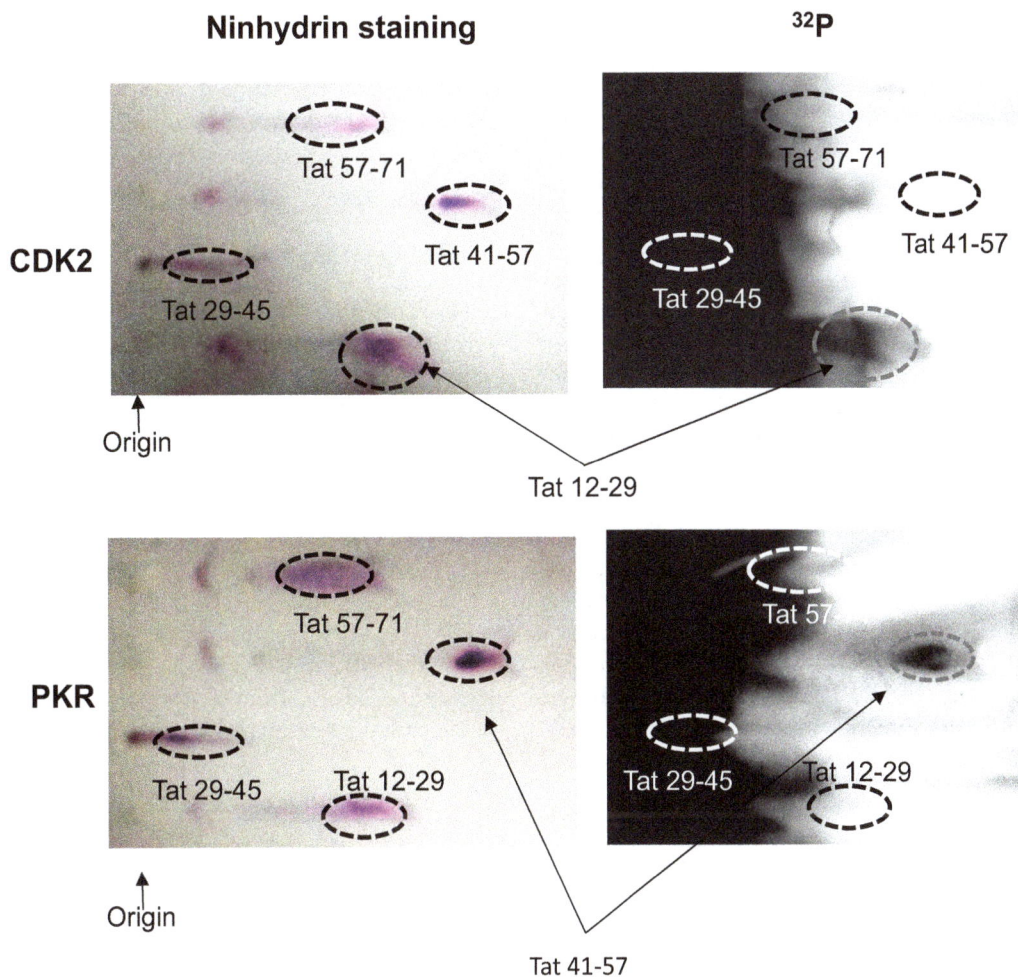

Fig. 3 Hunter peptide mapping analysis of Tat phosphorylation by CDK2 and PKR. Tat-derived peptides were phosphorylated in vitro by CDK2/cyclin E or PKR, as indicated. The reactions were loaded on nitrocellulose plates and peptides were resolved by thin layer electrophoresis as described in Methods. Plates were dried and stained with ninhydrin (left panels) or exposed to Phospho Imager screen (right panels). Origin and peptide positions are indicated on figure. The results are representative from 2 experiments

either Ser-16 or Ser-46 reduced the overall Tat phosphorylation levels (Fig. 4a, compare lane 2 to lanes 3 and 4; see quantification in Fig. 4b), in accordance with our previous findings that alanine mutations of Tat Ser-16 and Tat Ser-46 prevented Tat phosphorylation [4].

As Tat Ser-16 can be phosphorylated by CDK2 as shown here and also by DNA-PK as determined by Tyagi's group [6], we tested the effect of CDK2 and DNA-PK small molecule inhibitors on Tat phosphorylation in cultured cells. Flag-Tat was expressed in 293T cells and the cells were treated overnight with SU 9516, an inhibitor of CDK2 (Tocris) or NU 7441, an inhibitor for PK DNA (Tocris). After the overnight treatment, all cells were also briefly treated with 0.1 M okadaic acid to induce Tat phosphorylation. Tat was immunoprecipitated from cellular lysates with anti-Flag antibodies and separated on SDS PAGE as described above. Tat containing gel pieces were in gel digested with trypsin and subjected to LC-MS/MS analysis. Mass spectra were analyzed with Proteome Discoverer 1.4 and quantified using a label-free approach. We used SIEVE 2.1 software which reanalyzes the original MS spectra and extracts selected ions (frames) with the highest ion current values and integrates their ion elution profiles. We focused on Tat Ser-16 peptide that was previously identified with high confidence. Using trend analysis, we detected over 700 frames which were matched by importing Proteome Discoverer 1.4 analysis results back into SIEVE 2.1. We detected eight Flag-Tat peptides (Fig. 4b) which were normalized using global normalization to equal ratios for each experimental group. Relative ratios of the Tat peptides (Fig. 4c) indicate that non-phosphorylated LEPWEHPGSQPK peptide containing Ser-16 was present at similar ratios in the control and the treatment samples. In contrast, ratios of Ser-16 phosphopeptide (LEPWEHPGSQPK + Phospho (9)) were decreased in the samples treated with CDK2 and DNA-PK inhibitors suggesting decreased Ser-16 phosphorylation. Quantification of the non-phosphorylated peptide (LEPWEHPGSQPK) and phospho Ser-16 peptide (LEPWEHPGSQPK + Phospho (9)) showed about 30% decrease in CDK2-inhibitor treated cells and about 15% decrease in DNA-PK inhibitor treated cells

(Fig. 4d). Thus both CDK2 and DNA-PK can phosphorylated Tat Ser-16 in vivo and CDK2 is likely to be the main contributor.

Effect of CDK2 and PKR knock downs on HIV-1 replication

To confirm that CDK2 and PKR were critical for HIV-1 replication, we generated stable shRNA-mediated knock downs (KD) for CDK2 (Fig. 5a, b) and PKR (Fig. 5c, d) in CEM T cells. Protein levels of CDK2 and PKR were reduced when measured by flow cytometry (Fig. 5a, c) or by Western blot (Fig. 5b, d). To test the effect of knockdowns on HIV-1 replication, CEM T cells were infected with Vesicular stomatitis virus G protein (VSV-G)-pseudotyped pNL4-3.Luc.R-E-virus (HIV-1-LUC-G). The CDK2 KD inhibited HIV-1 replication (Fig. 5e) in agreement with our recent report showing reduction of one round HIV-1 infection in CDK2 KD cells [15]. In contrast, one round of HIV-1 infection was induced in the PKR KD cells (Fig. 5e) in agreement with a recent study that showed inhibition of HIV-1 replication by PKR [11].

Tat Ser-16 alanine mutation inhibits HIV-1 transcription and Tat S16E mutation restores it

Next, we analyzed the effect of Tat Ser-16 and Ser-46 mutations on HIV-1 transcription from proviral DNA. We introduced Tat alanine and phosphorylation-mimicking glutamic acid mutations in pNL4-3 Luc proviral vector which was transfected in 293T cells along with EGFP expressing vector to monitor transfection efficiency. Both Tat S16A and Tat S46A mutations strongly reduced luciferase expression to 2 and 0.1% respectively, suggesting inhibition of HIV-1 transcription (Fig. 6a). Tat S16E mutation showed minimal effect (52%, Fig. 6a) suggesting that glutamic acid substitution supported HIV-1 transcription that was inhibited by the alanine mutation. In contrast, Tat S46E mutation only demonstrated minimal 4% transcription efficiency comparing to WT Tat (Fig. 6a) suggesting that any alteration of in Tat Ser-46 residue is inhibitory and that phosphorylation of Ser-46 is also likely to suppress HIV-1 transcription. To further analyze the effect of Tat Ser-16 and Ser-46 mutations, we generated pseudotyped HIV-1 viruses using pNL4-3

(See figure on next page.)

Fig. 4 Tat phosphorylation and the effect of CDK2 and PKR in cultured cells. **a** Mutation of Ser-16 or Ser-46 residue reduced HIV-1 Tat phosphorylation in cultured cells. Flag-tagged Tat, WT and S16A and S46A mutants were expressed in 293T cells and metabolically labeled with (^{32}P) orthophosphate. Tat protein was immunoprecipitated from cell lysates, resolved on 10% SDS-PAGE and exposed to Phosphor Imager screen. Tat expression was verified by Western blotting with anti-Flag antibodies. Lane 1, mock-transfected cells. Lane 2, WT Tat. Lane 3, Tat S16A mutant. Lane 4, Tat S46A mutant. The figure represents one of the three independent experiments. **b** Relative intensities of Tat and the mutants phosphorylation from three independent experiments. The mean ± SD are shown. *$p < 0.01$. **c** Label-free quantitative analysis of the high resolution MS spectra produced by Orbitrap MS scans for Tat by SIEVE 2.1 software. Average intensities of the indicated Tat peptide are shown with mean and standard deviations. **d** Quantification of non-phosphorylated and Ser-16 phosphorylated LEPWEHPGSQPK + Phospho(9) peptides derived from the data on **c**. Data are further adjusted to indicate the ratio of non-phosphorylated versus phosphorylated peptides. *$p < 0.05$

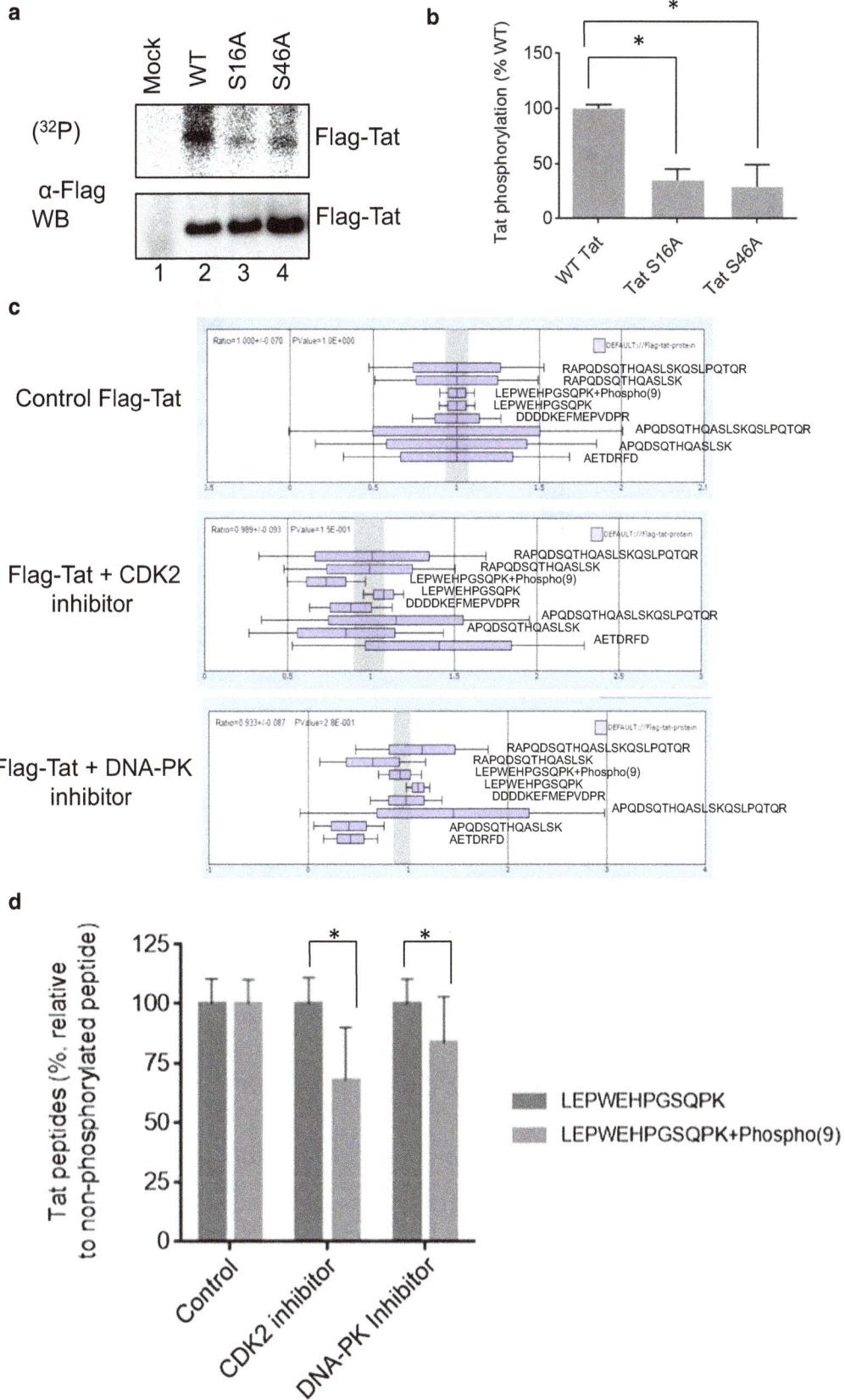

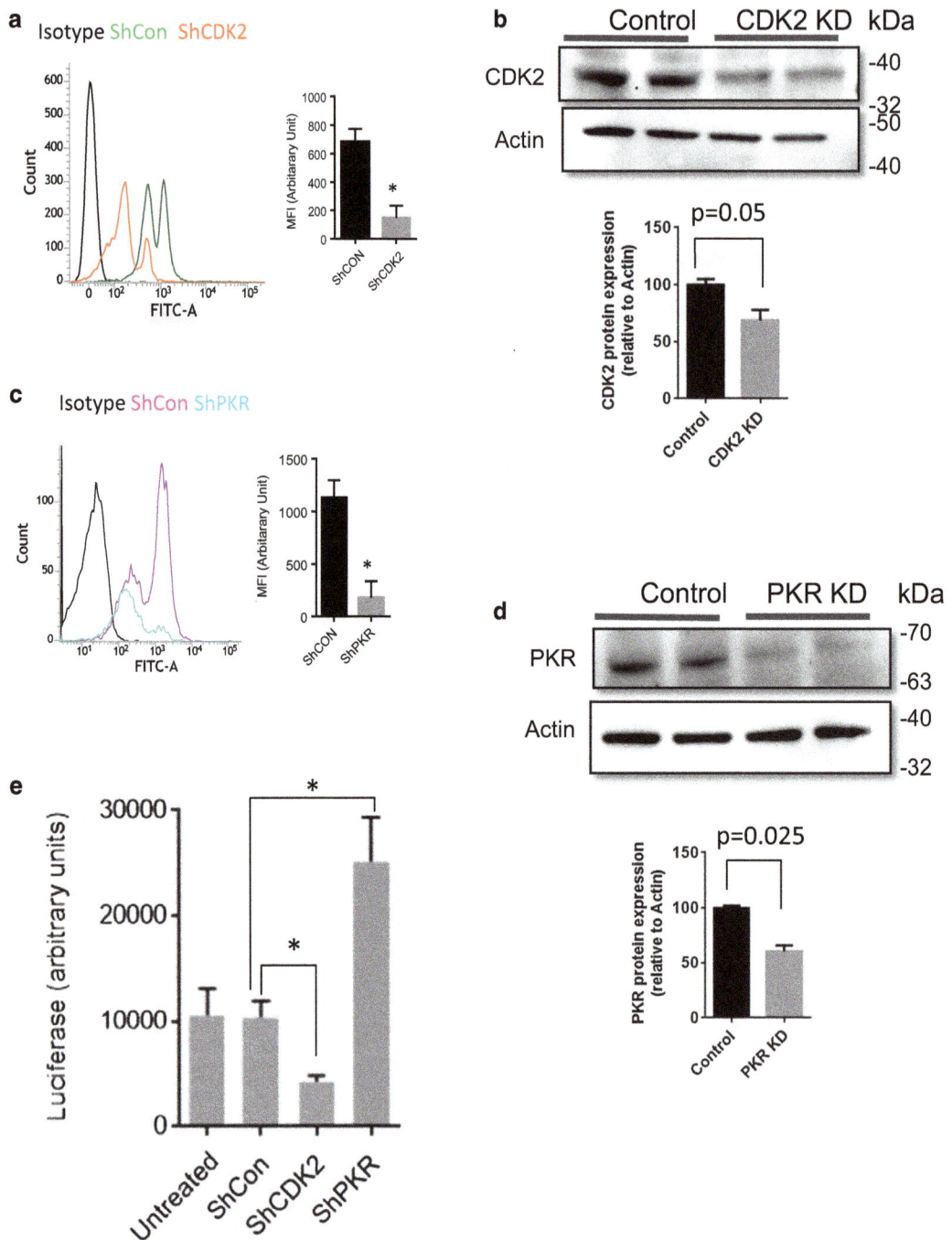

Fig. 5 Effect of CDK2 and PKR Knock downs on HIV-1 replication. **a–d** CDK2 and PKR knockdown were generated in CEM T cells stably transduced with lentiviruses expressing CDK2 or PKR-targeting shRNA, or control non-targeting shRNA. **a, c** Expression of PKR and CDK2 in CEM T cells respectively determined by FACS analysis. Representative histogram shows isotype antibody staining (black), shRNA control (green or purple respectively) and CDK2 or PKR-targeting shRNA (orange or blue respectively). Bar graph of mean fluorescent intensity (MFI, y axis starts at mean fluorescence intensity of the isotype control; n = 2 per group).Mean ± SD. **b, d** Protein expression levels of CDK2 and PKR in stable knock down cell lines. Actin was used as normalization control. Bar graphs show the extent of the corresponding protein knock outs normalized to actin. **e** CEM T cells were infected with HIV-1-LUC-G virus and luciferase activity was measured at 48 h post infection. The mean ± SD are shown. *$p \leq 0.01$

Luc proviral DNA and VSVG-expressing vector and then infected CEM T cells to analyze one round HIV-1 infection. We could only assemble viruses with Tat S16E or Tat S46E mutations and not with Tat S16A or Tat S46A mutations (Fig. 6b). Thus we normalized p24 levels for Tat S16E and Tat S46E viruses but not for Tat S16A and Tat S46S viruses that produced background levels of p24 (Fig. 6b, c). Thus, viruses assembled from proviral vectors with Tat S16E or Tat 46E mutations led to generation of replication capable viruses (Fig. 6b). The virus with Tat S16E mutation replicated well (61% comparing to WT Tat, Fig. 6b) and had a robust p24 production during the viral assembly (55%, Fig. 6c). In contrast, the virus with Tat S46E did not replicate well (11% comparing to WT, Fig. 6b) and also showed less robust p24 production during viral assembly (20%, Fig. 6c), suggesting that Tat Ser-46 phosphorylation can have a negative effect on viral replication. To analyze whether Tat mutants expressed well, WT and mutant Tat were expressed as Flag fusions in 293T cells. All tested mutants expressed well (Fig. 6d) suggesting that HIV-1 transcription and replication defects were not due to the deficiency in Tat production.

We next tested the effect of Tat mutations on Tat nuclear localization which was shown to be affected by Tat Ser-46 phosphorylation [11]. EGFP-fused WT Tat and mutants were expressed in 293T cells and examined under fluorescent microscope. WT Tat and all mutants except Tat S46E were localized in the nucleus (Fig. 6e). However, Tat S46E showed more diffused localization similar to EGFP suggesting that it may have a defect. Taken together, the phosphomimetic mutation of Tat Ser-16 restored HIV-1 transcription and viral replication, while alanine and phosphomimetic mutation in Tat Ser-46 led to a complete or partial inhibition of HIV-1 transcription and replication.

Effect of Tat phosphorylation on its ubiquitination

We next analyzed whether Tat phosphorylation had an effect on its ubiquitination, since Tat was previously shown to be monoubiquitinated [13] and because ubiquitination is generally mediated by protein phosphorylation [16]. To analyze ubiquitination of Tat, we expressed Flag-tagged Tat along with His-tagged Ubiquitin (His-Ub) in 293T cells (Fig. 7a). We separated His-Ub on a Ni column and quantified Tat ubiquitination using anti-Flag antibodies (Fig. 7b). None of the Tat mutations, except Tat S46D and previously reported Tat K71A mutant [13], showed reduced ubiquitination (Fig. 7b). However, we did not achieve statistical significance for Tat 46D in four separate experiments (Fig. 7c) suggesting that this reduction is moderate. Both Tat S16A and Tat S16D mutants remained monoubiquitinated (Fig. 7a, b) suggesting that Tat Ser-16 phosphorylation has no effect on ubiquitination. Collectively, Tat ubiquitination was mostly nonaffected by Ser-16 or Ser-46 mutations, suggesting no effect of Tat phosphorylation on Ubiquitination.

Tat S16A mutation reduced Tat binding to TAR RNA

Previously, Tat phosphorylation in vitro by PKR was shown to enhance [10] as well as inhibit [11] its interaction with TAR RNA. Thus, we analyzed the effect of Tat Ser-16 and Ser-46 mutations on the binding of Tat to TAR RNA. Biotinylated 58 nucleotides long TAR RNA was coupled to the avidin-containing agarose beads and incubated with cell lysates prepared from cells transfected with Flag-Tat expressing vectors. All mutants as well as WT Tat were well expressed (Fig. 8a). Tat associated with TAR RNA bound to the beads was resolved on SDS-PAGE and detected with anti-Flag antibodies. Tat did not bind to the mutant TAR RNA that lacked the bulge structure (Fig. 8b, lane 2). Tat S16A mutant had a reduced binding to TAR RNA (40% reduction, Fig. 8c). Tat S46D mutant showed some reduction in TAR RNA binding but it was not statistically significant (Fig. 8c). Both Tat S16D and Tat S46A mutants bound to TAR RNA (Fig. 8c). Thus, Tat Ser-16 phosphorylation enhanced binding of Tat binding to TAR RNA.

(See figure on next page.)

Fig. 6 Alanine mutations in Tat Ser-16 and Ser-46 reduced HIV-1 proviral DNA transcription replication. **a** Transcription activity of pNL4-3. Luc.R-E-vectors with WT and mutant Tat. 293T cells were transfected with the indicated proviral vectors and also co-transfected with EGFP expressing vector. At 48 h posttransfection, the cells were lysed and luciferase activity was detected. EGFP fluorescence was measured and used for normalization. Results are averages of quadruplicates from a typical experiment of 3 performed. Percent of activity relative to the WT Tat are shown above the bars. $*p \leq 0.001$. **b, c** Replication of VSVg pseudotyped pNL4-3.Luc.R-E-vectors with WT and mutant Tat S16A, S16E, S46A and S46E sequences. 293T cells were transfected with proviral vectors and VSVg-expressing plasmid. At 48 h posttransfection, media was collected and used to infect CEM T cells (**b**) and for p24 measurement (**c**). In **b**, luciferase activity for WT, S16E and S46E viruses was normalized to p24. Percent of activity relative to the WT Tat is shown above the bars. $*p \leq 0.001$. **d** Expression of Flag-tagged WT Tat and mutants. 293T cells were transfected with Flag-Tat vectors expressing WT Tat, Tat S16A, Tat S16D, Tat S46A and Tat S46D mutants. At 48 h posttransfection, the cells were lysed. The lysates were resolved on the 12% SDS-PAGE and immunoblotted with anti-Flag (upper panel) or anti-tubulin (low panel) antibodies. **e** 293T cells were transfected with vectors expressing EGFP, WT Tat-EGFP, Tat S16A-GEFP, Tat S16E-EGFP, Tat S46A-EGFP and Tat-S46E-EGFP. At 24 h posttransfection the cells were photographed on Olympus IX51 using a blue filter for EGFP fluorescence with × 300 magnification

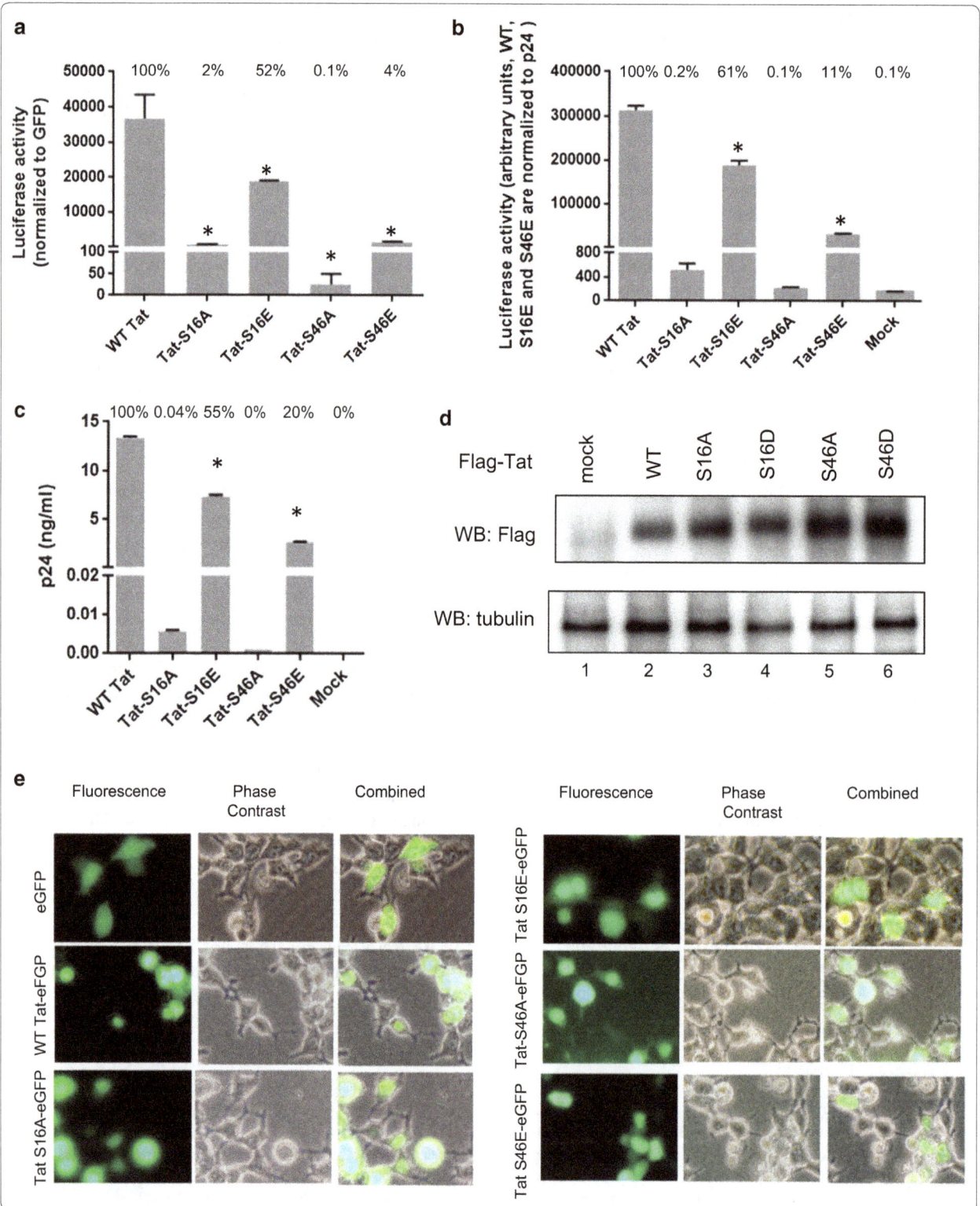

Tat S16D and Tat S46D mutations reduced Tat binding to CDK9/cyclin T1

To analyze the effect of Tat phosphorylation on the binding to CDK9/cyclin T1, we expressed Flag-tagged Tat and Tat S16A, S16D, S46A and S46D mutants along with cyclin T1 and then immunoprecipitated Tat with anti-Flag antibodies. All mutants bound less cyclin T1 (Fig. 8d, e), but Tat S16D and Tat S46D mutants showed the strongest reduction in cyclin T1 binding (Fig. 8d, lanes 4 and 6, and Fig. 8e). These results suggest that Ser-16 and Ser-46 phosphorylation might affect the interaction of Tat with CDK9/cyclin T1 complex.

Molecular dynamics analysis of the effect of Tat Ser-16 and Ser-46 phosphorylation on Tat/CDK9/cyclin T1 complex

To further understand how the Tat Ser-16 and Ser-46 residues influence Tat binding to CDK9/cyclin T1, computational approach was used in which the residues were modeled in CDK9/cyclin T1/Tat complex with ICM-Pro software package using the coordinates of PDB entry 3MIA [17] as the template. To elucidate structural consequences of Tat phosphorylation at Ser-16 and Ser-46, we performed 20 ns Molecular Dynamics (MD) simulations in a periodical water box for the CDK9/Cyclin T1/Tat protein complexes in which Tat was non-phosphorylated on Ser-16 and Ser-46 (S16&S46) or double phosphorylated (S16P&S46P). Since CDK9 Thr-186 is phosphorylated in the kinase active P-TEFb complex [18], a phosphate group was introduced into this residue as well in all cases (Tpo186). Initial conformations of all these complexes were identical, except for the side chains of phosphorylated Ser-16 and Ser-46 residues obtained by global energy minimization using standard ICM-Pro protocol.

Figure 9a shows spatial superposition of the S16&S46 and the S16P&S46P complexes at the final point of the 20 ns MD trajectory. Analysis of the CDK9/cyclin T1/Tat complex crystal structure (PDB: 3MIA) as well as the results of 20 ns MD showed that the side chain of Ser-16 is buried in the Tat-Cyclin T1 interface and its conformation is stabilized by the intermolecular hydrogen bond with the main chain oxygen of Cyclin T1's Val-54. This

hydrogen bond was found to be remarkably stable in the S16&S46 complex and preserved throughout the entire 20 ns of MD time.

Unlike Ser-16, Ser-46 is exposed to solvent in the crystal structure of the CDK9/cyclin T1/Tat complex. The C-terminal part of Tat (residues 49–86) is not resolved in the crystal structure indicating that this part of the Tat is likely to be unstructured and also exposed to solvent. This is further supported by the analysis of the last 37 C-terminal residues of Tat (RKKRRQRRRAHQNSQTHQVSLSKQPTSQPRGDPTGPKE) that showed no identifiable sequence motifs to form secondary structures and was predicted to be a random coil by two independent protein secondary structure prediction servers (AGADIR: http://agadir.crg.es/ and JPRED: http://www.compbio.dundee.ac.uk/www-jpred/). In contrast, the N-terminal part of Tat that includes Ser-16 and Ser-46 residues was found to be quite stable in the CDK9/cyclin T1/Tat complex during the 20 ns MD simulations, preserving overall fold and correct coordination of Zn^{2+} ions and therefore could be used as a template for comparative analysis of possible structural consequences of Ser-16 and Ser-46 phosphorylation.

Phosphorylation of Ser-16 residue resulted in the relocation of its side chain from the internal interface position to the external solvent exposed position, disruption of a hydrogen bond between Tat Ser-16 and cyclin T1 Val-54 (Fig. 9b) and formation of a hydrogen bond between Ser-16 phosphate group and the first methionine of Tat (Fig. 9c). The transition also led to the formation of a hydrogen bond between Tat Glu-9 and CDK9 Lys-144 (Fig. 9d, e). In order to quantitatively characterize the extent of this transition, we calculated Solvent Accessible Surface Area (SASA) of the PO_3 group of Tat Ser-16. The calculations showed that this transition takes only 5 ns when SASA of the PO_3 group changed from insignificant 3 $Å^2$ to a very significant 51.2 $Å^2$. During the rest of the 20 ns MD trajectory, SASA of the PO_3 group fluctuated around ~ 50 $Å^2$. This solvent exposed conformation of phosphorylated Ser-16 was stabilized by strong hydrogen bond that formed between Ser-16 PO_3 and Tat methionine (Fig. 9c) as mentioned above.

(See figure on next page.)

Fig. 7 Tat Ser-46 mutations on its ubiquitination. **a** Tat S46A mutation decreased Tat ubiquitination. 293T cells were co-transfected with pCI-His-hUbi plasmid and WT Flag-Tat, Flag-Tat S16A, Flag-Tat S46A expressing plasmids. The cells were lysed at 48 h posttransfection. His–Ub conjugated proteins were extracted in guanidine denaturing buffer and purified on Ni–NTA agarose beads as described in Methods. Proteins were eluted from the beads and resolved on 12% Tris-Tricine SDS-PAGE, transferred to polyvinylidene fluoride (PVDF) membranes and immunoblotted with anti-Flag antibodies which detected monoubiquitinated Tat. Loading controls were obtained by resolving a portion of the total lysate on 12% SDS-PAGE. Lower panel show quantification as a mean of three independent measurements ± SD. Unpaired *t* test was used to test statistical significance. *$p \leq 0.01$. **b** Tat S46D mutation decreased Tat ubiquitination. 293T cells were transfected and processed as in **a** except WT Flag-Tat, Flag-Tat S16D, Flag-Tat S46D and Flag-Tat K71A expressing plasmids were used. Lower panel show quantification

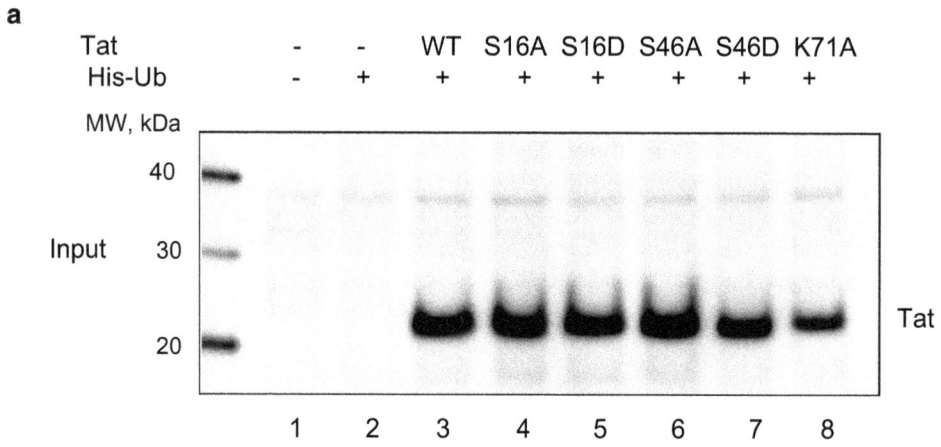

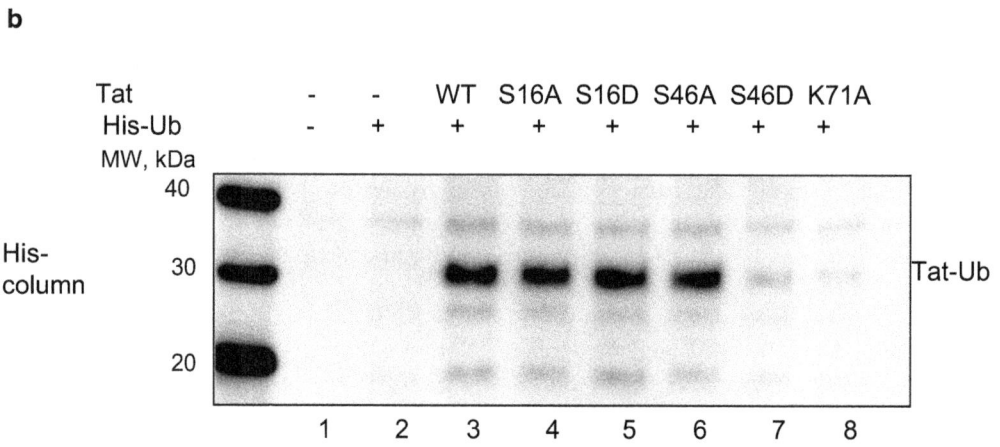

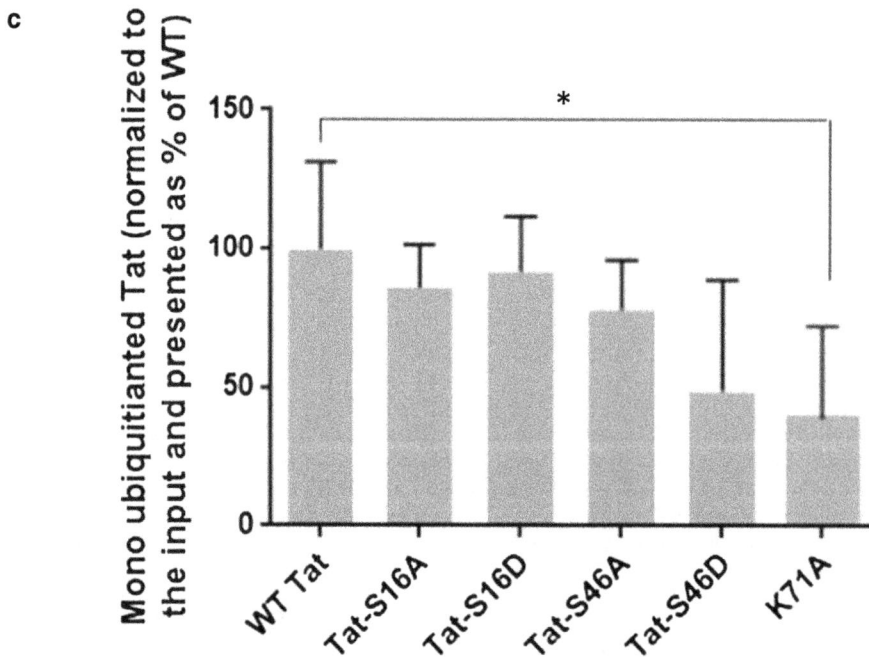

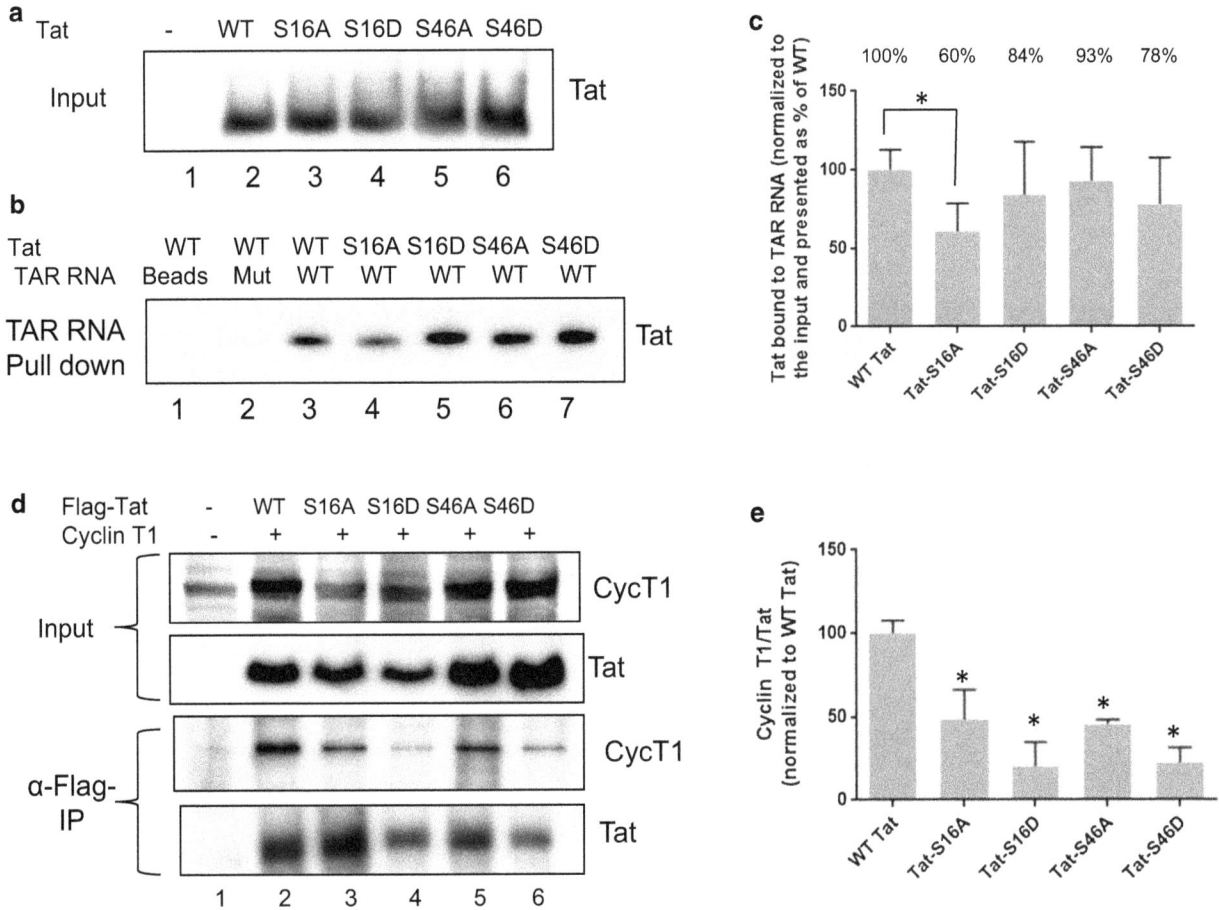

Fig. 8 Effect of Tat S16A, S16D, S46A and S46D mutations on the interaction with TAR RNA and association with cyclin T1. **a–c** Tat Ser-16 and Ser-46 mutations decrease the interaction of Tat with TAR RNA. 293T cells were transfected with plasmids expressing WT Flag-Tat, Flag-Tat S16A or Flag-Tat S46A. The cells were lysed at 48 h posttransfection and the lysates were incubated with WT TAR RNA and mutant TAR RNA lacking bulge and immobilized on streptavidin beads. The beads were washed and proteins were eluted with SDS loading buffer and resolved on the 12% SDS-PAGE. Tat and TAR RNA were detected with anti-Flag and anti-biotin antibodies, respectively. **a** Tat loading control. Lane 1, control minus Tat. **b** Tat bound to the TAR RNA beads. Lane 1, control beads with no TAR RNA. Lane 2, control with mutant TAR RNA. **c** Quantification of Tat bound to TAR RNA beads relative to the loading control with asterisk indicating $p \leq 0.01$. **d, e** Tat Ser-16 and Ser-46 mutations decreased Tat association with cyclin T1. 293T cells were transfected with plasmids expressing WT Flag-Tat, Flag-Tat S16A, Flag-Tat S16D, Flag-Tat S46A and Flag-Tat S46D and with cyclin T1 expressing vector. The cells were lysed at 48 h posttransfection. Tat was immunoprecipitated with anti-Flag antibodies from the lysates and proteins were resolved on the 12% SDS-PAGE. Tat and cyclin T1 were detected with anti-Flag and anti-cyclin T1 antibodies. **e** Quantification cyclin T1/Tat ratio adjusted to the WT Tat control. Mean of three independent measurements $\pm$ SD are shown.*$p \leq 0.001$

(See figure on next page.)

Fig. 9 Molecular dynamics analysis (MD) of CDK9/Cyclin T1/Tat complex with phosphorylated Tat Ser-16 and Ser-46. **a** Spatial superposition of the CDK9/Cyclin T1/Tat complexes with non-phosphorylated Tat (S16&S46) and Tat phosphorylated on Ser-16 and Ser-46 (S16P&S46P) at 20 ns MD time, protein main chains are shown as follows: Cyclin T1—in blue and grey colors, CDK9—in green and carrot colors and Tat—in yellow and cyan colors, respectively. CDK9 Thr-186 was phosphorylated in all the MD simulations. $ATP^{+}Mg2^{+}$ is shown in ball-and-stick presentation. Initial conformation of the complexes were built by homology with crystal structure (PDB: 3MIA) as described in Methods. Arrows indicates the position of Ser-16 and phosphorylated Ser-16 (Sep16) and phosphorylated Thr 186 (Tpo186). Phosphorylated Ser-46 is abbreviated as Sep46. b Enlarged picture showing interaction of Tat Ser-16 with Cyclin T1 Val-54. **b, c** Enlarged pictures showing conformational change of Tat protein due to its phosphorylation. Initial interaction of Tat Ser-16 with Cyclin T1 Val-54 (**b**) is lost upon Ser-16 phosphorylation and the interaction with Tat Met-1 is formed (**c**). **d, e** Enlarged pictures showing interaction of Tat Glu-9 with CDK9 Lys-144 when Tat was phosphorylated (**e**) and no interaction when Tat was not phosphorylation (**d**)

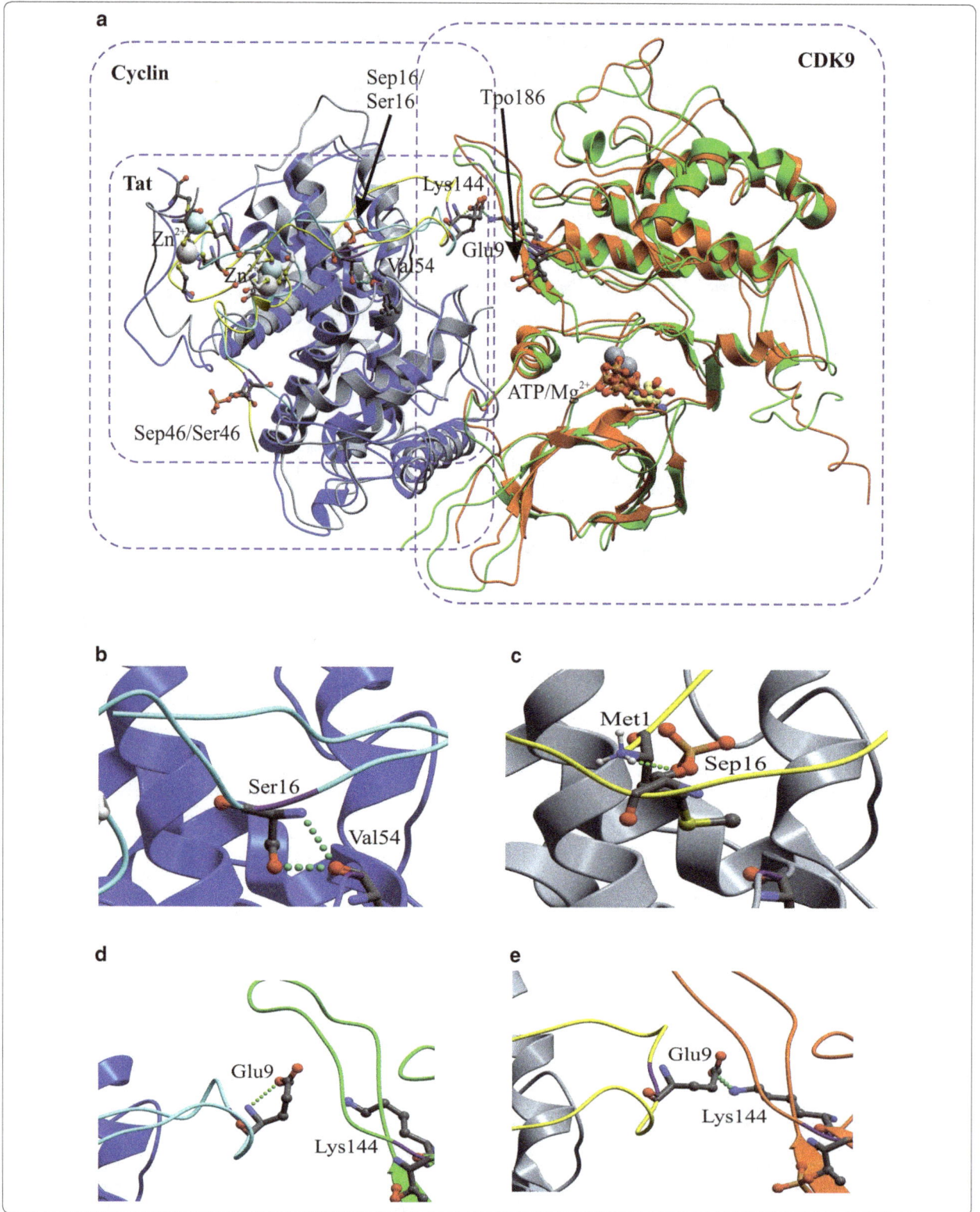

Another consequence of Ser-16 phosphorylation was the relocation of Tat segment (amino acid residues 17–34) that coordinates the two bound Zn^{2+} ions. As shown in Fig. 9, during this transition the Zn^{2+} ions preserved their coordination partners (Tat's Cys-22, Cys-25, Cys-30, Cys-34, Cys-37 and Cyclin T1's Cys-261), but changed their positions relative to CDK9 and cyclin T1. Although, Cα Root-Mean-Square Deviation (RMSD) of this segment at 20 ns MD time in comparison with the initial conformation is almost identical for S16&S46 and S16P&S46P complexes (0.7Å and 0.8Å respectively), the positions of the Zn^{2+} ions were shifted from their initial crystal structure positions by more than 4 Å indicating rigid body-like rotation of the Tat segment due to relocation of phosphorylated Ser-16 side chains from the internal to the external position. Analysis of large scale flexibility of the CDK9/cyclin T1/Tat complexes in non-phosphorylated and phosphorylated states conducted with Dyn-Dom v. 1.5 [19] showed the presence of two flexible domains in Tat structure (residues 5–17 and 18–25 & 29–37). During 20 ns MD the second flexible domain (residues 18–25 & 29–37) of Tat in S16P&S46P complex rotated as a rigid body by 33.2° as compared to the position of the domain in S16&S46 CCT complex. Tat's Gln-17 acted as a mechanical hinge residue of this flexible domain. Since the Zn^{2+} binding segment of Tat protein in the CDK9/cyclin T1/Tat complex is externally accessible, and it is likely to interact with other proteins involved in HIV-1 transcription activation such as the components of super elongation complex. Therefore its relocation in activated CDK9/cyclin T1/Tat complex might have a significant effect on HIV-1 transcription.

Conclusion

Overall, our findings showed that HIV-1 Tat is phosphorylated on Ser-16 residue in cultured cells (summarized in Fig. 10). CDK2/cyclin E and to a lesser extent DNA-PK is likely to phosphorylate Tat Ser-16 and induce HIV-1 transcription and replication. In contrast, PKR that phosphorylates primarily Tat Ser-46 inhibits HIV-1 replication, as shown previously [11] and as our PKR knock down experiment in this study pointed out. Thus, phosphorylated Tat Ser-16 and Tat Ser-46 residues seem to play distinct regulatory roles. Ser-16 phosphorylation can facilitate Tat binding to TAR RNA and may facilitate rearrangement of CDK9/cyclin T1/cyclin T1 complex and help to dissociate CDK9/cyclin T1 from TAR RNA bound Tat during transcription elongation. In contrast, Tat Ser-46 phosphorylation prevents Tat localization to the nucleus and reduces binding to TAR RNA and cyclin T1, thus imposing overall transcription block for Tat function. Our findings presented here indicate a novel regulatory mechanism of HIV-1 transcription mediated by Tat Ser-16 phosphorylation.

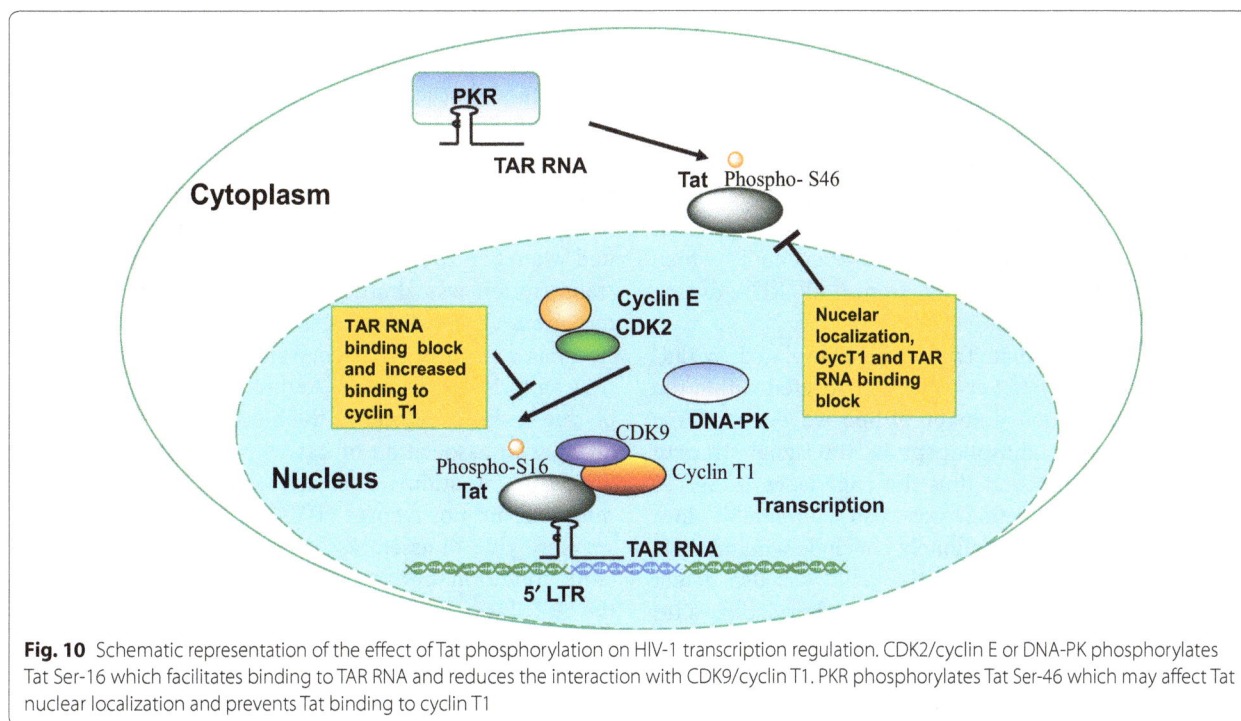

Fig. 10 Schematic representation of the effect of Tat phosphorylation on HIV-1 transcription regulation. CDK2/cyclin E or DNA-PK phosphorylates Tat Ser-16 which facilitates binding to TAR RNA and reduces the interaction with CDK9/cyclin T1. PKR phosphorylates Tat Ser-46 which may affect Tat nuclear localization and prevents Tat binding to cyclin T1

Discussion

Latent infection prevents complete HIV-1 eradication by antiretroviral drugs that are only effective against actively replicating HIV-1 virus. On the other hand, activation of HIV-1 transcription is not affected by the existing antiretroviral drugs and continuous virus expression in residual macrophages may lead to HIV-1 associated pathogenesis [20]. Many factors contribute to the establishment of latency, including inefficient transcription activation by Tat that may be the result of its insufficient expression, activity of cellular cofactors or absence or modification of Tat itself [1]. Tat recruits P-TEFb from the high molecular weight complex where kinase-inactive CDK9/cyclin T1 is bound to 7SK RNA, hexamethylene bis-acetamide-inducible protein 1 (HEXIM1) dimer, Lupus antigen-related protein 7 (LARP7) protein [21–23] and the methylphosphate capping enzyme (MePCE) [24, 25]. Tat also facilitates the formation of super elongation complex (SEC) that contains additional elongation factors and co-activators, including AFF4, ELL2, AF9, ENL [26–28]. AFF4 acts as a scaffold for SEC assembly interacting with cyclin T1 [26]. Tat, on the other hand, increases protein level of ELL2 that is targeted by Siah1 for polyubiquitination and degradation that stabilizes SEC [26–28]. Tat may also recruit ELL1 forming a distinct SEC complex [28]. In a future study, it will be interesting to determine whether Tat Ser-16 phosphorylation promotes Tat association with SEC and/or SEC stabilization. We found here that phosphorylated Tat Ser-16 residue may disrupt a hydrogen bond between Tat Ser-16 and cyclin T1 Val-54 and form a hydrogen bond between Tat Glu-9 and CDK9 Lys-144. Thus, Tat Ser-16 phosphorylation can potentially rearrange CDK9/cyclin T1/Tat complex that may affect the association with SEC. Interestingly, Tat Ser-16 phosphorylation also reduces cyclin T1 binding. One can speculate that non-phosphorylated Tat recruits CDK9/cyclin T1 to TAR RNA, where Ser-16 phosphorylation facilitates its binding to TAR RNA but also loosens the association with CDK9/cyclin T1 which may help to dissociate P-TEFb from TAR RNA during transcription elongation.

We showed here that Tat is phosphorylated in cultured cells primarily on Ser-16 residue located within the N-terminal activation domain. While we detected the presence of Ser-46 phosphopeptide, the signal strength was comparably low and thus the confidence of Ser-46 phosphorylation detection was also comparably low. Thus we are not able to definitely conclude whether Ser-46 is phosphorylated in cultured cells. We also detect with low confidence additional phosphorylation sites located in the C-terminus, so the importance of these additional sites needs to be further investigated. Hence, in vivo, the Tat Ser-16 residue is likely to be the major phosphorylation site. In vitro, Tat Ser-16 can be phosphorylated by CDK2/cyclin E as shown here and also by DNA-PK as shown previously by Tyagi's lab [6] whereas Ser-46 was phosphorylated by PKR. We also tested small molecule inhibitors of CDK2 and DNA-PK which led to ~30 and ~15% reduction in Ser-16 phosphorylation, correspondingly. Thus Tat Ser-16 is likely to be controlled by at least two distinct kinases in vivo. It will be interesting to combine CDK2 and DNA-PK inhibitors and test them in vivo, for example in humanized HIV-1 infected mice. All these observations are in agreement with our earlier study in which CDK2 was proposed to phosphorylate Ser-16 [4] and a recent study by Yong-Soo Bae and colleagues who showed that Tat is phosphorylated by PKR on Thr-23, Thr-40, Ser-46, Ser-62 and Ser-68 in vitro [11]. Also in agreement with our recent study we showed that CDK2 knock down inhibited HIV-1 replication [15], whereas PKR knock down induced it in agreement with Yong-Soo Bae and colleagues study [11].

Our previous work showed that CDK2/cyclin E plays a key role in HIV-1 transcription [3, 29]. We reported that CDK2 phosphorylates CDK9 on Ser-90 residue located within (^{90}SPYNR^{94}) consensus phosphorylation site and that alanine mutation of Ser-90 inhibited HIV-1 transcription [30]. Recently, CDK2 was also shown to phosphorylate SAM domain and HD domain-containing protein 1 (SAMHD1) that controls the cellular deoxyribonucleoside triphosphate (dNTP) pool sizes by hydrolyzing dNTP and inhibits HIV-1 reverse transcription [31–33]. Our recent study showed that CDK2 activity was inhibited in peripheral blood mononuclear cells obtained from patients with sickle cell disease, which led to the activation of SAMHD1 and inhibition of ex vivo HIV-1 infection [15]. Our current findings point to Tat Ser-16 as an additional relevant targets for CDK2 phosphorylation in HIV-1 replication. Thus, CDK2 remains to be a plausible kinase for future anti-HIV-1 therapeutics.

We showed here that HIV-1 transcription was inhibited when Ser-16 residue was mutated to alanine, but the transcription was almost fully recovered with Tat S16E mutation. This finding suggests that Ser-16 phosphorylation has a positive regulatory effect in HIV-1 transcription and viral replication. As pointed above, this could be due to enhancement of the binding to TAR RNA and changes in association of Tat with P-TEFb. In contrast, Tat S46A mutation was clearly inhibitory and Tat S46E mutation did not recover HIV-1 transcription. However, we were able to assemble a recombinant virus with Tat S46E mutation but it replicated poorly comparing to the WT Tat and Tat S16E viruses suggesting that Ser-46 phosphorylation can suppress viral replication. This conclusion is in agreement with Yong-Soo Bae and colleagues report who showed that Tat Ser-46 phosphorylation prevents Tat shuttling to the nucleus [11]. Accordingly, we observed retention of Tat S46E mutant in the cytoplasm. Thus, inhibitory mechanism of Ser-46 phosphorylation includes defects in Tat translocation and binding to TAR RNA and CDK9/cyclin T1 in the agreement with previous reports [11]. Tat is monoubiquitinated by Hdm2 in a non-proteolytic fashion on Lys-71 residue [13] which we explored here in conjunction to the Tat phosphorylation. However, we did not detect any strong effect of Tat Ser-16 mutations and only a weak effect of Tat S46D mutation on ubiquitination suggesting that Tat phosphorylation has no direct effect on Tat ubiquitination. The overall Tat phosphorylation was significantly reduced not only with Ser-16 mutation but also with Ser-46 alanine mutation. Thus it remains to be determined why Ser-46 affects the overall phosphorylation which primarily takes place on Ser-16.

Earlier studies showed that PKR phosphorylates C-terminus of Tat [7, 8, 10]. We previously demonstrated that short 57 nucleotide-long TAR RNA inhibited PKR, while the longer 82 nucleotide-length TAR RNA activated PKR [34]. Thus PKR can be both inhibited and activated in HIV-1 transcribing cells and thus might participate in Tat phosphorylation and deregulation of HIV-1 replication. Yong-Soo Bae and colleagues showed that p53 suppressed HIV-1 replication through the activation of PKR [11]. In their study, PKR-mediated phosphorylation prevented Tat from translocation to the nucleus and inhibited its interaction with TAR RNA and CDK9/cyclin T1, in agreement with our findings. Since Yong-Soo Bae and colleagues only analyze Tat phosphorylation by PKR in vitro and confirmed Tat phosphorylation with a mutation analysis and phospho-threonine and phospho-serine specific antibodies [11], it remains to be determined if Tat is phosphorylated in vivo by PKR under the conditions when PKR is activated. As mutations in both Tat Ser-16 and Tat Ser-46 downregulate the overall Tat phosphorylation level, mutation analysis is clearly not sufficient and direct phosphorylation analysis is needed to detect Ser-46 phosphorylation. PKR was shown to be inhibited by several mechanisms during HIV-1 replication that include the inhibition by TAR RNA, TRBP, adenosine deaminase ADAR1 and PKR regulatory factor PACT (see review [35]). PKR is also inactive in some cultured cell lines including Jurkat T cells [36], which were used in some experiments by Yong-Soo Bae and colleagues. While in their study binding of Tat to TAR RNA was reduced with 23–40–46–62–68 D mutations, single Tat S46D mutation had less pronounced effect on the binding of Tat to TAR RNA [11]. This is in agreement with our findings here that depicted a minimal effect of Tat S46D mutation on the binding to TAR RNA which was only strongly affected by Tat S16A mutation.

Yong-Soo Bae and colleagues showed that HIV-1 provirus with S46A mutation was defective in viral replication [11], providing a support to our current observations that pNL4-3 proviruses with Tat S16A or Tat S46A mutations were inactive.

Our analysis of Tat binding to cyclin T1 showed that both Ser-16 and Ser-46 aspartic acid mutations reduced the binding. While strong reduction of the binding for aspartic acid mutants was unexpected, the Tat S16E mutant is likely to retain some activity as it is able to replicate. It is also possible that phosphomimetic mutations do not fully capture the effect of physiological phosphorylation which can be dynamic.

The analysis of CDK9/cyclin T1/Tat complex in silico by MD simulations showed that Ser-16 was embedded in the Tat-cyclin T1 interface and formed a hydrogen bond with cyclin T1's Val- 54, thus potentially stabilizing the structure of CDK9/cyclin T1/Tat complex. This hydrogen bond was preserved during the MD simulation suggesting its high stability. Unlike Ser-16, the Ser-46 residue was found to be exposed to solvent in the crystal structure of the CDK9/cyclin T1/Tat complex. Phosphorylation of Ser-16 residue resulted in the disruption of a hydrogen bond between Tat Ser-16 and cyclin T1 Val-54 and formation of a hydrogen bond between Tat Glu-9 and CDK9 Lys-144. This relocation was relatively rapid taking only 5 ns out of the total 20 ns MD simulation. The solvent accessible surface area (SASA) was increased by more than factor 10 for the Ser-16 phosphate group. Also, Ser-16 phosphorylation was found to relocate the Zn^{2+} ions-binding Tat segment (amino acids 17–34), which is likely to affect the overall stability of the CDK9/cyclin T1/Tat complex. Large scale flexibility analysis of CDK9/cyclin T1/Tat complex showed that in S16P&S46P Tat, flexible domains (residues 18–25 and 29–37) were rotated along the Gln17 residue acting as a hinge by more than 30° resulting in a large shift of the Zn^{2+} ions. This rotation was not seen in the S16&S46 complex or S16&S46P complexes. Thus, the modeling data indicate that phosphorylated Ser-16 might stabilize CDK9/cyclin T1/Tat complex, while an alanine mutation of Ser-16 destabilized the CDK9/cyclin T1 interface.

Tat binds to the proteasome-associated PAAF1 factor, and modulates the proteasome function by switching it to the non-proteolytic mode [37]. Methylation of Tat's Arg-52 and Arg-53 located in the TAR RNA binding domain of Tat reduces its binding to TAR RNA and P-TEFb and inhibits HIV-1 transcription [38]. Affinity of Tat to TAR RNA and P-TEFb is also increased with the acetylation of Tat's Lys-28 [13]. We did not detect Tat methylation or acetylation as this domain of Tat is cleaved by trypsin and an additional enzyme is needed to recover this peptide for the MS analysis. Thus it remains to be determined whether Tat methylation or acetylation of its TAR RNA binding domain is related to Tat phosphorylation.

Taken together, our study identified Tat Ser-16 as a novel phosphorylation site that affected the overall Tat phosphorylation and regulated Tat interaction with TAR RNA and CDK9/cyclin T1. Thus, phosphorylation of Tat Ser-16 residue represents a novel mechanism of HIV-1 regulated transcription that may provide novel insights for a strategy to control HIV-1 transcription from latent HIV-1 provirus.

Methods
Materials
293T cells were purchased from ATCC (Manassas, VA). Anti-FLAG monoclonal antibodies were purchased from Sigma (St. Louis, MO) and protein A/G agarose beads from Santa Cruz Biotechnology (Santa Cruz, CA). Recombinant CDK9/cyclin T1 and CDK2/cyclin E were purchased from ProQinase (Freiburg, Germany). GST-tagged truncated recombinant human PKR (EIF2AK2, amino acids 252–551) was purchased from Thermo Fisher (Waltham, MA). Double-stranded RNA (polyinosinic-polycytidylic acid) was purchased from Sigma (St. Louis, MO). Horseradish peroxidase (HRP)-conjugated $F(ab)_2$ fragment was purchased from GE Healthcare (Piscataway, NJ). All other inorganic reagents were purchased from Fisher Scientific (Fair Lawn, NJ) or Sigma. Radioactive materials were purchased from Perkin-Elmer (Waltham MA).

Plasmids
The HIV-1 genomic vector, pNL4-3.Luc.R⁻E⁻ (Courtesy of Prof. Nathaniel Landau, NYU School of Medicine, New York, NY) was obtained from the NIH AIDS Research and Reference Reagent Program. pAd.CMV link 1 Tat plasmids expressing WT Tat, TatS16A, Tat S16D, Tat S46A and Tat S46D were generated as previously described [4]. pCI-His-hUbi plasmid was obtained from AddGene (Cambridge, MA).

Knockdown of PKR and CDK2
Lentiviruses expressing small hairpin RNA (shRNA)-targeting human PKR, CDK2, and control shRNA were purchased from Santa Cruz (Dallas, Texas). CEM T cells were infected at 1.1 MOI/1000 cells. Spinoculation was carried out at $800 \times g$ for 30 min. Cells were then incubated for 24 h prior to the addition of puromycin (0.75 µg/ml) for selection of the shRNA-expressing clones. Efficiency of knockdown was assessed by real-time PCR analysis. Total RNA was extracted using TRIzol reagent according to the manufacturer's protocol (Invitrogen, Grand Island, NY). Total RNA (100 ng) was reverse-transcribed to cDNA using Superscript™

RT-PCR kit (Invitrogen, Carlsbad, CA), hexamers and oligo-dT were used as primers. For real-time PCR analysis, cDNA was amplified using Roche LightCycler 480 and SYBR Green1 Master mix (Roche Diagnostics, Indianapolis, IN). PCR was carried out with denaturation at 95 °C for 10 s, annealing at 60 °C for 10 s, and extension at 72 °C for 10 s for 45 cycles. The 18S rRNA was used as a house keeping normalization standard for quantification of mRNA levels of PKR and CDK2. The following primers were used: PKR forward, CAAGTAAAGATT GGAGACTTTGGA; PKR reverse, TCAAATCTGTAC CGCCGAAT; CDK2 forward, TTTGCTGAGATGGTG ACTCG; CDK2 reverse, CTTCATCCAGGGGAGGTA CA; 18S rRNA forward, CTGTTGCTACATCGACCT TT; 18S rRNA reverse, CTCCAGGTTTTGCAACCA GT. Mean Cp values for target genes and 18S rRNA were determined and $\Delta\Delta$Ct method was used to calculate relative expression levels.

HIV-1 infection assays
Vesicular stomatitis virus G protein (VSV-G)-pseudotyped pNL4-3.Luc.R-E-virus (HIV-1-LUC-G) was prepared as previously described [39]. CEM-T cells were infected and cultured at 0.5×10^5 cells/ml in 96-well plate at 37 °C and 5% CO_2 for 48 h. The cells were collected, washed with PBS and resuspended in 100 µl PBS. Then, 100 µl reconstituted luciferase buffer (Luclite Kit, Perkin Elmer) was added to each well and after 10 min incubation, the lysates were transferred into white plates (Perkin Elmer) and luminescence measured using GloMax luminometer (Promega).

p24 ELISA
CEM T cells were infected with pseudotyped viruses pNL4-3.Luc.R-E with WT Tat and Tat S16A, S16E, S46A and S46E mutants. The supernatant was collected 48 h post- infection and p24 protein was detected using RETRO-TEK/ZeptoMetrix HIV-1 p24 ELISA kit (Cat. #0801200). HIV-1 p24 antibody coated microplate was prewashed with a washing buffer, then added 200 µl of samples and p24 antigen standards (125, 62.5, 31.3, 15.6, 3.9 and 0 pg/ml) and incubated overnight at 37 °C. The plate was then washed and 100 µl of HIV-1 p24 detector antibody was added to each well and incubated for 1 h at 37 °C. The plate was again washed, then added 100 µl of Streptavidin-Peroxidase and incubated for 30 min at 37 °C. A blue color was developed within 20 min at room temperature, following the addition of 100 µL of substrate solution. The color development was stopped and the optical density was read at 450 nm using the iMark microplate reader (Bio Rad). The standard curve derived

from the reading was used to interpolate the concentration of HIV-1 p24 protein in each sample.

TAR RNA design

Biotinylated WT TAR RNA (59 nt) and mutant TAR RNA with the deletions of stem-loop nucleotides 21–27 and 38–41 were synthesized by Integrated DNA Technologies (Coralville, Iowa).

Tat Mutagenesis in pNL4-3.Luc.R-E- and pCMV Link 1 Flag-Tat vectors

QuikChange XL site-directed mutagenesis kit (Agilent, Santa Clara, CA) was used to generate mutants of Tat. To mutagenize Tat in HIV-1 proviral pNL4-3.Luc.R⁻E vector, Sall-BamH1 fragments were excised and subcloned in pEGFP-N1 vector (Clontech, Mountain View, CA). Tat Ser-16 residue was mutated to alanine with GCCCTG GAAGCATCCAGGAGCTCAGCCTAAAACTGCTTG TACC (forward) and GGTACAAGCAGTTTTAGGCTG AGCTCCTGGATGCTTCCAGGGC (reverse) primers and to glutamic acid with the GCCCTGGAAGCATCC AGGAGAACAGCCTAAAACTGCTTGTACC (forward) primer and GGTACAAGCAGTTTTAGGCTG TTCTCCTGGATGCTTCCAGGGC (reverse) primer. Tat Ser-46 residue was mutated to alanine with GAC AAAAGCCTTAGGCATCGCCTATGGCAGGAAGAA GCGG (forward) and CCGCTTCTTCCTGCCATAGGC GATGCCTAAGGCTTTTGTC (reverse) primers and to glutamic acid with GACAAAAGCCTTAGGCATCGA ATATGGCAGGAAGAAGCGG (forward) and CCG CTTCTTCCTGCCATATTCGATGCCTAAGGCTTT TGTC (reverse) primers. PCR reactions were run for 18 cycles with the extension time of 8 min to allow the synthesis of the whole plasmid sequence. PCR products were digested with *Dpn I* to degrade the original template. The PCR products were transformed into XL-Gold cells. Colonies were picked, and DNA was isolated using High Pure Plasmid Isolation kit (Roche Applied Sciences, San Francisco, CA). The obtained clones were sequenced using service from Macrogen (Rockville, MD). To reconstruct HIV-1 provirus, Sall-BamH1 DNA fragments contacting Tat mutant sequences were subcloned back to pNL4-3.Luc.R⁻E vector.

Mutagenesis of Tat in expression pCMV Link 1 vector was done directly in the target vector using the same procedure described above. Tat Ser-16 residue was mutated to alanine with TGGGAGCATCCAGGAGCT CAGCCTAAGACTGCT (forward) and AGCAGTCTT AGGCTGATCTCCTGGATGCTCCCA (reverse) primers and to aspartic acid with the TGGGAGCATCCA GGAGATCAGCCTAAGACTGCT (forward) primer and AGCAGTCTTAGGCTGATCTCCTGGATGCTC CCA (reverse) primer. Tat Ser-46 residue was mutated

to alanine with AAGGCTTAGGCATCGCCTATGGCA GGAAGAAG (forward) and CTTCTTCCTGCCATA GTCGATGCCTAAGCCTT (reverse) primers and to aspartic acid with AAGGCTTAGGCATCGACTATG GCAGGAAGAAG (forward) and CTTCTTCCTGCC ATAGTCGATGCCTAAGCCTT (reverse) primers. To mutate Tat lysine 71 which is the subject of ubiquitination, an alanine mutant (K71A) was generated in pCMV Link 1 Tat vector using TCAGACTCATCAGGCTTC TCTATCAGCGCAATCCCTACCC (forward) and GGG TAGGGATTGCGCTGATAGAGAAGCCTGATGAGT CTGA (reverse) primers following the above mentioned procedure.

Transfections

293T cells were seeded in 6-well plates to achieve 50% confluence at the day of transfection. The cells were transfected with indicated plasmids using Lipofectamine and Plus reagents (Life Technologies) following manufacturer's protocol. The efficiency of transfection was verified using a plasmid encoding green fluorescent protein. The cells were cultured for 48 h posttransfection and then analyzed.

Immunoprecipitations

293T cells were lysed in whole cell lysis buffer (50 mM Tris–HCl, pH 7.5, 0.5 M NaCl, 1% NP-40, 0.1% SDS) supplemented with protease cocktail. Tat was precipitated as indicated with anti-Flag antibodies and as we previously described [4]. Briefly, 400 µg of lysate and 800 ng of antibodies were combined with 50 µl of 50% slurry of protein A/G agarose and incubated for 2 h at 4 °C in a TNN Buffer (50 mM Tris–HCl, pH 7.5, 150 mM NaCl and 1% NP-40). The agarose beads were precipitated and washed with TNN buffer, resolved on 12% Tris-Tricine SDS-PAGE, transferred to polyvinylidene fluoride (PVDF) membranes and immunoblotted with appropriate antibodies. In case of in vivo Tat phosphorylation experiments the gel was dried and exposed to Phosphor Imager screen.

Phosphorylation of Tat-derived peptides in vitro

Tat-derived peptides were synthesized by GenScript (Piscataway, NJ). About 2 µg of peptides Tat (12–29) ¹²HPGS¹⁶QPKTACTPCYCKK²⁹ containing Tat Ser-16 (dissolved in 1 mM DTT and sonicated prior to reaction); Tat (29–45) ²⁹KCCFHCQVCFTTKGLGI⁴⁵ (sonicated prior to reaction); Tat (41–57) ⁴¹KGLGIS̲⁴⁶YGRKKR-RQRRR⁵⁷ containing Tat Ser-46; and Tat (57–71) ⁵⁷RAPQDSQTHQASLSK⁷¹ (sonicated prior to reaction) were phosphorylated by recombinant human CDK2/cyclin E, CDK9/cyclin T1 and truncated recombinant human PKR (PKR reaction mix contained 10 ng of dsRNA) in a

10 μl reaction containing 50 mM Hepes–KOH buffer (pH 7.5), 10 mM MgCl$_2$, 6 mM EGTA, 2.5 mM DTT, 100 μM cold ATP and 5 μCi γ-(^{32}P)ATP and incubated for 30 min at 30 °C. The reactions were stopped with Laemmli sample buffer containing 6 M urea, resolved on 12% Tris-Tricine SDS-PAGE with 6 M urea, stained with SimplyBlue safe stain (Thermo Fisher) and subjected to autoradiography and quantification with Phosphor Imager (Packard Instruments, Wellesley, MA).

Hunter phosphopeptide mapping

Phosphopeptide mapping was conducted using Hunter thin layer peptide mapping electrophoresis system (C.B.S. Scientific, Del Mar, CA). Tat-derived peptides were phosphorylated by recombinant CDK2/cyclin E or recombinant PKR with (^{32}P)ATP as described above. Phosphorylated peptides were applied to thin layer cellulose plates (Boehringer Mannheim, Indianapolis, IN) and separated by electrophoresis at pH 1.9 (H$_2$O-acetic acid–formic acid, 900:78:22) conducted at 1000 V, 12 mA for 1 h. Cellulose plates were dried and stained with 0.25% ninhydrin in acetone. The plates were then exposed to Phosphor imager screen.

HIV-1 Tat phosphorylation in vivo

293T cells were transfected with pAd.CMV link 1 Flag-Tat WT, Tat S16A or Tat S46A mutant expressing plasmids using Lipofectamine and Plus reagents (Life Technologies). After 48 h incubation, the cells were placed in a phosphate-free and serum-free DMEM media (Life Technologies) for 2 h. Subsequently, the media was changed to phosphate-free DMEM media supplemented with 0.5 mCi/ml of (^{32}P)-orthophosphate and cells were further incubated for 3 h at 37 °C. To increase Tat phosphorylation, 0.1 μM okadaic acid (Sigma) was added to block cellular PPP-phosphatases. Cells were washed with PBS and lysed in whole cell lysis buffer containing 50 mM Tris–HCl, pH 7.5, 0.5 M NaCl, 1% NP-40, 0.1% SDS and protease inhibitors cocktail (Sigma). After 10 min on ice, cellular material was scraped, incubated at 4 °C for 30 min on a shaker and then centrifuged at 14,000 rpm, at 4 °C for 30 min. The supernatant was recovered and protein concentration was determined using Lowry protein assay (Bio-Rad). Tat was precipitated with monoclonal anti-Flag antibodies (Sigma) coupled to protein G-agarose for 2 h at 4 °C in a TNN Buffer (50 mM Tris–HCl, pH 7.5, 0.15 M NaCl, 1% NP-40). Tat was resolved on 12% Tris-Tricine SDS-PAGE. Tat containing bands were excised and subjected to in gel reduction, alkylation and digestion with trypsin as previously described [40].

To analyze the effect of CDK2 and DNA-PK inhibitors on Tat phosphorylation, 293T cells were grown to 40% confluence and transfected with Flag-Tat expression vector using Lipofectamine 3000/PLUS in OPTI-MEM media as directed by manufacturer. At 24 h posttransfection, the cells were treated overnight with 5 μM SU9516 (Tocris), which is an inhibitor of CDK2 with estimated in vitro IC$_{50}$ = 22 nM. Parallel samples were also treated overnight with 2.5 μM NU7441 (Tocris), an inhibitor for PK DNA with estimated in vitro IC50 = 14 nM. Control cells were treated with DMSO. At 16 h posttreatment, all cells were additionally treated with 100 nM okadaic acid for 2 h. Tat was purified and processed for mass spectrometry analysis as describe above.

Mass spectrometry

Samples were loaded onto in-house prepared nano C18 column and eluted for 60 min with 2–30% gradient of acetonitrile and flow rate 300 nl/min using Shimadzu Prominence Nano HPLC. The 1 FT MS scan and 3 data dependent FT MS/MS scans were performed on Thermo LTQ Orbitrap XL mass spectrometer on major multi-charged MS peaks with resolution 60,000 in each event set. Samples from each patient were run in triplicate. The resulting set of MS/MS spectra were analyzed by Proteome Discoverer 2.1 with SEQUEST (Thermo) search engine (precursor tolerance 30 ppm and fragments tolerance 0.1 Da). These high resolution data and search criteria reduce amount of false positives and dramatically decrease the search time. Protein identifications were carried out using Proteome Discoverer 1.4 software in combination with the SEQUEST protein database search engine and International Protein Index (IPI) Human Protein Database (version 1.79) to which HIV-1 proteins were added. A sequential database search was performed using the human FASTA database. Only peptides with a cross-correlation (XCorr) cutoff of 2.6 for $[M+2H]^{2+}$, 3.0 for $[M+3H]^{3+}$ and a higher charge state were considered. These SEQUEST criteria typically result in a 1–2% false discovery rate (FDR). The FDR was determined by searching on a decoy database. We used SIEVE 2.1 software (Thermo Fisher, Waltham, MA, USA) which is compatible with Proteome Discoverer 1.4 for label-free quantitative analysis of the high resolution MS spectra produced by Orbitrap MS scans.

Flow cytometry

Cell suspensions were fixed and permeabilized using BD Biosciences kit (554714) followed by staining with primary antibodies against CDK2 (Santa Cruz, sc6248) or PKR (Santa Cruz, sc393038) and secondary anti-rabbit IgG antibody (FITC) from Invitrogen. Stained cells were analyzed with FACSCalibur instrument (Becton–Dickinson) and CellQuest software. Three independent experiments were carried out for each sample.

Analysis of Tat–TAR RNA interaction

A slurry (40 µl) of streptavidin agarose beads (Invitrogen) was blocked for 30 min with 64 µg yeast tRNA and 100 µg BSA in Binding buffer (20 mM Tris–HCl pH 7.5, 2.5 mM MgCl$_2$, 100 mM NaCl) and then incubated with 10 µg of biotinylated TAR RNA or biotinylated mutant TAR RNA on a rotating platform at 4 °C. Whole cell lysates from 293T cells grown in 6-well plates and transfected with 2 µg/well of plasmids expressing WT Flag-Tat, Flag-Tat S16A or Flag-Tat S46A were added to the beads in TAK buffer (50 mM Tris–HCl pH 8.0, 5 mM MgCl$_2$, 5 mM MnCl$_2$, 10 µM ZnSO$_4$, 1 mM DTT, 100 mM NaCl) and rotated for 2 h at 4 °C. Beads were washed in TNN Buffer (50 mM Tris–HCl, pH 7.5, 0.15 M NaCl, 1% NP-40) and eluted in 2x SDS-loading buffer to resolve on 12% SDS-PAGE. Immunoblots were probed with anti-Flag and anti-biotin antibodies.

Analysis of Tat ubiquitination

To analyze Tat ubiquitination in vivo, 293T cells grown in 6-well plates were co-transfected with 1 µg/well of pCI-His-hUbi plasmid (Addgene) and 1.5 µg/well of WT Flag-Tat, Flag-Tat S16A, Flag-Tat S16D, Flag-Tat S46A, Flag-Tat S46D or Flag-Tat K71A plasmid using Lipofectamine as described above. At 48 h posttransfection, the cells were washed twice in PBS, and resuspended in Guanidine denaturing buffer (6 M Guanidium-HCl, 100 mM Na$_2$HPO$_4$, 10 mM Imidazole and Sigma protease inhibitors). Cell lysates were sonicated and cleared by centrifugation. His–Ub conjugated proteins were purified on Ni–NTA agarose beads (Novagen, Madison, WI). Each sample lysate (400 µl) was combined with 50% slurry of Ni–NTA agarose beads (50 µl) and incubated at 4 °C for 4 h. The agarose beads were washed twice in Urea-containing buffer (100 mM NaH$_2$PO$_4$, 10 mM Tris Base, 8 M Urea and 10 mM Imidazol) and eluted with 2x SDS-loading buffer. Proteins were resolved on 12% Tris-Tricine SDS-PAGE, transferred to polyvinylidene fluoride (PVDF) membranes and immunoblotted with anti-Flag antibodies.

Building a homology model of CDK9/Cyclin T1/Tat complex

Regularized models of the spatial structures of the CDK9/Cyclin T1/Tat complex were built based on the available crystal structures (PDB: 3MI9, 3MIA [17]) using homology modeling tools included in the standard protocols of the ICM-Pro software package (Molsoft LLC, USA) [41]. Loops absent in the crystal structures were built using the Monte-Carlo energy minimization protocol with the loop-modeling tools of ICM-Pro as described previously [30]. Only standard torsion angles (ϕ, ψ, ω and χi) of amino acids were allowed to vary during the energy minimization. The ICM default set of energy parameters

(ECEPP/3 potential) for van der Waals, electrostatic, torsion energy interactions and hydrogen bonding were used in these calculations. Missing hydrogen and heavy atoms were added and atom types and partial charges were assigned. The protein models were adjusted so that the optimal positions of polar hydrogens were identified. Steric clashes were removed by the energy minimization. Amino acid point mutations in the protein structures and as well as phosphorylation of Ser and Thr residues were done using standard protocols of the ICM-Pro software package.

MD simulations

MD simulations were performed using the double precision version of AMBER 12 (University of California, San Francisco), the widely used software package for molecular and dynamic modeling of proteins [42] running on the multiprocessor clusters of National Research Centre "Kurchatov Institute". MD simulations involve several standard steps including: (a) creation of the protein topology file and preparation of input data for AMBER 12 using the TLEAP tool; (b) construction of hydration models for the protein complex under investigation in a periodic water box with a minimal distance to the water box border of 12 Å; (c) energy minimization and thermodynamic equilibration of hydrated proteins and surrounding solvent; (d) MD simulations at a constant temperature using the Amber99SB parameter set and the TIP3P water model [43, 44]. The thermodynamically equilibrated system was used to perform MD simulations at 310 °K using the Langevin thermostat with constant pressure (1 atm) and an MD duration of 20 ns with time steps of 2 fs. States of the model system were recorded after every 10 ps of MD time for analysis. Neighbor searching was performed every 10 steps. The PME algorithm was used for electrostatic interactions with a cut-off of 1.0 nm as implemented in AMBER. A cut-off of 1.0 nm was used for van der Waals interactions. SHAKE algorithm was used to constrain bonds involving hydrogen [45]. Large-scale flexibility of model proteins was analyzed using the DynDom v.1.5 software package [19].

Authors' contributions
AI, XL, TA, NK, HL, XN and NA conducted experiments, discussed and analyzed data. AVI and MGP conducted modeling and discussed data. AI, TA and SN designed the study, discussed the results and wrote the manuscript. SN performed overall design, general control and coordination of the study. All authors read and approved the final manuscript.

Author details

[1] Center for Sickle Cell Disease, Howard University, 1840 7th Street, N.W. HURB1, Suite 202, Washington, DC 20001, USA. [2] Department of Medicine, Howard University, Washington, DC, USA. [3] Yakut Science Center for Complex Medical Problems, Yakutsk, Russia. [4] Division of Molecular and Radiation Biophysics, Petersburg Nuclear Physics Institute, Gatchina, Russia. [5] Research Center for Nanobiotechnologies, Peter the Great St. Petersburg Polytechnic University, St. Petersburg, Russia.

Acknowledgements

This study was supported by NIH Research Grants 1P50HL118006 (to SN), 1R01HL125005 (to SN), 5G12MD007597 (to SN), U19AI109664 (to SN), P30AI117970 (to SN), 1UM1AI26617 (to SN), Russian Foundation for Basic Research (No. 12-04-91444-NIZ to MP and AVI) and Russian Ministry of Education and Science (No. 2012-1.5-12-000-1001-030 to AVI). This research was also funded by the District of Columbia Center for AIDS Research, an NIH funded program (AI117970), which is supported by the following NIH Co-Funding and Participating Institutes and Centers: NIAID, NCI, NICHD, NHLBI, NIDA, NIMH,NIA, FIC, NIGMS, NIDDK, and OAR. The content is solely the responsibility of the authors and does not necessarily represent the official views of the NIH. We thank NIH AIDS Research and Reference Reagent Program for pHEF-VSVG expression vector (courtesy of Dr. Lung-Ji Chang) and pNL4-3.Luc.R⁻E⁻ (Courtesy of Dr. Nathaniel Landau). The authors thank Molsoft LLC for providing academic license for the ICM-Pro software package. The work was conducted using computing resources of the Federal Collective Usage Center Complex for Simulation and Data Processing for Mega-science Facilities at NRC "Kurchatov Institute" and scientific equipment of the Center of Shared Usage "The analytical center of Nano- and Biotechnologies of SPbPU"

Competing interests

The authors declare that they have no competing interests.

References

1. Lafeuillade A, Stevenson M. The search for a cure for persistent HIV reservoirs. AIDS Rev. 2011;13(2):63–6.
2. Nekhai S, Jeang KT. Transcriptional and post-transcriptional regulation of HIV-1 gene expression: role of cellular factors for Tat and Rev. Future Microbiol. 2006;1(4):417–26.
3. Deng L, Ammosova T, Pumfery A, Kashanchi F, Nekhai S. HIV-1 Tat interaction with RNA polymerase II C-terminal domain (CTD) and a dynamic association with CDK2 induce CTD phosphorylation and transcription from HIV-1 promoter. J Biol Chem. 2002;277(37):33922–9.
4. Ammosova T, Berro R, Jerebtsova M, Jackson A, Charles S, Klase Z, Southerland W, Gordeuk VR, Kashanchi F, Nekhai S. Phosphorylation of HIV-1 Tat by CDK2 in HIV-1 transcription. Retrovirology. 2006;3:78.
5. Debebe Z, Ammosova T, Jerebtsova M, Kurantsin-Mills J, Niu X, Charles S, Richardson DR, Ray PE, Gordeuk VR, Nekhai S. Iron chelators ICL670 and 311 inhibit HIV-1 transcription. Virology. 2007;367(2):324–33.
6. Tyagi S, Ochem A, Tyagi M. DNA-dependent protein kinase interacts functionally with the RNA polymerase II complex recruited at the human immunodeficiency virus (HIV) long terminal repeat and plays an important role in HIV gene expression. J Gen Virol. 2011;92(Pt 7):1710–20.
7. McMillan NA, Chun RF, Siderovski DP, Galabru J, Toone WM, Samuel CE, Mak TW, Hovanessian AG, Jeang KT, Williams BR. HIV-1 Tat directly interacts with the interferon-induced, double-stranded RNA-dependent kinase, PKR. Virology. 1995;213(2):413–24.
8. Brand SR, Kobayashi R, Mathews MB. The Tat protein of human immunodeficiency virus type 1 is a substrate and inhibitor of the interferon-induced, virally activated protein kinase, PKR. J Biol Chem. 1997;272(13):8388–95.
9. Holmes AM. In vitro phosphorylation of human immunodeficiency virus type 1 Tat protein by protein kinase C: evidence for the phosphorylation of amino acid residue serine-46. Arch Biochem Biophys. 1996;335(1):8–12.
10. Endo-Munoz L, Warby T, Harrich D, McMillan NA. Phosphorylation of HIV Tat by PKR increases interaction with TAR RNA and enhances transcription. Virol J. 2005;2:17.
11. Yoon CH, Kim SY, Byeon SE, Jeong Y, Lee J, Kim KP, Park J, Bae YS. p53-derived host restriction of HIV-1 replication by protein kinase R-mediated Tat phosphorylation and inactivation. J Virol. 2015;89(8):4262–80.
12. Ott M, Geyer M, Zhou Q. The control of HIV transcription: keeping RNA polymerase II on track. Cell Host Microbe. 2011;10(5):426–35.
13. Bres V, Kiernan RE, Linares LK, Chable-Bessia C, Plechakova O, Treand C, Emiliani S, Peloponese JM, Jeang KT, Coux O, et al. A non-proteolytic role for ubiquitin in Tat-mediated transactivation of the HIV-1 promoter. Nat Cell Biol. 2003;5(8):754–61.
14. Ammosova T, Obukhov Y, Kotelkin A, Breuer D, Beullens M, Gordeuk VR, Bollen M, Nekhai S. Protein phosphatase-1 activates CDK9 by dephosphorylating Ser175. PLoS ONE. 2011;6(4):e18985.
15. Kumari N, Ammosova T, Diaz S, Lin X, Niu X, Ivanov A, Jerebtsova M, Dhawan S, Oneal P, Nekhai S. Increased iron export by ferroportin induces restriction of HIV-1 infection in sickle cell disease. Blood Adv. 2016;1(3):170–83.
16. Lu Z, Hunter T. Ubiquitylation and proteasomal degradation of the p21(Cip1), p27(Kip1) and p57(Kip2) CDK inhibitors. Cell Cycle. 2010;9(12):2342–52.
17. Tahirov TH, Babayeva ND, Varzavand K, Cooper JJ, Sedore SC, Price DH. Crystal structure of HIV-1 Tat complexed with human P-TEFb. Nature. 2010;465(7299):747–51.
18. Chen R, Yang Z, Zhou Q. Phosphorylated positive transcription elongation factor b (P-TEFb) is tagged for inhibition through association with 7SK snRNA. J Biol Chem. 2004;279(6):4153–60.
19. Hayward S, Lee RA. Improvements in the analysis of domain motions in proteins from conformational change: DynDom version 1.50. J Mol Graph Model. 2002;21(3):181–3.
20. Honeycutt JB, Thayer WO, Baker CE, Ribeiro RM, Lada SM, Cao Y, Cleary RA, Hudgens MG, Richman DD, Garcia JV. HIV persistence in tissue macrophages of humanized myeloid-only mice during antiretroviral therapy. Nat Med. 2017;23(5):638–43.
21. Krueger BJ, Jeronimo C, Roy BB, Bouchard A, Barrandon C, Byers SA, Searcey CE, Cooper JJ, Bensaude O, Cohen EA, et al. LARP7 is a stable component of the 7SK snRNP while P-TEFb, HEXIM1 and hnRNP A1 are reversibly associated. Nucleic Acids Res. 2008;36(7):2219–29.
22. Markert A, Grimm M, Martinez J, Wiesner J, Meyerhans A, Meyuhas O, Sickmann A, Fischer U. The La-related protein LARP7 is a component of the 7SK ribonucleoprotein and affects transcription of cellular and viral polymerase II genes. EMBO Rep. 2008;9(6):569–75.
23. He N, Jahchan NS, Hong E, Li Q, Bayfield MA, Maraia RJ, Luo K, Zhou Q. A La-related protein modulates 7SK snRNP integrity to suppress P-TEFb-dependent transcriptional elongation and tumorigenesis. Mol Cell. 2008;29(5):588–99.
24. Barboric M, Lenasi T, Chen H, Johansen EB, Guo S, Peterlin BM. 7SK snRNP/P-TEFb couples transcription elongation with alternative splicing and is essential for vertebrate development. Proc Natl Acad Sci USA. 2009;106(19):7798–803.
25. Jeronimo C, Forget D, Bouchard A, Li Q, Chua G, Poitras C, Therien C, Bergeron D, Bourassa S, Greenblatt J, et al. Systematic analysis of the protein interaction network for the human transcription machinery reveals the identity of the 7SK capping enzyme. Mol Cell. 2007;27(2):262–74.
26. He N, Liu M, Hsu J, Xue Y, Chou S, Burlingame A, Krogan NJ, Alber T, Zhou Q. HIV-1 Tat and host AFF4 recruit two transcription elongation factors into a bifunctional complex for coordinated activation of HIV-1 transcription. Mol Cell. 2010;38(3):428–38.
27. Yokoyama A, Lin M, Naresh A, Kitabayashi I, Cleary ML. A higher-order complex containing AF4 and ENL family proteins with P-TEFb facilitates oncogenic and physiologic MLL-dependent transcription. Cancer Cell. 2010;17(2):198–212.
28. Sobhian B, Laguette N, Yatim A, Nakamura M, Levy Y, Kiernan R, Benkirane M. HIV-1 Tat assembles a multifunctional transcription elongation complex and stably associates with the 7SK snRNP. Mol Cell. 2010;38(3):439–51.
29. Nekhai S, Zhou M, Fernandez A, Lane WS, Lamb NJ, Brady J, Kumar A. HIV-1 Tat-associated RNA polymerase C-terminal domain kinase, CDK2, phosphorylates CDK7 and stimulates Tat-mediated transcription. Biochem J. 2002;364(Pt 3):649–57.
30. Breuer D, Kotelkin A, Ammosova T, Kumari N, Ivanov A, Ilatovskiy AV, Beullens M, Roane PR, Bollen M, Petukhov MG, et al. CDK2 regulates HIV-1

transcription by phosphorylation of CDK9 on serine 90. Retrovirology. 2012;9:94.

31. Goldstone DC, Ennis-Adeniran V, Hedden JJ, Groom HC, Rice GI, Christodoulou E, Walker PA, Kelly G, Haire LF, Yap MW, et al. HIV-1 restriction factor SAMHD1 is a deoxynucleoside triphosphate triphosphohydrolase. Nature. 2011;480(7377):379–82.

32. Hrecka K, Hao C, Gierszewska M, Swanson SK, Kesik-Brodacka M, Srivastava S, Florens L, Washburn MP, Skowronski J. Vpx relieves inhibition of HIV-1 infection of macrophages mediated by the SAMHD1 protein. Nature. 2011;474(7353):658–61.

33. Laguette N, Sobhian B, Casartelli N, Ringeard M, Chable-Bessia C, Segeral E, Yatim A, Emiliani S, Schwartz O, Benkirane M. SAMHD1 is the dendritic- and myeloid-cell-specific HIV-1 restriction factor counteracted by Vpx. Nature. 2011;474(7353):654–7.

34. Nekhai S, Kumar A, Bottaro DP, Petryshyn R. Peptides derived from the interferon-induced PKR prevent activation by HIV-1 TAR RNA. Virology. 1996;222(1):193–200.

35. Clerzius G, Gelinas JF, Gatignol A. Multiple levels of PKR inhibition during HIV-1 replication. Rev Med Virol. 2011;21(1):42–53.

36. Li S, Koromilas AE. Dominant negative function by an alternatively spliced form of the interferon-inducible protein kinase PKR. J Biol Chem. 2001;276(17):13881–90.

37. Lassot I, Latreille D, Rousset E, Sourisseau M, Linares LK, Chable-Bessia C, Coux O, Benkirane M, Kiernan RE. The proteasome regulates HIV-1 transcription by both proteolytic and nonproteolytic mechanisms. Mol Cell. 2007;25(3):369–83.

38. Xie B, Invernizzi CF, Richard S, Wainberg MA. Arginine methylation of the human immunodeficiency virus type 1 Tat protein by PRMT6 negatively affects Tat Interactions with both cyclin T1 and the Tat transactivation region. J Virol. 2007;81(8):4226–34.

39. Debebe Z, Ammosova T, Breuer D, Lovejoy DB, Kalinowski DS, Kumar K, Jerebtsova M, Ray P, Kashanchi F, Gordeuk VR, et al. Iron chelators of the di-2-pyridylketone thiosemicarbazone and 2-benzoylpyridine thiosemicarbazone series inhibit HIV-1 transcription: identification of novel cellular targets–iron, cyclin-dependent kinase (CDK) 2, and CDK9. Mol Pharmacol. 2011;79(1):185–96.

40. Ilinykh PA, Tigabu B, Ivanov A, Ammosova T, Obukhov Y, Garron T, Kumari N, Kovalskyy D, Platonov MO, Naumchik VS, et al. Role of protein phosphatase 1 in dephosphorylation of Ebola virus VP30 protein and its targeting for the inhibition of viral transcription. J Biol Chem. 2014;289(33):22723–38.

41. Abagyan R, Totrov M. Biased probability Monte Carlo conformational searches and electrostatic calculations for peptides and proteins. J Mol Biol. 1994;235(3):983–1002.

42. Case DA, Cheatham TE 3rd, Darden T, Gohlke H, Luo R, Merz KM Jr, Onufriev A, Simmerling C, Wang B, Woods RJ. The Amber biomolecular simulation programs. J Comput Chem. 2005;26(16):1668–88.

43. Hornak V, Abel R, Okur A, Strockbine B, Roitberg A, Simmerling C. Comparison of multiple Amber force fields and development of improved protein backbone parameters. Proteins. 2006;65(3):712–25.

44. Lindorff-Larsen K, Piana S, Palmo K, Maragakis P, Klepeis JL, Dror RO, Shaw DE. Improved side-chain torsion potentials for the Amber ff99SB protein force field. Proteins. 2010;78(8):1950–8.

45. van Gunsteren WF, Berendsen HJC. Algorithms for macromolecular dynamics and constraint dynamics. Mol Phys. 1977;34:1311–27.

14

Aged Chinese-origin rhesus macaques infected with SIV develop marked viremia in absence of clinical disease, inflammation or cognitive impairment

Stephanie J. Bissel[1*], Kate Gurnsey[1], Hank P. Jedema[1,3], Nicholas F. Smith[1], Guoji Wang[1], Charles W. Bradberry[1,2,3] and Clayton A. Wiley[1]

Abstract

Background: Damage to the central nervous system during HIV infection can lead to variable neurobehavioral dysfunction termed HIV-associated neurocognitive disorders (HAND). There is no clear consensus regarding the neuropathological or cellular basis of HAND. We sought to study the potential contribution of aging to the pathogenesis of HAND. Aged (range = 14.7–24.8 year) rhesus macaques of Chinese origin (RM-Ch) (n = 23) were trained to perform cognitive tasks. Macaques were then divided into four groups to assess the impact of SIVmac251 infection (n = 12) and combined antiretroviral therapy (CART) (5 infected; 5 mock-infected) on the execution of these tasks.

Results: Aged SIV-infected RM-Ch demonstrated significant plasma viremia and modest CSF viral loads but showed few clinical signs, no elevations of systemic temperature, and no changes in activity levels, platelet counts or weight. Concentrations of biomarkers of acute and chronic inflammation such as soluble CD14, CXCL10, IL-6 and TNF-α are known to be elevated following SIV infection of young adult macaques of several species, but concentrations of these biomarkers did not shift after SIV infection in aged RM-Ch and remained similar to mock-infected macaques. Neither acute nor chronic SIV infection or CART had a significant impact on accuracy, speed or percent completion in a sensorimotor test.

Conclusions: Viremia in the absence of a chronic elevated inflammatory response seen in some aged RM-Ch is reminiscent of SIV infection in natural disease resistant hosts. The absence of cognitive impairment during SIV infection in aged RM-Ch might be in part attributed to diminishment of some facets of the immunological response. Additional study encompassing species and age differences is necessary to substantiate this hypothesis.

Keywords: HIV, Simian immunodeficiency virus, HIV-associated neurocognitive disorder, Cognition, Aging, Rhesus macaque

Background

Combined antiretroviral therapy (CART) has completely or almost completely suppressed HIV replication translating to significant reductions in mortality and morbidity in infected individuals. Along with better long-term outcomes and decreased frequency of AIDS-related illness among HIV-infected patients taking suppressive CART, deaths attributable to HIV infection have decreased by 48% since the peak in 2005 [1]. Nevertheless, non-AIDS defining illnesses including neurocognitive deficits normally associated with aging are often observed in the HIV-infected population.

The term HIV-Associated Neurocognitive Disorders (HAND) is used to describe a spectrum of clinical disorders ranging from asymptomatic neurocognitive

*Correspondence: stephaniebissel@pitt.edu
[1] University of Pittsburgh, 3550 Terrace Street, S758 Scaife Hall, Pittsburgh, PA 15261, USA
Full list of author information is available at the end of the article

impairment to mild neurocognitive disorder to HIV-associated dementia (HAD), the clinical correlate of HIV encephalitis [2]. Although CART has been found to prevent or delay these neurocognitive sequelae, less severe neurocognitive dysfunction remains a common comorbidity. Anywhere from 25 to 50% of the HIV-infected population on successful long-term CART experience mild-moderate HAND [3–9] and as this population ages, they are two to seven times more likely to have mild cognitive impairment than their seronegative peers [10–14]. Other comorbidities and behavioral traits have been reported to be risk factors for HAND such as cardiovascular-related conditions [15, 16], obesity [17], diabetes [16, 17], hyperlipidemia [16], tobacco use [16], hepatitis C co-infection [18], alcohol and substance abuse [14, 19], education [20, 21], poverty [21], sleep disorders [14], and psychiatric comorbidities [14]. Many of these conditions are typically associated with aging and contribute to the assumption that HIV-infected individuals undergo a premature aging process. This theory has much traction, but it has been questioned whether available data support the theory of accelerated aging [22]. Regardless, the risk of developing HAND is likely confounded by many of these variables and will be challenging to tease apart, especially with older age.

We know little about the pathogenesis of HAND and why it persists in the presence of CART [23]. Before CART was introduced, HAD was associated with increased HIV RNA in the cerebrospinal fluid (CSF) in patients with severe immunosuppression, arguing for a direct effect due to viral replication in the central nervous system (CNS) [24–27]. However, in populations with access to CART, there is no strong correlation between HIV RNA in the CSF and neurocognitive impairment [28, 29]. Together, these observations suggest that a constellation of immune and viral processes contributes to cognitive dysfunction. Potential mechanisms include comorbidities, "hit and run" effect of HIV entering the CNS early and causing long term neurodegenerative damage [30–34], chronic inflammation in the periphery and/or CNS, substance abuse, age and CART neurotoxicity.

HIV-infected individuals experience complications associated with age earlier than non-infected individuals [35]. Treated HIV-infected individuals experience chronic inflammation, hypercoagulation, and an increased risk of non-AIDS-related morbidity and mortality [36]. There are few preclinical models that can address the cellular and system bases of age-related neurocognitive dysfunction during HIV infection. Since non-human primate (NHP) brains are highly concordant with cortical and subcortical architecture of humans,

they can be employed to study neurological abnormalities and neuropathogenesis in conjunction with aging. Human and NHP have different but comparable lifespans where the effects of aging on complex immune and nervous system function can be studied. Thus, SIV infection of NHPs offers a valid model to study the effects of aging and chronic lentiviral infection.

To model the less severe forms of HAND, we trained aged Chinese-origin rhesus macaques (RM-Ch) to perform cognitive tests and then assigned them to four performance-matched experimental groups. Half of the RM-Ch were then infected with SIVmac251. Cognitive function along with clinical and virological assessments were followed for 8 months, at which point half of the infected and half of the mock-infected RM-Ch were administered CART for an additional 6 months. Since RM-Ch are reported to have lower viremic peaks and set points, greater maintenance of CD4 T cell counts, and significantly longer survival times than rhesus macaques of Indian origin [37–39], we anticipated a slow disease progression that could recapitulate neurological abnormalities observed during HIV infection.

Methods

Subjects

Aged (13.5–23.5 year at beginning of study) female rhesus macaques of Chinese origin ($n = 23$) (RM-Ch) with no previous behavioral training were used for the present study. Macaques were housed and maintained according to American Association of Laboratory Animal Care standards. The University of Pittsburgh's Institutional Animal Care and Use Committee approved all experimentation. Following acquisition, animals were habituated to pole and collar handling and placement in a behavioral primate chair (Primate Products, Immokalee, FL). Collars were fitted with compact accelerometers (Actical, Philips Respironics, Murrysville, PA) to detect sleep and activity patterns. Temperature sensor monitors (DST micro-T temperature logger, Star-Oddi, Iceland) were implanted in the mid-scapular region. To learn to accept water reinforcement rewards, subjects were trained to use a sipper tube attached to the chair. Water was regulated 7 days/week and supplemented (weekly average of 20 ml/kg/d) at the end of each day after training and testing and over the weekend.

For antibody response determination, additional plasma from 9 young adult rhesus macaques (3–11 year old) infected with SIVmac251 for a median of 153 days post-infection was used. Five of these macaques were classified as controllers of infection, while four macaques were classified as progressors.

Water reinforcement rewards

During cognitive testing, water rewards were given to reinforce positive responses to stimuli. Animals with > 20% weight loss from commencement of water regulation were removed from water restriction until weights rebounded to acceptable levels before continuing water regulation. During the study period, nine animals (5 SIV-infected; 4 mock-infected) required temporary removal from water restriction lasting from 18 to 89 days in duration. These animals were not dehydrated or losing weight because of SIV infection, rather the animals were overweight when water regulation was initiated. Four SIV-infected macaques were also removed from water restriction due to illness prior to euthanasia for SIV-related (n = 1) or other (n = 3) reasons. Cognitive assessment data was not obtainable during these periods.

Cognitive assessments

Cognitive assessments took place in a sound attenuated chamber (model AB4240, Eckel Industries, Cambridge, MA) fitted with a 40 W light and white-noise generator. The E-prime software suite (Psychology Software Tools, Sharpsburg, PA) coupled with a CarrollTouch infrared touch screen (Elo Touch Solutions, Milpitas, CA) was used for all stimulus presentation, response recording, and data processing. Baseline measures for cognitive tasks were evaluated at the end of the training period to establish performance and age-matched experimental groups using a grade assessment statistic as indicated in Table 1. Cognitive assessments were conducted Monday through Thursday.

Speeded motor task

On each cognitive assessment day, a stimulus was presented on a touchscreen to start each trial of a 200 trial session. After pressing and holding the stimulus, the trial was advanced to presentation of a new stimulus. Attending correctly to the new stimulus resulted in a water reward and removal of the stimulus (scored a correct response). No water reward was offered upon an incorrect response and the stimulus was removed. Reward levels were amplified with speed of response. Accuracy, response time and percent completion were recorded. Eight animals did not acquire the ability to hold the stimulus to advance the trial, so their task was modified. For these animals, each trial began with presentation of the second stimulus, and a successful touch of that stimulus was scored as accurate, with the response time determined as the duration between presentation of the stimulus and an accurate touch. Analyses were binned by every 2 weeks post-infection (wpi).

Plasma and CSF draws

Plasma and CSF draws were performed/attempted prior to SIV inoculation and every 2 wpi. Samples were drawn at the conclusion of the week's cognitive tasks to provide for recovery before tasks were resumed. Samples were aliquoted and stored at − 80 °C.

SIV inoculation

Macaques were inoculated with SIVmac251 (obtained from the Vaccine and Prevention Research Program, Division of AIDS, National Institute of Allergy and Infectious Diseases and Quality Biological Inc., Gaithersburg, MD from Dr. Ronald Desrosiers) by intravenous injection at 0 wpi. Macaques were observed daily for clinical signs of anorexia, weight loss, lethargy, or diarrhea. When deemed necessary by an examining veterinarian, animals with poor health were euthanized before completing the study. Due to age-related conditions such as congestive heart failure, kidney disease, and obstructive blood clots, euthanasia was necessary in both SIV-infected (5/12 animals) and mock-infected macaques (2/11 animals).

Antiretroviral therapy

Beginning 38 wpi, animals in the antiretroviral treatment groups received daily subcutaneous injections of reverse transcriptase inhibitors bis{[(isopropoxycarbonyl)oxy]methyl}({[(2R)-1-(6-amino-9H-purin-9-yl)-2 propanyl]oxy}methyl)phosphonate (TDF,Tenofovir disoproxil; 5.1 mg/kg) and 4-amino-5-fluoro-1-[(2R,5S)-2-(hydroxymethyl)-1,3-oxathiolan-5-yl]-1,2-dihydropyrimidin-2-one (FTC, emtricitabine, 50 mg/kg). Animals in no treatment groups received saline injections. TDF and FTC were generously provided by Gilead Sciences, Inc. (Foster City, CA) through Material Transfer Agreements.

Quantitation of SIV RNA in plasma and CSF

Virions from 1 ml of plasma or 200–500µl of CSF were pelleted by centrifugation at 23,586×g for 1 h, 4 °C. Total RNA was extracted from the pellet using Trizol reagent (Invitrogen, ThermoFisher Scientific, Waltham, MA). A standard quantitative RT-PCR was performed with 10µl RNA for each sample based on amplification of conserved sequences in *gag* [40].

Tissue collection and processing

At the conclusion of the study, animals were euthanized and perfused with phosphate buffered saline. Brain, spinal cord, spleen, liver, thymus, mesenteric and axial lymph nodes, lung, small bowel, colon, heart, ovary, quadriceps muscles, and kidney were collected. Portions of each tissue were fixed in 10% buffered formalin

Table 1 Study groups, clinical outcomes, neuropathological and systemic pathological findings, and SIV infection in brain regions and systemic organs

Group	Primate #	Age (years)	# days infected	Completed study	Periods off study[a]	Grade/ assessment statistic	Neuropathological findings	Systemic pathological findings	mf ctx	cau/ put/ cc	insula/ bg	thal, hip	cb	occ ctx
SIV + CART−	205	22.8	442	Y	Y	A	Corticospinal tract microglial activation		−	−	−	−	−	−
	221	15.9	442	Y	N	A+		Bronchopneumonia, mild; nephritis, mild	−	−	−	−	−	−
	211	20.9	124	N	Y	B	SIV encephalomyelitis		$+ 3.5 \times 10^5$	+	+	+	+	+
	202	21.4	253	N	Y	C−	Bacterial meningitis; rare SIV + cell in spinal cord		$- 5.2 \times 10^1$	−	−	−	−	−
	209	22.3	275	N	Y	C−			−	−	−	−	−	−
	214	23.2	175	N	N	A−	CMV radiculitis; CMV meningoencephalitis; diffuse microglial activation WM > GM	CMV aspiration pneumonia	$- 1.4 \times 10^0$	−	−	−	−	−
SIV-CART-	220	20.5	442	Y	Y	F−			−					
	212	21.7	NA	Y	Y	A+		Nephritis, mild, focal						
	222	17.0	NA	Y	N	A+								
	204	22.0	NA	Y	Y	C		Medullary fibrosis						
	203	25.0	NA	Y	N	C−								
	216	18.5	NA	N	Y	D+	Global cortical contracted eosinophilic neurons	Splenic angiosarcoma; kidney angiosarcoma & hemorrhagic cyst; prominent macrophages in mes LNs, small bowel, & colon lamina propria						

Table 1 continued

Group	Primate #	Age (years)	# days infected	Completed study	Periods off study[a]	Grade/assessment statistic	Neuropathological findings	Systemic pathological findings	mf ctx	cau/put/cc	insula/bg	thal/hip	cb	occ ctx
	218	18.1	NA	N	N	B+		Benign liver cyst; pancreatic islet cells have cleared cytoplasm; inflamed coronary plaque; chronic inflammation of fallopian tubes; type II fiber atrophy in quadriceps muscles; interstitial inflammation in left kidney; metaplastic tubules in right kidney						
SIV-CART+	213	26.0	NA	Y	N	A+								
	217	18.8	NA	Y	N	B		Diffuse myocardial fibrosis, mild						
	210	19.8	NA	Y	Y	C	Secondary demyelination in lateral column							
	200	21.8	NA	Y	N	D+								
	219	18.7	NA	Y	N	D+		Papillary muscle infarction, chronic						
SIV+CART+	207	19.8	442	Y	N	A+		Chronic bronchitis, low level; macrophage infiltration of cardiac muscle, very mild	−	−	−	−	−	−
	201	18.6	342	N	Y	B	SIV meningoencephalitis, mild; SIV + microglial nodules; SIV myelitis; vacuolar myelitis	Consolidating pneumonia (non-SIV-related), severe	$+ 8.7 \times 10^2$	+	+	+	+	+
	208	19.7	441	Y	N	C+	Menigitis, mild, unknown etiology		$- 3.7 \times 10^{-1}$	−	−	−	−	−
	215	18.7	442	Y	Y	D+	PVCI	Alveolar macrophage infiltration, moderate, pigmented	−	R	−	−	−	−
	224	18.1	441	Y	Y	F	Cerebellar infarct, chronic	Chronic inflammation of striated muscle adventitia	−	−	−	−	−	−

Table 1 continued

Group	Spleen	Liver	Spinal cord	Thymus	mes LN	Lung	Small bowel	Colon	Heart	Ovary	ax LN	Quad muscle	Kidney	Other
SIV + CART−	+	−	−	−	+	−	−	+	−	−	+	−	+	
	+	R	−	−	−	−	−	−	−	−	R	−	−	
	+	R	+	−	+	+	+	+	R	−	+	−	+	
	+	−	R	R	+	−	+	+	−	−	+	−	+	
	+	−	−	R	+	+	+	+	−	−	+	−	−	Peritracheal LN, adrenal gland
	+	−	−	+	+	+	+	+	−	+	+	−	−	Peripheral nerves
	−	−	−	−	−	−	+	−	−	−	−	−	−	
SIV-CART−														
SIV-CART+														
SIV + CART+	−	−	−	−	−	−	−	−	−	−	−	−	−	
	+	R	+	−	+	−	+	+	−	+	+	−	−	
	+	−	R	−	−	−	+	+	−	−	+	−	−	
	+	−	−	−	−	−	+	−	−	−	−	−	−	
	−	−	−	−	−	−	+	−	−	−	+	−	−	

Study groups were selected on basis of age and performance. Systemic and neuropathological findings are summarized for each animal. In situ hybridization for SIV RNA was perfromed in each area listed. Quantitation of SIV RNA in the midfrontal cortex was performed by RTPCR. Positive values are shown as copies/µg RNA

CMV cytomegalovirus, *WM* white matter, *GM* gray matter, *PVCI* perivascular chronic inflammation, *mf* midfrontal, *ctx* cortex, *cau* caudate, *put* putamen, *cc* corpus callosum, *bg* basal ganglia, *thal* thalamus, *hip* hippocampus, *cb* cerebellum, *occ* occipital, *mes* mesenteric, *LN* lymph node, *ax* axial, *quad* quadriceps, *musc* muscle

[a] Periods off study for weight loss, illness or quarantine for false positive TB test

and paraffin embedded. After making coronal sections (~ 5 mm), every other section of the right brain hemisphere was fixed, while remaining sections were snap frozen in ~ 100 mg pieces of midfrontal cortex, caudate, putamen, hippocampus and cerebellum.

Quantitation of SIV RNA in brain tissue

Approximately 100 mg midfrontal cortex was disrupted in Trizol reagent using a Mini BeadBeater (Glen Mills, Inc., Clifton, NJ) to isolate RNA. SIV gag copy numbers were determined as described previously [40, 41] except the total amount of RNA was used to normalize the samples. Total RNA was quantitated using Quant-iT Ribogreen RNA Assay Kit (Invitrogen, ThermoFisher Scientific).

Histological assessment

Formalin fixed paraffin embedded sections from brain and other organs were processed for hematoxylin and eosin staining and CD68 and GFAP immunohistochemistry as described before [42]. To assess distribution and abundance of SIV infected cells, in situ hybridization (ISH) was performed as previously described [43] using riboprobes targeting portions of *gag*, *pol*, and *env* of the molecular clone of SIVmacBK28 [44].

Flow cytometry

After overnight shipment, 100 ml aliquots of EDTA-anticoagulated whole blood were incubated with a mastermix of fluorochrome-conjugated antibodies against a lymphocyte panel or a monocyte panel. The lymphocyte panel included antibodies against the following surface molecules: CD20 (L27, AlexaFluor 700), CD45 (D058-1283, PerCP), CD4 (SK3, PE-Cy7), CD8 (SK1, AmCyan), CD3 (SP34-2, PE-CF594). The monocyte panel included antibodies against the following surface molecules: HLA-DR (L243, APC-Cy7), CD45 (D058-1283, PerCP), CD3 (SP34-2, PE-CF594), CD20 (L27, AlexaFluor 700), CD14 (M5E2, FITC), CD16 (3G8, PacificBlue). All antibodies were from BD Biosciences (San Jose, CA). After lysing red blood cells, samples were acquired on a BD LSRII at Immunology Services unit of the Wisconsin National Primate Research Center (University of Wisconsin, Madison, WI). Data analysis was performed using FlowJo version 9.6.2 (Tree Star, Inc., Ashland, OR).

sCD14 ELISA

Plasma soluble CD14 concentrations were measured in duplicate using the Human CD14 Quantikine ELISA kit (R&D Systems, Minneapolis, MN) according to the manufacturer's protocol.

Multiplex analysis of plasma inflammation markers

ProcartaPlex Multiplex Immunoassays (Affymetrix eBioscience, San Diego, CA) were used to detect non-human primate IL-6, IL-18, CXCL10 and TNF-α at the following time points: baseline (0 wpi), acute infection (2 and 4 wpi), and prior to initiation of CART (34/36 wpi). The 4 wpi time point was not measured in mock –infected macaques. Samples were read by the University of Pittsburgh Cancer Institute LUMINEX Facility using the Luminex 100 reader (Luminex Corporation, Austin, TX).

Humoral responses

ELISA analyses of the humoral immune responses to SIV envelope protein were tested at baseline, ~ 24 wpi, and necropsy as previously described [45] with modifications. A reference plasma with strong anti-Env antibody concentrations was aliquoted and stored at − 80 °C. A batch of EIA/RIA high binding plates were coated overnight with 0.08 μg/ml of rgp130 SIV mac251 (ImmunoDx, Woburn, MA) in PBS (pH 7.4) using 100 μl/well at 4 °C. Plates were blocked with 200 μl B3T buffer (150 mM NaCl, 50 mM Tris–HCl, 1 mM EDTA, 3.3% fetal bovine serum, 2% bovine serum albumin, 0.07% Tween 20) for 1 h at 37 °C. An aliquot of the reference plasma and test plasmas were serially diluted in B3T buffer and added to the plate in duplicate at 100 μl/well for 1 h at 37 °C. 100 μl of horseradish peroxidase-conjugated goat anti-monkey IgG (Rockland Immunochemicals, Inc., Limerick, PA) at 1:10,000 was added for 1 h at 37 °C. Plates were washed 6× with 0.1% Tween 20 in PBS after each step then developed using SureBlue TMB 1-Component Microwell Peroxidase Substrate (SeraCare Life Sciences, Milford, MA) for approximately 25 min. A TMB Stop Solution (SeraCare) was added and plates were read at 450 nm. The OD values for the reference plasma were used to interpolate relative values of anti-Env antibody concentrations using Prism 7 software (GraphPad Software, Inc.).

Statistical analysis

Mann–Whitney tests were used to compare mock-infected controls with SIV-infected macaques. For time course comparisons to baseline values, Kruskal–Wallis tests followed by Dunn's multiple comparison tests were performed. Statistical analyses were performed with Prism 6 (GraphPad Software, San Diego, CA).

Results
Modeling HAND in aged SIV-infected macaques

A group of 23 aged macaques (age range at time of infection = 14.7–24.8 year; median age = 18.6 year) underwent a cognitive training period of 18 months to acclimate and teach the following: pole and collar handling, placement in a behavioral primate chair, water rewards, and cognitive tasks. Initially, it was planned to train the animals for a sensorimotor speeded response task and two executive function tasks. However, within the 18-month training period, this was not possible due to difficulties in training aged animals that had never undergone behavioral training (subjects were retired former breeders). Subjects began training with the speeded motor task, which was continued for the remainder of the study. Behavioral performance was assessed as detailed in Fig. 1a.

Using baseline measurements for the speeded motor task (grade assessment statistic), four performance and aged-matched groups were established at the end of the training period (Table 1): SIV-infected, no treatment (initially n = 6); mock-infected, no treatment (initially n = 5); mock-infected CART treated (initially n = 6); and SIV-infected, CART treated (initially n = 6). Aged adults were difficult to train to interact with the touchscreens. Training techniques utilized in the past with younger animals, such as target training then bridging

into a new behavior were often unsuccessful with this cohort. Eight aged RM-Ch did not reach the final stage of training for the final task at the end of the training period, so the task was modified accordingly for these animals. For comparison with past younger animals, the number of training sessions to learn to interact with the touchscreen ranged from 18 to 90 sessions for the aged RM-Ch, while 100% of a group of 14 young adult males successfully learned the task in half the time (11–46 sessions).

Acute RM-Ch infected with SIV were clinically asymptomatic

Macaques were infected with SIVmac251 at the end of the 18-month training period. Similar to individuals with acute HIV infection, infection of macaques with SIV sometimes results in an acute febrile response accompanied by development of a maculopapular rash, lymphadenopathy, diarrhea, weight loss, transient platelet decrease, and changes in sleep and motor activity [38, 46–51]. Surprisingly, the aged SIV-infected RM-Ch exhibited minimal to no clinical

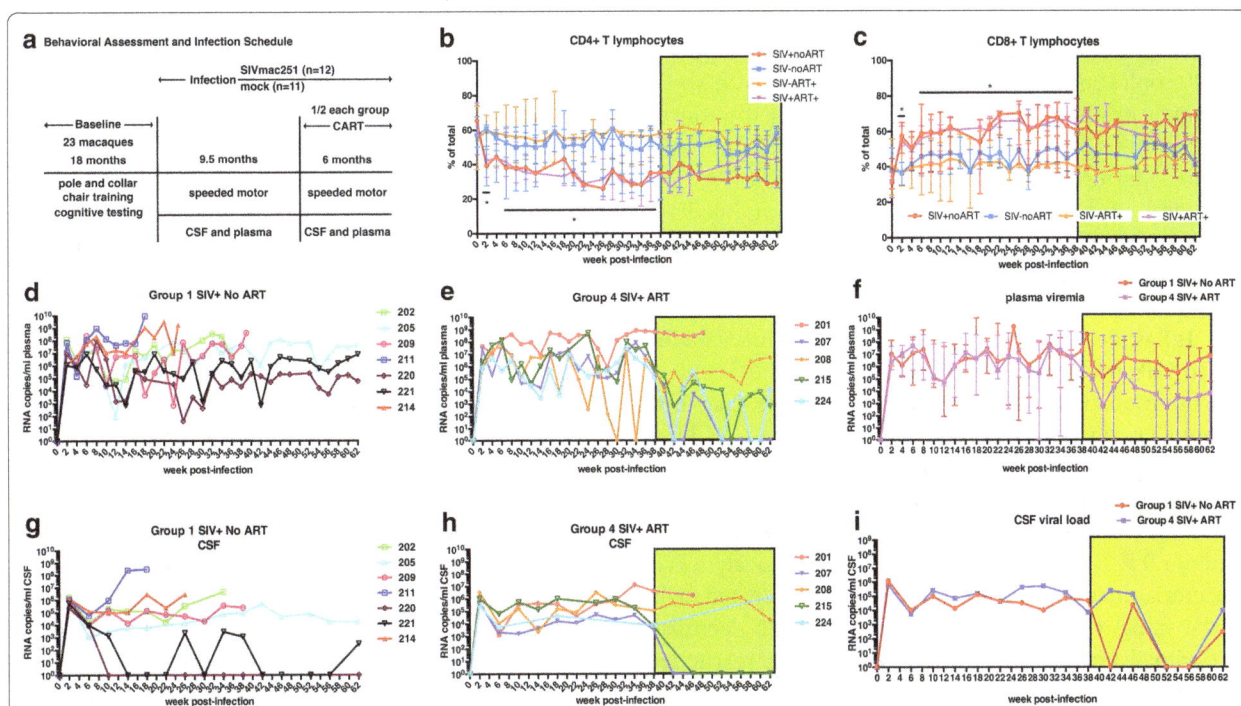

Fig. 1 SIV-infection of aged macaques of Chinese origin has significant viremia. Timeline of cognitive testing, infection and CART (**a**). The proportion of CD4+ lymphocytes declines slightly in aged macaques of Chinese origin but recovers after CART. Longitudinal median ± standard error of peripheral blood proportions for CD4+ lymphocytes (**b**) and CD8+ lymphocytes (**c**) in SIV-infected and mock-infected aged RM-Ch. Plasma (**d**) and CSF (**g**) SIV viral loads from 7 SIV-infected macaques that did not receive treatment show significant viral replication. Plasma (**e**) and CSF (**h**) SIV viral loads from 5 SIV-infected macaques that received CART at 38 wpi show decreased viral replication during the treatment period. Median plasma (**f**) and mean CSF (**i**) SIV viral load of SIV-infected macaques that received CART compared to macaques that did not. The bars in (f) represent the upper and lower values. Asterisks indicate $P < 0.05$ for indicated time points. Kruskal–Wallis tests were used for (**b**), (**c**), (**f**), and (**i**). The green shaded area represents the period macaques received CART

signs of infection; however, some other studies have observed that RM-Ch exhibit fewer clinical signs than RM of Indian origin [37]. Acute changes in weight from baseline after SIV-inoculation were similar to mock-infected animals for the first 2 wpi (Additional file 1: Fig. S1). At 3 and 4 wpi, SIV-infected animals showed greater weight loss than mock-infected RM-Ch, but since the variation in weight changes observed pre-infection was frequent and of similar amplitude, this change could not be attributed to SIV infection. There was no change in body temperature or platelet counts (Additional file 1: Figs. S2 and S3), and no lymphadenopathy was palpable. Comparison of temperature to plasma and CSF viral loads for individual SIV-infected animals are shown in Additional file 1: Fig. S6. Finally, activity counts and sleep patterns were similar to pre-infection levels and between the SIV-infected and mock-infected animals (data not shown).

Aged RM-Ch infected with SIV showed significant viremia

Despite absence of clinical signs during acute infection, aged SIV-infected RM-Ch had a median plasma viral load at 2 wpi of 9.65×10^6 copies/ml (range, 5.88×10^5–1.43×10^8 copies/ml) (Fig. 1). The viral load remained elevated in animals that did not receive CART through the remainder of the experiment with median viral loads at 10^7 copies/ml at several time points; however, some macaques exhibited significant variation over the course of infection. CART lowered median plasma viral load 2–3 logs during the 6-month treatment period (Fig. 1f). CSF viral load had an acute peak at 2 wpi (median, 1.23×10^6 copies/ml; range, 2.54×10^5–3.67×10^6 copies/ml) (Fig. 1i). Two SIV-infected macaques had undetectable to low levels of CSF virus after acute infection (Fig. 1g), while the remaining SIV-infected animals maintained CSF viral loads that ranged from 10^3 to 10^6 copies/ml. Three of the eight SIV-infected macaques that died before the end of the study showed elevated CSF viral load. Two of these animals demonstrated SIV encephalitis (#211; necropsy CSF viral load = 3.3×10^8 copies/ml) or SIV meningoencephalitis (#201; necropsy CSF viral load = 1.9×10^6 copies/ml), while the other macaque had a bacterial meningitis with infrequent SIV-infected cells in the spinal cord but not in the brain (#202; necropsy CSF viral load = 4.68×10^6 copies/ml). In macaques that received CART, detection of viral RNA in the CSF was completely eliminated in two macaques, decreased one log in one macaque, and showed a small decrease in one macaque that died a few weeks following CART initiation. One macaque showed increased viral RNA in the CSF with CART, but since few samples could be collected for this animal, effectiveness of CART throughout the treatment period was unknown.

Changes in peripheral blood cell populations in aged RM-Ch infected with SIV

The proportion of CD4+ T cells in SIV-infected macaques dropped from a median of 62–41% of T cells at 2 wpi, with a reciprocal increase in proportion of CD8+ T cells (Fig. 1a, b). This proportion decrease remained steady throughout the length of infection, although during the treatment period, animals receiving CART began to show T cell proportions similar to baseline and non-infected macaques. Absolute CD4+ T cell counts also decreased after infection, but the decrease was only significant at 32 and 34 wpi. Total CD8+ T cell counts were transiently increased during acute infection and at various time points thereafter ($P < 0.05$ at 22, 26, 40 and 52 wpi). NK cell counts followed a similar transient increase pattern ($P < 0.05$ at 26 and 52 wpi). Total cell counts for CD4+ and CD8+ T cells, NK cells and especially B cells showed transient fluctuations in the non-infected groups as well. T and NK cell counts tended to increase in non-infected macaques, while B cell counts decreased over time for all groups (Additional file 1: Fig. S4). Comparison of CD4+ T cell and CD8+ T-cell counts to plasma and CSF viral loads for individual SIV-infected animals are shown in Additional file 1: Fig. S7. Monocyte subset populations were also followed to examine expansion of inflammatory monocytes (Additional file 1: Fig. S5). The first few measurements after infection were not readable, so baseline cell counts of monocyte subsets were not available. There was little difference in median cell counts of classical monocyte populations (CD14 + CD16−). Intermediate or inflammatory monocytes (CD14 + CD16 +) showed transient increases at 12, 22, and 26 wpi, but the proportion of these cells was similar in SIV-infected and non-infected macaques.

Effect of age on survival and CNS infection

Five of the twelve (41%) aged SIV-infected macaques required euthanasia prior to the conclusion of the experiment, while two of the eleven (18%) non-infected macaques did not finish the study (Table 1). The SIV-infected macaques that did not complete the study had a higher median plasma viremia and CSF viral load at euthanasia than the SIV-infected macaques who completed the study (at the last time point prior to treatment, plasma: 5.3×10^8 copies/ml vs 1.82×10^7 copies/ml; CSF: 1.9×10^6 copies/ml vs 3.80×10^2 copies/ml). SIV-infection could be attributed as the reason for euthanasia in one macaque that developed SIV pneumonitis and encephalomyelitis. The other infected macaques succumbed to obstructed blood flow to the bowel, pneumonia, rhesus cytomegalovirus infection and bacterial meningitis. Using *in situ* hybridization, SIV infected cells were detected in the brains of three SIV-infected macaques at necropsy. Two macaques (#201 and #211) had infected lesions in every region examined, while one had infrequent infected cells in the caudate and putamen (#215) (Table 1). An additional two macaques (#202 and #208) also showed infrequent infected cells in the spinal cord. SIV RNA was detected in midfrontal cortex of four of the SIV-infected macaques that required euthanasia prior to the conclusion of the experiment and one that finished the study (median, 51.6 copies/μg RNA; range, $0.4–3.5 \times 10^5$ copies/μg RNA) (Table 1). Other neuropathological findings included mild to moderate deep white matter microgliosis, corticospinal tract degeneration, and chronic infarcts, but these findings were not exclusively associated with infection status. In the periphery, SIV-infected cells were detected in several organs of the non-treated SIV-infected macaques. While SIV infected cells were detected in treated SIV-infected macaques, the frequency and range was less than the non-treated macaques.

Neither SIV infection nor CART elicited changes in aged RM-Ch sensorimotor behavioral testing outcome

Baseline performances of each macaque were assigned a grade assessment statistic to create performance and age-matched groups. In these aged RM-Ch, there was a range of performance ability that did not correlate with age of the animal or any other observed variable. The median response time and percent accuracy in the speeded motor test was similar in SIV-infected and non-infected groups in the 12 weeks prior to infection (Fig. 2). During the acute infection period, both SIV-infected and non-infected groups showed improvements in response time and percent accuracy. This was attributed to the aged macaques slowly continuing to acquire proficiency/skill in the given task. After approximately 10 wpi, the response time and percent accuracy began to plateau. Neither infection or treatment had a significant effect on response time or percent accuracy (Fig. 2). Comparison of reaction time and accuracy to plasma and CSF viral loads for individual SIV-infected animals are shown in Additional file 1: Fig. S8, while the reaction time and accuracy of individual mock-infected macaques are shown in Additional file 1: Fig. S9. These results suggest that aged RM-Ch are capable of learning and improving tasks even during acute SIV-infection.

SIV-infection of aged RM-Ch was characterized by minimal inflammation

Pathogenic HIV/SIV infection is characterized by acute and persistent inflammation. To assess whether aged SIV-infected RM-Ch showed indications of a typical inflammatory response during infection, plasma sCD14, IL-6, IL-18, CXCL10 and TNF-α concentrations were assessed

during the acute time points and prior to initiation of therapy. sCD14 levels were similar in both SIV-infected and non-infected macaques at all time points examined (Fig. 3a). IL-6, CXCL10 and TNF-α concentrations were undetectable in many of the animals regardless of infection status. However, IL-18 was significantly increased in SIV-infected macaques at 2 wpi (Fig. 3c). Overall, these results suggest that aged macaques of Chinese origin do not respond to SIV infection in the inflammatory manner characteristic of younger macaques and patients with HIV infection [52–57].

To address an aspect of the adaptive immune response in SIV-infected aged RM-Ch, we compared anti-Env antibody responses to SIV-infected young RM of Indian origin. It has been reported that RM-Ch generate stronger antibody responses them RM of Indian origin [55]. The majority of SIV-infected aged macaques generated detectable anti-Env antibody responses (Fig. 4). Two aged SIV-infected RM-Ch (#211 and #201) that required euthanasia prior to completion of the study failed to generate detectable anti-Env antibodies similar to two young adult progressor macaques. Three of four of the young adult animals with disease progression generated minimal if any anti-Env responses. Two of the remaining three aged SIV-infected macaques that required euthanasia prior to the conclusion of the experiment also showed minimal anti-Env antibody responses, while the animal that succumbed to obstructed blood flow to the bowel developed substantial anti-Env antibody responses. The aged SIV-infected macaques that completed the study generated variable anti-Env antibody responses similar to the young adult controller macaques.

Discussion

To understand processes contributing to HAND and aging, our objective was to model HAND in aged NHP in order to dissect the pathological and eventually mechanistic basis of this range of neurocognitive disorders. SIV infection of aged RM-Ch was quite different than reported for young adults [37, 38, 51, 57–72]. They showed minimal to no clinical signs upon infection, with no elevations of systemic temperature and no changes in activity levels, platelet counts or weight. Yet, the aged macaques demonstrated significant plasma viremia and modest CSF viral loads. Neither acute nor chronic SIV infection nor CART had a significant impact on accuracy, speed or percent completion in a speeded motor test. Since this study did not include young adult RM-Ch, we have used historic data that were not generated in the same conditions for comparisons. Although this does not detract from the findings, it will be important to perform additional study encompassing species and age differences to substantiate our conclusions.

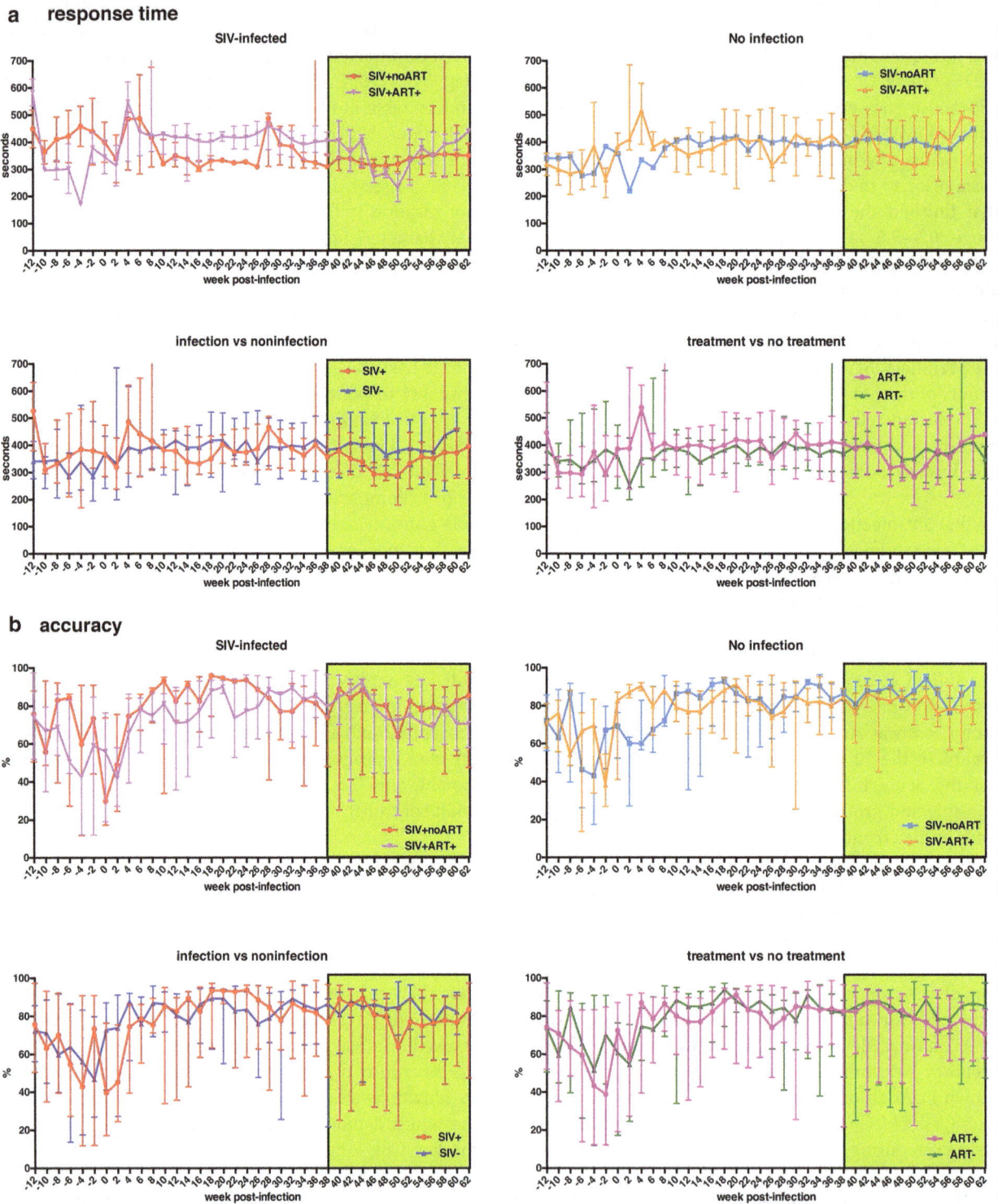

Fig. 2 Neither infection or CART impacted performance on a speeded motor task in aged Chinese macaques. Comparison of median response times and accuracy did not show significant differences. Shown here are between group comparisons of mean ± standard error speeded motor performance response time (**a**) and accuracy (**b**). Analyses for response time and accuracy were binned by every 2 wpi over the course of training period, SIVmac251 or mock infection and CART. Differences between SIV-infection without CART versus SIV-infection with CART (SIV-Infected), Mock-infection without CART versus Mock-infection with CART (No Infection), SIV-infected versus Mock-Infected (Infection vs Noninfection), and CART versus PBS (treatment vs no treatment) are shown for a and b. Kruskal–Wallis tests were used to compare results displayed in each graph, but no statistically significant differences were found. The green shaded area represents the period macaques received CART

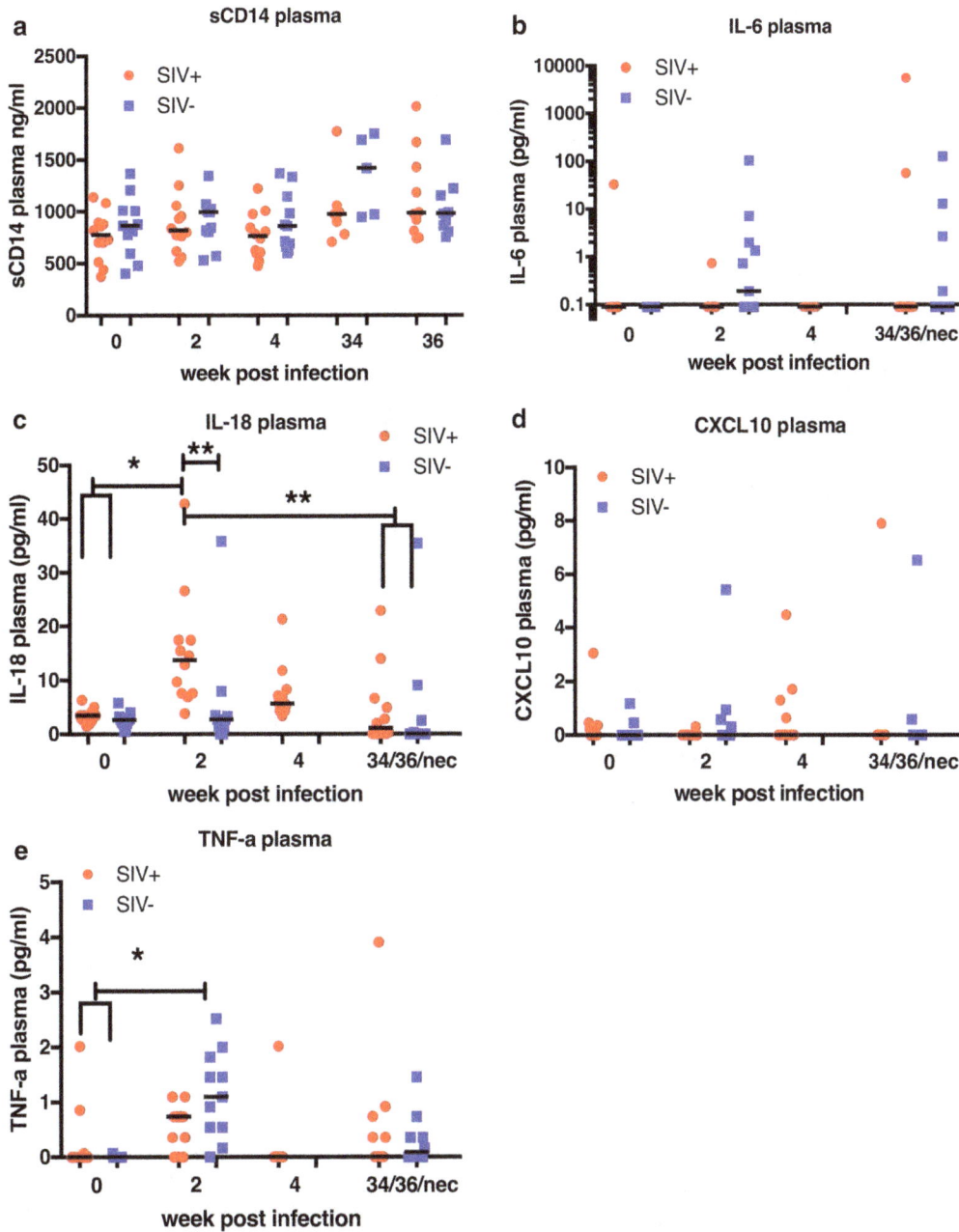

Fig. 3 No elevation of hallmarks of chronic inflammation during lentiviral infection in aged SIV-infected Chinese macaques. IL-18 is elevated in aged SIV-infected macaques of Chinese origin during acute infection, but other hallmarks of chronic inflammation during lentiviral infection remain stable. Median plasma concentrations of soluble CD14 (sCD14) (**a**), IL-6 (**b**), IL-18 (**c**), CXCL10 (**d**), and TNF-α (**e**) at 0, 2, 4 wpi and 34 or 36 wpi or necropsy (34/36/nec). 0 wpi represents baseline, 2 and 4 wpi represent acute infection and 34/36/nec represent chronic infection. Kruskal–Wallis tests were used to analyze differences between groups. *$P < 0.05$. **$P < 0.01$

Modeling human age-related neurological degeneration

Our study plan was to obtain macaques with brains similar in age to 50-year-old humans that could be trained for cognitive assessment and evaluated during chronic infection. Reasoning on the basis of proportional chronology, we estimated the 14–20-year-old macaques used in this study were roughly analogous to 50–60-year-old humans. It has been reported that macaques over 20 years of age show neuropathological changes of ageing analogous to those seen in humans over 60 years of age [73]. In our experience, only the most aged of nonhuman primates (~ 30 years old) have shown amyloid beta accumulation (a hallmark of pathological aging in humans commencing at 60–65 years of age but observed

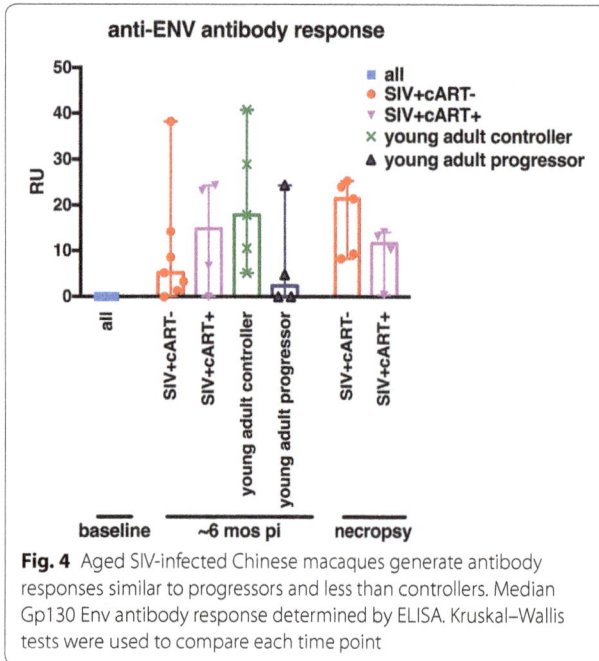

Fig. 4 Aged SIV-infected Chinese macaques generate antibody responses similar to progressors and less than controllers. Median Gp130 Env antibody response determined by ELISA. Kruskal–Wallis tests were used to compare each time point

at younger ages in early onset neurodegenerative disease).

As different macaque species have variable susceptibility to SIV disease progression, it was important to choose a macaque species that was resilient to rapid disease progression and thus permit long-term study. We reasoned this would enable the animals to survive the training and testing paradigm and mitigate conditions that would confound the behavioral studies. The RM-Ch subspecies best fit these requirements.

We had several difficulties modeling the current commonly described forms of HAND in aging individuals beginning with training the 14–20-year-old macaques to learn cognitive tasks. Compared to past young adults, the aged macaques were recalcitrant to training, and despite increasing the training period, the macaques were only able to reliably perform the speeded motor task. Then after SIV infection, the aged RM-Ch failed to show clinical signs and we could not discriminate differences in neurocognitive performance. Despite matching groups for baseline cognitive task performance, the heterogeneous responses of the small groups of outbred aged RM-Ch further limited the ability to sensitively discern cognitive impairment. This highlights the difficulty and limitations of experimentally modeling the issues facing aviremic HIV-infected patients on effective long-term CART, yet experiencing HAND, in aged macaques. Might a different experimental approach or model be more suitable? This will have to be interrogated systematically in order to develop a system to address how chronic inflammation impacts cognition in the face of effective viral suppression.

Aged SIV-infected RM-Ch showed marked levels of plasma viremia

Juvenile and adult RM-Ch are reported to have innate resistance to SIV infection compared to rhesus macaques of Indian origin [37, 38, 58]. Levels of viral replication in RM-Ch tend to be lower than in macaques of Indian origin, but significant inter-individual variation in disease progression has been reported [59, 60]. Surveying the literature for plasma viremia in younger SIV-infected RM-Ch, peak viremia ranges from 10^3 to 10^8 copies/ml with an approximate mean of 5×10^7 copies/ml, while set point viremia ranges from 10^3 to 10^7 copies/ml [37, 38, 51, 57, 59–72]. Although viral strain and route of inoculation influence direct comparison of viral loads, the median plasma viremia of the aged RM-Ch in this study was in line with these published values at 9.65×10^6 copies/ml; however, the set point viremia was maintained at a median of 10^7 copies/ml, which is similar to the high end of the reported set point range.

Aged RM-Ch showed minimal clinical signs of SIV infection

Despite this viral load, little clinical evidence of infection was apparent. Some investigators have made similar observations with young RM-Ch showing fewer clinical signs of infection than RM of Indian origin and little appreciable weight loss [37]. However, others have observed that approximately half of young RM-Ch present with lymphadenopathy and experience weight loss, wasting, and diarrhea [38, 51]. Weight in the SIV-infected aged RM-Ch was similar to non-infected macaques. Temperature also remained remarkably stable, even during acute infection. This is contrary to infection of younger rhesus macaques that demonstrate hyperthermia during acute infection that lasts approximately 3 months [50], though these RM were most likely of Indian origin. Declines in platelet counts are reported to be an indicator of disease progression in HIV and SIV infection [49, 74], yet the aged macaques in this study did not show any alterations in platelet counts. Activity and sleep disturbances are also associated with SIV infection [50, 75, 76], but activity counts during day and night periods were similar to pre-infection and mock-infected animals. The absence of change in these clinical parameters suggests that SIV infection of aged RM-Ch is more analogous to SIV infection in the natural host (e.g. sooty mangabeys and African green monkeys), potentially for the same reason that some aspects of the immunological response to SIV such as type I IFN expression is less robust in the natural host than observed in other macaques [77]. Yet, this is a complex hypothesis to test, especially with the considerable variability observed in clinical parameters and immune activation of SIV infection of young RM-Ch [38, 51, 57, 66, 77].

Supporting the hypothesis that aged RM-Ch are refractory to clinical SIV-related disease,

CD14 + CD16 + monocyte subset proportions and counts were similar in infected and non-infected macaques throughout the course of infection suggesting absence of an inflammatory environment that promotes this phenotype. Monocyte subsets are known to undergo dynamic changes as a function of duration of HIV/SIV infection and are variably reported to correlate or not with development of SIV encephalitis or HAND [78–82]. However, SIV-infected aged RM-Ch did show a decrease in the proportion of CD4+ T cells during acute infection. This population remained decreased throughout the length of infection (or until treatment). The absolute median CD4+ T cell count was also decreased but was not observed in every animal and was variable. There is no consensus reported for loss of CD4+ T cells in young adult RM-Ch. While a few reports observe stable CD4 counts [62, 68] or transient CD4 loss [70], several others detect significant CD4+ T cell loss [51, 59, 60, 71, 72].

Aged RM-Ch did not show significant sensorimotor deficits with SIV infection or CART

Despite our extensive experience training young adult rhesus macaques to perform a variety of complex neurobehavioral tasks, aged RM-Ch proved recalcitrant to training. Nevertheless, we were successful in training aged macaques for a speeded motor task where we could reliably assess their reaction time, touch screen accuracy and percent completion. Others have shown that young adult SIV-infected macaques show neurological abnormalities that can be documented through a variety of behavioral and neurophysiological tests. Motor skills, discrimination learning, discrimination retention, recognition, recency memory and attention impairments are observed early and during the chronic phase of SIV infection in adult rhesus macaques [83–88]. Some performance impairments were characterized by gradual deteriorations throughout the course of infection, while others showed sharp declines. In comparison, the aged RM-Ch did not show any significant changes on response time or percent accuracy during a speeded motor task. Why did SIV infection fail to induce neurological abnormalities in aged RM-Ch? Without the ability to test multiple realms of cognition, it is impossible to rule out deficits in other types of memory, e.g. executive function. As an alternative hypothesis, HAND could be a consequence of chronic inflammation, with the absence of sensorimotor impairment in aged RM-Ch being a reflection of the diminished clinical and immunological response.

Neuropathology of SIV infection and CART in aged RM-Ch

Neuropathological examination did not show any overt signs of neurodegeneration in SIV-infected or mock-infected aged macaques (Table 1). Remarkably, little fluctuation in the cognitive task was observed from baseline to chronic infection. This was also true in animals with CNS-related pathology; however, these animals typically required respite from cognitive testing shortly before succumbing to an illness. While SIV RNA in the midfrontal cortex was detectable in only a few animals, the CSF SIV RNA load remained moderate in the majority of animals, so there were presumably low levels of viral replication in the CNS. While non-quantitative neuropathological assessment did not demonstrate age-related differences between infected and mock-infected aged RM-Ch, more sensitive quantitative pathological and gene expression assessments are planned.

Virological responses of aged RM-Ch to CART

In SIV-infected animals, administration of TDF and FTC for 6 months was effective at decreasing plasma and CSF viral load in most animals. More interesting, treatment had neither a discernable positive or negative effect on neurobehavioral performance tasks for either infected or mock-infected animals. This is consistent with some human studies that have not documented neurobehavioral impairments in patients treated with CART [89]. However, it has been postulated that CART regimens potentially contribute to neurocognitive deficits by reducing dendritic arborization [90, 91].

SIV infection in aged RM-Ch shows lack of inflammatory environment

The lack of clinical signs and cognitive impairment drove us to examine the inflammatory response in aged SIV-infected Ch-RM. A hallmark of HIV and SIV infection is chronic inflammation and activated coagulation. This increased proinflammatory state is thought to drive alterations and senescence in immune cell populations [92] and increase availability of infectable cells [93]. Increased levels of D-dimer, IL-6, sCD14, CXCL10, TNF-α, IL-18, and CCL2 among others have been shown to be increased during acute infection or chronically increased throughout infection [52–54]. Many of these inflammatory markers are also increased in aged individuals, and it has been hypothesized that HIV infection accelerates aging [36, 94]. We did not discern any elevation in these markers during infection compared to baseline measurements and mock-infected aged RM-Ch. Plasma IL-18 (an IL-1 superfamily protein produced by activated macrophages) was elevated in SIV-infected RM-Ch during acute infection, but returned to baseline during the chronic phase of infection.

Interrogation of anti-Env antibody responses showed SIV infection was not inherently immunologically silent. Most of the young adult SIV-infected progressors generated minimal to no detectable anti-Env IgG suggesting antibody responses play a role in disease progression characteristics. Overall, the aged Ch-RM generated antibody responses similar to progressors or less than young adult controllers. SIV-neutralizing antibody titers were not determined, so it is unclear whether the binding IgG detected by ELISA was functional. A comprehensive investigation of innate and adaptive immune responses during the course of SIV infection in aged Ch-RM and controls deserves further exploration to examine potential causes for the lack of clinical signs.

The overall lack of an overt inflammatory response during either acute or chronic infection is similar to that observed during nonpathogenic SIV infections in their natural hosts [95–97]. Both natural hosts and macaques respond to SIV infection with strong upregulation of type I interferon-stimulated genes (ISG) [98]. Whereas ISG levels in natural hosts are quickly restored to baseline, upregulation of ISGs become chronic in younger Ch-RM. Although ISG expression was not assessed here, no increase in CXCL10 was observed suggesting lack of sustained ISG response in aged Ch-RM.

Another potential reason for the diminished immune response in aged RM-Ch could be immune senescence. Aged macaques have been reported to show characteristics of immune senescence with increased proinflammatory status and altered immune cell populations [92]. In fact, we have noted that aged macaques have variable, delayed, and significantly weaker anti-beta-amyloid IgG levels in response to beta-amyloid immunization [73].

An elevated inflammatory milieu, such as increased sCD14 and sCD163 along with low CD4 T-cell count nadirs are also reported to predict development of HAND [99–103]. It could be hypothesized that absence of robust inflammation during acute infection, absence of many clinical signs of infection or disease and lack of chronic inflammation in the face of substantive viral replication obviate neurological damage. Although these observations warrant verification with controls demonstrating cognitive impairment concurrently with inflammation, our data are consistent with the hypothesis that HAND may be related to a chronic immune response to infection rather than the infection itself.

Conclusions

We show that aged RM-Ch present with minimal clinical signs during SIV infection despite substantial viremia. Along with absence of indicators of disease, aged SIV-infected RM-Ch do not display deficits in cognitive tests and do not demonstrate chronic inflammation. SIV infection of aged RM-Ch did not bring about histological signs of neurodegeneration. Although these conclusions will need to be substantiated encompassing species and age differences, the observations suggest that these characteristics are reminiscent of SIV infection in natural disease resistant hosts.

Additional file

Additional file 1: Figure S1. Effect of age and SIV-infection on weight. In comparison to mock-infected macaques, SIV-infection of aged Chinese rhesus macaques does not impact weight. Animals were weighed on a weekly basis. Median longitudinal weight (kg) over the course of infection for each group (A). Change in median weight (kg) from baseline in SIV-infected (red) and mock-infected (blue) macaques during the acute phase of infection (B). Both SIV-infected and mock infected macaques lost weight at 2 and 3 wpi. At 4 wpi, SIV-infected macaques lost a small amount of mass while mock-infected macaques slightly gained mass. Change in median weight (kg) from baseline in SIV-infected (red) and mock-infected (blue) macaques at time of necropsy (C). Mock-infected macaques gained over 1 kg by the end of the study whereas SIV-infected macaques were similar to their starting weight. Figure S2. Effect of age, SIV-infection and cART on body temperature. There were no changes in body temperature after SIV-infection in aged Chinese rhesus macaques. Body temperature was recorded at least once a day and the median temperature determined in two week intervals. Baseline temperature (week 0 post-infection) was the average of 12 weeks of preinoculation measurements. Time course of body temperature in SIV-infected macaques and controls (A). Lines represent median values. Time course of change in temperature (Δ °C) from baseline (B). Change in temperature from baseline during the first 4 weeks post-infection (C). Change in temperature from baseline at necropsy (D). Figure S3. Effect of age, SIV-infection and cART on platelet counts. Platelet counts are not significantly altered during acute SIV infection in aged rhesus macaques of Chinese origin. Time course of median platelet counts during the duration of infection (A). Lines represent median values. Platelet counts of SIV-infected and mock-infected macaques during the first 4 weeks post-infection (B). Figure S4. Total cell counts during the course of SIV infection. Total CD4+ T-cell counts decrease during SIV infection in aged rhesus macaques of Chinese origin. Total CD8+ T-cell and NK-cell counts shown an elevation during acute infection then fall to similar levels as mock-infected macaques. Time course change in CD4+ T-cell (A), CD8+ T-cell (B), NK-cell (C), and B-cell counts (D) during SIV and mock infection. Lines represent median values. Figure S5. Total monocyte subset counts during the course of SIV infection. CD14+CD16- (A), CD14+CD16+ (B), CD14-CD16+ (C) monocyte subset counts during SIV infection in aged rhesus macaques of Chinese origin. Lines represent median values. Figure S6. Plasma and CSF viral load versus temperature in individual SIV-infected macaques. Each graph shows the time course of plasma SIV loads, CSF SIV loads and temperature in an individual aged Chinese rhesus macaque during SIV infection. Graphs of SIV-infected macaques that did not receive treatment (Group 1) are shown in (a) and graphs of SIV-infected macaques that were treated with CART (Group 4) are shown in (b). The green shaded area represents the period macaques received CART or saline.

Figure S7. Plasma and CSF viral load versus CD4+ and CD8+ T-cell count in SIV-infected macaques. Each graph shows the time course of plasma SIV loads, CSF SIV loads, CD4+ T-cell counts, and CD8+ T-cell counts in an individual aged Chinese rhesus macaque during SIV infection. Graphs of SIV-infected macaques that did not receive treatment (Group 1) are shown in (a) and graphs of SIV-infected macaques that were treated with CART (Group 4) are shown in (b). The green shaded area represents the period macaques received CART or saline. Figure S8. Plasma and CSF viral load versus reaction time and accuracy in SIV-infected macaques. Each graph shows the time course of plasma SIV loads, CSF SIV loads, reaction time (RT), and percent accuracy (Acc) in an individual aged Chinese rhesus macaque during SIV infection. Graphs of SIV-infected macaques that did not receive treatment (Group 1) are shown in (a) and graphs of SIV-infected macaques that were treated with CART (Group 4) are shown in (b). The green shaded area represents the period macaques received CART or saline. Figure S9. Time and accuracy in mock-infected macaques. Each graph shows the reaction time (RT) and percent accuracy (Acc) in a speeded motor task for an individual aged Chinese rhesus macaque over the study period. Graphs of mock-infected macaques that did not receive treatment (Group 2) are shown in (a) and graphs of mock-infected macaques that were treated with CART (Group 3) are shown in (b). The green shaded area represents the period macaques received CART or saline.

Abbreviations

AIDS: acquired immune deficiency syndrome; CART: combined antiretroviral therapy; CNS: central nervous system; CSF: cerebrospinal fluid; EDTA: ethylenediaminetetraacetic acid; EIA/RIA: enzyme immunoassay/radioimmunoassay; ELISA: enzyme-linked immunosorbent assay; FTC: emtricitabine; HAD: HIV-associated dementia; HAND: HIV-associated neurocognitive disorders; HIV: human immunodeficiency virus; ISG: interferon-stimulated genes; ISH: in situ hybridization; NHP: nonhuman primate; OD: optical density; rgp130: recombinant glycoprotein 130; RM-Ch: rhesus macaques of Chinese origin; sCD14: soluble CD14; SIV: simian immunodeficiency virus; SIVmac: SIV from macaques; TDF: Tenofovir disoproxil; TMB: tetramethylbenzidine; wpi: week(s) post-infection.

Authors' contributions

SJB designed the project, helped perform the experiments, consolidated and analyzed the data, prepared the figures and tables, interpreted the data, and wrote the manuscript; KG provided supervision, helped perform the experiments, consolidated and analyzed the data, and participated in the writing of the manuscript; HPJ analyzed and interpreted the data; NFS processed samples and generated, graphed and interpreted PCR data; GW helped perform the experiments; CWB designed the project, interpreted the data, provided supervision, and participated in the writing of the manuscript; CAW conceived and designed the project, provided supervision, interpreted the data, and participated in the writing of the manuscript. All authors read and approved the final manuscript.

Author details

[1] University of Pittsburgh, 3550 Terrace Street, S758 Scaife Hall, Pittsburgh, PA 15261, USA. [2] Veterans Affairs Pittsburgh Healthcare System, 4100 Allequippa Street, Pittsburgh, PA 15213, USA. [3] Present Address: National Institute on Drug Abuse, 251 Bayview Boulevard, Baltimore, MD 21224, USA.

Acknowledgements

We thank Nicole Nania for valuable veterinary assistance and Chris Janssen and Anita Trichel for veterinary care. We thank Simon M. Barratt-Boyes for rhesus macaque blood samples. We thank Arlene Carbone-Wiley, Mark Stauffer and Dana Weber for valuable technical assistance and preparation of histological specimens. We thank ABL Inc. and the Vaccine Research Program, Division of AIDS, NIAID for providing the viral inoculum. We thank Eva Rakasz at the Immunology Services unit of the Wisconsin National Primate Research Center for flow cytometry analysis.

Competing interests

The authors declare that they have no competing interests.

Funding

This work was supported by National Institutes of Health (NIH) grants MH097476 to S.J.B., C.B., and C.A.W. The viral inoculum was provided by ABL Inc. and the Vaccine Research Program, Division of AIDS, NIAID. Flow cytometry analysis was supported in part by an NIH grant to the Immunology Services unit of the Wisconsin National Primate Research Center (5P51OD011106).

Luminex analyses were supported in part by and NIH award P30CA047904 to the UPCI Cancer Biomarkers Facility: Luminex Core Laboratory. Tenofovir disoproxil and emtricitabine were generously provided by Gilead Sciences, Inc. (Foster City, CA) through Material Transfer Agreements. The funding bodies had no role in study design, data collection, analysis, and interpretation, or the decision to write up and submit the work for publication.

References

1. World Health Organization. Fact sheet—latest statistics on the status of the AIDS epidemic. http://www.unaids.org/en/resources/fact-sheet. Accessed 20 Nov 2017.
2. Achim CL, Wang R, Miners DK, Wiley CA. Brain viral burden in HIV infection. J Neuropathol Exp Neurol. 1994;53:284–94.
3. Boisse L, Gill MJ, Power C. HIV infection of the central nervous system: clinical features and neuropathogenesis. Neurol Clin. 2008;26:799–819.
4. Heaton RK, Clifford DB, Franklin DR Jr, Woods SP, Ake C, Vaida F, et al. HIV-associated neurocognitive disorders persist in the era of potent antiretroviral therapy: CHARTER Study. Neurology. 2010;75:2087–96.
5. Heaton RK, Franklin DR, Ellis RJ, McCutchan JA, Letendre SL, Leblanc S, et al. HIV-associated neurocognitive disorders before and during the era of combination antiretroviral therapy: differences in rates, nature, and predictors. J Neurovirol. 2011;17:3–16.
6. Tozzi V, Balestra P, Bellagamba R, Corpolongo A, Salvatori MF, Visco-Comandini U, et al. Persistence of neuropsychologic deficits despite long-term highly active antiretroviral therapy in patients with HIV-related neurocognitive impairment: prevalence and risk factors. J Acquir Immune Defic Syndr. 2007;45:174–82.
7. Ances BM, Clifford DB. HIV-associated neurocognitive disorders and the impact of combination antiretroviral therapies. Curr Neurol Neurosci Rep. 2008;8:455–61.
8. Simioni S, Cavassini M, Annoni JM, Rimbault Abraham A, Bourquin I, Schiffer V, et al. Cognitive dysfunction in HIV patients despite long-standing suppression of viremia. AIDS. 2010;24:1243–50.
9. Sacktor N, Skolasky RL, Seaberg E, Munro C, Becker JT, Martin E, et al. Prevalence of HIV-associated neurocognitive disorders in the Multi-center AIDS Cohort Study. Neurology. 2016;86:334–40.
10. Sheppard DP, Ludicello JE, Bondi MW, Doyle KL, Morgan EE, Massman PJ, et al. Elevated rates of mild cognitive impairment in HIV disease. J Neurovirol. 2015;21:576–84.
11. Valcour V, Shikuma C, Shiramizu B, Watters M, Poff P, Selnes O, et al. Higher frequency of dementia in older HIV-1 individuals: the Hawaii Aging with HIV-1 Cohort. Neurology. 2004;63:822–7.
12. Fazeli PL, Crowe M, Ross LA, Wadley V, Ball K, Vance DE. Cognitive functioning in adults aging with HIV: a cross-sectional analysis of cognitive subtypes and influential factors. J Clin Res HIV AIDS Prev. 2014;1:155–69.
13. Joska JA, Westgarth-Taylor J, Hoare J, Thomas KG, Paul R, Myer L, et al. Neuropsychological outcomes in adults commencing highly active anti-retroviral treatment in South Africa: a prospective study. BMC Infect Dis. 2012;12:39.
14. Saylor D, Dickens AM, Sacktor N, Haughey N, Slusher B, Pletnikov M, et al. HIV-associated neurocognitive disorder—pathogenesis and prospects for treatment. Nat Rev Neurol. 2016;12:234–48.
15. Becker JT, Kingsley L, Mullen J, Cohen B, Martin E, Miller EN, et al. Vascular risk factors, HIV serostatus, and cognitive dysfunction in gay and bisexual men. Neurology. 2009;73:1292–9.
16. Fabbiani M, Ciccarelli N, Tana M, Farina S, Baldonero E, Di Cristo V, et al. Cardiovascular risk factors and carotid intima-media thickness are associated with lower cognitive performance in HIV-infected patients. HIV Med. 2013;14:136–44.
17. McCutchan JA, Marquie-Beck JA, Fitzsimons CA, Letendre SL, Ellis RJ, Heaton RK, et al. Role of obesity, metabolic variables, and diabetes in HIV-associated neurocognitive disorder. Neurology. 2012;78:485–92.
18. Vivithanaporn P, Nelles K, DeBlock L, Newman SC, Gill MJ, Power C. Hepatitis C virus co-infection increases neurocognitive impairment severity and risk of death in treated HIV/AIDS. J Neurol Sci. 2012;312:45–51.
19. Weber E, Morgan EE, Iudicello JE, Blackstone K, Grant I, Ellis RJ, et al. Substance use is a risk factor for neurocognitive deficits and neuropsychiatric distress in acute and early HIV infection. J Neurovirol. 2013;19:65–74.

20. Becker JT, Kingsley LA, Molsberry S, Reynolds S, Aronow A, Levine AJ, et al. Cohort profile: recruitment cohorts in the neuropsychological substudy of the Multicenter AIDS Cohort Study. Int J Epidemiol. 2015;44:1506–16.

21. Tedaldi EM, Minniti NL, Fischer T. HIV-associated neurocognitive disorders: the relationship of HIV infection with physical and social comorbidities. Biomed Res Int. 2015;2015:641913.

22. Fisher M, Cooper V. HIV and ageing: premature ageing or premature conclusions? Curr Opin Infect Dis. 2012;25:1–3.

23. Gelman BB. Neuropathology of HAND with suppressive antiretroviral therapy: encephalitis and neurodegeneration reconsidered. Curr HIV/AIDS Rep. 2015;12:272–9.

24. Brew BJ, Pemberton L, Cunningham P, Law MG. Levels of human immunodeficiency virus type 1 RNA in cerebrospinal fluid correlate with AIDS dementia stage. J Infect Dis. 1997;175:963–6.

25. Ellis RJ, Moore DJ, Childers ME, Letendre S, McCutchan JA, Wolfson T, et al. Progression to neuropsychological impairment in human immunodeficiency virus infection predicted by elevated cerebrospinal fluid levels of human immunodeficiency virus RNA. Arch Neurol. 2002;59:923–8.

26. Ho DD, Rota TR, Schooley RT, Kaplan JC, Allan JD, Groopman JE, et al. Isolation of HTLV-III from cerebrospinal fluid and neural tissues of patients with neurologic syndromes related to the acquired immunodeficiency syndrome. N Engl J Med. 1985;313:1493–7.

27. Sonnerborg AB, Ehrnst AC, Bergdahl SK, Pehrson PO, Skoldenberg BR, Strannegard OO. HIV isolation from cerebrospinal fluid in relation to immunological deficiency and neurological symptoms. AIDS. 1988;2:89–93.

28. Brew BJ, Letendre SL. Biomarkers of HIV related central nervous system disease. Int Rev Psychiatry. 2008;20:73–88.

29. Tyler KL, McArthur JC. Through a glass, darkly: cerebrospinal fluid viral load measurements and the pathogenesis of human immunodeficiency virus infection of the central nervous system. Arch Neurol. 2002;59:909–12.

30. Nath A, Conant K, Chen P, Scott C, Major EO. Transient exposure to HIV-1 Tat protein results in cytokine production in macrophages and astrocytes. A hit and run phenomenon. J Biol Chem. 1999;274:17098–102.

31. Tansey MG, McCoy MK, Frank-Cannon TC. Neuroinflammatory mechanisms in Parkinson's disease: potential environmental triggers, pathways, and targets for early therapeutic intervention. Exp Neurol. 2007;208:1–25.

32. Langston JW, Forno LS, Tetrud J, Reeves AG, Kaplan JA, Karluk D. Evidence of active nerve cell degeneration in the substantia nigra of humans years after 1-methyl-4-phenyl-1,2,3,6-tetrahydropyridine exposure. Ann Neurol. 1999;46:598–605.

33. Jang H, Boltz D, Sturm-Ramirez K, Shepherd KR, Jiao Y, Webster R, et al. Highly pathogenic H5N1 influenza virus can enter the central nervous system and induce neuroinflammation and neurodegeneration. Proc Natl Acad Sci USA. 2009;106:14063–8.

34. Galloway DA, McDougall JK. The oncogenic potential of herpes simplex viruses: evidence for a 'hit-and-run' mechanism. Nature. 1983;302:21–4.

35. Desquilbet L, Jacobson LP, Fried LP, Phair JP, Jamieson BD, Holloway M, et al. HIV-1 infection is associated with an earlier occurrence of a phenotype related to frailty. J Gerontol A Biol Sci Med Sci. 2007;62:1279–86.

36. Deeks SG, Tracy R, Douek DC. Systemic effects of inflammation on health during chronic HIV infection. Immunity. 2013;39:633–45.

37. Trichel AM, Rajakumar PA, Murphey-Corb M. Species-specific variation in SIV disease progression between Chinese and Indian subspecies of rhesus macaque. J Med Primatol. 2002;31:171–8.

38. Ling B, Veazey RS, Luckay A, Penedo C, Xu K, Lifson JD, et al. SIV(mac) pathogenesis in rhesus macaques of Chinese and Indian origin compared with primary HIV infections in humans. AIDS. 2002;16:1489–96.

39. Joag SV, Stephens EB, Adams RJ, Foresman L, Narayan O. Pathogenesis of SIVmac infection in Chinese and Indian rhesus macaques: effects of splenectomy on virus burden. Virology. 1994;200:436–46.

40. Cline AN, Bess JW, Piatak M Jr, Lifson JD. Highly sensitive SIV plasma viral load assay: practical considerations, realistic performance expectations, and application to reverse engineering of vaccines for AIDS. J Med Primatol. 2005;34:303–12.

41. Venneti S, Bonneh-Barkay D, Lopresti BJ, Bissel SJ, Wang G, Mathis CA, et al. Longitudinal in vivo positron emission tomography imaging of infected and activated brain macrophages in a macaque model of human immunodeficiency virus encephalitis correlates with central and peripheral markers of encephalitis and areas of synaptic degeneration. Am J Pathol. 2008;172:1603–16.

42. Bissel SJ, Wang G, Ghosh M, Reinhart TA, Capuano S 3rd, Stefano Cole K, et al. Macrophages relate presynaptic and postsynaptic damage in simian immunodeficiency virus encephalitis. Am J Pathol. 2002;160:927–41.

43. Bonneh-Barkay D, Bissel SJ, Kofler J, Starkey A, Wang G, Wiley CA. Astrocyte and macrophage regulation of YKL-40 expression and cellular response in neuroinflammation. Brain Pathol. 2012;22:530–46.

44. Fuller CL, Choi YK, Fallert BA, Capuano S 3rd, Rajakumar P, Murphey-Corb M, et al. Restricted SIV replication in rhesus macaque lung tissues during the acute phase of infection. Am J Pathol. 2002;161:969–78.

45. Wu X, Yang ZY, Li Y, Hogerkorp CM, Schief WR, Seaman MS, et al. Rational design of envelope identifies broadly neutralizing human monoclonal antibodies to HIV-1. Science. 2010;329:856–61.

46. Baskin GB, Murphey-Corb M, Watson EA, Martin LN. Necropsy findings in rhesus monkeys experimentally infected with cultured simian immunodeficiency virus (SIV)/delta. Vet Pathol. 1988;25:456–67.

47. Benveniste RE, Morton WR, Clark EA, Tsai CC, Ochs HD, Ward JM, et al. Inoculation of baboons and macaques with simian immunodeficiency virus/Mne, a primate lentivirus closely related to human immunodeficiency virus type 2. J Virol. 1988;62:2091–101.

48. Letvin NL, Desrosiers RC. Simian immunodeficiency virus. Berlin: Springer; 1994.

49. Metcalf Pate KA, Lyons CE, Dorsey JL, Shirk EN, Queen SE, Adams RJ, et al. Platelet activation and platelet-monocyte aggregate formation contribute to decreased platelet count during acute simian immunodeficiency virus infection in pig-tailed macaques. J Infect Dis. 2013;208:874–83.

50. Horn TF, Huitron-Resendiz S, Weed MR, Henriksen SJ, Fox HS. Early physiological abnormalities after simian immunodeficiency virus infection. Proc Natl Acad Sci USA. 1998;95:15072–7.

51. Wei Q, Liu L, Cong Z, Wu X, Wang H, Qin C, et al. Chronic Δ(9)-tetrahydrocannabinol administration reduces IgE(+)B cells but unlikely enhances pathogenic SIVmac251 infection in male rhesus macaques of Chinese origin. J Neuroimmune Pharmacol Off J Soc NeuroImmune Pharmacol. 2016;11:584–91.

52. Kuller LH, Tracy R, Belloso W, De Wit S, Drummond F, Lane HC, et al. Inflammatory and coagulation biomarkers and mortality in patients with HIV infection. PLoS Med. 2008;5:e203.

53. Paiardini M, Muller-Trutwin M. HIV-associated chronic immune activation. Immunol Rev. 2013;254:78–101.

54. Stacey AR, Norris PJ, Qin L, Haygreen EA, Taylor E, Heitman J, et al. Induction of a striking systemic cytokine cascade prior to peak viremia in acute human immunodeficiency virus type 1 infection, in contrast to more modest and delayed responses in acute hepatitis B and C virus infections. J Virol. 2009;83:3719–33.

55. Ling B, Veazey RS, Penedo C, Xu K, Lifson JD, Marx PA. Longitudinal follow up of SIVmac pathogenesis in rhesus macaques of Chinese origin: emergence of B cell lymphoma. J Med Primatol. 2002;31:154–63.

56. Ling B, Rogers L, Kaushal D, Morici L, Lackner A, Pahar B, et al. SIV specific immune responses and gene regulations in SIV-infected long-term nonprogressing rhesus macaques. http://www2.tulane.edu/asvpr/upload/Ling-Abstract-2010.pdf (2010) Accessed 15 Dec 2017.

57. Zhou Y, Bao R, Haigwood NL, Persidsky Y, Ho WZ. SIV infection of rhesus macaques of Chinese origin: a suitable model for HIV infection in humans. Retrovirology. 2013;10:89.

58. Trask JS, Garnica WT, Malhi RS, Kanthaswamy S, Smith DG. High-throughput single-nucleotide polymorphism discovery and the search for candidate genes for long-term SIVmac nonprogression in Chinese rhesus macaques (Macaca mulatta). J Med Primatol. 2011;40:224–32.

59. Cong Z, Xue J, Xiong J, Yao N, Wang W, Jiang H, et al. Correlation of central memory CD4+ T-Cell decrease in the peripheral blood with disease progression in SIVmac251-infected Chinese rhesus macaques. J Med Primatol. 2015;44:175–82.

60. Zhang LT, Tian RR, Zheng HY, Pan GQ, Tuo XY, Xia HJ, et al. Translocation of microbes and changes of immunocytes in the gut of rapid- and slow-progressor Chinese rhesus macaques infected with SIVmac239. Immunology. 2016;147:443–52.

61. Liu H, Xiao QH, Liu JB, Li JL, Zhou L, Xian QY, et al. SIV Infection Impairs the Central Nervous System in Chinese Rhesus Macaques. J Neuroimmune Pharmacol Off J Soc NeuroImmune Pharmacol. 2016;11:592–600.

62. Tian RR, Zhang MX, Zhang LT, Zhang XL, Zheng HY, Zhu L, et al. High immune activation and abnormal expression of cytokines contribute to death of SHIV89.6-infected Chinese rhesus macaques. Arch Virol. 2015;160:1953–66.

63. Ling B, Rogers L, Johnson AM, Piatak M, Lifson J, Veazey RS. Effect of combination antiretroviral therapy on Chinese rhesus macaques of simian immunodeficiency virus infection. AIDS Res Hum Retrovir. 2013;29:1465–74.

64. Monceaux V, Viollet L, Petit F, Cumont MC, Kaufmann GR, Aubertin AM, et al. CD4+ CCR5 + T-cell dynamics during simian immunodeficiency virus infection of Chinese rhesus macaques. J Virol. 2007;81:13865–75.

65. Elbim C, Monceaux V, Mueller YM, Lewis MG, Francois S, Diop O, et al. Early divergence in neutrophil apoptosis between pathogenic and nonpathogenic simian immunodeficiency virus infections of nonhuman primates. J Immunol. 2008;181:8613–23.

66. Cumont MC, Diop O, Vaslin B, Elbim C, Viollet L, Monceaux V, et al. Early divergence in lymphoid tissue apoptosis between pathogenic and nonpathogenic simian immunodeficiency virus infections of nonhuman primates. J Virol. 2008;82:1175–84.

67. Sanders-Beer B, Babas T, Mansfield K, Golightly D, Kramer J, Bowlsbey A, et al. Depo-Provera does not alter disease progression in SIVmac-infected female Chinese rhesus macaques. AIDS Res Hum Retrovir. 2010;26:433–43.

68. Marcondes MC, Penedo MC, Lanigan C, Hall D, Watry DD, Zandonatti M, et al. Simian immunodeficiency virus-induced CD4+ T cell deficits in cytokine secretion profile are dependent on monkey origin. Viral Immunol. 2006;19:679–89.

69. Xia HJ, Zhang GH, Ma JP, Dai ZX, Li SY, Han JB, et al. Dendritic cell subsets dynamics and cytokine production in SIVmac239-infected Chinese rhesus macaques. Retrovirology. 2010;7:102.

70. Ling B, Piatak M Jr, Rogers L, Johnson AM, Russell-Lodrigue K, Hazuda DJ, et al. Effects of treatment with suppressive combination antiretroviral drug therapy and the histone deacetylase inhibitor suberoylanilide hydroxamic acid; (SAHA) on SIV-infected Chinese rhesus macaques. PLoS ONE. 2014;9:e102795.

71. Bao R, Zhuang K, Liu J, Wu J, Li J, Wang X, et al. Lipopolysaccharide induces immune activation and SIV replication in rhesus macaques of Chinese origin. PLoS ONE. 2014;9:e98636.

72. Chen S, Lai C, Wu X, Lu Y, Han D, Guo W, et al. Variability of bio-clinical parameters in Chinese-origin Rhesus macaques infected with simian immunodeficiency virus: a nonhuman primate AIDS model. PLoS ONE. 2011;6:e23177.

73. Kofler J, Lopresti B, Janssen C, Trichel AM, Masliah E, Finn OJ, et al. Preventive immunization of aged and juvenile non-human primates to beta-amyloid. J Neuroinflamm. 2012;9:84.

74. Nicolle M, Levy S, Amrhein E, Schmitt MP, Partisani M, Rey D, et al. Normal platelet numbers correlate with plasma viral load and CD4+ cell counts in HIV-1 infection. Eur J Haematol. 1998;61:216–7.

75. Fox HS, Weed MR, Huitron-Resendiz S, Baig J, Horn TF, Dailey PJ, et al. Antiviral treatment normalizes neurophysiological but not movement abnormalities in simian immunodeficiency virus-infected monkeys. J Clin Invest. 2000;106:37–45.

76. Huitron-Resendiz S, Marcondes MC, Flynn CT, Lanigan CM, Fox HS. Effects of simian immunodeficiency virus on the circadian rhythms of body temperature and gross locomotor activity. Proc Natl Acad Sci USA. 2007;104:15138–43.

77. Campillo-Gimenez L, Laforge M, Fay M, Brussel A, Cumont MC, Monceaux V, et al. Nonpathogenesis of simian immunodeficiency virus infection is associated with reduced inflammation and recruitment of plasmacytoid dendritic cells to lymph nodes, not to lack of an interferon type I response, during the acute phase. J Virol. 2010;84:1838–46.

78. Bissel SJ, Wang G, Trichel AM, Murphey-Corb M, Wiley CA. Longitudinal analysis of activation markers on monocyte subsets during the development of simian immunodeficiency virus encephalitis. J Neuroimmunol. 2006;177:85–98.

79. Burdo TH, Soulas C, Orzechowski K, Button J, Krishnan A, Sugimoto C, et al. Increased monocyte turnover from bone marrow correlates with severity of SIV encephalitis and CD163 levels in plasma. PLoS Pathog. 2010;6:e1000842.

80. Pulliam L, Gascon R, Stubblebine M, McGuire D, McGrath MS. Unique monocyte subset in patients with AIDS dementia. Lancet. 1997;349:692–5.

81. Gama L, Shirk EN, Russell JN, Carvalho KI, Li M, Queen SE, et al. Expansion of a subset of CD14highCD16negCCR2low/neg monocytes functionally similar to myeloid-derived suppressor cells during SIV and HIV infection. J Leukoc Biol. 2012;91:803–16.

82. Kim WK, Sun Y, Do H, Autissier P, Halpern EF, Piatak M Jr, et al. Monocyte heterogeneity underlying phenotypic changes in monocytes according to SIV disease stage. J Leukoc Biol. 2010;87:557–67.

83. Weed MR, Gold LH, Polis I, Koob GF, Fox HS, Taffe MA. Impaired performance on a rhesus monkey neuropsychological testing battery following simian immunodeficiency virus infection. AIDS Res Hum Retrovir. 2004;20:77–89.

84. Prospero-Garcia O, Gold LH, Fox HS, Polis I, Koob GF, Bloom FE, et al. Microglia-passaged simian immunodeficiency virus induces neurophysiological abnormalities in monkeys. Proc Natl Acad Sci USA. 1996;93:14158–63.

85. Weed MR, Hienz RD, Brady JV, Adams RJ, Mankowski JL, Clements JE, et al. Central nervous system correlates of behavioral deficits following simian immunodeficiency virus infection. J Neurovirol. 2003;9:452–64.

86. Murray EA, Rausch DM, Lendvay J, Sharer LR, Eiden LE. Cognitive and motor impairments associated with SIV infection in rhesus monkeys. Science. 1992;255:1246–9.

87. Gold LH, Fox HS, Henriksen SJ, Buchmeier MJ, Weed MR, Taffe MA, et al. Longitudinal analysis of behavioral, neurophysiological, viral and immunological effects of SIV infection in rhesus monkeys. J Med Primatol. 1998;27:104–12.

88. Marcario JK, Raymond LA, McKiernan BJ, Foresman LL, Joag SV, Raghavan R, et al. Motor skill impairment in SIV-infected rhesus macaques with rapidly and slowly progressing disease. J Med Primatol. 1999;28:105–17.

89. Winston A, Vera JH. Can antiretroviral therapy prevent HIV-associated cognitive disorders? Curr Opin HIV AIDS. 2014;9:11–6.

90. Robertson K, Liner J, Meeker RB. Antiretroviral neurotoxicity. J Neurovirol. 2012;18:388–99.

91. Tovar-y-Romo LB, Bumpus NN, Pomerantz D, Avery LB, Sacktor N, McArthur JC, et al. Dendritic spine injury induced by the 8-hydroxy metabolite of efavirenz. J Pharmacol Exp Ther. 2012;343:696–703.

92. Willette AA, Coe CL, Birdsill AC, Bendlin BB, Colman RJ, Alexander AL, et al. Interleukin-8 and interleukin-10, brain volume and microstructure, and the influence of calorie restriction in old rhesus macaques. Age (Dordr). 2013;35:2215–27.

93. Haase AT. Targeting early infection to prevent HIV-1 mucosal transmission. Nature. 2010;464:217–23.

94. Singh T, Newman AB. Inflammatory markers in population studies of aging. Ageing Res Rev. 2011;10:319–29.

95. Pandrea I, Apetrei C. Where the wild things are: pathogenesis of SIV infection in African nonhuman primate hosts. Curr HIV/AIDS Rep. 2010;7:28–36.

96. Evans DT, Silvestri G. Nonhuman primate models in AIDS research. Curr Opin HIV AIDS. 2013;8:255–61.

97. Pandrea I, Silvestri G, Apetrei C. AIDS in african nonhuman primate hosts of SIVs: a new paradigm of SIV infection. Curr HIV Res. 2009;7:57–72.

98. Jacquelin B, Mayau V, Targat B, Liovat AS, Kunkel D, Petitjean G, et al. Nonpathogenic SIV infection of African green monkeys induces a strong but rapidly controlled type I IFN response. J Clin Invest. 2009;119:3544–55.

99. Beck SE, Queen SE, Witwer KW, Metcalf Pate KA, Mangus LM, Gama L, et al. Paving the path to HIV neurotherapy: predicting SIV CNS disease. Eur J Pharmacol. 2015;759:303–12.

100. Burdo TH, Weiffenbach A, Woods SP, Letendre S, Ellis RJ, Williams KC. Elevated sCD163 in plasma but not cerebrospinal fluid is a marker of neurocognitive impairment in HIV infection. AIDS. 2013;27:1387–95.

101. Lyons JL, Uno H, Ancuta P, Kamat A, Moore DJ, Singer EJ, et al. Plasma sCD14 is a biomarker associated with impaired neurocognitive test performance in attention and learning domains in HIV infection. J Acquir Immune Defic Syndr. 2011;57:371–9.

15

The role of follicular helper CD4 T cells in the development of HIV-1 specific broadly neutralizing antibody responses

Eirini Moysi, Constantinos Petrovas*⊙ and Richard A. Koup

Abstract

The induction of HIV-1-specific antibodies that can neutralize a broad number of isolates is a major goal of HIV-1 vaccination strategies. However, to date no candidate HIV-1 vaccine has successfully elicited broadly neutralizing antibodies of sufficient quality and breadth for protection. In this review, we focus on the role of follicular helper CD4 T-cells (Tfh) in the development of such cross-reactive protective antibodies. We discuss germinal center (GC) formation and the dynamics of Tfh and GC B cells during HIV-1/SIV infection and vaccination. Finally, we consider future directions for the study of Tfh and offer perspective on factors that could be modulated to enhance Tfh function in the context of prophylactic vaccination.

Keywords: Germinal center, Tfh, Broadly neutralizing antibody, Vaccines

Background

A sterilizing HIV-1 vaccine would greatly facilitate the fight against the HIV-1 epidemic. Research efforts over the past 35 years have afforded unique insights into the biology, virology and immunology of HIV-1 infection including a better appreciation of the importance of cross-clade reactive, broadly neutralizing antibodies (bnAbs) [1, 2]. HIV-1 is a highly diverse pathogen and successfully evades immunity by constantly shifting its antigenicity through evolution [3]. The failure of the Merck adenovirus type 5 (Ad5)-based vaccine in the STEP trial to induce robust protective cell-mediated immunity (CMI) responses to either prevent HIV-1 infection or suppress viral load in infected individuals refocused vaccine development efforts on humoral immunity [4]. bnAbs are antibodies that recognize highly conserved sites of vulnerability in many different circulating strains of HIV-1 [5, 6]. As such, they hold great promise for HIV-1 vaccine development. Studies of passive bnAb transfer in non-human primates and humans have been shown to prevent infection and reduce viral loads,

suggesting that combinations of durable bnAb levels could be used prophylactically as well as therapeutically [1, 2, 7–13]. However to date, despite the use of potent immunogens and delivery strategies, efficacy in HIV-1 vaccine trials remains either very low or absent [14–17]. This apparent disconnect between potent immunogen delivery and optimal response elicitation has sparked a renewed interest in the tissue-specific dynamics of bnAb development, including the selection and expansion of specific germline BCR precursors in B cell follicles, and the immunological correlates of those dynamics. Such topics have traditionally been hard to study in lymph node (LN) samples due to the difficulty in obtaining LN material from HIV-1+ individuals. More recently however, the availability of longitudinal biopsies from non-human primates in combination with the advancement of multi-parameter imaging and flow cytometry techniques have opened new avenues for tissue-specific immunity exploration [18, 19]. Here, we review the recent literature on Tfh cells and bnAbs in the context of chronic HIV-1/SIV infection and vaccination and offer perspective on open questions that need to be addressed in order to design vaccine strategies that will optimally engage the humoral arm of the adaptive immune system.

*Correspondence: petrovasc@mail.nih.gov
Immunology Laboratory, Vaccine Research Center, NIAID, NIH, Bethesda, USA

Tfh cells and their role in GC responses

Tfh are cells that localize to the lymph nodes, within well-defined structures called B-cell follicles (Fig. 1) [20, 21]. They are critical for the maturation, isotype switching, and somatic hypermutation (SHM) of B cells as well as for the survival of memory B cells and antibody-secreting plasma cells [20, 22, 23]. Their role thus is instrumental for the generation of high affinity antibodies. Tfh cells express low levels of CCR7 and are classically defined by the expression of the surface receptors CXCR5 and costimulatory receptors PD-1 and ICOS [20]. Their unique phenotype is preserved among different species including mice [24], non-human primates [25] and humans [21]. Although their ontogeny is not entirely clear, Tfh cells share characteristics with other CD4 T-cell lineages [26, 27]. However, their transcriptional regulation and gene expression profiles are distinct from all other lineages such as Th1, Th2, Th17 and regulatory T cells [28, 29]. Maturation of Tfh cells begins with antigen priming by DCs in the T cell zones surrounding the lymphoid follicles [30] and continues at the follicular T-B border with cognate interactions between Tfh and B-cells [31, 32]. These events lead to the induction of the transcription factor Bcl-6 as well as c-Maf that control lineage commitment to the Tfh fate [33, 34]. These early Tfh-B cell interactions require expression of the surface receptors ICOS, OX40 and CD40-ligand as well as expression of the cytokines IL-4 and IL-21 and have been shown to influence both Tfh fate commitment and the survival and ability of B cells to enter the GC response [29, 35–37]. B-cells activated during these early Tfh-B cell cognate interactions can subsequently move in extrafollicular areas for proliferation and differentiation into short-lived, antibody-secreting plasma cells or migrate into B cell follicles to establish a GC [38]. What determines either fate is not entirely clear but evidence exists to suggest that the decision might be contingent on the affinity of the B cell receptor (BCR) for the foreign antigen [39, 40], the density of antigen-MHC class II complex engagement [41], and the costimulatory signals received from T cells [38]. In these early steps of GC formation, the relative density of MHC class II expression on B cells appears to reflect the affinity of a given BCR precursor for antigen and the efficiency of BCR-mediated antigen uptake [42]. Thus, early cognate Tfh-B cell interactions may represent an important bottleneck in the ability of Tfh to recruit B cells of a given specificity into the response [43]. The follicular recruitment, frequency and function of Tfh, is additionally influenced by the relative abundance of antigen and availability of chemokines such as CXCL13 and SDF-1 [44]. In the GC, B cells constantly migrate between the light zone (LZ) and the dark zone (DZ) and thus the process of GC selection is highly regulated spatiotemporally [45]. T cell help in the LZ has been shown to activate the mTORC1 pathway, promoting a phase of anabolic growth that precedes and sustains the successive cycles of DZ proliferation [46]. Thus, Tfh in the LZ determine the cycling speed and number of cell divisions that a GC B cell will undergo as well as the associated number of B cell receptor (BCR) mutations in the GC per round of selection [43, 47, 48]. These data suggest that optimal GC reactivity and bnAb development depend on the phenotype of Tfh, as well as their spatiotemporal localization.

HIV-1/SIV infection and bnAb development
Role of Tfh cell quality

HIV-1/SIV infection and the resulting viremia influence the signals and mechanisms that regulate the dynamics of Tfh cells as well as the dynamics of Tfh-GC B cell interaction in LN follicles. Tfh induction can be traced as early as 14 days post-infection in NHPs challenged with SIV [49] and studies in humans and NHPs show that despite CD4 T cells being depleted during chronic HIV-1/SIV infection, the frequency of CXCR5+ PD-1[hi] CD4 T cells significantly increases both in the blood as well as in the LNs [50–53]. However, the increase in the frequencies of Tfh is not directly translated into higher bnAb levels. Only 20–30% of infected individuals are capable of mounting broadly neutralizing antibodies with HIV-1-specificities that have the potential to bind multiple HIV-1 envelope spikes of heterologous lineage during the first three years of infection [54]. Why some individuals and animals are able to develop bnAbs in the context of viremia whereas others do not is not entirely clear but both virologic, genetic and immunologic factors seem to influence this outcome. Virologic parameters that have been linked to bnAb production include characteristics of the infecting strain (ie viral loop length) [55–57] and degree of viral diversity [56]. For instance, exposure to multiple variants, as in the case of superinfection, has been shown to predict the development of bnAbs [56, 58] and studies in NHP and humans point to antigenic diversity (ie Env) being an important parameter with high viral loads and greater sequence evolution predicting a greater breadth of neutralization [56, 58, 59]. Host genetic factors, such as expression of specific HLA alleles have also been associated with bnAb activity in some cohorts [60, 61] whereas from an immunological stand-point, two parameters considered important are the ability of Tfh cells to provide help to B cells [62] and level of T-cell regulation [63].

CD4 T cells in the LN are a major target for HIV-1 infection. CXCR5+ PD-1[hi] cells in infected LNs have been shown to harbor a significantly increased frequency of HIV-1 DNA compared with non-Tfh cells [52] and

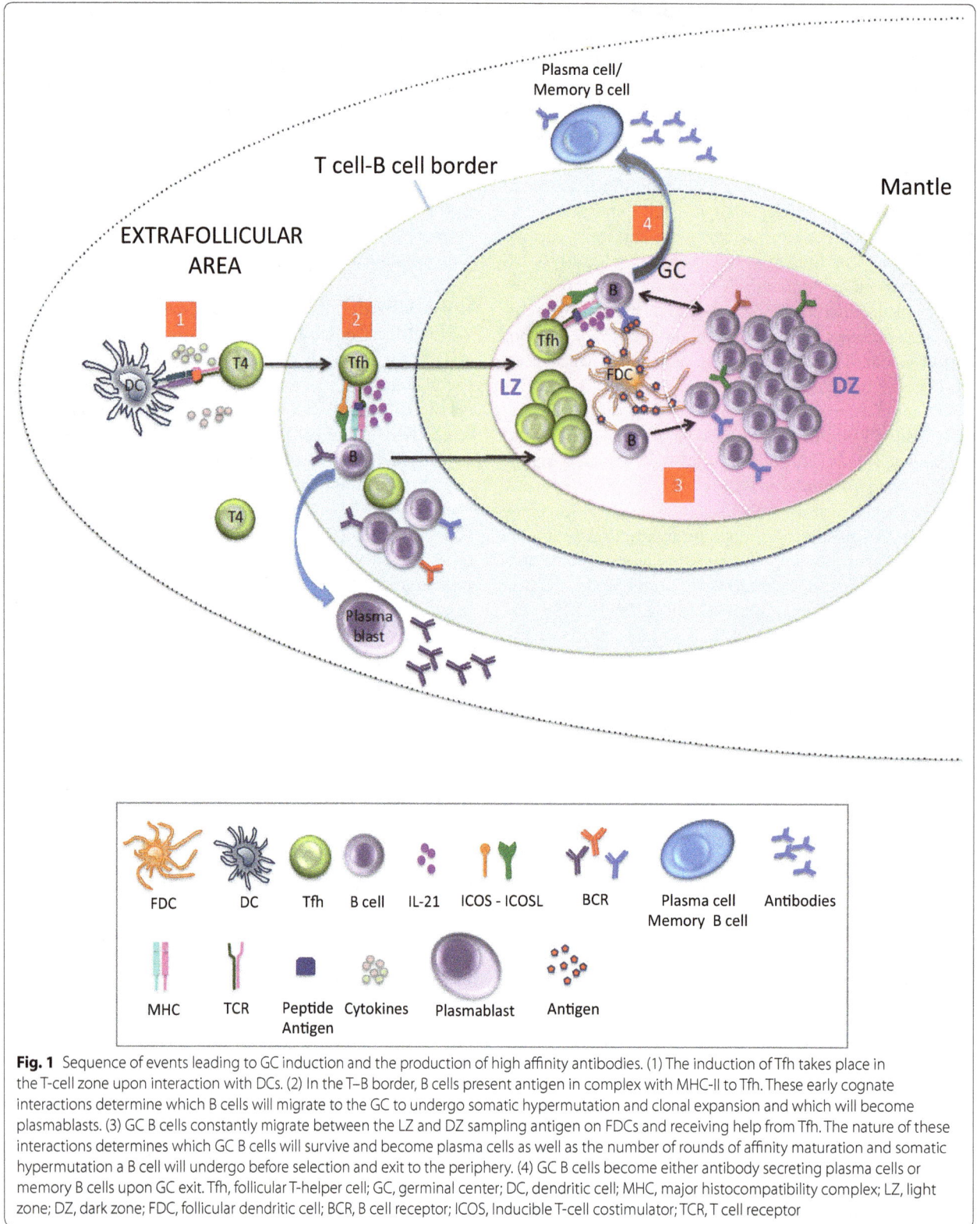

Fig. 1 Sequence of events leading to GC induction and the production of high affinity antibodies. (1) The induction of Tfh takes place in the T-cell zone upon interaction with DCs. (2) In the T–B border, B cells present antigen in complex with MHC-II to Tfh. These early cognate interactions determine which B cells will migrate to the GC to undergo somatic hypermutation and clonal expansion and which will become plasmablasts. (3) GC B cells constantly migrate between the LZ and DZ sampling antigen on FDCs and receiving help from Tfh. The nature of these interactions determines which GC B cells will survive and become plasma cells as well as the number of rounds of affinity maturation and somatic hypermutation a B cell will undergo before selection and exit to the periphery. (4) GC B cells become either antibody secreting plasma cells or memory B cells upon GC exit. Tfh, follicular T-helper cell; GC, germinal center; DC, dendritic cell; MHC, major histocompatibility complex; LZ, light zone; DZ, dark zone; FDC, follicular dendritic cell; BCR, B cell receptor; ICOS, Inducible T-cell costimulator; TCR, T cell receptor

to represent a major reservoir of latent virus in humans receiving antiretroviral therapy [64, 65]. In addition, their localization in close proximity to virion-ladden follicular dendritic cells (FDCs) in B cell follicles makes them increasingly susceptible to infection (Fig. 2) [66, 67]. Tfh cells isolated from HIV-1-infected patients produce less IL-21, a critical cytokine for GC formation, GC B cell proliferation and B cell maturation [68]. Exogenous administration of IL-21 has been shown to improve memory B cell frequencies, which suggests that IL-21 deficiency may, at least in part, impair the formation of memory B cell responses [69, 70]. HIV-1/SIV infection also imparts defects in the PD-1/PD-L1 axis. GC B cells from HIV-1 infected individuals express elevated levels of PD-L1 and have been shown to reduce ICOS and IL-21 expression in Tfh cells upon PD-1 ligation which could further compromise their ability to provide help to B cells [62]. The in vivo cycling capacity of Tfh cells is also compromised compared with other CD4 T-cell populations within the lymph nodes of infected NHP [53]. Moreover, in chronic untreated HIV-1+ infection Tfh become functionally skewed and oligoclonally restricted [71] Thus, HIV-1/SIV infection potentially alters the ability of Tfh to provide help to GC B-cells through a number of mechanisms. However, to what extend tissue-specific Tfh responses, including ICOS, CD40L expression and cytokine secretion differ between broadly neutralizers and non-neutralizers remains poorly understood. More recently, a number of studies have pointed to the heterogeneity of the Tfh population within the GC but less is known about the exact ontogeny of these individual phenotypes [72–74]. For instance, Tfh cells expressing CD57, show a significantly higher frequency of HIV-1 infection compared with extrafollicular CD4 T cells [75, 76] and

transcriptional signatures that show differences when compared to CD57- [72]. Moreover, chronic SIV infection has been shown to promote expansion of CXCR3+ expressing, IFN-γ producing GC Tfh cells (Th1-like) which are functionally distinct from CXCR3− Tfh in terms of phenotype and cytokine production [77]. To what extend these alterations affect the development of bnAbs is not currently known. Differences in the antigen-specificity or clonality of Tfh cells may also account for differences in the HIV-1-specific GC B-cell responses [71]. Even though the in vitro quantification of antigen-specific Tfh cells has been challenging [78] data supporting different roles for phenotypically distinct Tfh cells are available. In one study, IL-4 producing Env-specific Tfh but not those producing IFN-γ favored the development of Env-specific IgG+ GC B cells in NHP challenged with SHIV$_{AD8}$ in the chronic phase [59]. Further research is needed to understand how viral infection modulates the ability of Tfh cells to provide help to B cells, their positioning, Tfh subtype transcriptional differences as well as the factors that contribute to Tfh persistence in the face of chronic viremia.

Role of antigen and immune inflammation

Broadly neutralizing antibodies have been shown to develop after several years of infection in HIV-1+ individuals, with the first cross-neutralizing antibody responses appearing on average at 2.5 years post- infection [79]. Such bnAbs are characterized by a number of unusual features; they possess high-levels of somatic hypermutation reaching, in some cases, frequencies of 32% and 20% in heavy- and kappa- chain V genes respectively [5], extraordinarily long CDR3 antigen-contacting sites [5, 80, 81] and are poly- or autoreactive [82].

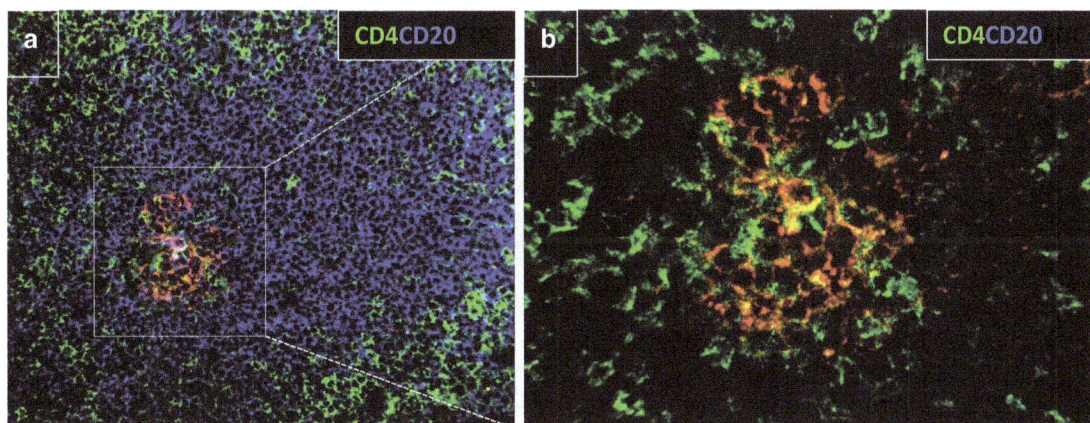

Fig. 2 Convergence of CD4+ T cells, B cells and FDC in a B cell follicle. Confocal imaging microscopy showing the convergence of immune populations contributing to the development of bnAbs in a lymph node B cell follicle derived from a HIV- individual. CD4 T cells are shown in green, CD20 in blue and FDCs in red. Images were acquired at ×40 (NA 1.3). Captions are **a** 50 μm and **b** 15 μm respectively

Their unique characteristics, potency and breadth arise through a continuous process of B cell adaptation and affinity maturation which may be fueled by a prolonged exposure to antigen [83, 84]. Antigenic persistence and antigen dose both determine the size and duration of the Tfh response and GC reaction [85] and Tfh cell accumulation in the chronic phase of HIV-1 infection is substantially decreased by ART [51–53]. Therefore, prolonged antigen availability within GCs in the context of HIV-1/SIV may be contributing to bnAb development by affecting both Tfh and B cell dynamics.

Role of GC B cell quality

Another hallmark of HIV-1/SIV infection is B cell dysregulation [86]. Several B cell abnormalities manifest during HIV-1 infection including phenotypic changes, polyclonal B cell activation and hypergammaglobulinaemia, as well as B cell unresponsiveness to T-cell independent and T-cell dependent B cell activation, all of which might affect the ability of HIV-1 infected individuals to develop bnAbs and respond to therapeutic vaccination or prophylactic vaccination against other infectious diseases such as hepatitis B and influenza [86–91]. The accumulation of Tfh cells in chronic HIV-1 [51, 52] and SIV [53] is associated with expansion of GC B cells and plasma cells. Maturation however into memory B cells is reduced [92]. In addition, B cells from patients with HIV-1 have low expression of the CXCL13 receptor CXCR5 compared with healthy controls and secrete large amounts of CXCL13 upon polyclonal stimulation which could, under physiological conditions alter the homing of B-cells [93]. Currently, there is little information on how B cell impairment affects the bnAb response in HIV-1/SIV infection. A better understanding of (1) the antigen-specific LN B cell responses, (2) the molecular profile and of GC B cell maturation process and (3) the spatial organization of GC immune reactions in the context of HIV-1/SIV are warranted in order to successfully design future vaccination strategies.

Role of follicular regulatory T-cells (Tfr)

FoxP3+ CD4+ Treg cells play an important role in the regulation of B cell responses as in their absence the levels of circulating antibodies increase [94]. T follicular regulatory (Tfr) cells, are a subset of FoxP3+ CD4+ Treg cells that localize to the GC during immune responses to control the magnitude of the response [95]. Phenotypically, Tfr express CXCR5+ alongside the classical Treg marker CD25 [96] but their exact function in the GC, especially in the context of HIV-1 is not yet clear. Given that FoxP3 is expressed in memory non-Treg CD4 T cells too, further phenotypic characterization of LN Tregs is necessary. Under physiological conditions, a skewed

presence of Tfr cells in extrafollicular areas compared to follicles has been shown [97]. In chronic HIV-1/SIV infection, the absolute number of Tfr cells within total LN CD4 T cells is increased [98, 99]. However how this may be impacting upon neutralizing B- cell development remains to be found. Studies in LNs of NHP, have shown an inverse correlation of the frequency of LN Tfh cells with Tfr frequency and the avidity of antibodies recognizing the SIV gp120 protein in plasma. Hence, Tfr could act to limit the maturation of antigen-specific responses [100] with bnAb development during HIV-1/SIV infection being favored by a relaxation in the regulatory control of GC antibody production [101, 102]. Further research in NHP LN biopsies and human FNA samples are thus warranted to address in more detail the role of Tfr responses in the expansion of B cells with neutralizing and non-neutralizing reactivities.

Lessons from vaccination

The realization that many individuals harbor bnAb precursors in their naïve B cell repertoires has reignited the hope that a bnAb-based HIV-1 vaccine might be attainable. Precursor frequency for bnAbs in the naïve repertoire is usually low, with those of the VRC-01 class estimated at ~1 out of 400,000 naïve B cells [103]. In addition, the affinity of such germline precursors for antigen is also low [104]. Thus, one critical question is how to optimally engage these precursors at tissue-level. The introduction of germline-targeting immunogens, namely immunogens aiming at activating B cells that express specific germline BCRs, represents one strategy to tackle low precursor frequencies [105, 106]. Furthermore, immunization studies indicate that for optimal vaccine efficacy the following conditions must be met: (1) B cell precursors must be present in the repertoire at sufficient frequencies [106, 107] (2) B cell precursors must have sufficient affinity for antigen for recruitment into the GC and competitive success [106, 107] (3) B cells and memory B cells must express a favorable antibody class [108] (4) the right structural context and T-B cell stoichiometry must occur in GC for optimal engagement and somatic hypermutation [107] (Table 1).

Tfh cells are central to GC formation and therefore their quantity and quality play a major role. In the absence of T cells, GCs formed in response to T-independent antigens collapse shortly after compartmentalization into the DZ and LZ [38]. To date, most of the data investigating Tfh quality and phenotype in the context of prophylactic vaccination come from circulating Tfh cells (pTfhs). Although the latter are often used as biomarkers of GC activity the lineage relationship between bona fide Tfh in LN and circulating Tfh is not clear [109–111]. The high heterogeneity of pTfh cell phenotypes and gene

Table 1 Parameters linked to the development of broadly neutralizing antibodies

Parameter	References
Tfh	
Frequency	[50]
Quality	[50, 52, 61, 69]
Phenotype / specificity	[50, 61, 69]
B-cells	
Precursor frequency	[40, 94, 95, 97, 106, 107, 116]
BCR affinity for antigen	[37, 40, 107]
Isotype class	[98]
Amount of help received by Tfh	[36, 40, 44, 52]
Antigen	
Persistence	[76, 106]
Diversity	[69]
Tregs/Tfr	
Frequency	[53, 90, 91]

expression profiles further complicates the interpretation of relevant studies [74, 112, 113]. Of all subsets, PD-1+ CXCR3− CXCR5+ CD4 T cells found in the blood have been found to be the population most related to GC Tfh cells by gene expression, cytokine expression profile and ability to provide help to B cells in vitro [110]. Higher expression of Tfh-associated genes, including CD40L, IL-21 and ICOS has been observed in animals mounting strong neutralizing antibody responses [43] and in the RV144 trial that produced some efficacy in humans, HIV-1-specific IL-21 producing pTfh cells were elevated [102, 110, 114, 115]. In addition, HIV-1 infected individuals with strong neutralizing responses harbor higher frequencies of pTfh [102, 110]. However, an association between pTfh and bnAb development is not always present [109]. Further research is needed to delineate the relationship between GC Tfh, pTfh and bnAbs in the context of prophylactic and therapeutic vaccination.

Antigen presentation and recognition are central to Tfh cell induction [30, 116] Therefore, increasing antigen availability has emerged as a rational approach to enhance Tfh responses for neutralizing antibody production in the context of vaccination [117]. Different strategies are under investigation targeting an effective delivery of immunogens, including (a) the continuous immunogen infusion whereby soluble native antigen degradation is reduced [118, 119], (b) the formation of immuno-complexes and deposition of antigen on monocytes, DCs or FDCs [120, 121], (c) the use of delivery platforms such as nanoparticles, liposomes, viral particles and use of adjuvants that can prolong antigen retention [122]. In parallel,

approaches to induce affinity maturation of bnAb-class specific naïve B-cell precursors (ie VRC01 or PGT121-class naïve B-cells) by delivering structurally optimized immunogens in sequential immunization protocols are also being tested [104, 123–125]. Combining such protocols with Tfh-boosting strategies will most likely be necessary for optimal vaccine efficacy. The type of prime-boost strategy also affects ensuing Tfh responses. Prime-boost strategies employing pure DNA instead of protein at priming, have been shown to increase Tfh differentiation, GC reactivity and antigen-specific antibody titers in mice [126] although to what extend they increase specifically broadly neutralizing antibodies remains to be determined. The interval between priming and boosting is also important for optimal Tfh and B-cell kinetics as an early boost, at the time when Tfh and B-cell maturation are still ongoing, could lead to suboptimal responses [127].

Understanding recall responses is also critical. GC B cell sequencing data indicate that memory B cells actively re-circulate after each immunization and reseed new GCs, with moderately mutated memory B cell lineages being more likely to participate in this reseeding. [128]. In a study by Havenar- Daughton et al, GC B cell frequencies in the draining LN in response to the final immunization were found to be the most predictive factor for the development of autologous nAbs with the top neutralizers having three fold more responding GC B cells than animals that only made non-neutralizing Ab responses [128]. Thus, understanding the recall kinetics of Tfh and B-cells in the context of serial immunizations will be key to developing prophylactic and therapeutic HIV-1 vaccines.

Conclusion

Much progress has been made over recent years in understanding Tfh cells and their implication in GC B cell responses. It is now clear that Tfh cells are instrumental for the generation of high affinity antibodies. Hence, manipulation of this subset and its microenvironment will be necessary for optimal vaccine efficacy. Tfh cell induction and optimal antigen-specific Tfh- B cell interaction will most likely necessitate a combination of more than one strategy. Deeper insights into the dynamics of Tfh cell induction, function and memory are also warranted. To this end, longitudinal studies in individuals with and without neutralizing activity with fine needle aspirates (FNA) could surpass the current limitations of LN biopsies and the need for complete removal of a LN at the site of induction. Powerful system immunology approaches, including bioinformatics and next-generation sequencing to uncover innate signatures and immune mechanisms that correlate with protection and that can improve vaccine induced long-lived neutralizing antibody responses will also be needed to guide the rational development of HIV-1 vaccines. A better understanding of those tissue-specific correlates that lead to robust GC B cell expansion, SHM and neutralization breadth will be key to achieving the goal of sterilizing HIV-1 immunity.

Authors' contributions

EM and CP discussed the paper, EM wrote the paper, CP and AK edit and approved the paper. All authors read and approved the final manuscript.

Acknowledgements

Authors would like to thank the personnel of Tissue Analysis Core at VRC, NIAID for helpful discussions and suggestions.

Competing interests

The authors declare that they have no competing interests.

Funding

This research was supported by the Intramural Research Program of the Vaccine Research Center, NIAID, National Institutes of Health and CAVD grant (#OP1032325) from the Bill and Melinda Gates Foundation (R.A.K.).

References

1. Hessell AJ, Rakasz EG, Poignard P, Hangartner L, Landucci G, Forthal DN, Koff WC, Watkins DI, Burton DR. Broadly neutralizing human anti-HIV antibody 2G12 is effective in protection against mucosal SHIV challenge even at low serum neutralizing titers. PLoS Pathog. 2009;5:e1000433.
2. Hessell AJ, Rakasz EG, Tehrani DM, Huber M, Weisgrau KL, Landucci G, Forthal DN, Koff WC, Poignard P, Watkins DI, Burton DR. Broadly neutralizing monoclonal antibodies 2F5 and 4E10 directed against the human immunodeficiency virus type 1 gp41 membrane-proximal external region protect against mucosal challenge by simian-human immunodeficiency virus SHIVBa-L. J Virol. 2010;84:1302–13.
3. Coffin J, Swanstrom R. HIV pathogenesis: dynamics and genetics of viral populations and infected cells. Cold Spring Harb Perspect Med. 2013;3:a012526.
4. Watkins DI, Burton DR, Kallas EG, Moore JP, Koff WC. Nonhuman primate models and the failure of the Merck HIV-1 vaccine in humans. Nat Med. 2008;14:617–21.
5. Kwong PD, Mascola JR. Human antibodies that neutralize HIV-1: identification, structures, and B cell ontogenies. Immunity. 2012;37:412–25.
6. Walker LM, Huber M, Doores KJ, Falkowska E, Pejchal R, Julien JP, Wang SK, Ramos A, Chan-Hui PY, Moyle M, et al. Broad neutralization coverage of HIV by multiple highly potent antibodies. Nature. 2011;477:466–70.
7. Lynch RM, Boritz E, Coates EE, DeZure A, Madden P, Costner P, Enama ME, Plummer S, Holman L, Hendel CS, et al. Virologic effects of broadly neutralizing antibody VRC01 administration during chronic HIV-1 infection. Sci Transl Med. 2015;7:319ra206.
8. Scheid JF, Horwitz JA, Bar-On Y, Kreider EF, Lu CL, Lorenzi JC, Feldmann A, Braunschweig M, Nogueira L, Oliveira T, et al. HIV-1 antibody 3BNC117 suppresses viral rebound in humans during treatment interruption. Nature. 2016;535:556–60.
9. Shingai M, Nishimura Y, Klein F, Mouquet H, Donau OK, Plishka R, Buckler-White A, Seaman M, Piatak M Jr, Lifson JD, et al. Antibody-mediated immunotherapy of macaques chronically infected with SHIV suppresses viraemia. Nature. 2013;503:277–80.
10. Mascola JR. Passive transfer studies to elucidate the role of antibody-mediated protection against HIV-1. Vaccine. 2002;20:1922–5.
11. Mascola JR, Lewis MG, Stiegler G, Harris D, VanCott TC, Hayes D, Louder MK, Brown CR, Sapan CV, Frankel SS, et al. Protection of Macaques against pathogenic simian/human immunodeficiency virus 89.6PD by passive transfer of neutralizing antibodies. J Virol. 1999;73:4009–18.
12. Caskey M, Klein F, Lorenzi JC, Seaman MS, West AP Jr, Buckley N, Kremer G, Nogueira L, Braunschweig M, Scheid JF, et al. Viraemia suppressed in HIV-1-infected humans by broadly neutralizing antibody 3BNC117. Nature. 2015;522:487–91.
13. Cohen YZ, Caskey M. Broadly neutralizing antibodies for treatment and prevention of HIV-1 infection. Curr Opin HIV AIDS. 2018;13:366–73.
14. Gray GE, Allen M, Moodie Z, Churchyard G, Bekker LG, Nchabeleng M, Mlisana K, Metch B, de Bruyn G, Latka MH, et al. Safety and efficacy of the HVTN 503/Phambili study of a clade-B-based HIV-1 vaccine in South Africa: a double-blind, randomised, placebo-controlled test-of-concept phase 2b study. Lancet Infect Dis. 2011;11:507–15.
15. Hammer SM, Sobieszczyk ME, Janes H, Karuna ST, Mulligan MJ, Grove D, Koblin BA, Buchbinder SP, Keefer MC, Tomaras GD, et al. Efficacy trial of a DNA/rAd5 HIV-1 preventive vaccine. N Engl J Med. 2013;369:2083–92.
16. Nicholson O, DiCandilo F, Kublin J, Sun X, Quirk E, Miller M, Gray G, Pape J, Robertson MN, Mehrotra DV, et al. Safety and immunogenicity of the MRKAd5 gag HIV type 1 vaccine in a worldwide phase 1 study of healthy adults. AIDS Res Hum Retrovir. 2011;27:557–67.
17. Rerks-Ngarm S, Pitisuttithum P, Nitayaphan S, Kaewkungwal J, Chiu J, Paris R, Premsri N, Namwat C, de Souza M, Adams E, et al. Vaccination with ALVAC and AIDSVAX to prevent HIV-1 infection in Thailand. N Engl J Med. 2009;361:2209–20.
18. Moysi E, Padhan K, Fabozzi G, Petrovas C. Novel advances on tissue immune dynamics in HIV/simian immunodeficiency virus: lessons from imaging studies. Curr Opin HIV AIDS. 2018;13:112–8.
19. Moysi E, Estes JD, Petrovas C. Novel imaging methods for analysis of tissue resident cells in HIV/SIV. Curr HIV/AIDS Rep. 2016;13:38–43.
20. Breitfeld D, Ohl L, Kremmer E, Ellwart J, Sallusto F, Lipp M, Forster R. Follicular B helper T cells express CXC chemokine receptor 5, localize to B cell follicles, and support immunoglobulin production. J Exp Med. 2000;192:1545–52.
21. Schaerli P, Willimann K, Lang AB, Lipp M, Loetscher P, Moser B. CXC chemokine receptor 5 expression defines follicular homing T cells with B cell helper function. J Exp Med. 2000;192:1553–62.
22. Ma CS, Deenick EK, Batten M, Tangye SG. The origins, function, and regulation of T follicular helper cells. J Exp Med. 2012;209:1241–53.
23. Kim CH, Rott LS, Clark-Lewis I, Campbell DJ, Wu L, Butcher EC. Subspecialization of CXCR5+ T cells: B helper activity is focused in a germinal center-localized subset of CXCR5+ T cells. J Exp Med. 2001;193:1373–81.
24. Iyer SS, Latner DR, Zilliox MJ, McCausland M, Akondy RS, Penaloza-Macmaster P, Hale JS, Ye L, Mohammed AU, Yamaguchi T, et al. Identification of novel markers for mouse CD4(+) T follicular helper cells. Eur J Immunol. 2013;43:3219–32.
25. Onabajo OO, George J, Lewis MG, Mattapallil JJ. Rhesus macaque lymph node PD-1(hi)CD4+ T cells express high levels of CXCR5 and IL-21 and display a CCR7(lo)ICOS+Bcl6+ T-follicular helper (Tfh) cell phenotype. PLoS ONE. 2013;8:e59758.
26. Crotty S. Do memory CD4 T cells keep their cell-type programming: plasticity versus fate commitment? Complexities of interpretation due to the heterogeneity of memory CD4 T cells, including T follicular helper cells. Cold Spring Harb Perspect Biol. 2018. https://doi.org/10.1101/cshperspect.a032102.
27. Vinuesa CG, Linterman MA, Yu D, MacLennan IC. Follicular helper T cells. Annu Rev Immunol. 2016;34:335–68.

28. Liu X, Nurieva RI, Dong C. Transcriptional regulation of follicular T-helper (Tfh) cells. Immunol Rev. 2013;252:139–45.

29. Nurieva RI, Chung Y, Hwang D, Yang XO, Kang HS, Ma L, Wang YH, Watowich SS, Jetten AM, Tian Q, Dong C. Generation of T follicular helper cells is mediated by interleukin-21 but independent of T helper 1, 2, or 17 cell lineages. Immunity. 2008;29:138–49.

30. Ballesteros-Tato A, Randall TD. Priming of T follicular helper cells by dendritic cells. Immunol Cell Biol. 2014;92:22–7.

31. Garside P, Ingulli E, Merica RR, Johnson JG, Noelle RJ, Jenkins MK. Visualization of specific B and T lymphocyte interactions in the lymph node. Science. 1998;281:96–9.

32. Okada T, Miller MJ, Parker I, Krummel MF, Neighbors M, Hartley SB, O'Garra A, Cahalan MD, Cyster JG. Antigen-engaged B cells undergo chemotaxis toward the T zone and form motile conjugates with helper T cells. PLoS Biol. 2005;3:e150.

33. Nurieva RI, Chung Y, Martinez GJ, Yang XO, Tanaka S, Matskevitch TD, Wang YH, Dong C. Bcl6 mediates the development of T follicular helper cells. Science. 2009;325:1001–5.

34. Hiramatsu Y, Suto A, Kashiwakuma D, Kanari H, Kagami S, Ikeda K, Hirose K, Watanabe N, Grusby MJ, Iwamoto I, Nakajima H. c-Maf activates the promoter and enhancer of the IL-21 gene, and TGF-beta inhibits c-Maf-induced IL-21 production in CD4+ T cells. J Leukoc Biol. 2010;87:703–12.

35. Belanger S, Crotty S. Dances with cytokines, featuring TFH cells, IL-21, IL-4 and B cells. Nat Immunol. 2016;17:1135–6.

36. Bossaller L, Burger J, Draeger R, Grimbacher B, Knoth R, Plebani A, Durandy A, Baumann U, Schlesier M, Welcher AA, et al. ICOS deficiency is associated with a severe reduction of CXCR5+CD4 germinal center Th cells. J Immunol. 2006;177:4927–32.

37. Brocker T, Gulbranson-Judge A, Flynn S, Riedinger M, Raykundalia C, Lane P. CD4 T cell traffic control: in vivo evidence that ligation of OX40 on CD4 T cells by OX40-ligand expressed on dendritic cells leads to the accumulation of CD4 T cells in B follicles. Eur J Immunol. 1999;29:1610–6.

38. Allen CD, Okada T, Cyster JG. Germinal-center organization and cellular dynamics. Immunity. 2007;27:190–202.

39. Shih TA, Meffre E, Roederer M, Nussenzweig MC. Role of BCR affinity in T cell dependent antibody responses in vivo. Nat Immunol. 2002;3:570–5.

40. Paus D, Phan TG, Chan TD, Gardam S, Basten A, Brink R. Antigen recognition strength regulates the choice between extrafollicular plasma cell and germinal center B cell differentiation. J Exp Med. 2006;203:1081–91.

41. Yeh CH, Nojima T, Kuraoka M, Kelsoe G. Germinal center entry not selection of B cells is controlled by peptide-MHCII complex density. Nat Commun. 2018;9:928.

42. Fleire SJ, Goldman JP, Carrasco YR, Weber M, Bray D, Batista FD. B cell ligand discrimination through a spreading and contraction response. Science. 2006;312:738–41.

43. Havenar-Daughton C, Lee JH, Crotty S. Tfh cells and HIV bnAbs, an immunodominance model of the HIV neutralizing antibody generation problem. Immunol Rev. 2017;275:49–61.

44. Petrovas C, Koup RA. T follicular helper cells and HIV/SIV-specific antibody responses. Curr Opin HIV AIDS. 2014;9:235–41.

45. Mesin L, Ersching J, Victora GD. Germinal center B cell dynamics. Immunity. 2016;45:471–82.

46. Ersching J, Efeyan A, Mesin L, Jacobsen JT, Pasqual G, Grabiner BC, Dominguez-Sola D, Sabatini DM, Victora GD. Germinal center selection and affinity maturation require dynamic regulation of mTORC1 kinase. Immunity. 2017;46(1045–1058):e1046.

47. Gitlin AD, Mayer CT, Oliveira TY, Shulman Z, Jones MJ, Koren A, Nussenzweig MC. HUMORAL IMMUNITY. T cell help controls the speed of the cell cycle in germinal center B cells. Science. 2015;349:643–6.

48. Gitlin AD, Shulman Z, Nussenzweig MC. Clonal selection in the germinal centre by regulated proliferation and hypermutation. Nature. 2014;509:637–40.

49. Hong JJ, Amancha PK, Rogers KA, Courtney CL, Havenar-Daughton C, Crotty S, Ansari AA, Villinger F. Early lymphoid responses and germinal center formation correlate with lower viral load set points and better prognosis of simian immunodeficiency virus infection. J Immunol. 2014;193:797–806.

50. Hong JJ, Amancha PK, Rogers K, Ansari AA, Villinger F. Spatial alterations between CD4(+) T follicular helper, B, and CD8(+) T cells during simian immunodeficiency virus infection: T/B cell homeostasis, activation, and potential mechanism for viral escape. J Immunol. 2012;188:3247–56.

51. Lindqvist M, van Lunzen J, Soghoian DZ, Kuhl BD, Ranasinghe S, Kranias G, Flanders MD, Cutler S, Yudanin N, Muller MI, et al. Expansion of HIV-specific T follicular helper cells in chronic HIV infection. J Clin Invest. 2012;122:3271–80.

52. Perreau M, Savoye AL, De Crignis E, Corpataux JM, Cubas R, Haddad EK, De Leval L, Graziosi C, Pantaleo G. Follicular helper T cells serve as the major CD4 T cell compartment for HIV-1 infection, replication, and production. J Exp Med. 2013;210:143–56.

53. Petrovas C, Yamamoto T, Gerner MY, Boswell KL, Wloka K, Smith EC, Ambrozak DR, Sandler NG, Timmer KJ, Sun X, et al. CD4 T follicular helper cell dynamics during SIV infection. J Clin Invest. 2012;122:3281–94.

54. van Gils MJ, Sanders RW. Broadly neutralizing antibodies against HIV-1: templates for a vaccine. Virology. 2013;435:46–56.

55. Hraber P, Korber BT, Lapedes AS, Bailer RT, Seaman MS, Gao H, Greene KM, McCutchan F, Williamson C, Kim JH, et al. Impact of clade, geography, and age of the epidemic on HIV-1 neutralization by antibodies. J Virol. 2014;88:12623–43.

56. Moore PL, Williamson C, Morris L. Virological features associated with the development of broadly neutralizing antibodies to HIV-1. Trends Microbiol. 2015;23:204–11.

57. Rademeyer C, Moore PL, Taylor N, Martin DP, Choge IA, Gray ES, Sheppard HW, Gray C, Morris L, Williamson C, Team Hs. Genetic characteristics of HIV-1 subtype C envelopes inducing cross-neutralizing antibodies. Virology. 2007;368:172–81.

58. Piantadosi A, Panteleeff D, Blish CA, Baeten JM, Jaoko W, McClelland RS, Overbaugh J. Breadth of neutralizing antibody response to human immunodeficiency virus type 1 is affected by factors early in infection but does not influence disease progression. J Virol. 2009;83:10269–74.

59. Yamamoto T, Lynch RM, Gautam R, Matus-Nicodemos R, Schmidt SD, Boswell KL, Darko S, Wong P, Sheng Z, Petrovas C, et al. Quality and quantity of TFH cells are critical for broad antibody development in SHIVAD8 infection. Sci Transl Med. 2015;7:298ra120.

60. Landais E, Huang X, Havenar-Daughton C, Murrell B, Price MA, Wickramasinghe L, Ramos A, Bian CB, Simek M, Allen S, et al. Broadly neutralizing antibody responses in a large longitudinal sub-Saharan HIV primary infection cohort. PLoS Pathog. 2016;12:e1005369.

61. Rouers A, Klingler J, Su B, Samri A, Laumond G, Even S, Avettand-Fenoel V, Richetta C, Paul N, Boufassa F, et al. HIV-specific B cell frequency correlates with neutralization breadth in patients naturally controlling HIV-infection. EBioMedicine. 2017;21:158–69.

62. Cubas RA, Mudd JC, Savoye AL, Perreau M, van Grevenynghe J, Metcalf T, Connick E, Meditz A, Freeman GJ, Abesada-Terk G Jr, et al. Inadequate T follicular cell help impairs B cell immunity during HIV infection. Nat Med. 2013;19:494–9.

63. Miles B, Miller SM, Folkvord JM, Kimball A, Chamanian M, Meditz AL, Arends T, McCarter MD, Levy DN, Rakasz EG, et al. Follicular regulatory T cells impair follicular T helper cells in HIV and SIV infection. Nat Commun. 2015;6:8608.

64. Banga R, Procopio FA, Noto A, Pollakis G, Cavassini M, Ohmiti K, Corpataux JM, de Leval L, Pantaleo G, Perreau M. PD-1(+) and follicular helper T cells are responsible for persistent HIV-1 transcription in treated aviremic individuals. Nat Med. 2016;22:754–61.

65. Boritz EA, Darko S, Swaszek L, Wolf G, Wells D, Wu X, Henry AR, Laboune F, Hu J, Ambrozak D, et al. Multiple origins of virus persistence during natural control of HIV infection. Cell. 2016;166:1004–15.

66. Haase AT, Henry K, Zupancic M, Sedgewick G, Faust RA, Melroe H, Cavert W, Gebhard K, Staskus K, Zhang ZQ, et al. Quantitative image analysis of HIV-1 infection in lymphoid tissue. Science. 1996;274:985–9.

67. Heath SL, Tew JG, Tew JG, Szakal AK, Burton GF. Follicular dendritic cells and human immunodeficiency virus infectivity. Nature. 1995;377:740–4.

68. Porichis F, Kaufmann DE. HIV-specific CD4 T cells and immune control of viral replication. Curr Opin HIV AIDS. 2011;6:174–80.

69. Pallikkuth S, Rogers K, Villinger F, Dosterii M, Vaccari M, Franchini G, Pahwa R, Pahwa S. Interleukin-21 administration to rhesus macaques chronically infected with simian immunodeficiency virus increases cytotoxic effector molecules in T cells and NK cells and enhances B cell function without increasing immune activation or viral replication. Vaccine. 2011;29:9229–38.

70. Vaccari M, Franchini G. T cell subsets in the germinal center: lessons from the macaque model. Front Immunol. 2018;9:348.

71. Wendel BS, Del Alcazar D, He C, Del Rio-Estrada PM, Aiamkitsumrit B, Ablanedo-Terrazas Y, Hernandez SM, Ma KY, Betts MR, Pulido L, et al. The receptor repertoire and functional profile of follicular T cells in HIV-infected lymph nodes. Sci Immunol. 2018;3(22):eaan8884. https://doi.org/10.1126/sciimmunol.aan8884

72. Alshekaili J, Chand R, Lee CE, Corley S, Kwong K, Papa I, Fulcher DA, Randall KL, Leiding JW, Ma CS, et al. STAT3 regulates cytotoxicity of human CD57+ CD4+ T cells in blood and lymphoid follicles. Sci Rep. 2018;8:3529.

73. Asrir A, Aloulou M, Gador M, Perals C, Fazilleau N. Interconnected subsets of memory follicular helper T cells have different effector functions. Nat Commun. 2017;8:847.

74. Wong MT, Chen J, Narayanan S, Lin W, Anicete R, Kiaang HT, De Lafaille MA, Poidinger M, Newell EW. Mapping the diversity of follicular helper T cells in human blood and tonsils using high-dimensional mass cytometry analysis. Cell Rep. 2015;11:1822–33.

75. Thacker TC, Zhou X, Estes JD, Jiang Y, Keele BF, Elton TS, Burton GF. Follicular dendritic cells and human immunodeficiency virus type 1 transcription in CD4+ T cells. J Virol. 2009;83:150–8.

76. Hufert FT, van Lunzen J, Janossy G, Bertram S, Schmitz J, Haller O, Racz P, von Laer D. Germinal centre CD4+ T cells are an important site of HIV replication in vivo. AIDS. 1997;11:849–57.

77. Velu V, Mylvaganam GH, Gangadhara S, Hong JJ, Iyer SS, Gumber S, Ibegbu CC, Villinger F, Amara RR. Induction of Th1-biased t follicular helper (Tfh) cells in lymphoid tissues during chronic simian immunodeficiency virus infection defines functionally distinct germinal center Tfh cells. J Immunol. 2016;197:1832–42.

78. Havenar-Daughton C, Reiss SM, Carnathan DG, Wu JE, Kendric K, Torrents de la Pena A, Kasturi SP, Dan JM, Bothwell M, Sanders RW, et al. Cytokine-independent detection of antigen-specific germinal center T follicular helper cells in immunized nonhuman primates using a live cell activation-induced marker technique. J Immunol. 2016;197:994–1002.

79. Mikell I, Sather DN, Kalams SA, Altfeld M, Alter G, Stamatatos L. Characteristics of the earliest cross-neutralizing antibody response to HIV-1. PLoS Pathog. 2011;7:e1001251.

80. Yu L, Guan Y. Immunologic basis for Long HCDR3 s in broadly neutralizing antibodies against HIV-1. Front Immunol. 2014;5:250.

81. McLellan JS, Pancera M, Carrico C, Gorman J, Julien JP, Khayat R, Louder R, Pejchal R, Sastry M, Dai K, et al. Structure of HIV-1 gp120 V1/V2 domain with broadly neutralizing antibody PG9. Nature. 2011;480:336–43.

82. Liu M, Yang G, Wiehe K, Nicely NI, Vandergrift NA, Rountree W, Bonsignori M, Alam SM, Gao J, Haynes BF, Kelsoe G. Polyreactivity and autoreactivity among HIV-1 antibodies. J Virol. 2015;89:784–98.

83. Bonsignori M, Zhou T, Sheng Z, Chen L, Gao F, Joyce MG, Ozorowski G, Chuang GY, Schramm CA, Wiehe K, et al. Maturation pathway from germline to broad HIV-1 neutralizer of a CD4-mimic antibody. Cell. 2016;165:449–63.

84. Sather DN, Armann J, Ching LK, Mavrantoni A, Sellhorn G, Caldwell Z, Yu X, Wood B, Self S, Kalams S, Stamatatos L. Factors associated with the development of cross-reactive neutralizing antibodies during human immunodeficiency virus type 1 infection. J Virol. 2009;83:757–69.

85. Baumjohann D, Preite S, Reboldi A, Ronchi F, Ansel KM, Lanzavecchia A, Sallusto F. Persistent antigen and germinal center B cells sustain T follicular helper cell responses and phenotype. Immunity. 2013;38:596–605.

86. Moir S, Fauci AS. Insights into B cells and HIV-specific B-cell responses in HIV-infected individuals. Immunol Rev. 2013;254:207–24.

87. Cagigi A, Nilsson A, Pensieroso S, Chiodi F. Dysfunctional B-cell responses during HIV-1 infection: implication for influenza vaccination and highly active antiretroviral therapy. Lancet Infect Dis. 2010;10:499–503.

88. De Milito A. B lymphocyte dysfunctions in HIV infection. Curr HIV Res. 2004;2:11–21.

89. De Milito A, Nilsson A, Titanji K, Thorstensson R, Reizenstein E, Narita M, Grutzmeier S, Sonnerborg A, Chiodi F. Mechanisms of hypergammaglobulinemia and impaired antigen-specific humoral immunity in HIV-1 infection. Blood. 2004;103:2180–6.

90. Lane HC, Masur H, Edgar LC, Whalen G, Rook AH, Fauci AS. Abnormalities of B-cell activation and immunoregulation in patients with the acquired immunodeficiency syndrome. N Engl J Med. 1983;309:453–8.

91. Shirai A, Cosentino M, Leitman-Klinman SF, Klinman DM. Human immunodeficiency virus infection induces both polyclonal and virus-specific B cell activation. J Clin Invest. 1992;89:561–6.

92. Colineau L, Rouers A, Yamamoto T, Xu Y, Urrutia A, Pham HP, Cardinaud S, Samri A, Dorgham K, Coulon PG, et al. HIV-infected spleens present altered follicular helper T cell (Tfh) subsets and skewed B cell maturation. PLoS ONE. 2015;10:e0140978.

93. Cagigi A, Mowafi F, Phuong Dang LV, Tenner-Racz K, Atlas A, Grutzmeier S, Racz P, Chiodi F, Nilsson A. Altered expression of the receptor-ligand pair CXCR5/CXCL13 in B cells during chronic HIV-1 infection. Blood. 2008;112:4401–10.

94. Eggena MP, Barugahare B, Jones N, Okello M, Mutalya S, Kityo C, Mugyenyi P, Cao H. Depletion of regulatory T cells in HIV infection is associated with immune activation. J Immunol. 2005;174:4407–14.

95. Linterman MA, Pierson W, Lee SK, Kallies A, Kawamoto S, Rayner TF, Srivastava M, Divekar DP, Beaton L, Hogan JJ, et al. Foxp3+ follicular regulatory T cells control the germinal center response. Nat Med. 2011;17:975–82.

96. Maceiras AR, Fonseca VR, Agua-Doce A, Graca L. T follicular regulatory cells in mice and men. Immunology. 2017;152:25–35.

97. Amodio D, Cotugno N, Macchiarulo G, Rocca S, Dimopoulos Y, Castrucci MR, De Vito R, Tucci FM, McDermott AB, Narpala S, et al. Quantitative multiplexed imaging analysis reveals a strong association between immunogen-specific B cell responses and tonsillar germinal center immune dynamics in children after influenza vaccination. J Immunol. 2018;200:538–50.

98. Andersson J, Boasso A, Nilsson J, Zhang R, Shire NJ, Lindback S, Shearer GM, Chougnet CA. The prevalence of regulatory T cells in lymphoid tissue is correlated with viral load in HIV-infected patients. J Immunol. 2005;174:3143–7.

99. Estes JD, Li Q, Reynolds MR, Wietgrefe S, Duan L, Schacker T, Picker LJ, Watkins DI, Lifson JD, Reilly C, et al. Premature induction of an immunosuppressive regulatory T cell response during acute simian immunodeficiency virus infection. J Infect Dis. 2006;193:703–12.

100. Blackburn MJ, Zhong-Min M, Caccuri F, McKinnon K, Schifanella L, Guan Y, Gorini G, Venzon D, Fenizia C, Binello N, et al. Regulatory and helper follicular T cells and antibody avidity to simian immunodeficiency virus glycoprotein 120. J Immunol. 2015;195:3227–36.

101. Borrow P, Moody MA. Immunologic characteristics of HIV-infected individuals who make broadly neutralizing antibodies. Immunol Rev. 2017;275:62–78.

102. Moody MA, Pedroza-Pacheco I, Vandergrift NA, Chui C, Lloyd KE, Parks R, Soderberg KA, Ogbe AT, Cohen MS, Liao HX, et al. Immune perturbations in HIV-1-infected individuals who make broadly neutralizing antibodies. Sci Immunol. 2016;1:aag0851.

103. Jardine JG, Kulp DW, Havenar-Daughton C, Sarkar A, Briney B, Sok D, Sesterhenn F, Ereno-Orbea J, Kalyuzhniy O, Deresa I, et al. HIV-1 broadly neutralizing antibody precursor B cells revealed by germline-targeting immunogen. Science. 2016;351:1458–63.

104. Jardine J, Julien JP, Menis S, Ota T, Kalyuzhniy O, McGuire A, Sok D, Huang PS, MacPherson S, Jones M, et al. Rational HIV immunogen design to target specific germline B cell receptors. Science. 2013;340:711–6.

105. Stamatatos L, Pancera M, McGuire AT. Germline-targeting immunogens. Immunol Rev. 2017;275:203–16.

106. Dosenovic P, Kara EE, Pettersson AK, McGuire AT, Gray M, Hartweger H, Thientosapol ES, Stamatatos L, Nussenzweig MC. Anti-HIV-1 B cell responses are dependent on B cell precursor frequency and antigen-binding affinity. Proc Natl Acad Sci U S A. 2018;115:4743–8.

107. Abbott RK, Lee JH, Menis S, Skog P, Rossi M, Ota T, Kulp DW, Bhullar D, Kalyuzhniy O, Havenar-Daughton C, et al. Precursor frequency and affinity determine B cell competitive fitness in germinal centers, tested with germline-targeting HIV vaccine immunogens. Immunity. 2018;48(133–146):e136.

108. Dogan I, Bertocci B, Vilmont V, Delbos F, Megret J, Storck S, Reynaud CA, Weill JC. Multiple layers of B cell memory with different effector functions. Nat Immunol. 2009;10:1292–9.

109. Boswell KL, Paris R, Boritz E, Ambrozak D, Yamamoto T, Darko S, Wloka K, Wheatley A, Narpala S, McDermott A, et al. Loss of circulating CD4 T cells with B cell helper function during chronic HIV infection. PLoS Pathog. 2014;10:e1003853.

110. Locci M, Havenar-Daughton C, Landais E, Wu J, Kroenke MA, Arlehamn CL, Su LF, Cubas R, Davis MM, Sette A, et al. Human circulating PD-1+CXCR3-CXCR5+ memory Tfh cells are highly functional and correlate with broadly neutralizing HIV antibody responses. Immunity. 2013;39:758–69.

111. He J, Tsai LM, Leong YA, Hu X, Ma CS, Chevalier N, Sun X, Vandenberg K, Rockman S, Ding Y, et al. Circulating precursor CCR7(lo)PD-1(hi) CXCR5(+) CD4(+) T cells indicate Tfh cell activity and promote antibody responses upon antigen reexposure. Immunity. 2013;39:770–81.

112. Schmitt N, Bentebibel SE, Ueno H. Phenotype and functions of memory Tfh cells in human blood. Trends Immunol. 2014;35:436–42.

113. Schmitt N, Ueno H. Blood Tfh cells come with colors. Immunity. 2013;39:629–30.

114. Chahroudi A, Silvestri G. HIV and Tfh cells: circulating new ideas to identify and protect. Immunity. 2016;44:16–8.

115. Schultz BT, Teigler JE, Pissani F, Oster AF, Kranias G, Alter G, Marovich M, Eller MA, Dittmer U, Robb ML, et al. Circulating HIV-specific interleukin-21(+)CD4(+) T cells represent peripheral Tfh cells with antigen-dependent helper functions. Immunity. 2016;44:167–78.

116. Deenick EK, Chan A, Ma CS, Gatto D, Schwartzberg PL, Brink R, Tangye SG. Follicular helper T cell differentiation requires continuous antigen presentation that is independent of unique B cell signaling. Immunity. 2010;33:241–53.

117. Linterman MA, Hill DL. Can follicular helper T cells be targeted to improve vaccine efficacy? [version 1; referees: 3 approved]. F1000Research. 2016;5(F1000 Faculty Rev):88. https://doi.org/10.12688/f1000 research.7388.1.

118. Pauthner M, Havenar-Daughton C, Sok D, Nkolola JP, Bastidas R, Boopathy AV, Carnathan DG, Chandrashekar A, Cirelli KM, Cottrell CA, et al. Elicitation of robust tier 2 neutralizing antibody responses in nonhuman primates by hiv envelope trimer immunization using optimized approaches. Immunity. 2017;46(1073–1088):e1076.

119. Tam HH, Melo MB, Kang M, Pelet JM, Ruda VM, Foley MH, Hu JK, Kumari S, Crampton J, Baldeon AD, et al. Sustained antigen availability during germinal center initiation enhances antibody responses to vaccination. Proc Natl Acad Sci U S A. 2016;113:E6639–48.

120. Flamar AL, Contreras V, Zurawski S, Montes M, Dereuddre-Bosquet N, Martinon F, Banchereau J, Le Grand R, Zurawski G, Levy Y. Delivering HIV Gagp24 to DCIR induces strong antibody responses in vivo. PLoS ONE. 2015;10:e0135513.

121. Park HY, Tan PS, Kavishna R, Ker A, Lu J, Chan CEZ, Hanson BJ, MacAry PA, Caminschi I, Shortman K, et al. Enhancing vaccine antibody responses by targeting Clec9A on dendritic cells. NPJ Vaccines. 2017;2:31.

122. Gao Y, Wijewardhana C, Mann JFS. Virus-like particle, liposome, and polymeric particle-based vaccines against HIV-1. Front Immunol. 2018;9:345.

123. Escolano A, Steichen JM, Dosenovic P, Kulp DW, Golijanin J, Sok D, Freund NT, Gitlin AD, Oliveira T, Araki T, et al. Sequential immunization elicits broadly neutralizing anti-HIV-1 antibodies in Ig knockin mice. Cell. 2016;166(1445–1458):e1412.

124. Briney B, Sok D, Jardine JG, Kulp DW, Skog P, Menis S, Jacak R, Kalyuzhniy O, de Val N, Sesterhenn F, et al. Tailored Immunogens direct affinity maturation toward HIV neutralizing antibodies. Cell. 2016;166(1459–1470):e1411.

125. Tian M, Cheng C, Chen X, Duan H, Cheng HL, Dao M, Sheng Z, Kimble M, Wang L, Lin S, et al. Induction of HIV neutralizing antibody lineages in mice with diverse precursor repertoires. Cell. 2016;166(1471–1484):e1418.

126. Hollister K, Chen Y, Wang S, Wu H, Mondal A, Clegg N, Lu S, Dent A. The role of follicular helper T cells and the germinal center in HIV-1 gp120 DNA prime and gp120 protein boost vaccination. Hum Vaccin Immunother. 2014;10:1985–92.

127. Sallusto F, Lanzavecchia A, Araki K, Ahmed R. From vaccines to memory and back. Immunity. 2010;33:451–63.

128. Havenar-Daughton C, Carnathan DG, Torrents de la Pena A, Pauthner M, Briney B, Reiss SM, Wood JS, Kaushik K, van Gils MJ, Rosales SL, et al. Direct probing of germinal center responses reveals immunological features and bottlenecks for neutralizing antibody responses to HIV Env trimer. Cell Rep. 2016;17:2195–209.

16

Total HIV DNA: a global marker of HIV persistence

Christine Rouzioux[1,2*] and Véronique Avettand-Fenoël[1,2]

Abstract

Among the different markers of HIV persistence in infected cells, total HIV DNA is to date the most widely used. It allows an overall quantification of all viral forms of HIV DNA in infected cells, each playing a different role in HIV replication and pathophysiology. The real-time PCR technology is to date, a precise, sensitive and reproducible technology that allows the description of the distribution of HIV infected cells in blood and tissues. The objective of this review is to present some examples which show the interest to quantify total HIV DNA levels. This marker brought an undeniable and considerable contribution to reservoir studies. Many results, both in clinical and basic research, allowed to get a large overview of the distribution of infected cells in the body, at all stages of HIV disease and during therapy. Future clinical studies aiming at reducing HIV reservoirs will benefit from HIV DNA quantification in blood and tissues, in association with other markers of HIV reservoir activity.

Keywords: Total HIV DNA, Real time PCR, Reservoirs, CD4+T cell subsets

Background

Among the different markers of HIV persistence in infected cells, total HIV-1 DNA is to date the most widely used marker. This marker is often considered as imperfect. However, it is the one that has brought and will bring the most results in HIV reservoir studies. The major criticism is that this marker makes it possible to quantify all forms of HIV-DNA, without differentiating the defective forms from the latent ones that can produce infectious viruses. This drawback can also be considered an advantage because it therefore allows an overall quantification of all viral forms of HIV DNA, each playing a different role in HIV replication and pathophysiology. In fact, defective proviruses participate in HIV pathogenesis, as they can produce viral antigens, incomplete viruses, can induce activation/inflammation in infected tissues, thereby maintaining viral replication and facilitating the persistence of HIV reservoirs throughout the body [1]. Clearly, all reservoir cells represent the engine of the viral infection and merit to be measured. The

pathophysiology of HIV-1 reservoirs is complex and different in infected compartments and tissues, that justifies to explore multiple markers together, each one having a different meaning. The question is not what is the best marker, but rather what is the best association of reservoir markers for each program [2]. Among all reservoir markers, total HIV DNA represents one of the master pieces to build the puzzle.

Technical aspects of total HIV DNA quantification

Total HIV DNA, also called cell-associated HIV DNA (CA-HIV DNA), is a marker of HIV reservoirs that permits the quantification of all forms of HIV DNA including stable integrated proviruses and unintegrated forms, including extrachromosomal 2-LTR, 1-LTR forms and linear forms. All these forms co-exist in infected cells during viral replication and their levels may vary among patients, according to the stages of HIV disease [3].

The most frequently used method for measuring total HIV DNA is the quantitative real-time PCR based assay [4]. HIV-1 DNA PCR assays are performed on total DNA extracts from cells. Amplification has to be done with primers and probe, targeting conserved regions of the viral genome. LTR, *pol* and *gag* genes are the most often selected, but the high viral genetic diversity has to be

*Correspondence: christine.rouzioux@aphp.fr
[1] Laboratoire de Virologie, APHP Hôpital Necker Enfants Malades, Paris, France
Full list of author information is available at the end of the article

taken into account, especially in countries where there are high numbers of various CRF and non-B subtypes. The quantification of the copy number is based on a standard curve prepared by serial dilutions of a standard, such as 8E5 cell line containing one genome per cell. The initial quantification of total DNA by the measurement of the optical density at 260 nm (OD_{260}), or by quantifying a cellular gene in parallel by PCR (such as CCR5 or albumin), is necessary to assess the cell number tested in a PCR and to calculate the frequency of infected cells per one million cells [5]. It is generally assumed that there is one copy per infected cell, in particular in latently infected cells which are dominant, especially among patients receiving a prolonged and effective antiretroviral treatment. The frequency of infected cells being very low, the objective is to quantify a rare event. Such quantification follows the Poisson probability distribution. So, whatever the technique used, it is necessary to test high numbers of cells, in order to reach low detection levels. Since the amount of total DNA is limited per PCR well, it is often necessary to test several replicates, in order to increase the number of cells tested and to estimate the frequency of infected cells, as well as possible (especially in case of very low frequency). The Boston patients and the Mississippi baby cases confirmed that the latent reservoir can persist at a level below the limit of detection of current assays, allowing the rebound of HIV infection months later. An ultra-sensitive protocol could be used by testing six to eight replicates, to explore a high number of cells and detect low levels as it has been done for Elite controllers and Post Treatment Controllers (also called VISCONTI patients) [6–8]. The same technology has been also developed for HIV-2 infected patients, having usually low reservoir levels. A new assay for HIV-2 DNA quantification based on the same technology has also been developed [9].

The quantitative real-time PCR offers a number of technical advantages, making the total HIV DNA the most widely used marker for exploring HIV reservoirs. There are multiple reasons for this situation: the assay is the most feasible and reproducible, it is quick, easy to perform, precise, accurate, sensitive and with a large dynamic range of quantification. Compared to other assays, such as QVOA which may need more than 100 ml of fresh blood, small amounts of blood or tissue can be tested and samples can be stored frozen before testing. Moreover, it is less expensive and time consuming. The technique has a good reproducibility, as shown with the intra-laboratory control reported in a recent review [10], the Inter-assay coefficient of variation was at 0.07, in the same range than a recent one at 0.15 [11]. Lastly, the results obtained, within inter-laboratories control,

has confirmed that this technique could be implemented within multi-centric protocols and clinical trials [12].

One standardized quantitative assay based on real-time PCR has been commercialized (Biocentric, Bandol, France). This has enabled access to both basic research and clinical research teams to use the same quantitative tool, making possible comparisons between studies [13].

Similarly to assays which have been developed for HIV RNA quantification, the total HIV DNA real-time PCR assay is easy to be adapted to automated nucleic acid extractors and real time-PCR machines. It takes around 4 h to test more than 80 samples within one run, making this technique well adapted to test large series of samples. This has provided good statistical power, which was very helpful to demonstrate that the total HIV DNA level in Peripheral Blood Mononuclear Cells (PBMC) predicts disease progression and to explore the dynamics of this marker, using mathematical models [14, 15].

Some teams also propose to use the digital droplet PCR (ddPCR) technology, which can precisely quantify with accuracy and reproducibility nucleic acids such as total HIV DNA [16, 17]. Jones et al. demonstrated that a six logs linear dynamic range of ddPCR is approaching the seven logs, achievable by real-time PCR. Its drawbacks include the cost of equipment and the complexity of the assay, while real-time PCR is widely used in research and clinical laboratories [18]. This technique has been mainly applied to blood samples, and results obtained are very close to those obtained with real-time PCR [19]. On the whole, ddPCR gives accurate quantification of low levels of HIV DNA, but false positive results with ddPCR may occur [17, 19, 20]. Less frequently, other technologies have been proposed to quantify total HIV-DNA, such as seminested real-time PCR, nested PCR assays [21–24]. Furthermore, PCR with amplification of extracts, at limiting dilution, and detection by real-time fluorescence confirmed by melt curve, is also commonly used [25].

Lastly, in order to explore the consistency between blood reservoir markers, a comparative analysis of measures of markers, in acute and chronic patients, reported correlations between markers. This includes correlations between total HIV DNA and integrated HIV DNA and HIV DNA in rectal CD4+T cells [26]. Of course, the correlations cannot be perfect, each marker having a different meaning and playing a different role in HIV reservoir persistence.

Total HIV DNA quantification applied to many kinds of samples
The quantification of total HIV DNA permits to estimate of the total number of all infected cells, resting or activated, present in blood, in tissues and biopsies.

Quantification in peripheral blood Total HIV DNA level is mainly quantified within pellets of PBMC, usually separated from plasma on Ficoll–Hypaque density gradient. The technique can also be readily adapted to quantify total HIV DNA directly on whole blood samples, the frequency of infected cells is then obtained by taking into account the blood formula. The predictive value of total HIV DNA has been reported, whatever the mode of expression of the results, per million CD4 + T cells, per million PBMC, or per ml of whole blood [27].

Because blood is the most accessible and easily quantifiable compartment, the majority of other reservoir markers, whether exploring the number of producing cells or measuring transcriptional activity, are also done mostly from the peripheral blood. So, the majority of studies have explored blood reservoirs, despite criticism that the majority of infected cells are in tissues and that the blood contains only a small number of infected cells. It would therefore be unrepresentative. It is true that the normal distribution of lymphocytes is 2% in the blood, while it is 98% in tissues. However, such a criticism does not seem to take into account the fact that the same criticism could apply to the quantification of blood CD4 + T lymphocytes and HIV RNA in plasma, whereas they are routinely used and they represent clinical markers definitely considered essential. The peripheral blood reservoir quantification is the most logical and clinically feasible approach, as are the use of CD4 + T cell count and plasma HIV RNA level for patient monitoring. In addition, the total level of HIV DNA in PBMC is the only marker of HIV reservoirs for which the predictive value of the risk of progression to AIDS and death has been well demonstrated [14, 28]. This confirms that the level of HIV DNA in peripheral blood level is representative of the total reservoir. However, it is true that infected blood cells may not adequately reflect all critical events occurring outside the bloodstream, neither the whole story of HIV reservoirs.

Quantification from sorted cells This assay has also been developed and largely applied to the quantification of infected cells within fractions of sorted blood or tissue cells, such as CD4 + T lymphocytes, CD4 + T cell subsets, including naïve (TN) central memory (TCM), transitional memory (TTM) and effector memory (TEM). Resting T and activated T cells are also informative to the pathophysiology of HIV infection. It is also interesting to combine assays, such as total HIV DNA quantification and capacity to produce HIV RNA in cell culture, using cell sorter such as FacsAria on the same living fractions [7, 29].

Quantification in tissue biopsies Total HIV DNA has proved very useful to describe the distribution of infected cells in tissues and anatomic reservoirs. That also allowed to document infected areas in which the distribution of medicinal products must be particularly important [30], including anatomic compartments, such as CNS that may also act as sanctuaries. The assay could be performed on small fragments, using a specific method for nucleic acid extraction [31]. Studies performed in non-human primate models have also benefitted from this marker with extensive quantifications in many tissues. This includes autopsies, showing the high number of infected cells, and more specifically the major role of lymph-nodes at the origin of viral dissemination throughout the organism [32, 33].

Total HIV DNA at different stages of HIV disease

The spectrum of total HIV DNA levels in PBMC during HIV infection have been presented in a recent and extensive review, confirming the major impact of this marker to get a global overview of HIV reservoir levels in different groups of infected patients. Of note, we used the same assay in all studies, that permits to compare patient groups [10].

During the natural history of HIV infection The data showed that the reservoir is seeded very early in infection, with high levels in primary infection at the peak, then the HIV DNA set point is rapidly established [34, 35]. Total HIV DNA in blood and gut levels are significantly lower in patients with primary infection, at stage Fiebig I, versus Fiebig II–IV [23]. Total HIV DNA level in PBMC were also described in children [36], at the AIDS stage [37] and was found strongly associated with HIV-associated neurocognitive disorders, independent of plasma HIV RNA, indicating the neurologic impact of a larger reservoir [38, 39]. Elite controllers are characterized by a very low reservoir level, especially those bearing HLA protective alleles [8, 40].

Interestingly, total HIV DNA levels in PBMC correlate positively with plasma HIV RNA and negatively with CD4 + T cell count [14]. There is a link between HIV reservoir levels and activation [41, 42]. Lastly, several reports confirmed the high predictive value of the total HIV-DNA level in PBMC during natural history [14, 28, 43–45]. HIV reservoirs play a major role within lymph-nodes, including in the B cell follicle sanctuary [32, 33]. The distributions of HIV DNA and HIV RNA differ between gut and blood [46], and in gut associated lymphoid tissue of controllers and non-controllers [47]. Quantification of HIV DNA in kidney, as well as in adipose tissue, indicates that they can be considered as anatomical reservoirs [48, 49]. Measuring HIV DNA in genital compartments may indicate the presence of infected cells and may help to explore this risk of sexual transmission [50, 51].

Under antiretroviral therapy The impact of antiretroviral therapy on HIV DNA is less than that on plasma HIV RNA. The decay of the total HIV DNA in blood is faster in acute infected patients receiving early treatment, compared to a slow decrease in patients treated at the chronic stage, in whom the kinetics shows a first phase of decay in the first year, then followed by a sort of plateau [52]. On the contrary, among acutely infected patients, the decrease continues beyond 4 years of primary infection treatment, while no further decay is noted in chronic treated patients [15, 35]. The earlier the treatment is initiated, the more prominent is the total HIV DNA decrease [34]. Studies of the total HIV DNA decay dynamics in blood, during more than a decade of suppressive antiretroviral therapy, indicates a slow decline during these last years, with a remarkable stability of a plateau, balanced by homeostatic proliferation [52–55]. High total HIV DNA levels in PBMC are informative when measured at treatment interruption, as they predict a shorter time to treatment resumption, independently of the CD4 nadir [56], while low levels predict a higher probability of maintaining viral control [57, 58].

This marker has proved to be particularly useful and has shown interest in immuno- pathophysiological studies. First, the results showed that HIV DNA level in PBMC is predominantly composed of T CD4 + Central Memory Cells (TCM) in patients at the chronic stage [59]. These TCM are preserved from infection by early treatment initiated in primary infection [29, 60], while HIV DNA subspecies persist in both activated and resting memory CD4 + T cells during therapy [61]. Early antiretroviral treatment maintains the distribution with protection of the TCM [62, 63]. So, the measurement of total HIV DNA levels in PBMC contributed to show that early treatment initiation remains, so far, the best way to limit the size of the reservoirs.

Interestingly, the distribution pattern in CD4 + T cell subsets of VISCONTI patients seems to have also been frozen by early treatment, with TCM that contributes minimally to the total blood reservoir. Moreover, HIV DNA levels decrease over time in some of them: all this suggesting that the protection of TCM compartment might be necessary, and/or participates to the control of HIV replication [5, 7].

Interestingly, this marker was the only positive marker of HIV infection in the first VISCONTI child, who still presents a long-term remission with a sustained control of HIV replication since more than 12 years [64]. This marker permitted to estimate the impact of cytoreductive chemotherapy on HIV reservoir persistence [65], and

the long-term impact in children and adolescents receiving treatment [66, 67]. The impact of treatments in different anatomical compartments, such as genital tract, to explore the residual risk of sexual transmission is important in the context of various levels of drug diffusion in tissues. Blips of viral replication in semen correlate with the level in PBMC, among men having sex with men on successful antiretroviral regimen [50, 68]. Levels of HIV reservoirs have been also estimated in patients receiving suppressive antiretroviral therapy, showing a true impact on different tissues and compartments, such as rectal tissue [24] and gut [46, 69, 70].

A particular context deserves to be discussed: the diagnosis of HIV infection in babies born to HIV positive mothers. For a long time, the detection of total HIV DNA in PBMCs has been the preferred technique, especially before access to viral load assays [69]. At present, the positive diagnosis of infection remains more difficult, particularly in cases of child infection despite maternal treatment. In such cases, the level of HIV is very low, because the viral replication is relatively blocked by the residual maternal treatment present in the child. So, HIV-DNA level in PBMC could be the only positive marker. In this actual context, there is a need for very sensitive and specific HIV DNA assays [13].

Lastly, total HIV DNA has been a useful marker in many clinical trials, for example, in primary infection [62, 71], in case of treatment with IL2, IL7 or alpha interferon [72–75]. Looking ahead to future clinical interventions aiming at reducing HIV reservoirs, the marker is also suitable, or even indispensable to the first step to select patients and to follow the impact of drugs and combinations [76–79].

The question that arises now is whether this marker could provide information to clinicians for therapeutic management. There are several clinical situations where it can be informative [10]: for example, in patients with long-term efficient treatment, low levels of total HIV-DNA indicate a low risk of disease progression, a low risk of viral rebound and development of drug resistance. On the contrary, in patients with a high level of total HIV-DNA, it is important to explain to them the high risk of viral rebound in case of non-adherence to treatment.

Conclusions

Among the different markers of HIV persistence, total HIV DNA has a special place because it is by far the most studied, and because the measurement is simple, precise and specific. It can reliably characterize the global size of HIV reservoirs. This marker has already had an undeniable and considerable contribution to reservoir studies, resulting in numerous insights, both in clinical and basic research. This is giving the opportunity to get a large overview of the distribution of HIV reservoir cells in the body, at all stages of HIV disease. Despite its drawback to quantify everything, including defective proviruses, total HIV DNA has enabled major advances, in particular in clinical research. However, there is an urgent need for other standardized markers of HIV reservoirs, in order to complete a panel of accurate tools that can constitute references. The debate should take into account all practical and clinical aspects, and should not sterilize the research, but rather sustain the use of complementary markers, to better explore the mechanisms of viral persistence.

Authors' contributions
CR and VAF discussed and wrote the paper together. Both authors read and approved the final manuscript.

Author details
[1] Laboratoire de Virologie, APHP Hôpital Necker Enfants Malades, Paris, France.
[2] EA 7327, Université Paris Descartes, Sorbonne Paris-Cité, Paris, France.

Acknowledgements
We thank ANRS for funding, patients for their participation and clinicians for their long-term involvement in the ANRS Cohort studies.

Competing interests
Both authors declares that they have no competing interests.

Funding
Grants of ANRS (Agence Nationale de Recherches sur le Sida et les Hépatites virales).

References
1. Imamichi H, Dewar RL, Adelsberger JW, Rehm CA, O'Doherty U, Paxinos EE, Fauci AS, Lane HC. Defective HIV-1 proviruses produce novel protein-coding RNA species in HIV-infected patients on combination antiretroviral therapy. Proc Natl Acad Sci USA. 2016;113:8783–8.
2. Rouzioux C, Richman D. How to best measure HIV reservoirs? Curr Opin HIV AIDS. 2013;8:170–5.
3. O'Doherty U, Swiggard WJ, Jeyakumar D, McGain D, Malim MH. A sensitive, quantitative assay for human immunodeficiency virus type 1 integration. J Virol. 2002;76:10942–50.
4. Massanella M, Richman DD. Measuring the latent reservoir in vivo. J Clin Invest. 2016;126:464–72.
5. Rouzioux C, Melard A, Avettand-Fenoel V. Quantification of total HIV1-DNA in peripheral blood mononuclear cells. Methods Mol Biol. 2014;1087:261–70.
6. Lambotte O, Boufassa F, Madec Y, Nguyen A, Goujard C, Meyer L, Rouzioux C, Venet A, Delfraissy JF. HIV controllers: a homogeneous group of HIV-1-infected patients with spontaneous control of viral replication. Clin Infect Dis. 2005;41:1053–6.
7. Saez-Cirion A, Bacchus C, Hocqueloux L, Avettand-Fenoel V, Girault I, Lecuroux C, Potard V, Versmisse P, Melard A, Prazuck T, et al. Post-treatment HIV-1 controllers with a long-term virological remission after the interruption of early initiated antiretroviral therapy. PLoS Pathog. 2013;9(e1003211):1003211–2.
8. Canoui E, Lecuroux C, Avettand-Fenoel V, Gousset M, Rouzioux C, Saez-Cirion A, Meyer L, Boufassa F, Lambotte O. Noel N, and the ACOCSG: a subset of extreme human immunodeficiency virus (HIV) controllers is characterized by a small HIV blood reservoir and a weak T-cell activation level. Open Forum Infect Dis. 2017;4:ofx064.
9. Bertine M, Gueudin M, Melard A, Damond F, Descamps D, Matheron S, Collin F, Rouzioux C, Plantier JC, Avettand-Fenoel V. New highly sensitive real-time PCR assay for HIV-2 group A and group B DNA quantification. J Clin Microbiol. 2017;55:2850–7.
10. Avettand-Fenoel V, Hocqueloux L, Ghosn J, Cheret A, Frange P, Melard A, Viard JP, Rouzioux C. Total HIV-1 DNA, a marker of viral reservoir dynamics with clinical implications. Clin Microbiol Rev. 2016;29:859–80.
11. Hong F, Aga E, Cillo AR, Yates AL, Besson G, Fyne E, Koontz DL, Jennings C, Zheng L, Mellors JW. Novel assays for measurement of total cell-associated HIV-1 DNA and RNA. J Clin Microbiol. 2016;54:902–11.
12. Gantner P, Melard A, Damond F, Delaugerre C, Dina J, Gueudin M, Maillard A, Saune K, Rodallec A, Tuaillon E, et al. Interlaboratory quality control of total HIV-1 DNA load measurement for multicenter reservoir studies. J Med Virol. 2017;89:2047–50.
13. Avettand-Fenoel V, Chaix ML, Blanche S, Burgard M, Floch C, Toure K, Allemon MC, Warszawski J, Rouzioux C. LTR real-time PCR for HIV-1 DNA quantitation in blood cells for early diagnosis in infants born to seropositive mothers treated in HAART area (ANRS CO 01). J Med Virol. 2009;81:217–23.
14. Rouzioux C, Hubert JB, Burgard M, Deveau C, Goujard C, Bary M, Sereni D, Viard JP, Delfraissy JF, Meyer L. Early levels of HIV-1 DNA in peripheral blood mononuclear cells are predictive of disease progression independently of HIV-1 RNA levels and CD4 + T cell counts. J Infect Dis. 2005;192:46–55 **(Epub 2005 May 2031)**.
15. Hocqueloux L, Avettand-Fenoel V, Jacquot S, Prazuck T, Legac E, Melard A, Niang M, Mille C, Le Moal G, Viard JP, Rouzioux C. Long-term antiretroviral therapy initiated during primary HIV-1 infection is key to achieving both low HIV reservoirs and normal T cell counts. J Antimicrob Chemother. 2013;68:1169–78.
16. Trypsteen W, Kiselinova M, Vandekerckhove L, De Spiegelaere W. Diagnostic utility of droplet digital PCR for HIV reservoir quantification. J Virus Erad. 2016;2:162–9.
17. Strain MC, Lada SM, Luong T, Rought SE, Gianella S, Terry VH, Spina CA, Woelk CH, Richman DD. Highly precise measurement of HIV DNA by droplet digital PCR. PLoS ONE. 2013;8:e55943.
18. Jones GM, Busby E, Garson JA, Grant PR, Nastouli E, Devonshire AS, Whale AS. Digital PCR dynamic range is approaching that of real-time quantitative PCR. Biomol Detect Quantif. 2016;10:31–3.
19. Kiselinova M, De Spiegelaere W, Buzon MJ, Malatinkova E, Lichterfeld M, Vandekerckhove L. Integrated and total HIV-1 DNA predict ex vivo viral outgrowth. PLoS Pathog. 2016;12:e1005472.
20. Bosman KJ, Nijhuis M, van Ham PM, Wensing AM, Vervisch K, Vandekerckhove L, De Spiegelaere W. Comparison of digital PCR platforms and semi-nested qPCR as a tool to determine the size of the HIV reservoir. Sci Rep. 2015;5:13811.
21. Pasternak AO, Adema KW, Bakker M, Jurriaans S, Berkhout B, Cornelissen M, Lukashov VV. Highly sensitive methods based on seminested real-time reverse transcription-PCR for quantitation of human immunodeficiency virus type 1 unspliced and multiply spliced RNA and proviral DNA. J Clin Microbiol. 2008;46:2206–11.
22. Vandergeeten C, Fromentin R, Merlini E, Bramah-Lawani M, DaFonseca S, Bakeman W, McNulty A, Ramgopal M, Michael N, Kim JH, et al. Cross-clade ultrasensitive PCR-based assays to measure HIV persistence in large cohort studies. J Virol. 2014;88:12385–96.
23. Ananworanich J, Sacdalan CP, Pinyakorn S, Chomont N, de Souza M, Luekasemsuk T, Schuetz A, Krebs SJ, Dewar R, Jagodzinski L, et al. Virological and immunological characteristics of HIV-infected individuals at the earliest stage of infection. J Virus Erad. 2016;2:43–8.

24. Khoury G, Anderson JL, Fromentin R, Hartogenesis W, Smith MZ, Bacchetti P, Hecht FM, Chomont N, Cameron PU, Deeks SG, Lewin SR. Persistence of integrated HIV DNA in CXCR3 + CCR6 + memory CD4 + T cells in HIV-infected individuals on antiretroviral therapy. AIDS. 2016;30:1511–20.

25. Boritz EA, Darko S, Swaszek L, Wolf G, Wells D, Wu X, Henry AR, Laboune F, Hu J, Ambrozak D, et al. Multiple origins of virus persistence during natural control of HIV infection. Cell. 2016;166:1004–15.

26. Eriksson S, Graf E, Dahl V, Strain MC, Yukl SL, Lysenko E, Bosch RJ, Lai J, Chioma S, Emad F, et al. Comparative analysis of measures of viral reservoirs in HIV-1 eradication studies. PLoS Pathog. 2013;9:e1003174.

27. Avettand-Fenoel V, Boufassa F, Galimand J, Meyer L, Rouzioux C. HIV-1 DNA for the measurement of the HIV reservoir is predictive of disease progression in seroconverters whatever the mode of result expression is. J Clin Virol. 2008;42:399–404.

28. Goujard C, Bonarek M, Meyer L, Bonnet F, Chaix ML, Deveau C, Sinet M, Galimand J, Delfraissy JF, Venet A, et al. CD4 cell count and HIV DNA level are independent predictors of disease progression after primary HIV type 1 infection in untreated patients. Clin Infect Dis. 2006;42:709–15.

29. Descours B, Avettand-Fenoel V, Blanc C, Samri A, Melard A, Supervie V, Theodorou I, Carcelain G, Rouzioux C, Autran B, Group AACS. Immune responses driven by protective human leukocyte antigen alleles from long-term nonprogressors are associated with low HIV reservoir in central memory CD4 T cells. Clin Infect Dis. 2012;54:1495–503.

30. Fletcher CV, Staskus K, Wietgrefe SW, Rothenberger M, Reilly C, Chipman JG, Beilman GJ, Khoruts A, Thorkelson A, Schmidt TE, et al. Persistent HIV-1 replication is associated with lower antiretroviral drug concentrations in lymphatic tissues. Proc Natl Acad Sci USA. 2014;111:2307–12.

31. Avettand-Fenoel V, Prazuck T, Hocqueloux L, Melard A, Michau C, Kerdraon R, Agoute E, Rouzioux C. HIV-DNA in rectal cells is well correlated with HIV-DNA in blood in different groups of patients, including long-term non-progressors. Aids. 2008;22:1880–2.

32. Hey-Nguyen WJ, Xu Y, Pearson CF, Bailey M, Suzuki K, Tantau R, Obeid S, Milner B, Field A, Carr A, et al. Quantification of residual germinal center activity and HIV-1 DNA and RNA levels using fine needle biopsies of lymph nodes during antiretroviral therapy. AIDS Res Hum Retroviruses. 2017;33:648–57.

33. Fukazawa Y, Lum R, Okoye AA, Park H, Matsuda K, Bae JY, Hagen SI, Shoemaker R, Deleage C, Lucero C, et al. B cell follicle sanctuary permits persistent productive simian immunodeficiency virus infection in elite controllers. Nat Med. 2015;21:132–9.

34. Laanani M, Ghosn J, Essat A, Melard A, Seng R, Gousset M, Panjo H, Mortier E, Girard PM, Goujard C, et al. Impact of the timing of initiation of antiretroviral therapy during primary HIV-1 infection on the decay of cell-associated HIV-DNA. Clin Infect Dis. 2015;60:1715–21.

35. Ananworanich J, Chomont N, Eller LA, Kroon E, Tovanabutra S, Bose M, Nau M, Fletcher JL, Tipsuk S, Vandergeeten C, et al. HIV DNA set point is rapidly established in acute HIV infection and dramatically reduced by early ART. EBioMedicine. 2016;11:68–72.

36. Boulle C, Rouet F, Fassinou P, Msellati P, Debeaudrap P, Chaix ML, Rouzioux C, Avettand-Fenoel V. HIV-1 DNA concentrations and evolution among African HIV-1-infected children under antiretroviral treatment (ANRS 1244/1278). J Antimicrob Chemother. 2014;69:3047–50.

37. Avettand-Fenoel V, Bouteloup V, Melard A, Fagard C, Chaix ML, Leclercq P, Chene G, Viard JP, Rouzioux C. Higher HIV-1 DNA associated with lower gains in CD4 cell count among patients with advanced therapeutic failure receiving optimized treatment (ANRS 123–ETOILE). J Antimicrob Chemother. 2010;65:2212–4.

38. Jumare J, Sunshine S, Ahmed H, El-Kamary SS, Magder L, Hungerford L, Burdo T, Eyzaguirre LM, Umlauf A, Cherner M, et al. Peripheral blood lymphocyte HIV DNA levels correlate with HIV associated neurocognitive disorders in Nigeria. J Neurovirol. 2017;23:474–82.

39. Valcour VG, Shiramizu BT, Sithinamsuwan P, Nidhinandana S, Ratto-Kim S, Ananworanich J, Siangphoe U, Kim JH, de Souza M, Degruttola V, et al. HIV DNA and cognition in a Thai longitudinal HAART initiation cohort: the SEARCH 001 Cohort Study. Neurology. 2009;72:992–8.

40. Noel N, Pena R, David A, Avettand-Fenoel V, Erkizia I, Jimenez E, Lecuroux C, Rouzioux C, Boufassa F, Pancino G, et al. Long-term Spontaneous control of HIV-1 relates to low frequency of infected cells and inefficient viral reactivation. J Virol. 2016;90:6148–58.

41. Hatano H, Jain V, Hunt PW, Lee TH, Sinclair E, Do TD, Hoh R, Martin JN, McCune JM, Hecht F, et al. Cell-based measures of viral persistence are associated with immune activation and programmed cell death protein 1 (PD-1)-expressing CD4 + T cells. J Infect Dis. 2013;208:50–6.

42. Cockerham LR, Siliciano JD, Sinclair E, O'Doherty U, Palmer S, Yukl SA, Strain MC, Chomont N, Hecht FM, Siliciano RF, et al. CD4 + and CD8 + T cell activation are associated with HIV DNA in resting CD4 + T cells. PLoS ONE. 2014;9:e110731.

43. Minga AK, Anglaret X, d'Aquin Toni T, Chaix ML, Dohoun L, Abo Y, Coulibaly A, Duvignac J, Gabillard D, Rouet F, Rouzioux C. HIV-1 DNA in peripheral blood mononuclear cells is strongly associated with HIV-1 disease progression in recently infected West African adults. J Acquir Immune Defic Syndr. 2008;48:350–4.

44. Hatzakis AE, Touloumi G, Pantazis N, Anastassopoulou CG, Katsarou O, Karafoulidou A, Goedert JJ, Kostrikis LG. Cellular HIV-1 DNA load predicts HIV-RNA rebound and the outcome of highly active antiretroviral therapy. AIDS. 2004;18:2261–7.

45. Tsiara CG, Nikolopoulos GK, Bagos PG, Goujard C, Katzenstein TL, Minga AK, Rouzioux C, Hatzakis A. Impact of HIV type 1 DNA levels on spontaneous disease progression: a meta-analysis. AIDS Res Hum Retrovir. 2012;28:366–73.

46. Yukl SA, Shergill AK, Ho T, Killian M, Girling V, Epling L, Li P, Wong LK, Crouch P, Deeks SG, et al. The distribution of HIV DNA and RNA in cell subsets differs in gut and blood of HIV-positive patients on ART: implications for viral persistence. J Infect Dis. 2013;208:1212–20.

47. Hatano H, Somsouk M, Sinclair E, Harvill K, Gilman L, Cohen M, Hoh R, Hunt PW, Martin JN, Wong JK, et al. Comparison of HIV DNA and RNA in gut-associated lymphoid tissue of HIV-infected controllers and noncontrollers. AIDS. 2013;27:2255–60.

48. Canaud G, Dejucq-Rainsford N, Avettand-Fenoel V, Viard JP, Anglicheau D, Bienaime F, Muorah M, Galmiche L, Gribouval O, Noel LH, et al. The kidney as a reservoir for HIV-1 after renal transplantation. J Am Soc Nephrol. 2014;25:407–19.

49. Damouche A, Lazure T, Avettand-Fenoel V, Huot N, Dejucq-Rainsford N, Satie AP, Melard A, David L, Gommet C, Ghosn J, et al. Adipose tissue is a neglected viral reservoir and an inflammatory site during chronic HIV and SIV infection. PLoS Pathog. 2015;11:e1005153.

50. Ghosn J, Leruez-Ville M, Blanche J, Delobelle A, Beaudoux C, Mascard L, Lecuyer H, Canestri A, Landman R, Zucman D, et al. HIV-1 DNA levels in peripheral blood mononuclear cells and cannabis use are associated with intermittent HIV shedding in semen of men who have sex with men on successful antiretroviral regimens. Clin Infect Dis. 2014;58:1763–70.

51. Prazuck T, Chaillon A, Avettand-Fenoel V, Caplan AL, Sayang C, Guigon A, Niang M, Barin F, Rouzioux C, Hocqueloux L. HIV-DNA in the genital tract of women on long-term effective therapy is associated to residual viremia and previous AIDS-defining illnesses. PLoS ONE. 2013;8:e69686.

52. Besson GJ, Lalama CM, Bosch RJ, Gandhi RT, Bedison MA, Aga E, Riddler SA, McMahon DK, Hong F, Mellors JW. HIV-1 DNA decay dynamics in blood during more than a decade of suppressive antiretroviral therapy. Clin Infect Dis. 2014;59:1312–21.

53. Viard JP, Burgard M, Hubert JB, Aaron L, Rabian C, Pertuiset N, Lourenco M, Rothschild C, Rouzioux C. Impact of 5 years of maximally successful highly active antiretroviral therapy on CD4 cell count and HIV-1 DNA level. AIDS. 2004;18:45–9.

54. Tierney C, Lathey JL, Christopherson C, Bettendorf DM, D'Aquila RT, Hammer SM, Katzenstein DA. Prognostic value of baseline human immunodeficiency virus type 1 DNA measurement for disease progression in patients receiving nucleoside therapy. J Infect Dis. 2003;187:144–8.

55. Avettand-Fenoel V, Flandre P, Chaix ML, Ghosn J, Delaugerre C, Raffi F, Ngovan P, Cohen-Codar I, Delfraissy JF, Rouzioux C. Impact of 48 week lopinavir/ritonavir monotherapy on blood cell-associated HIV-1-DNA in the MONARK trial. J Antimicrob Chemother. 2010;65:1005–7.

56. Piketty C, Weiss L, Assoumou L, Burgard M, Melard A, Ragnaud JM, Bentata M, Girard PM, Rouzioux C, Costagliola D. A high HIV DNA level in PBMCs at antiretroviral treatment interruption predicts a shorter time to treatment resumption, independently of the CD4 nadir. J Med Virol. 2010;82:1819–28.

57. Assoumou L, Weiss L, Piketty C, Burgard M, Melard A, Girard PM, Rouzioux C, Costagliola D. A low HIV-DNA level in peripheral blood mononuclear cells at antiretroviral treatment interruption predicts a higher probability of maintaining viral control. AIDS. 2015;29:2003–7.

58. Williams JP, Hurst J, Stohr W, Robinson N, Brown H, Fisher M, Kinloch S, Cooper D, Schechter M, Tambussi G, et al. HIV-1 DNA predicts disease progression and post-treatment virological control. Elife. 2014;3:e03821.

59. Chomont N, El-Far M, Ancuta P, Trautmann L, Procopio FA, Yassine-Diab B, Boucher G, Boulassel MR, Ghattas G, Brenchley JM, et al. HIV reservoir size and persistence are driven by T cell survival and homeostatic proliferation. Nat Med. 2009;15:893–900.

60. Bacchus C, Cheret A, Avettand-Fenoel V, Nembot G, Melard A, Blanc C, Lascoux-Combe C, Slama L, Allegre T, Allavena C, et al. A single HIV-1 cluster and a skewed immune homeostasis drive the early spread of HIV among resting CD4 + cell subsets within one month post-infection. PLoS ONE. 2013;8:e64219.

61. Murray JM, Zaunders JJ, McBride KL, Xu Y, Bailey M, Suzuki K, Cooper DA, Emery S, Kelleher AD, Koelsch KK. HIV DNA subspecies persist in both activated and resting memory CD4 + T cells during antiretroviral therapy. J Virol. 2014;88:3516–26.

62. Cheret A, Nembot G, Melard A, Lascoux C, Slama L, Miailhes P, Yeni P, Abel S, Avettand-Fenoel V, Venet A, et al. Intensive five-drug antiretroviral therapy regimen versus standard triple-drug therapy during primary HIV-1 infection (OPTIPRIM-ANRS 147): a randomised, open-label, phase 3 trial. Lancet Infect Dis. 2015;15:387–96.

63. Cheret A, Bacchus-Souffan C, Avettand-Fenoel V, Melard A, Nembot G, Blanc C, Samri A, Saez-Cirion A, Hocqueloux L, Lascoux-Combe C, et al. Combined ART started during acute HIV infection protects central memory CD4 + T cells and can induce remission. J Antimicrob Chemother. 2015;70:2108–20.

64. Frange P, Faye A, Avettand-Fenoel V, Bellaton E, Descamps D, Angin M, David A, Caillat-Zucman S, Peytavin G, Dollfus C, et al. HIV-1 virological remission lasting more than 12 years after interruption of early antiretroviral therapy in a perinatally infected teenager enrolled in the French ANRS EPF-CO10 paediatric cohort: a case report. Lancet HIV. 2016;3:e49–54.

65. Henrich TJ, Hobbs KS, Hanhauser E, Scully E, Hogan LE, Robles YP, Leadabrand KS, Marty FM, Palmer CD, Jost S, et al. Human immunodeficiency virus type 1 persistence following systemic chemotherapy for malignancy. J Infect Dis. 2017;216:254–62.

66. Luzuriaga K, Tabak B, Garber M, Chen YH, Ziemniak C, McManus MM, Murray D, Strain MC, Richman DD, Chun TW, et al. HIV type 1 (HIV-1) proviral reservoirs decay continuously under sustained virologic control in HIV-1-infected children who received early treatment. J Infect Dis. 2014;210:1529–38.

67. Avettand-Fenoel V, Blanche S, Le Chenadec J, Scott-Algara D, Dollfus C, Viard JP, Bouallag N, Benmebarek Y, Riviere Y, Warszawski J, et al. Relationships between HIV disease history and blood HIV-1 DNA load in perinatally infected adolescents and young adults: the ANRS-EP38-IMMIP study. J Infect Dis. 2012;205:1520–8.

68. Gantner P, Assoumou L, Leruez-Ville M, David L, Suzan-Monti M, Costagliola D, Rouzioux C, Ghosn J, Group EAES. HIV-1-RNA in seminal plasma correlates with detection of HIV-1-DNA in semen cells, but not with CMV shedding, among MSM on successful antiretroviral regimens. J Antimicrob Chemother. 2016;71:3202–5.

69. Yukl SX, Gianella S, Sinclair E, Epling L, Li Q, Duan L, Choi AX, Girling V, Ho T, Li P, et al. Differences in HIV burden and immune activation within the gut of HIV-positive patients receiving suppressive antiretroviral therapy. J Infect Dis. 2010;202:1553–61.

70. Ananworanich J, Schuetz A, Vandergeeten C, Sereti I, de Souza M, Rerknimitr R, Dewar R, Marovich M, van Griensven F, Sekaly R, et al. Impact of multi-targeted antiretroviral treatment on gut T cell depletion and HIV reservoir seeding during acute HIV infection. PLoS ONE. 2012;7:e33948.

71. Hoen B, Dumon B, Harzic M, Venet A, Dubeaux B, Lascoux C, Bourezane Y, Ragnaud JM, Bicart-See A, Raffi F, et al. Highly active antiretroviral treatment initiated early in the course of symptomatic primary HIV-1 infection: results of the ANRS 053 trial. J Infect Dis. 1999;180:1342–6.

72. Levy Y, Gahery-Segard H, Durier C, Lascaux AS, Goujard C, Meiffredy V, Rouzioux C, Habib RE, Beumont-Mauviel M, Guillet JG, et al. Immunological and virological efficacy of a therapeutic immunization combined with interleukin-2 in chronically HIV-1 infected patients. AIDS. 2005;19:279–86.

73. Levy Y, Lacabaratz C, Weiss L, Viard JP, Goujard C, Lelievre JD, Boue F, Molina JM, Rouzioux C, Avettand-Fenoel V, et al. Enhanced T cell recovery in HIV-1-infected adults through IL-7 treatment. J Clin Invest. 2009;119:997–1007.

74. Boue F, Reynes J, Rouzioux C, Emilie D, Souala F, Tubiana R, Goujard C, Lancar R, Costagliola D. Alpha interferon administration during structured interruptions of combination antiretroviral therapy in patients with chronic HIV-1 infection: INTERVAC ANRS 105 trial. AIDS. 2011;25:115–8.

75. Morlat P, d'experts G. Prise en charge médicale des personnes vivant avec le VIH. Recommandations du groupe d'experts. Paris: La documentation Française; 2015.

76. Bouchat S, Delacourt N, Kula A, Darcis G, Van Driessche B, Corazza F, Gatot JS, Melard A, Vanhulle C, Kabeya K, et al. Sequential treatment with 5-aza-2'-deoxycytidine and deacetylase inhibitors reactivates HIV-1. EMBO Mol Med. 2015;8:117–38.

77. Darcis G, Kula A, Bouchat S, Fujinaga K, Corazza F, Ait-Ammar A, Delacourt N, Melard A, Kabeya K, Vanhulle C, et al. An in-depth comparison of latency-reversing agent combinations in various in vitro and ex vivo HIV-1 latency models identified bryostatin-1 + JQ1 and ingenol-B + JQ1 to potently reactivate viral gene expression. PLoS Pathog. 2015;11:e1005063.

78. Rasmussen TA, Tolstrup M, Brinkmann CR, Olesen R, Erikstrup C, Solomon A, Winckelmann A, Palmer S, Dinarello C, Buzon M, et al. Panobinostat, a histone deacetylase inhibitor, for latent-virus reactivation in HIV-infected patients on suppressive antiretroviral therapy: a phase 1/2, single group, clinical trial. Lancet HIV. 2014;1:e13–21.

79. Elliott JH, McMahon JH, Chang CC, Lee SA, Hartogensis W, Bumpus N, Savic R, Roney J, Hoh R, Solomon A, et al. Short-term administration of disulfiram for reversal of latent HIV infection: a phase 2 dose-escalation study. Lancet HIV. 2015;2:e520–9.

Permissions

The contributors of this book come from diverse backgrounds, making this book a truly international effort. This book will bring forth new frontiers with its revolutionizing research information and detailed analysis of the nascent developments around the world.

We would like to thank all the contributing authors for lending their expertise to make the book truly unique. They have played a crucial role in the development of this book. Without their invaluable contributions this book wouldn't have been possible. They have made vital efforts to compile up to date information on the varied aspects of this subject to make this book a valuable addition to the collection of many professionals and students.

This book was conceptualized with the vision of imparting up-to-date information and advanced data in this field. To ensure the same, a matchless editorial board was set up. Every individual on the board went through rigorous rounds of assessment to prove their worth. After which they invested a large part of their time researching and compiling the most relevant data for our readers.

The editorial board has been involved in producing this book since its inception. They have spent rigorous hours researching and exploring the diverse topics which have resulted in the successful publishing of this book. They have passed on their knowledge of decades through this book. To expedite this challenging task, the publisher supported the team at every step. A small team of assistant editors was also appointed to further simplify the editing procedure and attain best results for the readers.

Apart from the editorial board, the designing team has also invested a significant amount of their time in understanding the subject and creating the most relevant covers. They scrutinized every image to scout for the most suitable representation of the subject and create an appropriate cover for the book.

The publishing team has been an ardent support to the editorial, designing and production team. Their endless efforts to recruit the best for this project, has resulted in the accomplishment of this book. They are a veteran in the field of academics and their pool of knowledge is as vast as their experience in printing. Their expertise and guidance has proved useful at every step. Their uncompromising quality standards have made this book an exceptional effort. Their encouragement from time to time has been an inspiration for everyone.

The publisher and the editorial board hope that this book will prove to be a valuable piece of knowledge for researchers, students, practitioners and scholars across the globe.

List of Contributors

Delia M. Pinto-Santini
Division of Basic Sciences, Fred Hutchinson Cancer Research Center, Seattle, WA, USA

Carolyn R. Stenbak
Biology Department, Seattle University, Seattle, WA, USA

Maxine L. Linial
Division of Basic Sciences, Fred Hutchinson Cancer Research Center, 1100 Fairview Ave.N., A3-205, Seattle, WA 98109, USA

Robert J. Gifford
MRC-University of Glasgow Centre for Virus Research, Glasgow, UK

Jonas Blomberg
Department of Medical Sciences, Uppsala University, Uppsala, Sweden

John M. Coffin
Department of Molecular Biology and Microbiology, Tufts University, Boston, MA, USA

Hung Fan
Department of Molecular Biology and Biochemistry and Cancer Research Institute, University of California, Irvine, CA 92697, USA

Thierry Heidmann
Department of Molecular Physiology and Pathology of Infectious and Endogenous Retroviruses, CNRS UMR 9196, Institut Gustave Roussy, 94805 Villejuif, France

Jens Mayer
Department of Human Genetics, Center of Human and Molecular Biology, Medical Faculty, University of Saarland, Homburg, Germany

Jonathan Stoye
The Francis Crick Institute, Mill Hill Laboratory, The Ridgeway, Mill Hill, London, UK

Michael Tristem
Imperial College London, Silwood Park Campus, Buckhurst Road, Ascot, Berkshire SL5 7PY, UK

Welkin E. Johnson
Biology Department, Boston College, Chestnut Hill, Massachusetts 02467, USA

Fu-Hsien Yu and Chin-Tien Wang
Department of Medical Research, Taipei Veterans General Hospital and Institute of Clinical Medicine, National Yang-Ming University School of Medicine, 201, Sec. 2, Shih-Pai Road, Taipei 11217, Taiwan

Meijuan Niu and Abdelkrim Temzi
HIV-1 RNA Trafficking Laboratory, Lady Davis Institute at the Jewish General Hospital, Montreal, QC H3T 1E2, Canada

Andrew J. Mouland
HIV-1 RNA Trafficking Laboratory, Lady Davis Institute at the Jewish General Hospital, Montreal, QC H3T 1E2, Canada
Department of Microbiology and Immunology, McGill University, Montreal, QC H3A 2B4, Canada
Department of Medicine, McGill University, Montreal, QC H3A 0G4, Canada

Shringar Rao
HIV-1 RNA Trafficking Laboratory, Lady Davis Institute at the Jewish General Hospital, Montreal, QC H3T 1E2, Canada
Department of Microbiology and Immunology, McGill University, Montreal, QC H3A 2B4, Canada.

Raquel Amorim
HIV-1 RNA Trafficking Laboratory, Lady Davis Institute at the Jewish General Hospital, Montreal, QC H3T 1E2, Canada
Department of Medicine, McGill University, Montreal, QC H3A 0G4, Canada

Harini Subbaraman, Merle Schanz and Alexandra Trkola
Institute of Medical Virology, University of Zurich, Zurich, Switzerland

Amy E. Baxter and Daniel E.Kaufmann
CR-CHUM, Université de Montréal, Montréal, QC, Canada
Scripps CHAVI-ID, La Jolla, CA, USA

Una O'Doherty
Department of Pathology and Laboratory Medicine, Division of Transfusion Medicine and Therapeutic Pathology, University of Pennsylvania, Philadelphia, PA, USA

Elise Landais
International AIDS Vaccine Initiative Neutralizing Antibody Center, The Scripps Research Institute, La Jolla, CA 92037, USA
Department of Immunology and Microbiology, The Scripps Research Institute, La Jolla, CA 92037, USA
International AIDS Vaccine Initiative, New York, NY 10004, USA

Penny L. Moore
Centre for HIV and STIs, National Institute for Communicable Diseases of the National Health Laboratory Service, Johannesburg, South Africa
Faculty of Health Sciences,University of the Witwatersrand, Johannesburg, South Africa
Centre for the AIDS Programme of Research in South Africa (CAPRISA), University of KwaZulu-Natal, Durban, South Africa

Joris Paris, Joëlle Tobaly-Tapiero, Marie-Lou Giron, Pascale Lesage and Ali Saïb
CNRS UMR7212, Hôpital St Louis, Inserm U944, Institut Universitaire d'Hématologie, Université Paris Diderot, Sorbonne Paris Cité, Paris, France

Alessia Zamborlini
CNRS UMR7212, Hôpital St Louis, Inserm U944, Institut Universitaire d'Hématologie, Université Paris Diderot, Sorbonne Paris Cité, Paris, France
CNRS UMR7212, Hôpital St Louis, Inserm U944, Institut Universitaire d'Hématologie, Université Paris Diderot, Sorbonne Paris Cité, Laboratoire PVM, Conservatoire National des Arts et Métiers (Cnam), Paris, France

Julien Burlaud-Gaillard and Philippe Roingeard
Plateforme IBiSA de Microscopie Electronique, Université François Rabelais and CHRU de Tours, Tours, France
INSERM U1259, Université François Rabelais and CHRU de Tours, Tours, France

Florence Buseyne
Institut Pasteur, Unité d'Epidémiologie et Physiopathologie des Virus Oncogènes, Paris, France
CNRS UMR3569,Insitut Pasteur, Paris, France

Elizabeth M. Anderson and Frank Maldarelli
HIV Dynamics and Replication Program, NCI, NIH, Frederick, MD 21702, USA

Steven J. Smith and Stephen H. Hughes
HIV Dynamics and Replication Program, National Cancer Institute-Frederick, National Institutes of Health, Frederick, MD, USA

Xue Zhi Zhao and Terrence R. Burke Jr
Chemical Biology Laboratory, National Cancer Institute-Frederick, National Institutes of Health, Frederick, MD, USA

Axel Fun, Pauline J. Schipper and Monique Nijhuis
Department of Medical Microbiology, Virology, University Medical Center Utrecht, Heidelberglaan 100, HP G04.614, 3584 CX Utrecht, The Netherlands.

Annemarie M. J. Wensing
Department of Medical Microbiology, Virology, University Medical Center Utrecht, Heidelberglaan 100, HP G04.614, 3584 CX Utrecht, The Netherlands
Department of Internal Medicine and Infectious Diseases, University Medical Center Utrecht, Utrecht, The Netherlands

Thomas Leitner
Theoretical Biology and Biophysics, Los Alamos National Laboratory, Los Alamos, NM, USA.

Linos Vandekerckhove
Department of General Internal Medicine and Infectious Diseases, Ghent University Hospital, Ghent, Belgium

Martin Däumer
Institute of Immunology and Genetics, Kaiserslautern, Germany

Alexander Thielen
Max Planck Institute for Informatics, Saarbrücken, Germany

Bernd Buchholz
Pediatric Clinic, University Medical Center Mannheim, Mannheim, Germany

Andy I. M. Hoepelman
Department of Internal Medicine and Infectious Diseases, University Medical Center Utrecht, Utrecht, The Netherlands

Elizabeth H. Gisolf
Department of Internal Medicine, Rijnstate Hospital, Arnhem, The Netherlands

Catalina Méndez, Scott Ledger, Kathy Petoumenos, Chantelle Ahlenstiel and Anthony D. Kelleher
Department of Immunovirology and Pathogenesis, Level 5, Wallace Wurth Building, The Kirby Institute for Infection and Immunity, UNSW Sydney, Kensington, Sydney, NSW 2052, Australia

Andrey Ivanov, Xionghao Lin, Namita Kumari, Hatajai Lassiter, Nowah Afangbedji and Xiaomei Niu
Center for Sickle Cell Disease, Howard University, 1840 7th Street, N.W. HURB1, Suite 202, Washington, DC 20001, USA

Sergei Nekhai
Center for Sickle Cell Disease, Howard University, 1840 7th Street, N.W. HURB1, Suite 202, Washington, DC 20001, USA
Department of Medicine, Howard University, Washington, DC, USA

Tatiana Ammosova
Center for Sickle Cell Disease, Howard University, 1840 7th Street, N.W. HURB1, Suite 202, Washington, DC 20001, USA
Department of Medicine, Howard University, Washington, DC, USA
Yakut Science Center for Complex Medical Problems, Yakutsk, Russia

Andrey V. Ilatovskiy and Michael G. Petukhov
Division of Molecular and Radiation Biophysics, Petersburg Nuclear Physics Institute, Gatchina, Russia
Research Center for Nanobiotechnologies, Peter the Great St. Petersburg Polytechnic University, St. Petersburg, Russia

Stephanie J. Bissel, Kate Gurnsey, Nicholas F. Smith, Guoji Wang and Clayton A. Wiley
University of Pittsburgh, 3550 Terrace Street, S758 Scaife Hall, Pittsburgh, PA 15261, USA

Charles W. Bradberry
University of Pittsburgh, 3550 Terrace Street, S758 Scaife Hall, Pittsburgh, PA 15261, USA
Veterans Affairs Pittsburgh Healthcare System, 4100 Allequippa Street, Pittsburgh, PA 15213, USA
Present Address: National Institute on Drug Abuse, 251 Bayview Boulevard, Baltimore, MD 21224, USA

Hank P. Jedema
University of Pittsburgh, 3550 Terrace Street, S758 Scaife Hall, Pittsburgh, PA 15261, USA
Present Address: National Institute on Drug Abuse, 251 Bayview Boulevard, Baltimore, MD 21224, USA

Eirini Moysi, Constantinos Petrovas and Richard A. Koup
Immunology Laboratory, Vaccine Research Center, NIAID, NIH, Bethesda,USA

Christine Rouzioux and Véronique Avettand-Fenoël
Laboratoire de Virologie, APHP Hôpital Necker Enfants Malades, Paris, France.
EA 7327, Université Paris Descartes, Sorbonne Paris-Cité, Paris, France

Index

www.ingramcontent.com/pod-product-compliance
Lightning Source LLC
Chambersburg PA
CBHW061301190326
41458CB00011B/3732